BOUCHER'S

Clinical Dental
Terminology

*A Glossary of Accepted Terms
in all Disciplines of Dentistry*

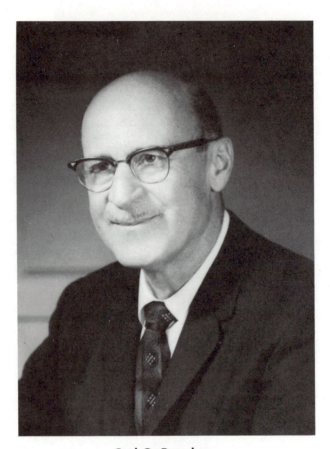

Carl O. Boucher

A man whose ideas, deeds, and words
live after him and enrich us all

BOUCHER'S

Clinical Dental

Terminology

A Glossary of Accepted Terms in all Disciplines of Dentistry

Thomas J. Zwemer, D.D.S., M.S.D., F.A.C.D., F.I.C.D.

Vice President for Academic Affairs, Emeritus,
Professor of Orthodontics, Emeritus,
School of Dentistry, Medical College of Georgia,
Augusta, Georgia;
Diplomate, American Board of Orthodontics

FOURTH EDITION

With 65 illustrations

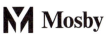 Mosby

St. Louis Baltimore Boston Chicago London Philadelphia Sydney Toronto

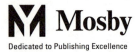

Dedicated to Publishing Excellence

Publisher: George Stamathis
Editor: Robert W. Reinhardt
Assistant Editor: Melba Steube
Project Manager: Carol Sullivan Wiseman
Senior Production Editor: Pat Joiner
Designer: Julie Taugner

FOURTH EDITION
Copyright © 1993 by Mosby–Year Book, Inc.

Previous editions copyrighted 1963, 1974, 1982

Printed in the United States of America

Mosby–Year Book, Inc.
11830 Westline Industrial Drive
St. Louis, Missouri 63146

Library of Congress Cataloging in Publication Data

Boucher's clinical dental terminology : a glossary of accepted terms
  in all disciplines of dentistry / [edited by] Thomas J. Zwemer.—
  4th ed.
      p.   cm.
    Includes bibliographical references.
    ISBN 0-8016-6706-2
    1. Dentistry—Dictionaries.   I. Zwemer, Thomas J.   II. Boucher,
  Carl O.   III. Title: Clinical dental terminology.
    [DNLM: 1. Dictionaries, Dental.   WU 13 B753]
  RK27.B63   1993
  617.6′003—dc20
  DNLM/DLC   92-24903
  for Library of Congress   CIP

93 94 95 96 97 CL/MY 9 8 7 6 5 4 3 2 1

NWST
1 ADD 7117

To

Dentists and their staffs

Dental educators and their students

Medical record administrators and their associates

Health insurance underwriters and their agents

Health planners and their constituencies

Preface

This book is designed to improve communication among those involved in dental health care delivery. The editor and publisher have attempted to present the consensus on the meaning and proper use of dental terms. The book is intended as a learning resource and as an aid to the precise use of the written and spoken word in dentistry.

This revision reflects the dramatic, changing nature of dental practice. Twenty-one contemporary reference works have been consulted in the preparation of the fourth edition of *Boucher's Clinical Dental Terminology*. The impact of the human innunodeficiency virus on the language, social policy, governmental guidelines, the practice of dentistry, and lifestyle has been captured in this edition. The growing fields of esthetic dentistry, implant dentistry, and pain management are strongly represented. The expanding discipline of dental pharmacology has been recognized and is included for the first time. The field of dental practice management has been expanded to include terms of basic investment instruments. The body of the work contains the American Dental Association's *Glossary of Dental Benefit Terms*.

In addition to the body of the work, the appendixes have been enlarged and expanded. The list of abbreviations in Appendix B has been expanded to include a broad range of federal and public health agency designations and human immunodeficiency virus–generated terms. Appendix C contains the American Dental Association's *Code on Dental Procedures*. Appendix D contains an explanation of the American Dental Association's tooth numbering systems, as well as the preferred method for mounting dental radiographs. Appendix E is the American Dental Association's suggested dental claim form. Appendix F is a new atlas section of selected illustrations of craniofacial anatomy. Appendixes G and H, containing information about biochemical profiling and laboratory values, have been expanded and updated. Appendix I is a directory of the American Dental Association, its constituent societies, and the national and state boards of examiners. All of the salient features of the American Dental Association's *CDT-1, Current Dental Terminaology* have been incorporated, under contract, in the fourth edition.

The editor and publisher believe that this updated and expanded edition will be a rich and ready source of information for the student, the dental staff, the practicing dentist, and all of those associated with dental health care delivery.

Thomas J. Zwemer

Acknowledgements, ed. 4

American jurisprudence, desk book, ed 2, Rochester, NY, 1979, Lawyers Cooperative.

American jurisprudence, desk book cumulative supplement, Rochester, NY, 1991, Lawyers Cooperative.

Avery JK: *Essentials of oral histology and embryology: a clinical approach,* St Louis, 1992, Mosby–Year Book.

Bhaskar SN: *Synopsis of oral pathology* ed 7, St Louis, 1986, Mosby–Year Book.

Brand RW, Isselhard DE: *Anatomy of orofacial structures,* ed 4, St Louis 1990, Mosby–Year Book.

CDT-1: a users manual, Chicago, 1991, American Dental Association.

Clark JW, consulting ed: *Clark's clinical dentistry,* Philadelphia, 1990, Lippincott.

Cohen S, Burns RC: *Pathways of the pulp,* ed 5, St Louis, 1991, Mosby–Year Book.

Cunnan N, ed: *Dun and Bradstreet's guide to your investments,* New York, 1987, Harper & Row.

Facts about AIDS for the dental team, ed 3, Chicago, American Dental Association.

Genco RJ et al: *Contemporary periodontics,* St Louis, 1990, Mosby–Year Book.

Goaz PW, White SC: *Oral radiology,* St Louis, 1987, Mosby–Year Book.

McDonald RE, Avery DR: *Dentistry for the child and adolescent,* ed 5, St Louis, 1988, Mosby–Year Book.

McGivney GP, Castleberry DJ: *McCracken's removable partial prosthodontics,* ed 8, St Louis, 1989, Mosby–Year Book.

The Merck Manual, ed 15, Rahway, NJ, 1987, Merck Sharp and Dohme Research Laboratories.

Mosby's medical and nursing dictionary, St Louis, 1983, Mosby–Year Book.

Okeson JP: *Fundamentals of occlusion and temporomandibular disorders,* ed 1, St Louis, 1985, Mosby–Year Book.

Peterson LJ et al: *Contemporary oral and maxillofacial surgery,* St Louis, 1988, Mosby–Year Book.

Physicians desk reference, ed 45, Oradell, NJ, Medical Economic.

Proffit WR: *Contemporary orthodontics,* St Louis, 1986, Mosby–Year Book.

Rosenstiel SF et al: *Contemporary fixed prosthodontics,* St Louis, 1988, Mosby–Year Book.

Stedman's medical dictionary, ed 25, Baltimore, 1990, Williams & Wilkins.

Sturdevant CM: *The art and science of operative dentistry,* ed 2, St Louis, 1985, Mosby–Year Book.

Webster's encyclopedic unabridged dictionary of the English language, New York, 1989, Portland House.

Acknowledgments, ed. 3

Associate Editors for the Third Edition

Thomas R. Dirksen, D.D.S., Ph.D., F.A.C.D.

Associate Dean for Biological Sciences; Professor and Chairman, Department of Oral Biology, School of Dentistry; Professor of Cell and Molecular Biology, School of Medicine; and Professor of Oral Biology and Cell and Molecular Biology, School of Graduate Studies, Medical College of Georgia, Augusta, Georgia

Leon A. Leonard, B.S. D.D.S., M.S., F.A.C.D.

Associate Dean for Clinical Sciences; Professor of Endodontics; and Professor Emeritus, Department of Oral Medicine, School of Dentistry, Medical College of Georgia, Augusta, Georgia

Bruce H. Rice, D.D.S., M.S., Ph.D., F.A.C.D.

Professor and Chairman Emeritus, Department of Oral Medicine, School of Dentistry, Medical College of Georgia, Augusta, Georgia; Diplomate, American Board of Periodontics

Roberet F. Kaltenbach, Jr., B.A., M.A., Ph.D.

Associate Professor, Department of Psychiatry and Health Behavior, School of Medicine; and Associate Professor, Department of Restorative Dentistry, School of Dentistry, Medical College of Georgia, Augusta, Georgia

Contributors to the Third Edition

Nick J. Minden, M.Ed., M.B.A., D.M.D.

Assistant Professor, Department of Community Dentistry, School of Dentistry, University of Florida, Gainesville, Florida

Gerald W. Woods, J.D.

Vice President for Business Operations, Medical College of Georgia, Augusta, Georgia

Jack D. Zwemer, B.S., D.D.S., Ph.D.

Professor, Department of Community Dentistry, School of Dentistry, Medical College of Georgia, Augusta, Georgia

Grateful acknowledgment is made to the authors and publishers of the following publications used for reference sources by the various contributors and collaborators:

Accepted dental therapeutics, ed 3, 1977, American Dental Association.

Adopted terminology, American Academy of Pedodontics, 1961.

Adriani J: *The pharmacology of anesthetic drugs,* ed. 4, Springfield, Ill., 1960, Thomas.

Aita JA: *Congenital facial anomalies with neurologic defects,* Springfield, Ill, 1969, Thomas.

Allen EV, Barker H: *Peripheral vascular diseases,* Philadelphia, 1962, Saunders.

American Academy of Maxillofacial Prosthetics, Workshop on Nomenclature, 1971 Annual Meeting.

Anderson GM: *Practical orthodontics,* ed 9, St Louis, 1960, Mosby–Year Book.

Anderson WAD, ed: *Pathology,* ed 6 St Louis, 1971, Mosby–Year Book.

Angle EH: *Angle system of regulation and retention of the teeth and treatment of fractures of the maxillae,* ed 7, Philadelphia, 1902, White Dental Manufacturing.

Annotated glossary of terms used in endodontics, CG Maurice, Chairman, Nomenclature Committee, American Association of Endodontists, Oral Surgery, Oral Medicine, and Oral Pathology, St Louis, 1968, Mosby–Year Book.

Archer WH: *Oral surgery: a step-by-step atlas of operative techniques,* ed 3, Philadelphia, 1961, Saunders Co.

Ash Major M: *A handbook of differential oral diagnosis,* St Louis, 1961, Mosby–Year Book.

Bassett RW, Ingraham R, Koser JR: *An atlas of gold restorations,* Los Angeles, 1964, University of Southern California.

Behrman SJ: *The implantation of magnets in the jaw to aid denture retention. J Prosthet Dent* 10:807, 1960.

Bennett CR: *Monheim's general anesthesia in dental practice,* ed 4, St Louis, 1974, Mosby–Year Book.

Bennett CR: *Monheim's local anesthesia and pain control in dental practice,* ed 5, St Louis, 1974, Mosby–Year Book.

Bernier JL: *Management of oral disease,* ed 2, St Louis, 1959, Mosby–Year Book.

Berry MF, Eisenson J: *Speech disorders: principles and practices of therapy,* New York, 1956, Appleton-Century-Crofts.

Black HC: *Black's law dictionary,* St Paul, Minn, West.

Blackwell RE: *GV Black's operative dentistry,* ed 9, South Milwaukee, 1955, Medico-Dental.

Blakiston's new gould medical dictionary, ed 4, New York, 1979, McGraw-Hill.

Blass JL: *Motivating patients for more effective dental service,* Philadelphia, 1958, Lippincott.

Bodine RL Jr: *Implant dentures: prosthodontic-favorable, J Prosthet Dent* 10:1132, 1960.

Boucher CO, ed: *Swenson's complete dentures,* ed 6, St Louis, 1970, Mosby–Year Book.

Boyd, W: *A textbook of pathology,* ed 8, Philadelphia, 1970, Lea & Febiger.

Brauer JD et al: *Dentistry for children,* ed 3, New York, 1952, McGraw-Hill.

Brodnitz FS: *Keep your voice healthy,* New York, 1953, Harper & Row.

Bureau of Health Manpower, Division of Dentistry, *Department of Health, Education, and Welfare: Prepaid dental care: a glossary, No (HRA) 76-20, Bethesda, Md, 1975, The Bureau.*

Burnett GW, Scherp HW, Schuster GS: *Oral microbiology and infectious disease,* ed 4, Baltimore, 1976, Williams & Wilkins.

Carnahan CW: *The dentist and the law,* St Louis, 1955, Mosby–Year Book.

Chusid JG, McDonald JJ: *Correlative neuroanatomy and functional neurology,* ed 11, Los Altos, Calif, 1962, Lange.

Cohen MM: *Pediatric dentistry,* ed 2, St Louis, 1961, Mosby–Year Book.

Collins VJ: *Principles of anesthesiology,* Philadelphia, 1966, Lea & Febiger.

Committee on Hospital Oral Surgery Service: Oral surgery glossary, 1971, American Society of Oral Surgeons.

Cooper HK: Integration of services in the treatment of cleft lip and cleft palate. *J Am Dent Assoc* 47:27, 1953.

Cooper HK: Oral aspects of rehabilitation, *J Am Coll Dent* 27:52, 1960.

Cooper HK et al: Psychological, orthodontic, and prosthetic approaches in rehabilitation of the cleft palate patient, *Dent Clin North Am* 4:381, 1960.

Cranin AN: Nomenclature, *J Implant Dent* 2:41, 1956.

Cranin AN: Some philosophic comments on the endosseous implant, *Dent Clin North Am* 14:173, 1970.

Cranin AN, Dennison TA: Blade and anchor construction technics, *J Am Dent Assoc* 83:833, 1971.

Dawson PE: *Evaluation, diagnosis, and treatment of occlusal problems,* St Louis, 1974, Mosby–Year Book.

Denton GB: *The vocabulary of dentistry and oral science,* Chicago, 1958, American Dental Association.

Dorland's *American illustrated medical dictionary,* Philadelphia, 1977, Saunders.

English WB, English AC: *A comprehensive dictionary of psychological and psychoanalytical terms,* New York, 1958, McKay.

Etter E: *Glossary of words and phrases used in radiology and nuclear medicine,* Springfield, Ill, 1960, Thomas.

Fairbanks G: *Voice and articulation drill book,* New York, 1940, Harper & Row.

Finn SB, Volker JF, Cheraskin E: *Clinical pedodontics,* Philadelphia, 1957, Saunders.

Fischer B: *Orthodontics,* ed 2, Philadelphia, 1957, Saunders.

Gabel AB: *American textbook of operative dentistry* ed 9, Philadelphia, 1954, Lea & Febiger.

Gellhorn E: *Physiological foundations of neurology and psychiatry,* Minneapolis, 1953, University of Minnesota Press.

Gilmore HW, Lund MR: *Operative dentistry,* ed 2, St Louis, 1973, Mosby–Year Book.

Glasser O: *Medical physics,* Chicago, 1944, Mosby–Year Book.

Glossary of terms used in dental radiology, 1964, American Academy of Oral Roentgenology.

Glossary of dental prepayment terms, *J Am Dent Assoc* 98:601, 1979.

Goldberg NL, Gershhoff A: The implant lower denture, *Dent Dig* 55:490, 1949.

Goldman HM, Cohen DW: *Periodontal therapy,* ed 4, St Louis, 1968, Mosby–Year Book.

Goldman HM, Cohen DW: *An introduction to periodontia,* ed 4, St Louis, 1969, Mosby–Year Book.

Goldman HM et al: *An introduction to periodontia,* ed 3, St Louis, 1966, Mosby–Year Book.

Goldman HM et al: *Periodontal therapy,* ed 2, St Louis, 1960, Mosby–Year Book.

Goodman LS, Gilman A: *The pharmacological basis of therapeutics,* ed 5, New York, 1975, Macmillan.

Gorlin RJ, ed: Summary of the Workshop on Ulcerative and Bullous Disorders of the Orofacial Region, *J Dent Res* 50:795, 1971.

Gorlin RJ, Goldman HM: *Thoma's oral pathology,* ed 6, St Louis, 1970, Mosby–Year Book.

Gorlin RJ, Pindborg JJ: *Syndromes of the head and neck,* New York, 1964, McGraw-Hill.

Graber TM: *Orthodontics, principles and practice,* Philadelphia, 1961, Saunders.

Grant DA, Stern IB, Everett FG: *Orban's periodontics,* ed 4, St Louis, 1972, Mosby–Year Book.

Gray GW, Wise CM: *Bases of speech,* ed 3, New York, 1958, Harper & Row.

Gregory WK: *Evolution emerging,* vol 1, New York, 1957, Macmillan.

Grossman LI: *Endodontic practice,* ed 7, Philadelphia, 1970, Lea & Febiger.

Gruebbel AO, consulting ed Symposium on practice administration, *Dent. Clin. North Am,* vol 5, March 1961.

Guide to dental materials and devices, ed 6, Chicago, 1972-1973, American Dental Association.

Healey HJ: *Endodontics,* St Louis, 1960, Mosby–Year Book.

Heartwell CM Jr, Rahn AO: *Syllabus of complete dentures,* ed 2, Philadelphia, 1974, Lea & Febiger.

Henderson D, Steffel VL: *McCracken's partial denture construction,* ed 3, St Louis, 1969, Mosby–Year Book.

Hickey JC, Zarb GA: *Boucher's prosthodontic treatment for edentulous patients,* ed 8, St Louis, Mosby–Year Book.

Hine MK, ed: *Review of dentistry,* ed 5, St Louis, 1970, Mosby–Year Book.

Hinsie LE, Campbell RJ: *Psychiatric dictionary,* New York, 1974, Oxford University Press.

Howard WW: *An atlas of operative dentistry,* St Louis, 1968, Mosby–Year Book.

Ingle JI, Beveridge EE: *Endodontics,* ed 2, Philadelphia, 1976, Lea & Febiger.

Ingraham R, Koser JR, Quint H: *An atlas of gold foil and rubber dam.* Buena Park, Calif, 1961. Uni-Tro College Procedures.

Jermyn AC: Peri-implantoclasia—cause and treatment, *J Implant Dent* 5:25, 1958.

Johnston JF, Phillips RW, Dykema R: *Modern practice in crown and bridge prosthodontics,* Philadelphia, 1960, Saunders.

Kantner CE, West R: *Phonetics,* New York, 1941, Harper & Row.

Kazanjian VH, Converse JM: *The surgical treatment of facial injuries,* ed 2, Baltimore, 1959, Williams & Wilkins.

Kerr DA, Ash MM Jr, Millard HD: *Oral diagnosis,* ed 3, St Louis, 1970, Mosby–Year Book.

Kilpatrick HC: *High speed and ultraspeed in dentistry,* Philadelphia, 1959, Saunders.

Kreps C, Wacht RF: *Financial administration,* Hinsdale, Ill, 1975, Dryden.

Kruger GO, ed: *Textbook of oral surgery,* ed, 4, St Louis, 1974, Mosby–Year Book.

Langley LL, Cheraskin E: *The physiological foundation of dental practice,* St Louis, 1956, Mosby–Year Book.

Lehninger AL: *Biochemistry,* ed 2, 1975, New York, Worth Publishers.

Levy IR: *Textbook for dental assistants,* ed 2 Philadelphia, 1942, Lea & Febiger.

Loechler PS, Mueller MW: Successful implant dentures, *Northwest Dent* 31:134, 1952.

Longacre JJ, ed: *Craniofacial anomalies,* Philadelphia, 1968, Lippincott.

Lynch MA: *Burket's oral medicine: diagnosis and treatment,* ed 7, Philadelphia, 1977, Lippincott.

Mann WR, Easlick KA: *Practice administration for the dentist,* St Louis, 1955, Mosby–Year Book.

McCall JO: *Practical dental assisting,* Brooklyn, 1948, Dental Items of Interest.

McCoy JD, Shepard, EE: *Applied orthodontics,* ed 7, Philadelphia, 1956, Lea & Febiger.

McDonald RE: *Dentistry for the child and adolescent,* ed 2, St Louis, 1974, Mosby–Year Book.

McGehee WHO, True HA, Inskipp EF: *A textbook of operative dentistry.* ed 4, New York, 1956. McGraw-Hill.

Metals handbook, Metals Park, Ohio, 1961, American Society for Metals.

Mitchell DF, Standish SM, Fast TB: *Oral diagnosis/oral medicine,* Philadelphia, 1971, Lea & Febiger.

Morrey LW, Nelsen RJ: *Dental science handbook,* Washington, DC, 1970, US Department of Health, Education, and Welfare.

Morrison GA: *In the dentist's office,* Philadelphia, 1959, Lippincott.

Moyers RE: *Handbook of orthodontics,* Chicago, 1958, Mosby–Year Book.

Nagle RJ, Sears VH: *Dental prosthetics,* St Louis, 1959, Mosby–Year Book.

National Bureau of Standards Handbook 59, *Permissible dose from external sources of ionizing radiation,* Washington, DC, 1954, US Government Printing Office.

National Dental Quality Assurance Advisory Commitee: *Dental quality assurance terminology: a glossary,* Chicago, 1980, American Fund for Dental Health.

Nomenclature Committee, The Academy of Denture Prosthetics: *Glossary of prosthodontic terms,* ed 3, St Louis, 1968, Mosby–Year Book.

Nomenclature Committee, American Association for Cleft Palate Rehabilitation: *Proposed morphological classification of congenital cleft lip and cleft palate, Cleft Palate Bull* 10:11, 1960.

Orban B: Oral histology and embryology, ed 2, St Louis, 1949, Mosby–Year Book.

Orban B, Wentz FM: *Atlas of clinical pathology of the oral mucous membrane,* St Louis, 1960, Mosby–Year Book.

Orten JM, Neuhaus OW: *Human biochemistry,* ed 10, St Louis, 1982, Mosby–Year Book.

Peyton FA, Craig RG: *Restorative dental materials,* ed 4, St Louis, 1971, Mosby–Year Book.

Phillips RW: *Skinner's science of dental materials,* ed 7, Philadelphia, 1973, Saunders.

Poppel MH, ed *Radiopaque diagnosis agents, Ann NY Acad Sci* 78:705, 1959.

Ramfjord SP, Ash M Jr: *Occlusion,* ed 2, Philadelphia, 1971, Saunders.

Robbins SL, Cotran RS: *Pathologic basis of disease,* ed 2, Philadelphia, 1979, Saunders.

Salzmann JA: *Principles of orthodontics,* ed 3, Philadelphia, 1950, Saunders.

Salzmann JA: *Orthodontics: principles and prevention,* vol 1, Philadelphia, 1957, Lippincott.

Salzmann JA: *Orthodontics: practice and techniques,* vol 2, Philadelphia, 1957, Lippincott.

Sarnat BG: *The temporomandibular joint.* Springfield, Ill., 1951, Thomas.

Sassouni V, with the collaboration of Forrest EJ: *Orthodontics in dental practice,* St Louis, 1971, Mosby–Year Book.

Schlyger SR, Yuodelis RA, Page RC. *Periodontal disease,* Philadelphia, 1977, Lea & Febiger.

Schroeter C: *Dentition of man,* Seattle, 1966, University of Washington Press.

Schwartz JR: *Inlays and abutments,* Brooklyn, 1952, Dental Items of Interest.

Schwarzrock LH, Schwarzrock SP: *Effective dental assisting,* ed 2, Dubuque, Iowa, 1959, Brown.

Selzer S: *Endodontology,* New York, 1971, McGraw-Hill.

Selve H: *Stress of life,* New York, 1956, McGraw-Hill.

Services for children with cleft lip and cleft palate, New York, 1955, American Public Health Association.

Shafer WG, Hine MK, Levy BM: *A textbook of oral pathology,* ed 3, Philadelphia, 1974, Saunders.

Sharry JJ: *Complete denture prosthodontics,* ed 2, New York, 1968, McGraw-Hill.

Shaw JH et al: *Textbook of oral biology* Philadelphia, 1978, Saunders.

Shepard EE: *Technique and treatment with the twin-wire appliance,* St Louis, 1961, Mosby–Year Book.

Sicher H, DuBrul EL: *Oral anatomy,* ed 5, St Louis, 1970, Mosby–Year Book.

Slobody LB: *Survey of clinical pediatrics,* New York, 1959, McGraw-Hill.

Sodeman WA: *Pathologic physiology,* ed 2, Philadelphia, 1957, Saunders.

Sommer RF, Ostrander FD, Crowley MC: *Clinical endodontics,* ed 3, Philadelphia, 1966, Saunders.

Souder WH, Paffenbarger GC: *Physical properties of dental materials,* National Bureau of Standards Circular No. C433, Washington, DC, 1942, US Government Printing Office.

Stedman's medical dictionary, ed 22, Baltimore, 1972, Williams & Wilkins.

Stibbs GD: *Textbook of operative dentistry,* St Louis, 1967, Mosby–Year Book.

Stibbs GD: *Cavity preparations,* Seattle, 1969, University of Washington Press.

Stinaff RK: *Dental practice administration,* ed 3, St Louis, 1968, Mosby–Year Book.

Storch CB: *Fundamentals of clinical fluoroscopy,* New York, 1951, Grune & Stratton.

Swidler G: *Handbook of drug interactions,* New York and London, 1971, Wiley.

Tarpley BW: *Technique and treatment with the labiolingual appliance,* St Louis, 1961, Mosby–Year Book.

Terkla LG, Laney WR: *Partial dentures,* ed 3, St Louis, 1963, Mosby–Year Book.

Thoma KH: *Oral surgery,* ed 5, St Louis, 1969, Mosby–Year Book.

Thoma KH, Robinson HBB: *Oral and dental diagnosis,* ed 5, Philadelphia, 1960, Saunders.

Thurow RC: *Edgewise orthodontics,* ed 3, St Louis, 1973, Mosby–Year Book.

Tiecke RW, Stuteville OH, Calandra JC: *Pathological physiology of oral disease,* St Louis, 1959, Mosby–Year Book.

Tocchine JJ: *Restorative dentistry,* New York, 1967, McGraw-Hill.

Travis L, *Handbook of speech pathology,* New York, 1957, Appleton-Century-Crofts.

Tylman SD: *Theory and practice of crown and fixed partial prosthodontics (bridge),* ed 6, St Louis, 1970, Mosby–Year Book.

Van Riper C, Irwin JV: *Voice and articulation,* Englewood Cliffs, NJ, 1958, Prentice-Hall.

Weast RC, ed: *Handbook of chemistry and physics,* ed 56, Cleveland, 1975, CRC.

Webster's third new international dictionary of the English language (unabridged), Springfield, Mass, 1976, Merriam.

Weinmann JP, Sicher H: *Bone and bones,* St Louis, 1955, Mosby–Year Book.

West R, Ansberry M, Carr A: *The rehabilitation of speech,* New York, 1957, Harper & Row.

Wheeler RC: *A textbook of dental anatomy, physiology and occlusion,* ed 5, Philadelphia, 1974, Saunders.

Windholz M: *The Merck index,* ed 9, Rahway, NJ, 1976, Merck.

Wuehrmann AH: *Radiation protection and dentistry,* St Louis, 1960, Mosby–Year Book.

Wuehrmann AH, Manson-Hing LR: *Dental radiology,* ed 2, St Louis, 1969, Mosby–Year Book.

Contents

Pronunciation Guide

ā	as in wait
ă	as in bat
ah	as in ma
ē	as in me
ĕ	as in met
e	as in her
ī	as in my
ĭ	as in bit
ō	as in boat
ŏ	as in hot
o	as in or
oo	as in loose
ū	as in due
ŭ or uh	as in but
ul	as in full

Å Abbreviation for Ångström. *See* unit, Ångström.

a nativitate (nă-tĭv′i-tăt) A condition existing at birth or from infancy; denotes a congenital disability.

A point *See* point, A.

aa (ana) A Greek term used in prescription writing, meaning of each.

A-alpha fibers *See* fibers, nerve.

ab (antecedente) Beforehand; a notice given previously or a condition existing earlier.

abacterial (ā-băk-tĕ′rē-ăl) Nonbacterial; free from bacteria.

abandonment (of a patient) Withdrawing a patient from treatment without giving reasonable notice or providing a competent replacement.

abatement (ah-bāt′mĕnt) Decrease in severity of pain or symptoms.

Abbe-Estlander operation (ăb-ā′ ĕst′lănd-er) *See* operation, Abbe-Estlander.

abduce (ăb-doos′) To draw away; abduct.

abduct (ăb-dŭkt′) To draw away from the median line or from a neighboring part or limb.

abduction (ăb-dŭk′-shŭn) The process of abducting; opposite of adduction.

aberrant (ăb-ĕr′ănt) Deviation from the usual or normal course, location, or action.

A-beta fibers *See* fibers, nerve.

abnormal Departure from the norm, however defined; departure from the mean of a distribution (statistics); departure from the usual, from a state of integration or adjustment.

abrade (ah-brād′) To wear away by friction.

abrasion (ah-brā′zhŭn) **1:** The abnormal wearing away of a substance or tissue by a mechanical process. **2:** Grinding or wearing away of tooth substance by mastication, incorrect brushing methods, bruxism, or similar causes.

   a., dentifrice Wearing away of the cementum and dentin of an exposed root by an abrasive-containing dentifrice.

abrasive (ah-brā′sĭv) A substance used for grinding or polishing that will wear away a material or tissue.

   a. disk *See* disk, abrasive.

   a. point, rotary *See* point, abrasive, rotary.

   a. strip *See* strip, abrasive.

abscess (ăb′sĕs) Localized accumulation of pus in a cavity formed by tissue disintegration.

   a., alveolar *See* periapical abscess.

   a., apical *See* periapical abscess.

   a., dentoalveolar *See* periapical abscess.

   a., lateral *See* periodontal abscess.

   a., periapical An abscess involving the apical region of the root, alveolus, and surrounding bone as a sequela of pulpal disease.

   a., periodontal An abscess involving the attachment tissues and alveolar bone as a sequela of periodontal disease.

   a., pulpal An abscess occurring within pulpal tissue.

absorb (ab-sorb′) **1:** Etymological: to suck up. **2:** Incorporation or assimilation of a liquid or gas into tissue or cells.

absorbefacient (ăb-sor″bah-fā′shĕnt) Causing absorption, or an agent that promotes absorption.

absorbent (ăb-sorb′ĕnt) A substance that causes absorption of diseased tissue; taking up by suction.

absorption (ăb-sorp′shŭn) **1:** The passage of a substance into the interior of another by solution or penetration. **2:** Taking up of fluids or other substances by the skin, mucous surfaces, absorbent vessels, or dental materials. **3:** The process by which radiation imparts some or all of its energy to any material through which it passes.

   a. coefficient The ratio of the linear rate of change of intensity of roentgen rays in a given homogeneous material to the intensity at a given point within the same mass.

abstraction (ăb-străk′shŭn) Indicates teeth or other maxillary and mandibular stuctures that are inferior to (below) their normal position; away from the occlusal plane.

abuse Improper use of program benefits, resources, and/or services by either dentists, institutions, or patients.

abutment (ah-bŭt′mĕnt) A tooth, root, or implant used for support and retention of a fixed or removable prosthesis.

   a., intermediate An abutment located between the abutments that form the end of the prosthesis.

a., multiple Abutments splinted together as a unit to serve as support and retention of a fixed prosthesis.

a.c. (ante cibum) A Latin phrase used in prescription writing meaning "before eating."

acanthesthesia (ah-kăn″thĕs-thē′zē-ah) A form of paresthesia with the feeling of a sharp point.

acanthion (ah-kan′thē-on) The tip of the anterior nasal spine.

acantholysis The loosening, separation, or disassociation of individual prickle cells within the epithelium from their neighbor, often seen in conditions such as pemphigus vulgaris and keratosis follicularis.

acanthosis (ăk-ăn-thō′sĭs) An increase in the number of cells in the prickle cell layer of stratified squamous epithelium, with thickening of the entire epithelial cell layer and a broadening and fusing of rete pegs.

acapnia (ah-căp′nē-ah) A condition characterized by diminished carbon dioxide in the blood.

acarbia (ah-kar′bē-ah) A condition in which the blood bicarbonate is lowered.

acatalasemia (a″kăt-ah-lā-sē′mē-ah) A congenital lack of the enzyme catalase in blood and other tissues that leads to a progressive necrosis of the oral tissues (Takahara's disease).

accelerator (ăk-sĕl′ĕr-ā″tor) **1:** That which increases rapidity of action or function. **2:** A catalyst or other substance that hastens a chemical reaction (e.g., NaCl added to water and plaster to hasten the set).

a., platelet thrombin See factor, platelet 2.

a., prothrombin conversion, I (factor V, labile factor, plasma accelerator globulin, proaccelerin, serum accelerator globulin) Considered by some to be a factor in serum and plasma that catalyzes the conversion of inactive prothrombin to an active form.

a., prothrombin conversion, II (cothromboplastin, extrinsic thromboplastin, factor VII, serum prothrombin conversion accelerator [SPCA], stable factor) Considered by some to be one of the factors in the blood that accelerates the conversion of active prothrombin to thrombin by thromboplastin. Vitamin K deficiency reduces the activity of this factor.

a., serum See factor V.

accelerin See factor V.

acceptability Overall assessment of the dental care available to a person or group; includes accessibility, cost, quality, results, convenience, and attitudes of dentists and patients.

acceptance The act of a person to whom something is offered or tendered by another, whereby he receives that which is offered with the intention of retaining it. A contract is not valid without the acceptance of an offer by the party to whom the offer is made, either expressly or by conduct.

a., absolute An express and positive agreement to pay a bill according to its text.

a., conditional An agreement to pay a bill on the fulfillment of a condition.

a., implied An acceptance interpreted by law from the acts or conduct of the patient.

access (ăk′sĕs) **1:** Means of approach. **2:** Surgical preparation of hard or soft tissue to allow entrance to a treatment site and adequate space for visualization and instrumentation of the field.

a., cavity Coronal opening required for effective cleaning, shaping, and filling of the pulp space.

a., computer 1: The process of transferring information into or out of a storage location. **2:** The time required to begin and complete the read/write function of a specified piece of data.

a., form Surgical removal of tooth structure sufficient for visualization and instrumentation of a restorative preparation.

access flaps A periodontal surgical technique to provide visualization of the root in conjunction with curettage and root planning. Types of access flaps include supracrestal, subcrestal—full thickness, and partial thickness flaps.

accessory canal (ăk-sĕs′ō-rē) See canal, accessory root.

accident 1: An unusual, unforeseen event. **2:** An unusual or unexpected result attending the performance of a usual or necessary act or event. **3:** Occurring without intent or happening by chance. The term does not have a precise legal definition but is generally used to indicate that an occurrence was not the result of negligence.

a., cerebrovascular (CVA) Apoplexy resulting from hemorrhage into the brain or occlusion of the cerebral vessels resulting from embolism or thrombosis.

a., unavoidable An accident not occasioned, either remotely or directly, by the want of such care or skill as the law holds every person bound to exercise; occurring without fault or negligence.

account A basic storage unit in an accounting system. Individual accounts accept debit and credit entries that reflect the different types of transactions made by the practice.

a. book A book in which the financial transactions of a business or profession are entered. Such books may be admitted as evidence.

a., open A straightforward arrangement between the dentist and the patient for the handling of financial payments due the dentist and owed by the patient.

a., payable Dollar amount owed to creditors for items of services purchased from them.

accountability An obligation to periodically disclose appropriate information in adequate detail and consistent form to all contractually involved parties.

accreditation A process of formal recognition of a school or institution attesting to the required ability and performance in an area of education, training or practice.

accretions (ah-krē′shŭns) Accumulation of foreign material such as mucinous plaque, materia alba, and calculus on teeth.

accrual Continually recurring short-term liabilities. Examples are accrued wages, taxes, and interest.

accrued interest Interest accumulated on a bond since the last payment was made. The buyer of the bond pays the market price plus accumulated interest. Exceptions include bonds that are in default and income bonds.

accrued needs The amount of treatment needed by an individual or a group at any given time. In dental plans, usually refers to conditions present at the time of enrollment. Synonym: accumulated needs.

acenesthesia (ah-sĕn″ĕs-thē′-zē-ah) Loss, or lack, of the normal perception of one's own body; absence of the feelings of a physical existence, a symptom common in many psychiatric states.

acentric relation (ā-sĕn′trĭk) *See* relation, jaw, eccentric.

acetaminophen An analgesic and antipyretic containing no aspirin, often used for mild to moderate pain and fever (Tylenol).

acetate (ăs′ĕ-tāt) A salt of acetic acid.

acetone (ăs′ĕ-tōn) Dimethylketone; an organic solvent normally present in urine in small amounts but in increased amounts in diabetes.

acetylcholine (ăs″ĕ-tĭl-kō′lēn) **1:** An acetate ester of choline that serves as a neurohumoral agent in the transmission of an impulse in autonomic ganglia, parasympathetic postganglionic fibers, and somatic motor fibers. **2:** An ester of choline actively involved as a chemical mediator at the neuromuscular junction, at autonomic ganglia, and between parasympathetic nerve endings and visceral effectors.

achlorhydria (ah-klor-hī-′drē-ah) Absence of free hydrochloric acid in the stomach even with histamine stimulation.

achondroplasia (ah-kŏn-drō-plā′zē-ah) (chondrodystrophia fetalis) A hereditary disturbance of endochondral bone formation transmitted as a mendelian dominant factor and resulting in dwarfism. Malocclusion and prognathism may occur.

Achronmycin V A proprietary name for the antibiotic tetracycline hydrochloride.

achromatopsia (ah-krō-mah-tōp′sē-ah) Total color blindness.

achyia The absence or lack of hydrocholic acid and the enzyme pesinogen in the stomach.

acid (ăs′ĭd) A chemical substance that, in an aqueous solution, undergoes dissociation with the formation of hydrogen ions; pH levels range from 0 to 6.9.

  a., acetic The acid of vinegar, sometimes used as a solvent for the removal of calculus from a removable dental prosthesis. *See also* solvent.

  a., ascorbic *See* vitamin C.

a., carbolic *See* phenol.

a., cevitamic *See* vitamin C.

a. etching Treating the enamel, generally with phosphoric acid, by removal of approximately 40 μm of rod cross section to provide retention for resin sealant, restorative material, or orthodontic bracket.

a., folic *See* vitamin B complex.

a., hydroxypropionic *See* acid, lactic.

a., lactic (hydroxypropionic acid) A monobasic acid, $C_3H_6O_3$, formed as an end product in the intermediary metabolism of carbohydrates. The accumulation of lactic acid in the tissues is in part responsible for the lowering of pH levels during inflammatory states; e.g., it is believed that the drop in pH level hastens bone resorption in periodontitis because the minerals in the bone are stable within the matrix only at the normal tissue pH level of 7.4.

a., nicotinic (niacin, P.-P. factor, pyridine 3-carboxylic acid, vitamin P.-P.) 1: One of the vitamins of the B complex group and its vitamer, niacinamide, specific for the treatment of pellagra. Niacinamide functions as a constituent of coenzyme 1 (DPN) and coenzyme II (TPN). Nicotinic acid is found in lean meats, liver, yeast, milk, and leafy geen vegetables. **2:** An acid, C_5H_4N (COOH), that forms part of the B complex group of vitamins. It is present and necessary in the body as a cofactor in intermediary carbohydrate metabolism. It is a constituent of certain coenzymes that function in oxidative-reductive metabolic systems. With niacinamide, it is a pellagra-preventive factor.

a., orthophosphoric *See* acid, phosphoric.

a., pantothenic 1: One of the B complex vitamins whose importance in human nutrition has not been established. It is a constituent of coenzyme A and as such is presumed to be involved in adrenocortical function. **2:** A vitamin of the B complex, widely distributed in food and tissues and important for normal development in certain animals such as chicks and rats. Deficiency in rats produces retrograde changes in alveolar and supporting bone.

a., phosphoric (H_3PO_4, orthophosphoric acid) The principal ingredient of silicate and zinc phosphate cement liquids.

a., pteroylglutamic *See* vitamin B complex.

a. salt A salt containing one or more replaceable hydrogen ions.

a., strong An acid that is completely ionized in aqueous solution.

acid-base balance In metabolism, the balance of acid to base necessary to keep the blood pH level normal (between 7.35 and 7.43).

acidemia (ăs″ĭ-dē′mē-ah) Decreased pH level of the blood, irrespective of changes in the blood bicarbonate.

acidifier (ah-sĭd′ĭ-fi-er) A chemical ingredient (acetic acid) that maintains the required acidity of the fixer and stop-bath solutions.

acidophilic (as″ĭ-dō-fĭl′ĭk) **1:** Readily stained with acid dyes. **2:** Growing well in an acid medium.

acidosis (as″i-do′sis) A pathologic disturbance of the acid-base balance of the body characterized by an excess of acid or inadequate base. Causes include acid ingestion, increased acid production as in diabetes or starvation, or loss of base through the kidneys or intestine.

a., compensated A condition of acidosis in which the body pH level is maintained within the normal range through compensatory mechanisms involving the kidneys or lungs.

a., respiratory Acidemia resulting from retention of a excess CO_2 due to hypoventilation.

a., uncompensated Acidosis in which compensatory mechanisms are unable to maintain the body pH level within the normal range.

Ackerman-Proffit orthogonal analysis A taxonomy of malocclusion based on set theory or Boolean Algebra organized using combinations and permutations of malocclusions within the three planes of space. See Appendix F.

acoustic coupler A connection between a phone line and a data set (modem). It uses an ordinary telephone a headset and requires no modification to the normal phone.

acquired centric relation (sĕn′trĭk) *See* relation, centric; relation, jaw, eccentric.

acquired immunodeficiency syndrome (AIDS) A disease caused by a retrovirus known as human immunodeficiency virus type 1 (HIV-1). A related but distinct retrovirous (HIV-2) has recently appeared in a limited number of patients in the United States. Patients are considered to have AIDS when one or more indicator diseases (as defined by the CDC) are present. The Centers for Disease Control (CDC) has classified stages of the disease as follows:

Group I acute HIV infection Within one month of exposure, the first clinical evidence of HIV infection may appear as an acute retroviral syndrome. This is a mononucleosis-like syndrome with symptoms including fever, rash, diarrhea, lymphadenopathy, myalgia, arthralgia, and fatigue. Development of antibodies usually follows.

Group II asymptomatic HIV infection Most persons developantibodies to the HIV within 6 to 12 weeks after exposure. Although individual may remain asymptomatic for months or years, they can transmit the virus.

Group III persistent generalized lymphadenopathy (PGL) This group of HIV-infected persons will develop persistent generalized lymphadenopathy lasting more than 3 months.

Group IV HIV-associated diseases Patients in this group are clinically variable and have signs and symptoms of HIV infection other than or in addition to lymphadenopathy. Based on clinical findings, patients in Group IV may be assigned to one or more of the following subgroups: (A) constitutional disease, also known as *wasting syndrome.* (This subgroup is characterized by fever for more than one month, involuntary weight loss of greater than 10% for baseline, or diarrhea persisting more than one month); (B) neurological disease; (C) secondary infectious disease; (D) secondary cancers; and (E) other conditions resulting from HIV infections.

acroanesthesia (ăk″rō-ăn-ĕs-thē′zē-ah) Anesthesia of a the extremities.

acrocephalia (ăk-rō-sĕ-fā′lē-ah) A deformity of the head characterized by an upward and forward bulge of the frontal bones and a flat occiput. Synonym: oxycephalia.

acrodynia (ăk-rō-dĭn′ĭ-ah) **(erythredema polyneuropathy, Feer's syndrome, pink disease, Swift's syndrome, Selter's disease)** A disease of children in which manifestations occur with the eruption of the primary teeth. Syndrome includes raw-beef hands and feet, superficial sensory loss, photophobia, tachycardia, muscular hypotonia, changes in temperament, stomatitis, periodontitis, and premature loss of teeth. The etiology has been related to mercury and deficiency of vitamin B_6 and essential fatty acids. *See also* erythredema polyneuropathy.

acroestesia (ăk-rō-ĕs-thē′zē-ah) **1:** Increased sensitivity **2:** Pain in the extremities.

acromegaly (ăk-rō-mĕg′ah-lē) (Marie's disease) A condition caused by hyperfunction of the pituitary gland in adults. Characterized by enlargement of the skeletal extremities, including the feet, hands, mandible, and nose.

acrosclerosis (ăk-rō-sklĕ-rō′sĭs) A special form of scleroderma that affects the extremities, head, and face and is associated with Raynaud's phenomenon. There may be significant thickening of the periodontal membrane.

acrylic, *adj.* (ah-krĭl′ĭk) frequently improperly used as a noun. Should be used to modify nouns; e.g., acrylic resin, acrylic resin denture, and acrylic resin tooth. *See* resin, acrylic; denture, acrylic resin; tooth, acrylic resin.

a. resin *See* resin, acrylic.

ACTH (adrenocorticotropic hormone, adrenocorticotropin, adrenotropic hormone, codicotropic hormone, corticotropin) Adrenocorticotropic hormone, produced by basophilic cells of the anterior lobe of the pituitary gland, which exerts a reciprocal regulating influence on the production of corticosteroids by the adrenal cortex.

actinic cheilitis (ăk-tĭn′ĭk) *See* cheilitis, actinic.

actinomycetemcomitans **(H)** (ăk-tĭn-ō-mī-sē′tem-ō-com-ĭ-tins) A microorganism found in and considered responsible for some periodontal infections.

actinomycetes (ăk″tĭ-nō-mī-sē′tēz) filamentous microorganisms that have been implicated in the formation of dental calculus and serve as a mode of attachment of dental calculus to the tooth surface. They have also been found in pathologic lesions of the alveolar processes (actinomycosis).

actinomycosis (ăk″tĭ-nō-mī-kō′sĭs) (lumpy jaw, streptothricosis) An infection of humans and some animal species caused by species of *Actinomyces,* which are gram-positive, filamentous, microaerophilic microorganisms.

action potential The electrical potential developed in a muscle or nerve during activity.

activate (ăk′tĭ-vāt) To adjust an appliance so that it will exert effective force on the teeth and jaws.

activated resin *See* resin, autopolymer.

activator (ăk′tĭ-vā-tor) **1:** An alkali, sodium carbonate, which is a component of photographic developing solution that softens and swells the gelatin of the film emulsion and provides the necessary alkaline medium for the developing agents to react with the sensitized silver halide crystals. **2:** A removable orthodontic appliance intended to function as a passive transmitter and sometimes stimulator of the forces of the perioral muscles. One in the myofunctional category of appliances also known by such names as *Andresen, Bimler, Monobloc, Frankel,* etc.

active Pertaining to the condition of an orthodontic appliance that has been adjusted to apply effective force to the teeth or jaws.

   a. reciprocation *See* reciprocation, active.

acuity (ah-kū′ĭ-tē) Sharpness; clearness; keenness.

   a., auditory The sensitivity of the auditory apparatus; sharpness of hearing. It relates to the ability to hear a given tone with respect to the degree of intensity required to produce a sensation that is just perceptible.

   a., visual Sharpness, acuteness, or cleaness of vision. Visual acuity may be defective because of optical or neurologic dysfunction.

acute A traumatic, pathologic, or physiologic phenomenon or process having a short and relatively severe course; Antonym: chronic.

   a. phase reactions A phrase that refers to abnormalities in the blood associated with acute and chronic inflammatory and necrotic processes and detected by a variety of tests, including erythrocyte sedimentation rate, C-reactive protein, serum hexosamine, serum mucoprotein, and serum nonglucosamine polysaccharides.

acyclovir (ā′sigh-clō-veer) An antiviral drug active against herpes viruses. Used as a 5% ointment, may be used systemically. Drug of choice in immunocompromised patients with Candidasis. Brand name Zovirax.

ADA Abbreviation for the American Dental Association, the national professional organization for dentists in the United States.

ADA Abbreviation for the American Dairy Association.

ADA Abbreviation for adenosine deaminase, an enzyme that breaks down toxic biological products. This failure causes a rare disease called *severe combined immunodeficiency.*

adamantinoblastoma (ăd-ah-măn″tĭ-nō-blăs-tō′-mah) *See* ameloblastoma.

adamantinoma (ăd-ah-măn″tĭ-nō′mah) *See* ameloblastoma.

Adams' clasp A retention clasp designed by C. Philip Adams to stabilize removable appliances by engaging the mesiobuccal and distobuccal surfaces of buccal teeth.

Adams-Stokes disease *See* disease, Adams-Stokes.

adaptation 1: An alteration that an organ or organism undergoes to accommodate to its environment. **2:** A close approximation of a tissue flap, appliance, or restorative material to natural tissue. **3:** An accurate adjustment of a band or a shell to a tooth. **4:** A condition in reflex activity marked by a decline in the frequency of impulses when sensory stimuli are repeated several times.

adapter, band An instrument used as an aid in fitting an orthodontic band to a tooth.

A-delta fibers *See* fiber, nerve.

addict (ăd′ĭkt) One who has developed addiction to a drug.

addiction (a-′dik-shen) The state of being addicted. Although there is no universally accepted definition, addiction is generally considered a condition involving two factors: **1:** a compulsive behavior pattern and **2:** an altered physiologic state that requires continued use of the drug to prevent withdrawal symptoms.

addictive (ăd′ĭk-tĭv) Pertaining to a drug whose repeated use may produce addiction. Present federal regulations place greater emphasis on the broader designation of potential for abuse.

Addis' test *See* test, Addis'.

Addison-Biermer anemia (ad′ĭ-sŭn bēr′mer) *See* anemia, pernicious.

Addison's disease *See* disease, Addison's.

additive An ingredient added to a food, drug, or other preparation to produce a desired result (e.g., color or consistency) unrelated to the primary purpose of the preparation.

adduct (ah-dŭkt′) To draw toward the center or midline.

adduction (ah-dŭk′shŭn) The process of bringing toward each other; the opposite of abduction.

adenalgia (ăd-ē-năl′jē-ah) Pain in a gland, resulting usually from inflammation (adenitis).

adenoid facies An archaic term used to describe patients who exhibit a long narrow face, short upper lip, open-mouth breathing, and a hyperactive swallowing pattern.

adenitis (ăd″ĕ-nī′tis) Inflammation of glandular tissue, often accompanied by pain (adenalgia).

adenoameloblastoma (ăd″ĕ-nō-ah-mĕl″ō-blăs-tō′mah) An epithelial noeplasm with a basic structure resembling enamel organs and glandular (adenomatous) tissue. It is generally benign.

adenocarcinoma (ăd″ĕ-nō-kar-sĭ-nō′mah) A malignant epithelial neoplasm with a basic structure of glandular (acinar) pattern, suggesting derivation from glandular tissue.

   a., acinar cell A malignant tumor whose cells appear as glandular tissue.

adenoma (ăd″ĕ-nō′mah) A benign epithelial neoplasm or tumor with a basic glandular (acinar) structure, suggesting derivation from glandular tissue.

   a., acidophilic *See* oncocytoma.

   a., oxyphilic *See* oncocytoma.

adenomatosis oris (ăd″ĕ-nō-mah-tō′sĭs) An enlargement of the mucous glands of the lip without secretion or inflammation.

adenopathy (ăd″ĕ-nŏp′ah-thē) An enlargement or in crease in size of glandular organs or tissues usually resulting from disease processes.

adequacy, velopharyngeal A functional closure of the velum to the postpharyngeal wall that restricts air and sound from entering the nasopharyngeal and nasal cavities.

ADH *See* hormone, antidiuretic.

adhesion (ăd-hē′zhŭn) **1:** The attraction of unlike molecules for one another. **2:** The molecular attraction existing between surfaces in close contact. **3:** The condition in which a material sticks to itself or another material. **4:** The abnormal joining of tissues, generally by fibrous connective tissue, to each other, occurring after repair of an injury.

   a., sublabial The abnormal union of the sublabial mucosa of the upper lip to the alveolar process; usually present in a unilateral or bilateral cleft of the lip.

adhesive An intermediate material that causes two materials to stick together; a luting agent.

   a. foil *See* foil, adhesive.

adjudicate The final step in dental peer review at which the dental peer review committee renders a formal, nonlegal decision on a case before it.

adjunct (ăj′ŭngkt) A drug or other substance that serves a supplemental purpose in therapy.

adjust (ăd-jŭst′) To make correspondent, comfortable, or to fit.

adjustment (ad-jŭst′mĕnt) A modification of a restoration or of a denture after insertion in the mouth.

   a., occlusal A grinding of the occluding surfaces of teeth to develop harmonious relationships between each other, their supporting structures, muscles of mastication, and temporomandibular joints.

adjuvant (ăj′oo-vănt) In a prescription, an auxiliary active ingredient that supports the action of the basic drug. *See also* basis.

administration, sublingual Placing of a drug under the tongue to dissolve and to be absorbed through the mucous membrane.

administrative costs The overhead expenses incurred in the operation of a dental benefits program, exclusive of costs of dental services provided.

administrative services only (ASO) An arrangement under which a third party, for a fee, processes claims and handles paperwork for a self-funded group. This frequently includes all insurance company services (actuarial services, underwriting, benefit description. etc.) except assumption of risk.

admission The voluntary concession or admission that a fact or allegation is true.

   a., hospital 1: Full stay. The formal acceptance by a hospital or other inpatient health care facility of a patient who is to be provided with room, board, and continuous nursing service in an area of the hospital or facility where patients generally reside at least overnight. **2:** Surgicenter with short stays. Day bed only with nursing; patient does not stay overnight. **3:** Outpatient admission. Patient who enters the hospital but requires no bed; the patient enters for treatment and leaves after treatment.

administrator One who manages or directs a dental benefits program on behalf of the program's sponsor. *See also* third-party administrator; dental benefits organization.

adnexa (ăd-nĕk′sah) Conjoined anatomic parts. Tissues adjacent to or contained within a nearby space.

adolescence The period of human development between the onset of puberty and adulthood. It is generally marked by the appearance of secondary sex characteristic (11 to 13 years) and spans the teen years.

adrenal corticoid *See* corticoid, adrenal.

adrenal crisis *See* crisis, adrenal.

Adrenal steroids *See* Corticoid, adrenal.

Adrenalin (ah-drĕn′ah-lĭn) The trade name for epinephrine. *See* epinephrine.

adrenaline (ad-rĕn′ah-lĭn) The British name for epinephrine.

adrenergic (ăd-rĕn-ĕr′jĭk) **1:** Transmitted by norepinephrine or activated by norepinephrine or the other sympathomimetic agents. **2:** A term applied to nerve fibers that liberate epinephrine or norepinephrine at a synapse when a nerve impulse passes. **3:** A drug that mimics the action of adrenergic nerves.

a. blocking agent *See* agent, adrenergic blocking.

a. fibers *See* fibers, adrenergic.

a. receptors *See* receptors, adrenergic.

adrenic (ăd-rĕ′nĭk) Pertaining to the adrenal gland.

adrenocortical insufficiency (ah-drē″nō-kor′tĭ-kăl) *See* hypoadrenocorticalism.

adrenocorticotropin (ah-drē″nō-kor″tĭ-kō-trō′pin) *See* ACTH.

adrenolytic (ah-drē″nō-lĭt′ĭk) Capable of impeding the action of epinephrine, levarterenol (norepinephrine), or both (sympatholytic).

a. agent *See* agent, adrenergic blocking.

adrenotropic (ăd-rĕ′nō-trŏp′ik) Having a special affinity for the adrenal gland.

adsorb To attract molecules of a substance to the surface of another solid substance.

adsorbent A substance that adsorbs (e.g., activated charcoal, clay).

adumbration (ăd″ŭm-brā′shŭn) A geometric lack of sharpness of the x-ray shadow. *See* penumbra, geometric.

advances Monies paid before the proper time of payment.

adverse selection A statistical condition within a group when there is a greater demand for dental services and/or more services necessary than the average expected for that group.

advertising Any paid form of nonpersonal presentation and promotion of ideas, goods, or services by an identified sponsor.

aeration (ā-er-ā′shŭn) The passage of air or gases into liquid (e.g., the passage of oxygen from pulmonary alveoli into the blood).

aerodontalgia (ā″er-ō-dŏn-tăl′jē-ah) Pulpal pain with decreased barometric pressure.

aeroembolism (ā″er-ō-ĕm′bō-lĭzm) **(air embolism)** An obstruction of a blood vessel caused by the entrance of air into the bloodstream.

aerosinusitis (ā″er-ō-sī″nŭ-sī′tĭs) The painful symptoms related to the maxillary sinus resulting from a change in barometric pressure.

aerosol (ā′er-ō-sŏl) **1:** The suspension of materials in a gas or vapor (e.g., saliva vaporized in air-water spray from high-speed handpiece). **2:** A substance dispensed as constituent of gas or vapor suspension.

aesthetic factors *See* esthetic dentistry.

affect (af′ekt) **1:** The feeling of pleasantness or pleasantness produced by a stimulus **2:** The emotional complex influencing a mental state. **3:** The feeling experienced in connection with an emotion.

afferent (ăf′er-ĕnt) Conveying from a periphery to a center.

a. impulse An impulse that arises in the periphery and is carried into the central nervous system. An afferent nerve conducts the impulse from the site of origin to the central nervous system.

affiliation (ah-fĭl-ē-ā′shŭn) The incorporation or formation of a partnership by two or more dentists for the purpose of practicing the profession of dentistry.

afflux (ăf′lŭks) The rush of blood to a part.

affricative (ah-frĭk′ah-tĭv) A fricative speech sound initiated by a plosive.

aftercondensation *See* postcondensation.

afterperception *See* postperception.

aftersensation *See* postsensation.

A:G ratio *See* ratio, A:G.

agar (ah′găr) **1:** A polysaccharide derived from sea weed. **2:** The basic constituent of a reversible hydrocolloid. *See also* hydrocolloid, reversible.

a., hydrocolloid A reversible hydrocolloid made from agar-agar.

age hardening *See* hardening, age.

agenesis (ā-jĕn′ĕ-sĭs) The defective development or congenital absence of parts.

agent 1: A person or product that causes action. **2:** A person who acts for, or in place of, another by authority from him.

a., adrenergic blocking A drug that blocks the action of the neurohormones norepinephrine and/or epinephrine or of adrenergic drugs at sympathetic neuroeffectors.

a., adrenolytic blocking An uncertain term sometimes used in reference to adrenergic blocking agents.

a., anesthetic A drug that produces local or general loss of sensation.

a., antiinflammatory A drug that reduces inflammation.

a., bleaching An agent used in the modification or removal of discoloration.

a., blocking An agent that occupies or usurps the receptor site normally occupied by a drug or a biochemical internediary (e.g., acetylcholine or epinephrine).

a., chemotherapeutic A chemical of natural or synthetic origin used for its specific action against disease, generally against infection.

a., cholinergic blocking 1: A drug that inhibits the action of acetylcholine or cholinergic drugs at the postganglionic cholinergic neuroeffectors. **2:** An anticholinergic agent.

a., ganglionic blocking A drug that prevents passage of nerve impulses at the synapses between preganglionic and postganglionic neurons.

a., myoneural blocking A drug that prevents transmission of nerve impulses at the junction of the nerve and the muscle.

a., oxidizing An agent that provides oxygen in reaction with another substance or, in the broader and more definitive chemical sense, a chemical capable of accepting electrons and thereby decreasing the negative charge on an atom of the substance being oxidized.

a., polishing An abrasive that produces a smooth, lustrous finish.

a., wetting Any agent that will reduce the surface tension of water. Generally used in investing wax patterns.

agglutinin (ah-gloo′tĭ-nĭn) An antibody that agglutinates red blood cells or renders them agglutinable.

aging In human development, the process of growing old. Physically, aging is marked by the reduction in the ability of cells to function normally or to produce new body cells at an optimum rate.

aging schedule A report showing how long accounts receivable have been outstanding. It gives the percentage of receivables not past due and the percent past due by 1 month, 2 months, or other periods.

aglossia (ah-glos′ē-ah) A developmental anomaly in which a portion or all of the tongue is absent.

agnathia (ăg-nā′thē-ah) An absence of the lower jaw.

agnosia (ăg-nō′zē-ah) A loss of ability to recognize common objects (i.e., to understand the significance of sensory stimuli [e.g., tactile, auditory, or visual] resulting from brain damage).

agonist (ăg′ō-nĭst) An organ, gland, muscle, or nerve center that is so connected physiologically with another that the two function simultaneously in forwarding a given process (e.g., two muscles that pull on the same skeletal member and receive a nervous excitation at the same time). Antonym: antagonist.

agony 1: Severe pain or extreme suffering. **2:** The death struggle.

agranulocytopenia (ah-grăn″u-lō-sī-tō-pē′nē-ah) *See* agranulocytosis.

agranulocytosis (ah-grăn″u-lō-sī-tō′sĭs) A decrease in the number of granulocytes in peripheral blood resulting from bone marrow depression by drugs and chemicals or replacement by a neoplasm. Oral lesions are ulceronecrotic, involving the gingivae, tongue, buccal mucosa, or lips. Regional lymphadenopathy and lymphadenitis are prevalent.

agreement The coming together in accord of two minds on a given proposition; a concord of understanding and intention with respect to the effect on their relative rights and duties.

AH-26 An epoxy resin root-canal sealer.

AHF antihemophilic factor. *See also* factor VIII.

aid Assistance; support.

a. in physiotherapy An agent used by the patient to cleanse the teeth and oral tissues and provide pseudofunctional stimulation of the gingival tissues to maintain periodontal health.

a., prosthetic speech A restoration used to close a congenital or acquired cleft or other opening in the hard palate, soft palate, or both, or to replace lost or missing tissue necessary for the production of good speech.

a., speech therapy A restoration, appliance, or electronic device used to improve speech.

a., visual Any model, drawing, or photograph used to help the patient understand proposed treatment.

AIDS Abbreviation for acquired immunodeficiency syndrome.

AIDS-related complex (ARC) *See* acquired immunodeficiency syndrome.

air The invisible, odorless gaseous mixture that makes up the earth's atmosphere.

a. chamber *See* chamber, relief.

a. complemental *See* volume, inspiratory reserve.

a. functional residual *See* capacity, functional residual.

a., minimal The volume of air in the air sacs themselves (part of the residual air).

a. reserve *See* volume, expiratory reserve.

a., residual *See* volume, residual.

a., supplemental *See* volume, expiratory reserve.

a. syringe *See* syringe, air.

a., tidal *See* volume, tidal.

a. turbine handpiece *See* handpiece, air turbine.

airway 1: A clear passageway for air into and out of the lungs. **2:** A device for securing unobstructed respiration during general anesthesia or in states of unconsciousness.

ala (ā′lah) A winglike process; e.g., the ala of the nose is the cutaneous-covered cartilaginous structure on the lateral aspect of the external naris.

alarm reaction *See* reaction, alarm; syndrome, general adaptation.

Albers-Schönberg disease (ăl′berz shān′berg) *See* osteopetrosis.

Albright's syndrome *See* syndrome, Albright's.

albumin (ăl-bū′mĭn) The primary protein of plasma (4.5% Gm) that aids in maintaining capillar osmotic pressure.

albuminuria (ăl-bū″mĭ-nū′rē-ah) **(hyperproteinuria, proteinuria, proteuria)** The presence of clinically detectable amounts of protein in the urine (usually less than 100 mg/24 hr may be found normally by special methods). The usual protein is albumin, although globulins, Bence Jones protein, and fibrinogen may be present and may exceed albumin. The condition may be due to prerenal or renal disease or to inflammation of the urinary tract.

alcohol (ăl′kō-hŏl) A transparent liquid that is colorless, mobile, and volatile. Alcohols are organic compounds formed from hydrocarbons by the substitution of hydroxyl radicals for the same number of hydrogen atoms.

a., absolute Alcohol containing no more than 1% H_2O.

alcoholism The continued extreme dependence on excessive amounts of alcohol, accompanied by a cumulative pattern of deviant behaviors. The most frequent medical consequences of alcoholism are chronic gastritis, central nervous system depression, and cirrhosis of the liver.

aldosterone (ăl-dŏs′ter-ōn) **(electrocortin)** An adrenal corticosteroid hormone that acts primarily to accelerate the exchange of potassium for sodium in the renal tubules and other cells. It is a potent mineralocorticoid but also has some regulatory effect on carbohydrate metabolism.

aldosteronism, primary (ăl-dŏs′ter-ōn-ĭzm) A hyper adrenal syndrome caused by abnormal elaboration of aldosterone and characterized by excessive loss of potassium and resultant muscle weakness. The symptoms suggest tetany. The condition is often associated with an adenoma or cortical hyperplasia of the adrenal glands.

alganesthesia (ăl-găn″es-thē′zē-ah) The absence of a normal sense of pain.

algesia (ăl-jē′zē-ah) Sensitivity to pain; hyperesthesia; a sense of pain.

algesic (ăl-jē′sĭk) Painful.

algesimetry (ăl-jĕ-sĭm′ĕ-trē) The measurement of response to painful stimuli.

algetic (ăl-jĕt′ĭk) Painful.

alginate (ăl′jĭ-nāt) A salt of alginic acid (e.g., sodium alginate), which, when mixed with water in accurate proportions, forms an irreversible hydrocolloid gel used for making impressions. *See also* hydrocolloid, irreversible.

align (ah-līn′) To move the teeth into their proper positions to conform to the line of occlusion.

alignment, tooth (ah-līn′mĕnt) Arrangement of the teeth in relationship to their supporting bone (alveolar process), adjacent teeth, and opposing dentition.

alkali (ăl′kah-lī) A strong water-soluble base. A chemical substance that, in aqueous solution, undergoes dissociation, resulting in the formation of hydroxyl (OH) ions.

alkaline (ăl′kah-līn) Having the reductions of an alkali. A pH level of 7.1 to 14 designates an alkaline solution.

a. diet *See* diet, alkaline.

a. reserve *See* reserve, alkaline.

alkaloid (ăl′kah-loyd) Any one of the many nitrogen-containing organic bases derived from plants. The alkaloids are bitter and physiologically active. A number are useful therapeutic agents.

a., synthetic A synthetically prepared compound having the chemical characteristics of the alkaloids.

alkalosis (ăl-kah-lō′sĭs) A disturbance of acid-base balance and water balance, characterized by an excess of alkali or a deficiency of acids.

a., compensated A condition in which the blood bicarbonate is usually higher than normal, but in which the compensatory mechanisms have kept the pH level within normal range. *See also* alkalosis, uncompensated.

a., respiratory Alkalemia produced by hypoventilation. Plasma bicarbonate is therefore decreased in respiratory alkalosis but raised in metabolic alkalosis.

a., uncompensated Alkalemia usually accompanied by an increased blood bicarbonate.

allele (ah-lēl′) **(allelomorph)** One or more genes occupying the same location in a chromosome but differing because of a mutational change of one.

allelomorph (ah-lē′lō-morf) *See* allele.

allergen (ăl′er-jĕn) A substance capable of producing an allergic response. Common allergens are pollens, dust, drugs, and foods.

allergy (ăl′er-jē) A hypersensitivity reaction of the body to an allergen; an antigen-antibody reaction is manifested in several forms—anaphylaxis, asthma, hay fever, urticaria, angioedema, dermatitis, and stomatitis.

a., "spontaneous" clinical *See* atopy.

allochiria (ăl-ō-kī′rē-ah) Tactile sensation experienced at the side opposite its origin.

allografts Transplantation of tissue between genetically nonidentical individuals of the same species, also known as homoplastic grafts or homografts.

alloplast (ăl′ō-plăst) Transplant (implant) consisting of material originating from a nonliving source that is surgically inserted to replace missing tissue.

alloplastic (ăl″ō-plăs′tĭk) Nonbiologic (metal, ceramic, plastic) material.

alloplasty (ăl′ō-plăs″tē) Plastic surgical procedure in which use is made of material not from the human body.

allowable benefits Any necessary, reasonable, and customary item of service or treatment covered in whole or in part under an insurance plan.

allowable charge The maximum dollar amount on which benefit payment is based for each dental procedure.

allowable expenses The dollar amounts allowable for each dental procedure covered by a dental insurance policy.

alloxan (ah-lok′săn) A substance, mesoxalylurea, capable of producing experimental diabetes by destroying the islet cells of the pancreas.

alloy (ăl′oy) **1:** Metals that are mutually soluble in a liquid state. **2:** The product of the fusion of two or more metals.

a., amalgam The alloy or product of the fusion of several metals, usually supplied as filings, that is mixed with mercury to produce dental amalgam.

a., dental amalgam *See* amalgam.

a., cobalt-chromium (chrome-cobalt amalgam) Base metal alloys available commercially as Stellites. Used in dentistry for metallic denture bases and partial dentures.

a., dental gold An alloy in which the principal in gredient is gold.

a., eutectic Any combination of metals, the melting point of which is lower than that of any of the individual metals of which it consists. One in which the components are mutually soluble in the solid state. It has a nonhomogeneous grain structure and is therefore likely to be brittle and subject to tarnishing and corrosion.

a., nickel-chromium A stainless steel.

alopecia (ăl-ō-pē′shē-ah) Normal or abnormal deficiency of hair. Baldness.

alphabet, international phonetic A set of internationally agreed-on alphabetical symbols, one for each sound; supplements the existing alphabet to fill out needed representation of sounds.

alpha-estradiol (ăl″fah-ĕs-trah-dī′ŏl) An estrogenic steroid, prepared by dehydrogenation of estrone, which is one of the factors responsible for the maintenance of the epithelial integrity of the oral tissues. A deficiency results in epithelial desquamation.

alpha-hemihydrate (ăl″fah-hĕm-ē-hī′drāt) A physical form of the hemihydrate of calcium sulfate $(CaSO_4)_2 \cdot H_2O$; dental artificial stone.

alpha-interferon *See* interferon, Alpha.

alphanumeric Pertaining to a character set that contains letters and numerals and usually other special characters.

alpha-tocopherol (ăl″fah-tō-kŏf′er-ŏl) *See* vitamin E.

alternate benefit A provision in a dental plan contract that allows the third-party payer to determine the benefit based on an alternative procedure that is generally less expensive than the one provided or proposed.

alternate treatment Contract provisions that authorize the carrier to determine the amount of benefits payable, giving consideration to alternate procedures, services, or courses of treatment that may be performed to accomplish the desired result. The attending dentist and the patient have the option of which procedure to use, although payment for the procedure may be based on the "alternate treatment" principle.

alternative benefit plan A plan, other than a traditional (fee-for-service, freedom of choice) indemnity or service corporation plan for reimbursing a participating dentist for providing treatment to an enrolled patient population.

alternative delivery system An arrangement for the provision of dental services in other than the traditional (e.g., licensed dentist providing treatment in a fee-for-service dental office) way.

alternative plan A compromise plan of treatment deviating from the ideal plan in scope and financial investment.

alumina (ah-lū′mĭ-nah) Aluminum oxide, an abrasive sometimes used as a polishing agent.

Aluwax (ăl′ū-wăx) A commercially prepared wax wafer containing aluminum that is used to register jaw relationship.

alveolalgia (ăl″vē-ō-lahl′jē-ah) *See* socket, dry.

alveolar (ăl-vē′ō-lahr) Pertaining to an alveolus.

a. crest *See* crest, alveolar.

a. process *See* process, alveolar.

a. ridge *See* ridge, alveolar.

alveolectomy (ăl″vē-ō-lĕk′tō-mē) Excision of a portion of the alveolar process to aid in the removal of teeth, modification of the contour after the removal of teeth, and preparation of the mouth for dentures.

alveolitis In dentistry, the inflamation of a tooth socket.

alveololingual sulcus *See* sulcus, alveololingual.

alveolus (ăl-vē′ō-lŭs) **1:** An air sac of the lungs formed by terminal dilations of the bronchioles. **2:** The socket in the bone in which a tooth is attached by means of the periodontal ligament.

alveoplasty The surgical shaping and smoothing of the margins of the tooth socket after extraction of the tooth, generally in preparation for the placement of a prosthesis.

amalgam (ah-mal′găm) **(dental amalgam alloy)** An alloy, one of the constituents of which is mercury.

a. carrier *See* carrier, amalgam.

a. carver *See* carver, amalgam.

a. condenser *See* condenser, amalgam.

a., copper An alloy composed principally of copper and mercury. *See also* amalgam.

a., dental An amalgam used for dental restorations and dies.

a. matrix *See* matrix, amalgam.

a. plugger *See* condenser, amalgam.

a., silver A dental amalgam, the chief constituent of which is silver. The ADA composition specifications are as follows: silver, 65% minimum; tin, 25% minimum; copper, 6% maximum; zinc, 2% maximum.

a. squeeze cloth A piece of linen used to hold plastic amalgam from which excess mercury is to be squeezed.

a. tattoo A solitary discrete gray, blue, or black discoloration of tissue usually located in the gingiva, alveolar ridge, or buccal mucosa caused by the embedment of minute amounts of dental amalgam. The asymptomatic lesion is static and requires no treatment. If doubt exists about the lesion or if the lesion is unsightly, excisional biopsy is recommended.

amalgamation (ah-măl″gah-mā′shŭn) Formation of an

alloy by mixing mercury with another metal or other metals. *See also* trituration.

amalgamator (ah-măl′gah-mā-tor) A mechanical device used to triturate the ingredients of dental amalgam into a plastic mass.

ameloblastic fibroma *See* fibroma, ameloblastic.

ameloblastic sarcoma *See* sarcoma, ameloblastic.

ameloblastoma (ah-měl″ō-blăs-tō′mah) **(adamantino blastoma, adamantinoma)** An epithelial neoplasm with a basic structure resembling the enamel organ and suggesting derivation from ameloblastic cells. It is usually benign.

    a., acanthomatous An epithelial odontogenic tumor that differs from the simple ameloblastoma in that the central cells within the cell nests are squamous and may be keratinized rather than stellate. The peripheries of the cell nests are composed of ameloblastic cells. *See also* ameloblastoma.

amelogenesis impefecta (ah-měl″ō-jěn′ě-sĭs) A severe hypoplasia or agenesis of enamel that is inherited as a dominant characteristic.

amenorrhea (ah-měn-or-rē′ah) Absence or abnormal cessation of the menstrual cycle.

Americans with Disabilities Act A federal law enacted on July 26, 1990, that defines a private dental office as a place of public accommodation, thereby requiring as of January 26, 1992, that dentists serve persons with diabilities.

amino acid An organic acid in which one of the CH hydrogen atoms has been replaced by NH_2. Amino acids are the building blocks of proteins.

    essential a.a.'s Amino acids required by the organism that must be supplied by the diet. Isoleucine, leucine, lysine, methionine, pheylalanine, threonine, tryptophan, and valine are essential to adults; these eight plus arginine and histidine are considered essential to infants and children.

    nonessential a.a.'s Amino acids that can be synthesized by the organism and are not required in the diet.

ammeter (ăm′mē-ter) A contraction of amperemeter. An apparatus that measures the amperage of an electric current.

ammonia thiosulfate (ah-mō′nē-ah thī-ō-sŭl′fāt) An ingredient of the photographic fixing solution that acts as a solvent for silver halides.

ammoniacal silver nitrate *See* silver nitrate, ammoniacal.

amnesia (ăm-nē′zē-ah) Lack or loss of memory.

amnesiac (ăm-nē′zē-ăk) A person affected by amnesia.

amnesic (am-ne′zik) *See* sedative.

amnestic (ăm-něs′tĭk) Amnesic; causing amnesia.

amorphous (ah-mor′fŭs) A substance having no specific space lattice, the molecules being distributed at random.

amortization A generic term that includes various specific practices, such as depreciation, depletion, write off of intangibles, prepaid expenses, and deferred charges.

amoxicillin A generic semisynthetic penicillin antibiotic similar to ampicillin.

ampere (ăm′pēr) **(Amp)** Unit of quantity of electric current, equal to a flow of 1 coulomb per second or the flow of 6.25×10^{18} electrons per second. The current produced by 1 volt acting through a resistance of 1 ohm.

amperemeter (ăm′pēr-mēt″er) *See* ammeter.

amphotericin An antibiotic and antifungal agent used extensively in the treatment of systemc mycoses.

ampicillin An acid stable semisynthetic penicillin antibiotic with a broader spectrum of effectiveness than penicillin G.

amputation, pulp *See* pulpotomy.

amputation, root Removal of a root of a multirooted tooth.

amputation neuroma *See* neuroma, traumatic.

amyloidosis (ăm″ĭ-loi-dō′sĭs) A condition in which amyloid, a glycoprotein, is deposited intercellularly in tissues and organs. Four types of amyloidosis are recognized, two of which, primary amyloidosis and amyloid tumor, frequently produce nodules in the tongue and gingiva.

    a., primary Amyloidosis occurring without a known predisposing cause. Amyloid deposits are found in the tongue, lips, skeletal muscles, and other mesodermal structures. The disease may be manifested by polyneuropathy, purpura, hepatosplenomegaly, heart failure, and the nephrotic syndrome.

    a., secondary Amyloidosis occurring secondary to chronic diseases such as tuberculosis, leprosy, rheumatoid arthritis, multiple myeloma, and prolonged bacterial infections. Amyloid deposits are found in parenchymal organs. The disease is usually manifested by proteinuria and hepatosplenomegaly.

amyotonia (ah-mi″o-tō′nē-ah) Abnormal flaccidity or flabbiness of a muscle or group of muscles.

anabolism (ah-năb′ō-lĭzm) The constructive process by which substances are converted from simple to complex forms by living cells; constructive metabolism.

anaerobes (ăn-a′er-ōbs) Microorganisms that can exist and grow only in the partial or complete absence of molecular oxygen.

analeptic (ăn-ah-lěp′tĭk) **1:** An agent that acts to overcome depression of the central nervous system. **2:** A strong central nervous system stimulant that is used to restore consciousness, especially from a drug-induced coma.

analgesia (ăn″al-jē′zē-ah) Insensibility to pain without loss of consciousness; a state in which painful stimuli are not perceived or interpreted as pain; usually induced by a drug, although trauma or a disease process may produce a general or regional analgesia.

a., infiltration The arrest of the sensory responses of nerve endings at the surgical site by injections of an anesthetic at that site.

a., regional Reversible loss of pain sensation over an area of the body by blocking the afferent conduction of its innervation with a local anesthetic agent.

analgesic (ăn-al-jē′sĭk) (analgetic) **1:** The property of a drug that enables it to raise the pain threshold. **2:** An analgesic may be classified in one of two groups: an analgesic that blocks the sensory neural pathways of pain (e.g., procaine and its derivatives) or an an algesic that acts directly on the thalamus to raise the pain threshold.

analgetic (ăn-al-jĕt′ĭk) *See* analgesic.

analgia (ăn-al′jē-ah) An absence of pain.

analysis (ah-năl′ĭ-sĭs) A separation into component parts.

a., bite *See* analysis, occlusal.

a., cephalometric (sĕf″ah-lō-mĕ′trĭk) Evaluation of the growth pattern or morphologic conditions based on cephalometric tracings.

a., dietary Evaluation of a diet on the basis of caloric intake and dietary components.

a., occlusal A study of the relations of the occlusal surfaces of opposing teeth and their functional harmony.

a., radiochemical Determination of the absolute disintegration rate of a radionuclide in a mixture based on the counting rate of a sample that has been separated and purified, in measured yield, by appropriate chemical procedures.

a. of variance (ANOV) A powerful statistic that allows comparisons among more than two (multiple) means or groups to occur simultaneously. ANOV assumes a normal distributed variable, homogeneity of variance and independent samples and uses internal data. The results are compared using the f-test, and significance levels are found in a table under the appropriate degrees of freedom listing.

analyzing rod *See* rod, analyzing.

anamnesis (ăn-ăm-nē′sĭs) A past history of disease or injury based on the patient's memory or recall at the time of dental and/or medical interview and examination.

anaphylactic (an″ah-fĭ-lăk′tĭk) Pertaining to decreasing, rather than increasing, immunity.

a. hypersensitivity (Arthus' reaction) A local tissue response that is the result of an Ah-AB caused by repeated intradermal injections with one antigen, resulting in inflammation and necrosis.

anaphylactoid (ăn″ah-fĭ-lăk′toid) Resembling anaphylaxis; pertaining to a reaction, the symptoms of which resemble those of the anaphylactic produced by the injection of serum and other nonspecific proteins.

a. reaction *See* reaction, anaphylactoid.

anaphylaxis (ăn″ah-fĭ-lăk′sĭs) A violent allergic reaction characterized by sudden collapse, shock, or respiratory and circulatory failure after injection of an allergen.

anaplasia (ăn″ah-plā′zē-ah) A regressive change in cells toward a more primitive or embryonic cell type. Anaplasia is a prominent criterion of malignancy in tumors.

anasarca (ăn″ah-sar′kah) **(dropsy)** Generalized edema.

anastomosis The joining together of two blood vessels or other tubular structures to furnish a direct or indirect communication between the two structures.

a. grafts The connection of two autogenous tubular structures as a part of reconstructive surgery.

anatomic (ăn-ah-tŏm′ĭk) Pertaining to the anatomy of a structure.

a. crown *See* crown, anatomic.

a. dead space The actual capacity of the respiratory passages that extend from the nostrils to and including the terminal bronchioles.

a. form *See* form, anatomic.

a. height of contour *See* contour, height of.

a. impression *See* impression, anatomic.

a. landmark *See* landmark, anatomic.

a. teeth *See* tooth, anatomic.

anatomy (ah-năt′ō-mē) The science of the form, structure, and parts of animal organisms.

a., dental The science of the structure of the teeth and the relationship of their parts. The study involves macroscopic and microscopic components.

a., radiographic The images on a radiographic film of the combined anatomic structures through which the roentgen rays (x rays) have passed.

ANB angle A cephalometric measurement of the anterior-posterior relationship the maxilla with the mandible.

anchorage 1: The supporting base for orthodontic forces that are applied to stimulate tooth movement. **2:** The area of application of the reciprocal forces that are generated when corrective forces are applied to teeth. May be one tooth or more in the jaw, environmental musculature, neck, or cranium.

a. bends Bends placed in an orthodontic wire to enhance the resistance to the anterior displacement of teeth during orthodontic treatment; primarily used in the Tweed and Begg techniques.

a., cervical An extraoral anchorage based at the back of the neck.

a., cranial An extraoral anchorage based at the back of the skull.

a., extraoral An orthodontic anchorage based outside the mouth. Dental attachments are typically linked to a wire bow or hooks extending between the lips and attached elastically to a cap, a strap around the neck, or another extraoral device.

a., facial An extraoral anchorage based on the face, usually the chin and forehead.

a., intermaxillary An anchorage based in the opposite jaw.

a., intramaxillary An anchorage based on teeth within the same jaw.

a., intraoral An anchorage based within the mouth (intermaxillary, intramaxillary, or myofunctional).

a., occipital A cranial anchorage based in the occipital area.

a., reciprocal All anchorage is reciprocal; sometimes used to describe a force system in which the resistance units are similar.

a., simple The use of a tooth as a resistance unit without tipping control.

a., stationary The use of a tooth as an anchorage unit with tipping control.

Andresen appliance *See* appliance, Andresen.

androgen (ăn′drō-jĕn) Any substance that possesses masculinizing qualities, such as testosterone.

anemia (ah-nē′mē-ah) A term indicating that the concentration of hemoglobin or the number of red blood cells is below the accepted normal value with respect to age and sex. In true anemia the total concentration of hemoglobin or the total number of erythrocytes is below normal irrespective of concentration values. Symptoms, which may not be evident, include weakness, pallor, anorexia, and those related to the cause of the anemia.

a., Addison-Biermer *See* anemia, pernicious.

a., aplastic An anemia characterized by a decrease in all marrow elements, including platelets, red blood cells, and granulocytes.

a., Biermer's *See* anemia, pernicious.

a., Cooley's *See* thalassemia major.

a., displacement *See* anemia, myelophthisic.

a., erythroblastic *See* thalassemia major.

a., hemolytic An anemia characterized by an increased rate of destruction of red blood cells, reticulocytosis, hyperbilirubinemia and/or increased urinary and fecal urobilinogen, and, generally, splenic enlargement. Hereditary hemolytic anemias include congenital hemolytic jaundice, sickle cell anemia, oval cell anemia, and thalassemia. Acquired hemolytic anemias include paroxysmal nocturnal hemoglobinuria and those due to immune mechanisms (erythroblastosis fetalis), transfusions of in compatible blood, infections, drugs, and poisons. Autoimmune hemolytic anemias are aquired hemolytic anemias associated with antibody-like substances that may not be true autoantibodies or even antibodies; they may be primary (idiopathic), or they may be secondary to lymphoma, lymphatic leukemia, disseminated lupus erythematosus, or sensitization to drugs and pollens.

a., hemorrhagic A deficiency in red blood cells and/or hemoglobin resulting from excessive bleeding.

a., hyperchromic An anemia in which the erythrocytes are larger than normal in size so that the content but not the concentration of hemoglobin is increased.

a., hypochromic An anemia caused by impaired hemoglobin synthesis resulting from a deficiency of iron or pyridoxine and from chronic lead poisoning.

a., iron-deficiency An anemia resulting from a deficiency of iron, characterized by hypochromic microcytic erythrocytes and a normoblastic reaction of the bone marrow. Iron deficiency may result from an increased demand during growth or repeated pregnancies, chronic or recurrent hemorrhage (e.g., menstrual abnormalities, hemorrhoids, or peptic ulcer), a low intake of iron, or impaired absorption, as in chronic diarrhea.

a., macrocytic-normochromic An anemia related to a failure of nucleoprotein synthesis caused by a deficiency of vitamin B_{12}, folic acid, or related substances.

a., Mediterranean *See* thalassemia major.

a., megaloblastic An anemia characterized by hyperplastic bone marrow changes and maturation arrest resulting from a dietary deficiency, impaired absorption, impaired storage and modification, or impaired use of one or more hematopoietic factors. Included are pernicious anemia, nutritional macrocytic anemias associated with gastrointestinal disturbances, anemias associated with impaired liver function (e.g., macrocytic anemia of pregnancy), hypothyroidism, leukemia, and achrestic anemia.

a., microcytic hypochromic An anemia in which the mean corpuscular volume (MCV), mean corpuscular hemoglobin (MCH) content, and mean corpuscular hemoglobin concentration (MCHC) are all low (e.g., iron-deficiency anemia, hereditary leptocytosis, hemoglobin C anemia, and anemias resulting from pyridoxine deficiency and chronic lead poisoning. **a., myelophthisic (displacement anemia)** An anemia resulting from displacement or crowding out of erythropoietic cells of the bone marrow by foreign tissue, as in leukemia, metastatic carcinorna, lymphoblastoma, multiple myeloma, osteoradionecrosis, and xanthomatosis.

a., normocytic-normochromic An anemia associated with disturbances of red cell formation and related to endocrine deficiencies, chronic inflammation, and carcinomatosis.

a., nutritional macrocytic Macrocytic-normochromic anemia occurring as a result of a deficiency of substances necessary for deoxyribonucleic acid synthesis; e. g., vitamin B_{12} and folic acid deficiency may result from a lack of intrinsic factors, sprue, or regional enteritis. Folic acid deficiency may occur in chronic alcoholism, as a result of a diet deficient in meats and vegetables, and in diseases causing intestinal malabsorption.

a., oval cell *See* elliptocytosis.

a., pernicious (Addison-Biermer anemia) A macrocytic-normochromic (megaloblastic anemia associated with achlorhydria and a lack of a gastric intrinsic factor necessary for the binding and absorption of vitamin B_{12}, which is an erythrocyte maturing factor. In addition to hematologic findings, atrophic glossitis and gastrointestinal and nervous disorders occur.

a., physiologic An anemia characterized by lowered blood values resulting from an increase in plasma volume that occurs most markedly during the sixth and seventh months of pregnancy.

a., sickle cell (drepanocythemia, sicklemia) A hereditary hemolytic anemia in which the presence of an abnormal hemoglobin (hemoglobin S) results in distorted, sickle-shaped erythrocytes. Manifestations include episodic crises of muscle, joint, and abdominal pain; neurologic symptoms; and leg ulcers. It occurs almost exclusively in blacks. *See also* trait, sickle cell.

a., spherocytic *See* jaundice, congenital hemolytic.

anergy (ăn′er-jē) In terms of hypersensitivity, an inability to react to specific antigens (i.e., lack of reaction to intradermally injected antigens in measles, Hodgkin's sarcoma, and overwhelming tuberculosis).

anesthesia (ăn″ĕs-thē′zē-ah) The loss of feeling or sensation, especially loss of tactile sensibility, with or without loss of consciousness.

a., basal A state of narcosis, induced before the administration of a general anesthetic, that permits the production of states of surgical anesthesia with greatly reduced amounts of general anesthetic agents.

a., block An anesthesia induced by injecting the drug close to the nerve trunk, at some distance from the operative field. *See also* anesthesia, infiltration.

a., conduction An anesthesia induced by injecting the drug close to the nerve trunk, at some distance from the operative field.

a., general An irregular, reversible depression of the cells of the higher centers of the central nervous system that makes the patient unconscious and insensible to pain.

a., glove An anesthesia with a distribution corresponding to the part of the skin covered by a glove.

a., infiltration An anesthesia induced by injecting the anesthetic solution directly into or around the tissues to be anesthetized; used for operative procedures on the maxillary premolar, anterior teeth, and mandibular incisors. *See also* anesthesia, block.

a., intraosseous An anesthesia produced by the injec-

tion of an anesthetic agent into the cancellous portion of a bone.

a., intrapulpal The injection of a local anesthetic directly into pulpal tissue under pressure.

a., local (regional anesthesia) The loss of pain sensation over a specific area of the anatomy without loss of consciousness.

a., regional A term used for local anesthesia. *See also* anesthesia, local.

a., topical A form of local anesthesia whereby free nerve endings in accessible structures are rendered incapable of stimulation by applying a suitable solution directly to the surface of the area.

anesthesiologist (ăn″ĕs-thē″zē-ŏl′ō-jĭst) A specialist in anesthesiology.

anesthetic (ăn″ĕs-thĕt′ĭk) A drug that produces loss of feeling or sensation generally or locally.

a. agent *See* agent, anesthetic.

a., local A drug that, when injected into the tissues and absorbed into a nerve, will temporarily interrupt its property of conduction.

a., topical A drug applied to the surface of tissues that produces local insensibility to pain.

anesthetist (ah-nĕs′thĕ-tĭst) A person who administers anesthetics.

anesthetize (ah-nĕs′thĕ-tīz) To place under anesthesia.

aneurysm (ăn′ŭ-rĭzm) A localized dilation of an artery in which one or more layers of the vessel walls are distended.

a., arteriovenous *See* shunt, arteriovenous.

angiitis, visceral (ăn″jē-ī′tĭs) *See* disease, collagen.

angina (ăn-jī′nah) A spasmodic, choking pain. The term is sometimes applied to the disease producing the pain (e.g., Ludwig's angina).

a., agranulocytic *See* agranulocytosis.

a., Ludwig's A cellulitis involving the submaxillary, sublingual, and submental spaces and characterized clinically by a firm swelling of the floor of the mouth, with elevation of the tongue.

a., monocytic A "sore throat" associated with infectious mononucleosis.

a. pectoris Frequently a symptom of cardiovascular diseases; characterized by a severe, viselike pain behind the sternum that sometimes radiates to the arms, neck, or mandible. It may also consist of a sense of constriction or pressure of the chest. It is caused by exertion or excitement and is relieved by rest.

a., Vincent's An incorrect term for involvement of the pharynx by the spread of acute necrotizing ulceromembranous gingivitis.

angioedema (ăn″jē-ō-ĕ-dē′mah) *See* edema, angioneurotic.

angioma (ăn″jē-ō′mah) A benign tumor of vascular nature. *See also* hemangioma; lymphangioma.

angioneurotic edema (ăn″jē-ō-nū-raht′ĭk) *See* edema, angioneurotic.

angle The degree of divergence of two or more lines or planes that meet each other; the space between such lines. Measured in degrees of an arc.

a., Bennett The angle formed by the sagittal plane and the path of the advancing condyle during lateral mandibular movement, as viewed in the horizontal plane.

a. board A device used to facilitate the establishment of reproducible angular relationships between a patient's head, the x-ray beam, and the x-ray film.

a., cavosuface The angle in a prepared cavity, formed by the junction of the wall of the cavity with the surface of the tooth.

a., cranial base The angle formed by a line representing the floor of the anterior cranial fossa intersecting a line representing the axis of the clivus of the base of the skull.

a., cusp 1: The angle made by the slopes of a cusp with the plane that passes through the tip of the cusp and is perpendicular to a line bisecting the cusp; measured mesiodistally or buccolingually. Half of the included angle between the buccolingual or mesiodistal cusp inclines. **2:** The angle made by the slopes of a cusp with a perpendicular line bisecting the cusp; measured mesiodistally or buccolingually.

a., facial An anthropometric expression of the degree of protrusion of the lower face, assessed by measuring the inclination of the facial plane relative to a horizontal reference plane.

a., former One of a series of paired, hoe-shaped cutting instruments having the cutting edge at an angle other than a right angle in relation to the axis of the blade.

a., bayonet former A hoe-shaped, paired cutting instrument; binangled with the blade parallel with the axis of the shaft, the cutting edge is not perpendicular to the axis of the blade. Used to accentuate angles in an ″invisible″ class 3 cavity.

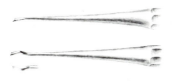

Angle former

a., Frankfort-mandibular incisor (FMIA) A procum procubency of mandibular incisor to the Frankfort horizontal plane. **a. incisal** (in-si′zal) The degree of slope between the axis-orbital plane and the palatal discluding skidway of the upper incisor.

a., incisal guidance The angle formed with the occlusal plane by drawing a line in the sagittal plane between the incisal edges of the maxillary and mandibular central incisors when the teeth are in centric occlusion.

a., incisal guide The inclination of the incisal guide on the articulator.

a., lateral incisal guide The inclination of the incisal guide in the frontal plane.

a., protrusive incisional guide The inclination of the incisal guide in the sagittal plane.

a., line An angle formed by the junction of the two walls along a line; designated by combining the names of the walls forming the angle.

a. of mandible The gonial angle. The relation existing between the body of the mandible and the ramus of the mandible.

a., occlusal rest The angle formed by the occlusal rest with the upright minor connector.

a., point An angle formed by the junction of three walls at a common point; designated by combining the names of the walls forming the angle.

a., rest *See* angle, occusal rest.

a., symphyseal The angle of the chin, which may be protruding straight, or receding, according to type.

Angle's classification modified A classification of the different forms of malocclusion set up by Edward Hartley Angle, American orthodontist (1855-1930).

Class I The normal anteroposterior relationship of the lower jar to the upper jaw. The mesiobuccal cusp of the maxillary first permanent molar occludes in the buccal groove of the mandibular first permanent molar; special class I—mutilated.

Type I All teeth in linguoversion.

Type II Narrow arches; labioversion of the maxillary anterior teeth and linguoversion of the mandibular lower anterior teeth.

Type III Linguoversion of the maxillary anterior teeth; bunched; lack of development in the proximal region.

Class II The posterior relationship of the lower jaw to the upper jaw. The mesiobuccal cusp of the maxillary first permanent molar occludes mesial to the buccal groove of the mandibular first permanent molar.

Division 1 Labioversion of the maxillary teeth.

Subdivision Signifies a unilateral condition.

Division 2 Linguoversion of the maxillary central incisor teeth.

Subdivision Signifies a unilateral condition.

Class III The anterior relationship of the lower jaw to the upper jaw, may have a subdivision. The mesiobuccal cusp of the maxillary first permanent molar occludes distal to the buccal groove of the mandibular first permanent molar.

Type I Good alignment general but abnormal arch relationship.

Type II Good alignment of the maxillary anterior teeth but linguoversion of the mandibular anterior teeth.

Type III Underdeveloped upper arch; linguoversion of maxillary anterior teeth; good mandibular alignment.

Ångström unit *See* unit, Ångström.

angular cheilosis *See* cheilosis, angular.

angulation (ăng″ū-la′shŭn) The direction of the primary beam of radiation in relation to object and film.

a., horizontal The angle measured within the occlusal plane at which the central ray of the x-ray beam is projected relative to a reference in the vertical or sagittal plane.

a., vertical The angle measured within the vertical plane at which the central ray of the x-ray beam is projected relative to a reference in the horizontal or occlusal plane.

anhidrosis (ăn″hĭ-drō′sĭs) An abnormal deficiency in the production of sweat; may be associated with an odontia in ectodermal dysplasia.

anhidrotic ectodermal dysplasia *See* hypohidrotic ectoderma dysplasia.

anhydremia (ăn-hĭ-drē′me-ah) A decrease in blood volume resulting from a decrease in the serum component of blood; occurs in shock or in any condition in which blood fluid is passed into the tissue and results in hemoconcentration.

anion (an′ī-ŏn) A negatively charged ion.

anionic detergent (ăn″ī-ahn′ĭk) *See* detergent, anionic.

anisocytosis (ăn-ī″sō-sī-tō′sĭs) An inequality in cell size, especially of red blood cells.

anisognathous (ăn″ī-sŏg′nah-thŭs) Maxillary and mandibular dental arches or jaws are of different sizes.

ankyloglossia (ăng″kĭ-lō-glahs′ē-ah) Tongue-tie; an abnormally short lingual frenum that limits movement of the tongue.

ankylosis (ăng″kĭ-lŏ′sĭs) An abnormal fixation and immobility of a joint.

a., false An inability to open the mouth because of trismus rather than disease of the joint.

a., fibrous Fixation of a joint by fibrous tissue.

a. of tooth *See* tooth, ankylosed.

anlage (ăn′lah-gĕh) The first cells in the embryo that form any distinct part or organ of the body.

anneal (ah-nēl′) **(homogenizing heat treatment, softening heat treatment)** The softening of a metal by controlled heating and cooling.

a. foil A process of subjecting noncohesive foil to heat to volatilize a protective gaseous coating on its surface, thus leaving the surface clean, making it cohesive.

a. glass A process of regulated heating and subsequent cooling to remove strain hardening or work hardening of glass.

a. metal A process of regulated heating and subsequent cooling to remove strain hardening or work hardening of metal.

announcement A communication (usually printed) that states office policies or practice limitations to the public and profession.

annual statement The report of an insurer or carrier showing assets and liabilities, receipts and disbursements, and other information for a specified 12-month period (fiscal or calendar year).

annuity A series of payments of a fixed amount for a number of years.

anochromasia (ăn″ō-krō-mā′sē-ah) A variation in the staining quality of cells, particularly of degenerating red blood cells.

anociassociation (ah-nō″sē-ah-sō-sē-ā′shŭn) The blocking of neuroses, fear, pain, and harmful influences or associations to prevent shock.

anode (ăn′ōd) The electrically positive terminal of a roentgen ray (x-ray) tube; a tungsten block embedded in a copper stem and set at an angle of 20 or 45 degrees to the cathode. The anode emits roentgen rays (x rays) from the point of impact of the electronic stream from the cathode.

a., rotating An anode that rotates during x-ray production to present a constantly different focal spot to the electron stream and to permit use of small focal spots or higher tube voltages without overheating the tube.

anode-film distance *See* distance, target-film.

anodontia (ăn-ō-dŏn′shē-ah) (aplasia of dentition) The failure of teeth to form; may be partial or complete.

a., partial Absence of parts of the dentition resulting from arrested tooth development.

a., total A complete absence of teeth resulting from arrested tooth development.

anodyne (ăn′ō-dīn) An agent or drug that relieves pain; milder than analgesia.

anomaly (ah-nŏm′ah-lē) An aberration or deviation from normal anatomic growth, development, or function.

a., dental An abnormality in which a tooth or teeth have deviated from normal in form, function, or position.

a., dentofacial Term indicating an oral or a dysgnathic anomaly.

a., dysgnathic An anomaly that extends beyond the teeth and includes the maxillae, the mandible, or both.

a., eugnathic An anomaly limited to the teeth and their immediate alveolar supports.

a., gestant *See* odontoma.

a., maxillofacial A distortion of normal development

of the face and jaws; a dysgnathic anomaly.

a., oral An abnormal structure other than of the teeth.

anophaxia (ăn-ō-făx′ē-ah) A tendency for one eye to turn upward.

anorexia (ăn-ō-rĕk′sē-ah) The partial or complete loss of appetite for food.

anorexia nervosa A psychoneurotic disorder characterized by a prolonged refusal to eat, resulting in emaciation, amenorrhea in women, emotional disturbance concerning body image, and an abnormal fear of becoming fat.

anoxemia (ăn-ahk-sē′mē-ah) A deficient aeration of the blood; a total lack of oxygen content in the blood.

anoxia (ăn-ahk′sē-ah) A condition of total lack of oxygen; a term frequently misused as a symptom of hypoxia.

anoxiate (ăn-ahk′sē-āt) To cause or produce anoxia.

anoxic hypoxia *See* hypoxia, anoxic.

antagonist 1: A drug that counteracts, blocks, or abolishes the action of another drug. **2:** A muscle that acts in opposition to the action of another muscle (e.g., flexor vs. extensor). **3:** A tooth in one jaw that occludes with a tooth in the other jaw.

a., insulin Circulating hormonal and nonhormonal substances that stimulate glyconeogenesis (e.g., 11-oxysteroids and S hormones).

a., narcotic A narcotic drug that acts specifically to reverse depression of the central nervous system.

antagonistic reflex *See* reflex, antagonistic.

ante cibum (ăn′tē sī′bum) *See* a.c.

antegonial notch The notch or concavity usually present at the junction between the ramus and body of the mandible, near the anterior margin of the masseter muscle attachment.

anterior 1: Situated in front of. **2:** A term used to denote the incisor and canine teeth or the forward region of the mouth. **3:** The forward position.

a. cranial base The anterior cranial fossa, sometimes identified by related landmarks such as the sella turcica and nasion.

a. determinants of occlusion *See* occlusion, anterior determinants of cusp.

a. guide *See* guide, anterior.

a. nasal spine *See* spine, anterior nasal.

a. palatal bar *See* connector, anterior palatal major.

a. tooth arrangement *See* arrangement, tooth, anterior.

anterior-posterior discrepancy An anterior-posterior morphologic imbalance between the maxilla and mandible and consequently between structures attached to either.

anteroclusion Malocclusion of the teeth in which the mandibular teeth are in a position anterior to their normal position relative to the teeth in the maxillary arch.

anteversion The tipping or tilting of teeth or other max-

illary and mandibular structures too far forward (anterior) from the normal or generally accepted standard.

anthelmintic (ăn″thĕl-mĭn′tĭk) A drug that acts against parasitic worms, especially intestinal worms.

anthrax (ăn′thraks) An infectious disease in herbivorous animals caused by a spore-forming bacillus. Primary lesions in human beings may be on the lips or cheeks.

anthropometry Measurement of the human body and its parts.

antibiotic (ăn-tĭ-bī-ŏt′ĭk) An organic substance produced by one of several microorganisms, especially certain molds, that is capable, in low concentration, of destroying or inhibiting the growth of certain other microorganisms.

a., oral reactions to Manifestations on the oral mucous membrane of reactions to antibiotics; characterized by glossitis, angular cheilosis, and/or a hairy tongue. Reactions may result from imbalance of oral flora produced by the antibiotics or to hypersensitivity to the antibiotics.

a. therapy *See* therapy, antibiotic.

antibody (ăn′tĭ-bŏd-ē) A specific substance that is produced by an animal as a reaction to the presence of an antigen and that reacts specifically with an antigen in some observable way.

anticholinergic (ăn″tĭ-kō″lĭn-er′jik) **(parasympatholytic, cholinolytic)** A drug that acts to inhibit the effects of the neurohormone acetylcholine or to inhibit the cholinergic neuroeffects. A cholinergic blocking agent.

anticholinesterase (ăn″tĭ-kō″lĭn-es′ter-ās) A drug or chemical that inhibits or inactivates the enzyme cholinesterase, resulting in the actions produced by the accumulation of acetylcholine at cholinergic sites.

anticoagulant (ăn″tĭ-kō-ăg′ū-lănt) A drug that delays or prevents coagulation of blood.

anticonvulsive (ăn″tĭ-kŏn-vul′sĭv) Relieving or preventing convulsion.

antidepressants Agents used to counteract or treat depression.

antidote (ăn′tĭ-dōt) A substance that acts to antagonize the toxic effects of a drug, especially in overdose, or of a poison.

antiemetic (ăn″tē-ē-mĕt′ĭk) A drug used to prevent, stop, or relieve nausea and emesis (vomiting).

antiepileptic drugs Agents that inhibit or control seizures associated with epilepsy.

antiflatulants Agents used relieve gastrointestinal gas.

antifungal agents Agents that inhibit, control or kill fungi. The most common yeast-like fungus occuring in or near the oral cavity is *Candida albicans*.

antiflux A material that prevents and confines the flow of solder (e.g., graphite).

antigen (ăn′tĭ-jĕn) A substance, usually a protein, that elicits the formation of antibodies that react with it when introduced parenterally into an individual or species to which it is foreign.

antihelmintics Agents used to destroy intestinal worms.

antihemophilic factor (an″tĭ-hē″mō-fĭl′ĭk) *See* factor VII.

antihistamine (ăn″tĭ-hĭs′tah-mĭn) A drug that counteracts the release of histamine (e.g., in allergic reactions); also has topical anesthetic and sedative effects, as well as a drying effect on the nasal mucosa.

antihistaminic (ăn″tĭ-hĭs-tah-mĭn′ĭk) Referring to a drug that acts to prevent or antagonize the pharmacologic effects of histamine released in the tissues.

antihypertensive drugs Agents that lower or reduce high blood pressure.

antihypnotic (ăn″tĭ-hĭp-not′ĭk) Preventing or hindering sleep.

antiinflammatory agents Compounds that counteract or reduce inflammation.

antileptic (ăn″tĭ-lĕp′tĭk) Assisting, supporting, revulsive.

anti-Monson curve *See* curve, reverse.

antineoplastic agent A drug the prevents the development, maturation, or spread of neoplastic cells.

antioxidants Agents that reduce or prevents oxidation, such as occurs in the deterioration of fats, oils, and nonprecious metals.

antiphlogistic (ăn″tĭ-flō-jĭs′tĭk) Obsolete term for antiinflammatory or antipyretic.

antiplaque agents Compounds the inhibit, control, or kill organisms associated with dental plaque formation.

antipruritic (ăn″tĭ-proo-rĭt′ĭk) Relieving or preventing itching.

antipyretic (ăn″tĭ-pī-rĕt′ĭk) A drug that reduces fever primarily through action on the hypothalamus, thereby resulting in increased heat dissipation through augmented peripheral blood flow and sweating.

antisepsis (ăn″tĭ-sĕp′sĭs) The prevention of infection of a body surface, usually skin or oral mucosa, through the application of an antimicrobial agent.

antiseptic (ăn″tĭ-sĕp′tĭk) An antimicrobial agent for application to a body surface, usually skin or oral mucosa, in an attempt to prevent or minimize infection at the area of application.

antisialagogue (ăn″tĭ-sī-ăl′ah-gawg) A drug that reduces, slows, or prevents the flow of saliva.

antisialic (ăn″tĭ-sī-ăl′ĭk) Checking or that which checks salivary secretions.

antispasmodic (ăn″tĭ-spăz-mod′ĭk) **(antispastic)** A drug that relieves muscle spasms.

antispastic *See* antispasmodic.

antistreptolysin O (ăn″tĭ-strĕp-tol′ĭ-sĭn) An antibody against streptolysin O, a hemolysin produced by group A streptococci. A high titer is supporting evidence of rheumatic fever.

antitarter dentifrice A toothpastes that contain antiplaque agents.

antithermic Reducing temperature. *See also* antipyretic.

antitussive (ăn″tĭ-tŭs′ĭv) A drug that relieves or prevents cough.

Antoni type tissue *See* tissue, Antoni types A and B.

antrodynia (ăn″trō-dĭn′ē-ah) Pain in the maxillary antrum.

antrostomy (ăn-trŏs′tō-mē) A surgical opening into an antrum, either through the medial wall into the nose or through the lateral wall into the oral cavity.

antrum (ăn′trŭm) A maxillary sinus. A cavity in the maxilla, lined by ciliated columnar epithelium, the inferior border of which approximates the apices of the roots of the maxillary posterior teeth.

  a. of Highmore *See* sinus, maxillary.

  a., maxillary *See* sinus, maxillary.

antuitrin S (ăn-tu′ĭ-trĭn) *See* hormone, pregnancy.

ANUG Abbreviation for acute necrotizing ulcerative gingivitis. A distinct, recurrent periodontal disease primarily involving the interdental papillae, which undergo necrosis and ulceration.

anxiety A condition of heightened and often disruptive tension accompanied by an ill-defined and distressing aura of impending harm or injury. Anxiety can disrupt physiologic functions through its effect on the autonomic nervous system. The patient may assume a tense posture, show excessive vigilance, move the hands and feet restlessly, and speak with a strained uneven voice. The pupils may be widely dilated, giving the appearance of unrestrained fright, and the hands and face may perspire excessively. In extremely acute forms the patient may have generalized visceral reactions of respiratory, cardiac, vascular, and gastrointestinal dysfunction. The dentist must recognize the existence of anxiety, seek its etiology and relation to dental treatment, and determine ways that the patient's defenses against anxiety can be used to facilitate rather than inhibit treatment.

  a. neurosis An extreme manifestation of anxiety characterized by acute anxiety attacks (sympathetic overreactivity), and phobias causing avoidance of the anxiety-provoking situations.

apathic (ah-păth′ĭk) Without sensation or feeling.

apathism (ăp′ah-thĭzm) The state of being slow in responding to stimuli.

apatite (ăp′ah-tīt) The inorganic mineral substance of teeth and bone. *See also* carbonate hydroxyapatite.

A-P discrepancy *See* anterior-posterior discrepancy.

APC *See* aspirin, phenacetin, caffeine.

apertognathia (ah-per″tō-năth′ē-ah) "Open-bite" deformity. An occlusion characterized by a vertical separation between the maxillary and mandibular anterior teeth. Incorrectly called an *open bite*.

Apert's syndrome *See* syndrome, Apert's.

aperture An opening.

apex The end of the root.

a. blunderbuss An open or everted apex of a tooth, resembling the divergent form of the barrel of a blunderbuss rifle.

apexification (ā-pĕk″sĭ-fĭ-kā′shŭn) The process of induced root development or apical closure of the root by hard tissue deposition.

apexigraph (ā-pĕks′ĭ-grăf) A device for determining the position of the apex of a tooth root.

APF Abbreviation for acidulated phosphate fluoride, an agent used as a dental caries preventive and suggested by some for the control of plaque.

aphagia (ah-fā′jē-ah) The inability to swallow.

aphasia (ah-fā′zē-ah) A loss of power of expression through speech, writing, or signs or of comprehension of spoken or written language resulting from disease or injury of the brain centers.

aphtha (ăf′thah) **(apthous stomatitis) 1:** A small ulcer on the mucous membrane. **2:** pl.**-hae** Vesicles that undergo subsequent ulceration and are surrounded by a raised erythematous area.

a., Bednar's (bĕd′narz) **(pterygoid ulcer)** An ulcer on the soft palate near the greater palatine foramen; seen in newborns.

a., Mikulicz' (mĭk′ū-lĭch) A recurrent ulceration of the oral mucosa, resembling herpes. *See also* periadenitis mucosa necrotica recurrens.

a., recurrent *See* stomatitis, herpetic; ulcer, aphthous, recurrent.

a., recurrent scarring *See* periadentitis mucosa necrotical recurrens.

aphthosis A clinical manifestation of apthae.

aphthous Characterized by aphthae or aphthosis.

a. fever A fever assoicated with a aphthosis.

a. pharyngitis Aphthosis of the pharynx.

a. Stomatitis *See* Stomatitis, herpetic.

aphthous stomatitis (ăf′thŭs) *See* aphtha; stomatitis, aphthous; stomatitis, herpetic.

apical (ăp′ĭ-kal) Pertaining to the end portion of the root.

a. curettage Surgical removal of diseased tissue surrounding a root apex.

a. fiber *See* fiber, apical.

apicectomy (ā″pĭ-sĕk′tō-mē) *See* apicoectomy.

apicoectomy (ā″pĭkō-ĕk′tō-mē) **(apicectomy, apiectomy, root amputation, root resection)** The surgical removal of the apex or apical portion of a root.

apiectomy (ā″pē-ĕk′tō-mē) *See* apicoectomy.

aplasia (ah-plā′zē-ah) A lack of origin or development (e.g., aplasia of dentition associated with ectodermal dysplasia).

a. of dentition *See* anodontia.

apnea (ăp′nē-ah) A temporary cessation of respiratory movements.

apneumatic (ăp-nū-măt′ĭk) Free from air; used to describe something accomplished with the exclusion of air (e.g., an apneumatic operation).

apoplexy (ăp′ō-plĕk″sē) A stroke caused by acute vascular lesions of the brain.

apostematosa, cheilitis glandularis *See* cheilitis glandularis apostematosa.

apothecaries' system *See* system, apothecaries.

apoxesis (ăp-ahk-sē′sĭs) *See* curettage, apical.

apparatus (ăp″ah-rā′tŭs) Arrangement of a number of parts that act together to perform some special function.

a., attachment The tissues that invest and support the teeth for function: the cementum, periodontal ligament, and alveolar bone.

a., masticating The structures involved in chewing (e.g., the teeth, mandibular musculature, mandible and its temporomandibular joints, accessory mandibular and facial musculature, and tongue, which are controlled by an exquisitely functioning neuromuscular mechanism). *See also* system, stomatognathic.

appellant (ah-pĕl′ănt) The party who, dissatisfied with the disposition of a case on the trial level, appeals to a higher court.

appliance (ah-pfī′ańs) A device used to provide function or therapeutic effect. *See also* restoration.

a., obturator *See* obturator.

a., orthodontic A device used for influencing tooth position. Orthodontic appliances may be classified as fixed or removable, active or retaining, and intraoral or extraoral.

a., extraoral orthodontic A device that uses a portion of the face, neck, or back of the head as a base from which to deliver traction force to the teeth or jaws.

a., chin cup extraoral orthodontic An extraoral traction appliance to restrain the forward positioning of the mandible and/or the forward growth of the mandible.

a., Kloehn cervical extraoral orthodontic The classical cervical extraoral traction appliance introduced by S.J. Kloehn. Uses a relatively light and flexible (0.045 inch; 1.15 mm) inner arch rigidly attached to a long outer bow.

a., fixed orthodontic An appliance that is cemented to the teeth or attached by an adhesive material.

a., Begg fixed orthodontic An appliance developed by P.R. Begg, based on a modified ribbon-arch attachment.

a., edgewise fixed orthodontic An orthodontic appliance, the last of those developed by E.H. Angle, characterized by attachment brackets with a rectangular slot for engagement of a round or rectangular arch wire.

a., labiolingual fixed orthodontic An appliance using the maxillary and mandibular first permanent molars as anchorage, with labial arches 0.036 to 0.040 inch (0.090 to 0.10 cm) in diameter introduced into horizontal buccal tubes attached to the anchor bands and lingual arches of the same diameter fitted into vertical or horizontal tubes fastened to the lingual side of the anchor bands.

a., pin and tube fixed orthodontic A labial arch with vertical posts that insert into tubes attached to bands on the teeth.

a., straight-wire fixed orthodontic A variation of the edgewise appliance in which an effort is made to obviate the need for many arch-wire adjustments by reorientation of the arch-wire slots. The first such modifications were introduced by E.H. Angle; L.M. Andrews first proposed such variations in all planes of space.

a., twin-wire fixed orthodontic An orthodontic appliance developed by J.E. Johnson, typically using a pair of 0.010-inch (0.25-mm) wires to form the midsection of the arch wire.

a., universal fixed orthodontic An orthodontic appliance developed by S.R. Atkinson, combining some of the principles of edgewise and ribbon-arch appliances with very light arch wires.

a., hay rake fixed orthodontic A device used to limit abnormal swallowing excursions of the tongue. In this manner, harmful effects of tongue thrusting are mitigated until the patient learns a new swallowing pattern.

a. fracture (biphase pin fixation, external pin fixation, Stader splint) Any one of the various devices for extraoral reduction and fixation of fractures in which pins, clamps, or screws are placed in the fractured segments, the fractured parts aligned, and then the pins, clamps, or screws joined with metal bars or rigid plastic connectors (e.g., the Stader splint or Roger-Anderson pin-fixation appliance).

a., intraoral orthodontic A device placed inside the mouth to correct or alleviate a malocclusion

a., removable orthodontic An appliance designed so that it can be removed and replaced by the patient.

a., Andresen removable orthodontic An appliance intended to function as a passive trans mitter and sometimes stimulator of the forces of the perioral muscles. One of the activator type of orthodontic appliances that induces or directs oral forces to contribute to improved tooth position and jaw relationship.

a., Bimler removable orthodontic An activator-type appliance.

a., Crozat removable orthodontic A wrought wire appliance originally introduced by George Crozat in VXX.

a., Frankel removable orthodontic An activator-type appliance developed by Rolf Frankel.

a., retaining orthodontic An orthodontic device used to hold the teeth in place, following orthodontic tooth movement, until the occlusion is stabilized.

a., Hawley retaining orthodontic See retainer.

a., obtruator See obturator.

a., prosthetic (archaic term; generally not used to refer to a prosthesis) A complete or partial denture for children when groups of teeth are lost or are congenitally missing. Used to maintain space or masticatory function or for esthetic reasons.

a., therapeutic A vehicle used to transport and retain some agent for therapeutic purposes (e.g., a radium carrier).

application program A standard and frequently used computer program tailored to medical and dental needs. It may be supplied to the user by the manufacturer, purchased from a software house, or written by the user.

applicator A device for applying medication; usually a slender rod of glass or wood, used with a pledget of cotton on the end.

appointment A mutually agreed-on time reserved for the patient to receive treatment.

a. book A ledger or table of workdays divided into segments of time to enable the dentist to reserve specified lengths of time for patient treatment.

a. card A small card given to the patient as a reminder of the time reserved for the appointment.

apposition (ăp-ō-sĭ′shŭn) The condition of being placed or fitted together; juxtaposition; coaptation.

appropriate 1: The determination that the service provided is suited for the condition. **2:** Suitable for a particular person, group, community, condition, occasion, and/or place. **3:** Proper.

approved services 1: All services provided in a dental plan. In some plans, authorization must be obtained before approved service is provided; other plans make exception for treatment of emergency needs; still others require no prior authorization for any treatment approved under the program. **2:** Dental services that meet quality standards maintained in a dental plan.

approximal (approximating) Contiguous; adjacent; next to each other.

approximating See approximal.

apraxia (ah-prăk′sē-ah) A loss of ability to execute a purposeful, goal-oriented, or skilled act resulting from selective damage to certain high-level brain centers, either sensory, motor, or both.

apron A piece of clothing worn in front of the body for protection.

a. band A labioincisal or gingival extension of an orthodontic band that aids in retention of the band and in proper positioning of the bracket.

a., lead An apron made of materials containing metallic lead or lead compounds used to reduce radiation hazards.

a., lingual *See* connector, linguoplate major.

a., rubber dam A small strip of rubber dam, perforated to fit over an implant abutment that is used to inhibit introduction of cement into the periimplant space.

ARC Abbreviation for AIDS-related complex. *See* acquired immunodeficiency syndrome.

arc, reflex A system of nerves used in a reflex or involuntary act, consisting primarily of an afferent nerve with sensory receptor, a nerve center, and an efferent nerve that stimulates the effector muscle or gland.

arch(es) A structure with a curved outline.

a., bar *See* bar, arch.

a., basal *See* base, apical.

a., dental The composite structure of the dentition and alveolar ridge or the remains thereof after the loss of some or all of the natural teeth.

a., dental, contraction *See* contraction.

a., dentulous dental A dental arch containing natural teeth.

a., edentulous dental A dental arch from which all natural teeth are missing. The residual alveolar ridge.

a., partially edentulous dental A dental arch from which one or more but not all teeth are missing.

a. expansion *See* expansion.

a. form *See* form, arch.

a., high labial A labial arch wire adapted so that it lies gingival to the anterior tooth crowns; it has auxiliary springs extending downward in contact with the teeth to be moved.

a. length The length of a dental arch, usually measured through the points of contact between adjoining teeth.

a. length, available The space available for all teeth.

a. length deficiency The difference between required and available arch length.

a. length, required The sum of the mesiodistal widths of all teeth.

a., ovoid An arch that curves continuously from the molars on one side to the molars on the opposite side so that two such arches placed back to back describe an oval.

a., palatine (glossopalatine arch) The pillars of the fauces; the two arches of mucous membrane enclosing the muscles at the sides of the passage from the mouth to the pharynx.

a., passive lingual An orthodontic appliance effective in maintaining space and preserving arch length when bilateral primary molars are prematurely lost.

a., pharyngeal The branchial arches of the fetus.

a., removable lingual An arch wire designed to fit the lingual surface of the teeth. It has two posts soldered on each end that fit snugly into the vertical tubes of the molar anchor bands.

a., stationary lingual An arch wire designed to fit the lingual surface of the teeth and soldered to the anchor bands.

a., tapering A dental arch that converges from molars to central incisors to such an extent that lines passing through the central grooves of the molars and premolars intersect within 1 inch (2.5 cm) anterior to the central incisors.

a., trapezoidal An arch that has the same convergence as a tapering arch but to a lesser degree. The anterior teeth are somewhat square to abruptly rounded from canine tip to canine tip. The canines act as corners of the arch.

a., U-shaped A dental arch in which there is little difference in diameter (width) between the first premolars and the last molars; the curve from canine to canine is abrupt, so a dental arch in the shape of a capital U is formed.

a. width The width of a dental arch. The width, which varies in all diameters between the right and left opposites, is determined by direct measurement between the canines, between the first molars, and between the second premolars. These intercanine, interpremolar, and intermolar distances can be cited as *arch width.*

a. wire A wire applied to two or more teeth through fixed attachments to cause or guide orthodontic tooth movement.

a. wire, full A wire extending from the molar region of one side of an arch to the other.

a. wire, sectional A wire extending to only a few teeth, usually on one side or in the anterior segment.

architecture, gingival *See* gingival architecture.

archiving The storage of older, rarely required data or patient information in a cheaper and/or more compact form.

arcus senilis (ar'kŭs sĕ-nǐ'lǐs) An opaque, grayish-white ring at the periphery of the cornea occurring in older adults.

area Region.

a., apical *See* base, apical.

a., basal seat (denture bearing area, denture-supporting area, stress-bearing area, stress-supporting area) The portion of the oral structures available to support a denture.

a., contact *See* point, contact.

a., denture-bearing *See* area, basal seat.

a., denture-supporting *See* area, basal seat.

a., impression The surface of the oral structures recorded in an impression.

a., pear-shaped *See* pad, retromolar.

a., post dam *See* area, posterior palatal seal.

a., posterior palatal seal The soft tissues along the junction of the hard and soft palates on which compression, within the physiologic limits of the tissues, can be applied by a denture to aid in its retention.

a., postpalatal seal *See* area, posterior palatal seal.

a., pressure An area of excessive displacement of soft tissue by a prosthesis.

a., recipient The portion of the body on which a skin, bone, tooth, or other graft is placed.

a., relief The portion of the surface of the mouth under prosthesis on which pressures are reduced or eliminated.

a., rest (rest seat) The prepared surface of a tooth or fixed restoration into which the rest fits, giving support to a removable partial denture.

a., rugae (rū′gī) **(rugae zone)** That portion of the hard palate in which rugae are found.

a., saddle *See* area, basal seat.

a., stress-bearing *See* area, basal seat.

a., stress-supporting *See* area, basal seat.

a., supporting The areas of the maxillary and mandibular edentulous ridges best suited to carry the forces of mastication when the dentures are in use. *See also* area, basal seat.

arginine One of the essential amino acids for infants and children. *See* amino acid.

Argyll Robertson pupil (ar-gĭl′) *See* pupil, Argyll Robertson.

argyria (ar-jĭr′ē-ah) A bluish color of the skin or mucous membranes produced by the deposition of silver salts in collagen fibers after prolonged use of silver salts.

a., local A localized blue pigmentation of the oral mucosa from the deposition of silver amalgam in the submucosal connective tissue.

argyrosis (ar-jĭ-rō′sĭs) A pathologic bluish black pigmentation in a tissue resulting from the deposition of an insoluble albuminate of silver.

ariboflavinosis (ah-rī″bō-flā-vĭ-nō′sĭs) A nutritional disease resulting from a deficiency of riboflavin (vitamin B$_2$); characterized by angular cheilosis, seborrheic dermatitis, a magenta tongue, and ocular disturbance.

Arkansas stone (ar′kan-saw) *See* stone, Arkansas.

arm A definitely shaped extension or projection of a removable partial denture framework.

a., reciprocal A clasp arm used on a removable partial denture to oppose any force arising from an opposing clasp arm on the same tooth. *See also* arm, retention.

a., retention An extension or projection that is part of a removable partial denture and is used to aid in the retention and stabilization of the restoration. *See also* retainer divet.

a., truss *See* connector, minor.

a., upright *See* connector, minor.

armamentarium (ar″mah-měn-tā′rē-ŭm) The equipment and materials of a practitioner.

arrangement The pattern into which a group of things is organized.

a., financial An agreement between the dentist and patient on the method of handling the patient's account.

a., tooth The placement of teeth on a denture or temporary base with definite objectives in mind.

arrhythmia (ah-rĭth′mē-ah) A variation from the normal rhythm of the heart.

arrow point tracer *See* tracer, needle point.

arteriole (ar-tē′rē-ōl) A minute arterial branch proximal to a capillary.

arteriosclerosis (ar-tē″rē-o-sklĕ-rō′sĭs) A term applied to a group of diseases that affect the elasticity of the blood vessels. It may refer to atherosclerosis, hyperplastic arteriosclerosis, or Monckeberg's sclerosis. These degenerative processes generally affect only the tunica media and tunica intima. The effect is narrowing of the lumen of a blood vessel, causing rupture of the blood vessel or ischemia of an area of tissue that the vessel supplies.

arteriosclerotic heart disease (ar-tē″rē-ō-sklĕ-rŏt′ĭk) *See* disease, heart, arteriosclerotic.

arteriovenous shunt (ar-tē″rē-ō-vē′nŭs) *See* shunt, arteriovenous.

arteritis, temporal (ar″ter-ī′tĭs) Inflammation of the temporal artery that produces a nodular, tortuous swelling of the temporal artery accompanied by a burning, throbbing pain, initially in the teeth, temporomandibular joint, and eye, but ultimately localized over the artery. This disorder occurs primarily in persons over 55 years of age.

artery A blood vessel through which the blood passes from the heart to the various structures of the body. There are three layers of tissue in every artery: the inner coat (tunica intima), composed of an inner endothelial lining, connective tissue, and an outer layer of elastic tissue (inner elastic membrane); the middle coat (tunica media), composed chiefly of muscle tissue; and the outer coat (tunica adventitia), composed chiefly of connective tissue. The structure of the three layers varies with the location, size, and purpose of the blood vessel.

a., large An elastic artery with an abundant supply of elastic tissue and a great reduction of smooth muscle. The tunica intima is thick, and the endothelial cells are round or polygonal. The tunica media is the thickest of the three layers. It contains few smooth muscle fibers, and its outer border has a special concentration of elastic fibers—the external elastic membrane. The tunica adventitia is relatively thin and ill defined and is continuous with the loose connective tissue surrounding the vessel.

a., medium-sized Most of the arteries in the body (e.g., facial, maxillary, radial, ulnar, and popliteal).

Thick muscular bands are found in the tunica media. Thin elastic fibers course circularly in the tunica media and run longitudinally in the tunica adventitia. The tunica adventitia is as thick as the tunica media, and its outer layer gradually blends with the connective tissue that supports the artery and surrounding structures.

arthograms An x-ray of a joint usually with the introduction of a contrast compound into the joint capsule. In dentistry, an arthogram usually involves the temporomandibular joint.

arthralgia (ar-thrăl′jē-ah) Pain in a joint or joints.

arthritis (ar-thrī′tĭs) Any of a number of types of inflammation of a joint or joints.

   a., allergic Arthralgia, swelling, and stiffness of joints associated with food and drug allergies and serum sickness.

   a., atrophic *See* arthritis, rheumatoid.

   a., bacterial *See* arthritis, infective.

   a., hypertrophic *See* osteoarthritis.

   a., infective (bacterial arthritis) A primary and secondary bacterial infection of the joints (e.g., by staphylococcal, gonococcal, streptococcal, or pneumococcal organisms).

   a., rheumatic (roo-măt′ik) An acute polyarticular and migratory arthritis of unknown cause but assumed to be related to group A streptococcal infection of the upper respiratory tract.

   a., rheumatoid (roo′mah-toid) A chronic destructive inflammation of the joints of unknown origin, with associated constitutional manifestations. Chronic synovitis and regressive changes in the articular cartilage occur with pain, swelling, deformity, limitation of motion, and occasionally ankylosis of the joints. Variable systemic manifestations include weakness, loss of weight, anemia, leukopenia, splenomegaly, lymphadenopathy, and the formation of subcutaneous nodules. Small joints are principally affected. In most instances, onset is in the third or fourth decade of life.

   a., senile Arthritis occurring in persons of advanced age.

   a., specific infectious Arthritis caused by direct invasion and subsequent infection of joint structures by microorganisms from the bloodstream. Nearly all pathogenic bacteria have been isolated as etiologic agents.

   a., traumatic An acute or chronic inflammation of a joint as a result of acute or chronic injury.

arthroplasty (ar′thrō-plăs″tē) The surgical correction of a joint abnormality.

   a., gap *See* gap arthroplasty.

   a., interposition *See* interposition arthroplasty.

arthoscope An instrument to view the inside of a joint.

arthrostomy (ar-thrŏs′tō-mē) The surgical formation of an opening into a joint.

articular cartilage *See* cartilage, articular.

articulare Point of intersection of the dorsal contour of the mandibular condyle and the temporal bone.

articulate, *v.* (ar-tĭk′ū-lāt) **1:** To arrange or place in connected sequence. *See also* arrangement, tooth. **2:** To connect by articulating strips, paper, or cloth coated with ink-containing or dye-containing wax, used for marking or locating occlusal contacts.

articulation (ar-tĭk″ū-lā′shŭn) **1:** A joint. *See also* joint. **2:** The relationship of cusps of teeth during jaw movement.

   a., anatomic A rigid or movable junction of a bony part.

   a., articulator The use of a device that incorporates artificial temporomandibular joints that permit the orientation of casts in a manner duplicating or simulating various positions or movements of the mandible.

   a., balanced The simultaneous contacting of the upper and lower teeth as they glide over each other when the mandible is moved from centric relation to the various eccentric relations. *See also* occlusion, balanced.

   a., mandibular *See* articulation, temporomandibular.

   a., temporomandibular (temporomandibular joint, mandibular joint) 1: The joint formed by the two condyles of the mandible. **2:** The bilateral articulation between the glenoid or mandibular fossae of the temporal bones and condyles (condyloid processes) of the mandible. The structures that make up the temporomandibular joint include the mandibular fossae of the temporal bones, articular disks, mandibular condyles, and articular tubercles of the zygomatic process of the temporal bone.

   a., temporomandibular, capsule The ligamentous covering of the temporomandibular joint.

   a., temporomandibular, collagen disease Rheumatoid arthritis in which the joint may be so involved because of bone changes that the mandibular condyle is fused to the articular fossa in the base of the cranium.

   a., temporomandibular, hormonal disturbances Hormonal disorders that frequently affect growth patterns of the skeleton, involving the temporomandibular joint (e.g., acromegaly).

   a., temporomandibular, neuromuscular disorders Neuromuscular disorders involving the temporomandibular joint, in which the patient is unable to maintain appropriate patterns of mandibular closure consistent with good dental occlusion. The natural teeth degenerate rapidly and are frequently lost prematurely; when dentures are substituted, they cause the residual tissues to deteriorate rapidly. In addition to the chronic masticatory disability, the deglutitive mechanism functions poorly because of incoordinated lip and tongue action.

a., temporomandibular pain-dysfunction syndrome *See* temporomandibular joint pain-dysfunction syndrome.

articulator (ar-tĭk′ū-lā-tor) A mechanical device that represents the temporomandibular joints and jaw members to which maxillary and mandibular casts may be attached.

a., adjustable An articulator that may be adjusted to permit movement of the casts into various recorded eccentric relationships.

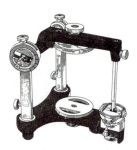

Adjustable articulator

artifact (ar′tĭ-făkt) A blemish or image in the radiograph that is not present in the roentgen image of the object.

artificial respiration *See* respiration, artificial.

artificial stone *See* stone, artificial.

aryepiglottic (ar″ē-ĕp″ĭ-glaht′ĭk) *See* arytenoepiglottic.

arytenoepiglottic (ar″ē-tē″nō-ĕp′ĭ-glaht′ĭk) **(aryepiglottic)** Pertaining to the arytenoid cartilage and the epiglottis.

Aschheim-Zondek test (ăsh′hĭm tsahn′dēk) *See* test, pregnancy.

ascites (ah-sī′tēz) An accumulation of serous fluid in the peritoneal cavity.

ascorbic acid *See* vitamin C.

asepsis (ah-sĕp′sĭs) Without infection; free of viable pathogenic microorganisms.

aseptic Not producing microorganisms or free from microorganisms.

asialia (ah″sē-ā′lē-ah) *See* asialorrhea.

asialorrhea (ah-sī″ah-lō-rē′ah) **(asialia)** A decrease in or lack of salivary flow. *See also* hyposalivation.

asjike (ahs-jī′kē) *See* beriberi.

aspartame A low-calarie sweetening agent about 200 times as sweet as sucrose.

aspect, buccal The facial surface or cheek side of posterior teeth.

asphyxia (ăs-fĭk′sē-ah) A condition of suffocation resulting from restriction of oxygen intake and interference with the elimination of carbon dioxide.

aspirate (ăs′pĭ-rāt) **1:** To draw or breathe in. **2:** To remove materials by vacuum. **3:** A phonetic unit whose identifying characteristic is the sound generated by the passage of air through a relatively open channel; the sound of ″h″; a sound followed by or combined with the sound of ″h.″

aspiration (ăs″pĭ-ra′shŭn) **1:** The act of breathing or drawing in. **2:** The removal of fluids, gases, or solids from a cavity by means of a vacuum pump.

a. biopsy *See* biopsy, aspiration.

a. pneumonia Pneumonia produced by aspiration of foreign material into the lungs.

aspirator (ăs′pĭ-rā-tor) An apparatus used for removal of fluids, gases, or solids from a cavity by vacuum.

aspirin burn *See* burn, aspirin.

aspirin, phenacetin, caffeine (APC, PAC) A pharmaceutical preparation used as an analgesic.

assault An intentional, unlawful offer of bodily injury to another by force or unlawfully directing force toward another person to create a reasonable fear of imminent danger, coupled with the apparent ability to do the harm threatened if not prevented. A completed assault is a battery. In a medical setting, the unconsented touching of the body would be an assault and battery.

assets Everything a business owns or is owned. Cash, investments, money due, materials, and inventories are current assets. Buildings and equipment are fixed assets. Goodwill is an intangible asset.

assignment of benefits A procedure whereby a beneficiary or patient authorizes the administrator of the program to forward payment for a covered procedure directly to the treating dentist.

assistant An agent or employee.

a., dental An auxiliary to the dentist. *See also* certified dental assistant.

asthenia (as-thē′nē-ah) The loss of vitality or strength; a condition of debility; weakness.

asthenic (ăs-thĕn′ĭk) A term describing an individual with a long, slender appearance who is thin and flat chested and has long limbs and a short trunk; comparable to the ectomorph in Sheldon's classification.

asthma (ăz′mah) Paroxysmal wheezing and difficulty in breathing resulting from bronchospasms frequently having an allergic basis and occasionally an emotional origin.

a., cardiac Shortness of breath (paroxysmal dyspnea), sonorous rales, and expiratory wheezes that resemble bronchial asthma; related to cardiac failure.

astigmatism (ah-stĭg′mah-tĭzm) A defective curvature of the refractive surfaces of the eye, resulting in a condition in which a ray of light is not focused sharply in the retina but is spread over a more or less diffuse area.

astringent (ah-strĭn′jĕnt) Styptic; an agent that checks the secretions of mucous membranes and contracts and hardens tissues, limiting the secretions of glands.

asymmetric (ā″sĭ-mĕ′trĭk) Unevenly arranged; out of balance; not the same on both sides; not a mirror image on both sides.

asynergy (ā-sĭn′er-jē) Lack of muscular coordination in special functions (e.g., hand-to-mouth movements for feeding).

asystole (ā-sĭs′tō-lē) The faulty contraction of the ventricles of the heart, resulting in incomplete or imperfect systole.

ataractic (ăt-ah-răk′tĭk) **(ataraxic, tranquilizer)** One of a poorly defined group of drugs designed to produce ataraxia. The former concept, that their use involved no mental or motor impairment, is subject to question.

ataraxia (ăt″ah-răk′sē-ah) A state of complete serenity without impairment of mental or physical functions.

ataraxic *See* ataractic.

ataxia (ah-tăk′sē-ah) A muscular incoordination characterized by irregular muscle activity.

    a., locomotor *See* tabes dorsalis.

atelectasis (ăt″ĕ-lek′tah-sĭs) The complete or partial collapse of a lung.

atherosclerosis (ăth″er-ō-sklĕ-rō′sĭs) A degenerative disease principally affecting the aorta and its major branches, the coronary artery, and the larger cerebral arteries. The arterial changes include narrowing of the lumen of the vessels; weakening of the arterioles, leading to rapture; an increased tendency toward development of atheromatous plaques; and thrombi. Atherosclerosis is a common cause of coronary thrombosis, congestive heart failure, aneurysms, hemorrhage, cerebral infarcts, and apoplexy.

athetosis (ăth″ĕ-tō′sĭs) A neuromuscular impairment in which extensive twisting and swaying spasms of the skeletal musculature interfere with voluntary control of movement; the spasms are especially conspicuous and disconcerting during emotional stress and on initiation of conscious voluntary acts.

athiaminosis (ah-thī″ah-mĭ-nō′sĭs) *See* beriberi.

athletic (ăth-lĕt′ĭk) Pertaining to a bodily constitution characterized by a strong, muscular, robust appearance.

atom (ăt′om) The smallest part of an element capable of entering into a chemical reaction.

atomic (ah-tom′ĭk) Pertaining to the atom.

    a. energy *See* energy, atomic.

    a. mass number (symbol A) The total number of nucleons (protons and neutrons) of which an atom is composed.

    a. number (Z) 1: The number of electrons outside the nucleus of a neutral atom. **2:** The number of protons in the nucleus.

    a. structure theory The theory that matter is composed of a vast number of particles, or atoms, bound together by a force of attraction of electrical charges.

    a. weight The weight of one atom of an element as compared with the weight of an atom of hydrogen. One atomic weight unit is equal to 1.660×10^{-24} Gm.

atomizer (ăt′ŭ-mī-zer) An apparatus for changing a jet of liquid into a spray.

atopy (ăt′ō-pē) **(atopic hypersensitivity, ″spontaneous″ clinical allergy)** A group of ″allergic″ disorders showing a marked familial distribution; although the susceptibility appears to be inherited, contact with the antigen must occur before hypersensitivity can develop. Disorders include asthma or hay fever resulting from pollens and gastrointestinal tract and skin reactions resulting from food.

atresia (ah-trē′zē-ah) The congenital absence or occlusion of a normal opening of one or more ducts in an organ.

    a., aural The absence of closure of the auditory canal.

atrophy (ăt′rō-fē) A progressive, acquired decrease in the size of a normally developed cell, tissue, or organ. It may result from a decrease in cell size, number of cells, or both.

    a., adipose Atrophy resulting from a reduction in fatty tissue.

    a., alveolar A depletion of the size of the alveolar process of the jaws from disuse, overuse, or pathologic disturbance of the bone.

    a., diffuse alveolar *See* periodontosis.

    a., bone 1: Bone resorption internally (in density) and externally (in form) (e.g., of residual ridges). **2:** A loss of bone substance or volume. Atrophy of bone ordinarily occurs without a corresponding change in the volume or external dimensions of bone, but the mass of bone tissue may be reduced as much as 75%. The internal architecture of the bone gradually becomes attenuated and finally disappears. Atrophied bone is brittle and has a more spongy consistency than normal bone. In cross section the cortex is thin, and the periosteal surface is smooth and unchanged, but the intramedullary substance is composed of a yellow, fatty, cancellous bone tissue. Bone atrophy may be systemic, regional, or local.

    a. of disuse Atrophy resulting from a lack of function of a tissue, organ, or body part.

    a., facial The failure of facial development. If it is bilateral, it may produce brachygnathia; unilateral types, although rare, are more common than the bilateral type. Causes include physical injury, neurovascular disease, and paralysis.

    a., muscular A wasting of muscle tissue, especially resulting from lack of use. There are numerous causes for simple atrophy of muscle, such as chronic malnutrition, immobilization, and denervation.

a., periodontal The quantitative degenerative changes that occur in the attachment apparatus and supporting bone of a tooth as a result of disease or disuse. When a tooth loses its antagonist, osteoporotic changes in the supporting bone, an afunctional change in the direction of periodontal fibers and narrowing of the periodontal membrane space occur.

a., postmenopausal A thinning of the oral mucosa after menopause.

a., pressure The tissue destruction and reduction in size as a consequence of prolonged or continued pressure on a local area or group of cells.

a., pressure, by epithelial attachment A theoretical type of atrophy. The theory, advanced to explain destruction of gingival fibers during gingival inflammation, states that gingival fiber degeneration is produced by pressure exerted by the proliferating pocket epithelium. It is now generally conceded that proteolytic substances produced in the tissues during inflammation are responsible for gingival fiber destruction; subsequently, the epithelium can proliferate apically.

a., senile The atrophy or diminution of all tissues characteristic of advanced age.

atropine (ăt′rō-pēn) An alkaloid that annuls parasympathetic effects and antagonizes the effects of pilocarpine. It acts directly on the effector cells, preventing the action but not the liberation of acetylcholine. It suppresses sweat and other glandular sections.

attached gingiva *See* gingiva, attached.

attachment 1: Means to fasten, connect, associate. **2:** A mechanical device for retention and stabilization of a dental prosthesis.

a., abnormal frenum (frē′nŭm) Aberrant insertions of labial, buccal, or lingual frena capable of initiating or perpetuating periodontal disease, such as creating diastemata between teeth, limiting lip or tongue movement.

a., epithelial The continuation of the sulcular epithelium that is joined to the tooth structure.

a., migration of epithelial The apical progression of the epithelial attachment along the tooth root.

a., gingival The fibrous attachment of the gingival tissues to the teeth.

a., intracoronal (precision attachment, slotted attachment) *See* intracoronal retainer.

a., orthodontic A device, secured to the crown of a tooth, that serves as a means of attaching the arch wire to the tooth.

a., parallel A prefabricated device for attaching a denture base to an abutment tooth. Retention is provided by friction between the parallel walls of the

two parts of the attachment.

a., precision *See* attachment, intracoronal.

a., slotted *See* attachment, intracoronal.

attack, heart *See* thrombosis, coronary.

attending dentist's statement A form used to report dental procedures to a third-party payer, the claim form was developed by the American Dental Association. Synonym: dental claim form.

attenuation (ah-těn″ū-ā′shŭn) The process by which a beam of radiation is reduced in energy when passing through some material.

attitude A person's mental set, opinion or disposition.

attraction The tendency of teeth or other maxillary or mandibular structures to become superior to (elevated above) the normal position.

attrition (ah-trish′ŭn) The normal loss of tooth substance resulting from friction caused by physiologic forces.

attritional occlusion *See* occlusion, attritional.

atypical (ā-tĭp′ē-kal) Pertaining to deviation from the basic or typical.

Au *See* unit, Ångström.

audiogram (aw′dē-ō-grăm) A graphic summary of the measurements of hearing loss showing the number of decibels lost at each frequency tested.

audiology (aw-dē-ahl′ō-jē) The study of the entire field of hearing, including the anatomy and function of the ear; impairment of hearing; and evaluation, education or reeducation, and treatment of persons with hearing loss.

audiometer (aw-dē-ahm′ě-ter) A device for testing hearing; calibrated to register hearing loss in terms of decibels.

audit 1: An examination of records or accounts to check their accuracy. **2:** A posttreatment record review or clinical examination to verify information reported on claims.

audit of treatment 1: An administrative or professional review of a participating dentist's treatment recommendations (per audit). **2:** The review of reimbursement claims for service performed (postaudit).

augmentation (awg″měn-tā′shŭn) **1:** Assistance to respiration by the application of intermittent pressure on inspiration. **2:** An increase of the size beyond the existing size, such as an implant placed over the mandibular or maxillary ridges.

Aureomycin (aw″rē-ō-mi′sĭn) Trade name for chlortetracycline.

auricle (aw′rĭ-kŭl) **1:** Pinna, the external part of the ear. **2:** Atrium, the chamber of the heart that receives the blood: on the right, from the general circulation, and on the left, from the pulmonary circulation.

auricular fibrillation *See* fibrillation, auricular.

auricular tags Rudimentary appendages of auricular tissue on the face along the line of union of the first branchial arch.

auriculotemporal syndrome *See* syndrome, auriculotemporal.

auscultation (aw″skul-tā′shŭn) The examination procedure of listening for sounds produced by the body to detect or judge an abnormal condition.

autoclave (aw′tō-klāv) An apparatus for effecting sterilization by steam under pressure.

autogenous bone graft *See* graft, autogenous bone.

autograft *See* graft, autogenous.

autoimmune disease (aw″tō-ĭ-mūn′) *See* disease, autoimmune.

automatic condenser *See* condenser, mechanical.

automatic mallet *See* condenser, mechanical.

automation Equipment that can perform a task repeatedly without human intervention.

automatism (aw-tŏm′ah-tĭzm) A tendency to take extra or superfluous doses of a drug when under its influence.

autonomic drugs Agents the act on the autonomic nervous system.

autopolymer (aw-tō-pol′ĭ-mer) A resin to which certain chemicals have been added to initiate and propagate polymerization without addition of heat.
  a. resin *See* resin, autopolymer.

autopolymerization (aw″tō-pol″ĭ-mer-ī-zā′shŭn) **(cold-curing)** The accomplishment of polymerization by chemical means without external application of heat or light.

autoprothrombin I (aw″tō-prō-thrŏm′bĭn) *See* factor VII.

autoprothrombin II *See* factor IX.

autoradiography (aw″tō-rā-dē-ŏg′rah-fē) A photographic recording of radiation from radioactive material, obtained by placing the surface of the radioactive material in close proximity to a photographic emulsion.

autosomal dominant disorders Genetic disorders that are transmitted by a dominate gene within an autosomal chromosome as opposed to a sex chromosome.

autosomal recessive disorders Genetic disorders carried by a recessive gene within an autosomal chromosome as opposed to a sex chromosome.

autotransformer A transformer with a single winding, having a large number of connections, or taps. Used to deliver a precise voltage to the high-tension primary circuit.

autotransplant *See* graft, autogenous.

auxiliary personnel Nonprofessional aides who assist the responsible professional in the provision of professional services. Dental hygienists are formally trained and may be licensed or certificated by state authorities. Dental assistants, laboratory technicians, and other auxiliaries may be formally trained.

auxiliary wires Orthodontic wires that support or augment the action of the main or primary arch wire in an orthodontic appliance. The Begg technique and the segmental technique make frequent and regular use of auxiliary wires.

AV Abbreviation for atrioventricular or auriculoventricular.

availability The supply in terms of type, volume, and location of health resources and services relative to the demands of a given individual or community.

average life (mean life) The average of the individual lives of all of the atoms of a particular radioactive substance; 1.443 times radioactive half-life. *See* halflife.

avitaminosis (ā-vī″tah-mǐ-nō′sǐs) A disease or condition resulting from a deficiency of one or more vitamins in the diet (e.g., scurvy, which results from ascorbic acid deficiency, and beriberi, which results from to thiamine deficiency).
  a., fat-soluble A disease resulting from deficiency of the fat-soluble vitamins (i.e., A, D, E, and K).

avoidance behavior A conscious or unconscious defense mechanism by which a person tries to escape from unpleasant situations or feelings, such as anxiety and pain.

avoirdupois system *See* system, avoirdupois.

avulse To tear off forcibly, as when a tooth is lost in an accident.

avulsed tooth *See* tooth, evulsed.

avulsion (ah-vŭl′shŭn) *See* evulsion.
  a., nerve *See* evulsion, nerve.

axial inclination (ăks′ē-ŭl) *See* inclination, axial.

axial plane *See* plane, axial.

axial wall plane *See* plane, axial wall.

axiopulpal (ăk″sē-o-pŭl′pŭl) Relating to the angle formed by the axial and pulpal walls of a prepared cavity.

axis (ăk′sĭs) A straight line around which a body may rotate.
  a., cephalometric *See* axis, Y.
  a., condylar An imaginary line through the two manidibular condyles around which the mandible may rotate during a part of the opening movement.
    a., condylar determination The location of the condylar axis by fixing a face-bow rigidly to the lower teeth, having the patient open and close the jaws, and recording the most posteriosuperior points of pure rotation with tattoo ink on the outer skin. *See also* face-bow; hinge-bow.
  a., condyle One of three axes of the jaw condyles: (1) the hinge axis, an intercondyle imaginary line across the face through both condyles; whenever either condyle is chosen to be a rotator, it will display (2) a vertical axis; and there is also (3) a sagittal axis. The hinge axis is a moving center for the opening and closing movements. The vertical axis is a center for the horizontal components of orbital movements. The sagittal axis is the center for the vertical components of orbital movements.
  a., hinge, -orbital plane A craniofacial plane deter-

mined by three tattooed points. Two are located one on each side of the face at the point of exit through the skin in front of the tragus of the imagined extended rearmost mandibular hinge axis. The third point is located on the right side of the nose at the level of the orbital rim just beneath the pupil when the patient is gazing directly forward. This plane corresponds to the anthropologic Frankfort plane.

a., horizontal *See* axis, hinge.

a., long An imaginary line passing longitudinally through the center of a body.

a., mandibular *See* axis, condylar.

a., opening *See* axis, condylar.

a., orbital movements of Movements projected on the axis-orbital plane in gathering the input data for an articulator.

a. of preparation The path taken by a restoration as it slides on or off of the preparation.

a., sagittal The imaginary line around which the working condyle rotates in the frontal plane during lateral mandibular movement. The sagittal and vertical axes function concurrently.

a. shift Imprecise term used before the nine different directionalized laterotrasions were discovered and named.

a., vertical The imaginary line around which the working condyle rotates in the horizontal plane during lateral mandibular movement. The sagittal and vertical axes function concurrently.

a., Y (cephalometric axis) The angle of a line connecting the sella turcica and the gnathion and related to a horizontal plane. An indicator of downward and forward growth of the mandible.

axon (ăk'son) An extension of a nerve cell body that conducts impulses away from the cell. Generally, there is only one axon to a cell, and it may extend up to 3 feet (0.9 m) in length.

azdiothymidine (AZT) A drug used to lengthen or extend the median incubation period of the human immunodeficiency virus. Brand name Retrovir.

AZT Abbreviation for azdiothymidine. *See* azdiothymidine.

B point *See* point, B.

Bacillus A genus of gram-positive, spore-producing bacteria in the family Bacillaceae, order Eubacteriales, including three that are pathogenic and the rest saprophytic soil forms. Many microorganisms formerly classified as *Bacillus* are now classified in other genera.

   B. anthracis A species of gram-positive facultative anaerobes that cause anthrax. The spores of this organism, if inhaled, can cause a pulmonary form of anthrax; spore can live for many years in animal products, such as hides and wool, and in the soil.

   B. subtilis The species found in grass or hay. Some strains produce the antibiotic bacillomycin.

bacitracin (băs-ĭ-trā′sĭn) An antibiotic produced by a gram-positive, spore-forming organism of the *Bacillus licheniformis* group; usually administered topically.

back-action clasp *See* clasp, back-action.

back pressure porosity *See* porosity, back pressure.

backing A metal support used to attach a facing to a prosthesis.

bacteremia (băk-ter-ē′mē-ah) **1:** Presence of bacteria in the bloodstream. It may be transient, intermittent, or continuous. Transient bacteremia may result from dental procedures such as root planing or tonsillectomy, or it may accompany the early phase of many infections. Continuous bacteremia is a feature of endocarditis. **2:** Presence of bacteria in the blood (e.g., it might occur during root planing of the tooth of a rheumatic patient who has not been prophylactically premedicated with antibiotics).

bacteria, resident (oral) The microorganisms constant in the oral flora of an individual.

bacterial culture *See* culture, bacterial.

bacteriolytic action (băk-tē-rē-ō-lĭt′ĭk) Breaking down of bacteria by an enzyme or other agent (e.g., by antibacterial factors in saliva).

Bacteroides (băk-tĕ-roi′dēz) A genus of Schizomycetes made up of rod-shaped, highly pleomorphic, gram-negative, non-spore-forming obligate anaerobic bacteria sometimes associated with periodontitis.

   B. endodontalis A strain of *B. melaninogenicus* associated with pupal infections.

B. forsythus A recently identified anaerobic gram-negative species of bacteroides found in periodontal pockets.

B. gingivalis A strain of *B. melaninogenicus* associated with acute periodontitis.

B. intermedius A strain of *B. melaninogenicus* associated with acute necrotizing ulcerative gingivitis.

B. melaninogenicus (Bacterium melaninogenicum) A small gram-negative diplobacillus found in the mouth and pharynx; an anaerobic organism sometimes associated with periodontitis.

bad-faith insurance practices 1: The failure to deal with a beneficiary of a dental benefits plan fairly and in good faith. **2:** An activity that impairs the right of the beneficiary to receive the appropriate benefits of a dental benefits plan or to receive them in a timely manner. Some examples of bad-faith insurance practices include evaluating claims based on standards significantly at variance with the standards of the community, failure to properly investigate a claim for benefits, and unreasonably and purposely delaying and/or withholding payment of a claim.

badge, film *See* film badge.

bailment The delivery of personal property by one person to another in trust for a specific purpose with an expressed or implied contract that after the purpose has been fulfilled the property shall be returned, duly accounted for, or kept until reclaimed.

balance To be in equilibrium or harmony. Frequently used as a adjective to describe occlusal equilibrium or facial esthetic harmony.

balance, acid-base In metabolism, the balance of acid to base necessary to keep the blood pH level normal (between 7.35 and 7.43).

balance billing Billing a patient for the difference between the dentist's actual charge and the amount reimbursed under the patient's dental benefits plan.

balance sheet A condensed statement showing the nature and amount of a company's assets, liabilities, and capital on a given date. In dollar amounts the balance sheet shows what the company owned, what it owed, and the ownership interest in the company of its stockholders.

balanced articulation *See* occlusion, balanced.

balanced bite *See* occlusion, balanced.

balanced occlusion *See* occlusion, balanced.

balancing contacts The contacts of teeth on the side opposite the bolus side. *See* contact, balancing.

balancing occlusal surfaces *See* surfaces, occlusa, balancing.

balancing side The side opposite the working side of the dentition or denture.

balloon, sinus A hollow rubber structure expandable with liquid or air that is used to support depressed fractures of the walls of the maxillary sinus.

balloon payment The final payment larger than the preceding payments when a debt is not fully amortized.

balsam (bawl′sŭm) Any of many viscous, sticky, aromatic fluids derived from plants; consists of resins plus oils.

BANA An acronym for benzol-arginine napthylamide *See* benzol-arginine napthylamide.

band 1: A cord, tie, chain, or metal collar by which something is bound. **2:** A contrasting strip or strip of material running through or along the edge of a material.

b. adapter *See* adapter, band.

b., apron *See* apron band.

b., orthodontic A thin metal ring, usually stainless steel, that secures orthodontic attachments to a tooth. The band, with orthodontic attachments welded or soldered to it, is closely adapted to fit the contours of the tooth and then is cemented into place.

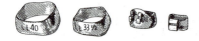

Preformed orthodontic bands

b., adjustable orthodontic A band provided with an adjusting screw to permit alteration in size.

b., pusher An instrument used to adapt the metal band to the tooth.

b. remover An instrument used to remove bands from the teeth.

b., rubber *See* elastic.

b., slip A band formed when a metal is placed under a load and one grain tends to slip or slide on another.

b., striated *See* striations, muscle.

bandage A strip of material wrapped about or applied to any body part.

b., Barton's A figure-of-eight bandage passing below the mandible and around the cranial bone to give upward support to the mandible.

b., thyroid A large bandage consisting principally of a

towel applied around the neck so that it exerts moderate pressure to the anterolateral part of the neck.

bank plan A financial arrangement made between the dentist, patient, and bank for financing dental accounts; the bank provides the capital for a rate of interest that enables the patient to pay the dental account over a longer period of time than would otherwise be possible—usually 12 to 18 months.

bar A metal segment of greater length than width. *See also* bar, connector.

b., anterior palatal *See* connector, major, anterior palatal.

b., arch Any one of several types of wires, bars, or splints conforming to the arch of the teeth and used for the treatment of fractures of the jaws and/or stabilization of injured teeth (e.g, Erich, Jelenko, Niro, Winter).

b., buccal An orthodontic appliance auxiliary consisting of a rigid, metal wire extending from the buccal side of the molar band anteriorly.

b. clasp *See* clasp, bar.

b., connector A connector of greater thickness and reduced width as compared with a plate-like connector, which has greater width and is thinner.

b., fixable-removable cross arch *See* connector, cross arch bar splint.

b., Gilson fixable-removable *See* connector, cross arch bar splint.

b., Kennedy *See* connector, minor, secondary lingual bar.

b., labial A major connector that is located labial (or buccal) to the dental arch and that joins bilateral parts of a mandibular removable partial denture.

b., lingual A major connector that is located lingual to the dental arch and that joins bilateral parts of a mandibular removable partial denture. *See also* connector, major, lingual bar.

b., secondary lingual *See* connector, minor, secondary lingual bar.

b., palatal A major connector that crosses the palate and unites bilateral parts of a maxillary removable partial denture. *See also* connector, major.

b., posterior palatal *See* connector, major, posterior palatal.

barbiturate (bar-bĭt′ŭ-rāt) A salt of barbituric acid.

barium sulfate (bă′rē-ŭm) A white, finely ground, tasteless powder that is insoluble in water, solvents, and solutions of acids and alkalis; used in radiography as a contrast medium because of its opacity to roentgen rays and as a protective barrier in plaster walls.

Barlow's disease *See* scurvy, infantile.

barrier, protective Material of a composition that will greatly absorb radiation (e.g., lead or concrete).

barrier techniques Protocols used in infection control to prevent cross-contamination between health care worker and patient, between patient and health care worker, or between patients. Strict barrier techniques are recommended by the CDC and the ADA to prevent the transmission of hepatitis B viral and human immunodeficiency viral types 1 and 2 infections. However, there are any number of bacterial, viral, and fungal microorganisms that can be transferred through improper or inadequate infection control procedures.

Barton's bandage *See* bandage, Barton's.

basal bone *See* bone, basal.

basal metabolic rate (bā′sel mĕt-ah-bal′ĭk) (BMR, basal metabolism) The basal rate, or energy exchange, determined by means of a clinical test of oxygen consumption in a subject who has had a good night's rest, has fasted for 12 to 14 hours, and has been physically, mentally, and emotionally at rest for 30 minutes; usually indicated as a percentage of the normal calorie production per surface area, the normal values ranging between ± 20%.

basal metabolism *See* basal metabolic rate.

basal seat The oral tissues and structures that support a denture.

  b. s. area *See* area, basal seat.

  b. s. outline An outline on the mucous membrane or on a cast of the entire area that is to be covered by a denture.

basal surface *See* surface, basal.

base 1: The foundation or support on which something rests; the point of attachment of a part; the principal ingredient of a material.   **2:** A compound that yields hydroxyl ions in water solution and causes neutralization of acid to form a salt and water.

  b., acrylic resin A denture base made of an acrylic resin.

  b., apical (basal arch) The portion of the jawbones that gives support to the teeth.

  b., cement A layer of insulated, sometimes medicated dental cement placed in the deep portions of a cavity preparation to protect the pulp, reduce the bulk of the metallic restoration, or eliminate undercuts in a tapered preparation.

  b., denture 1: The part of a denture that fits the oral mucosa of the basal seat, restores the normal contours of the soft tissues of the dentulous mouth, and supports the artificial teeth.   **2:** The portion of a denture that overlies the soft tissue, usually fabricated of resin or combinations of resins and metal.

  b., tinted denture A denture base that simulates the coloring and shading of natural oral tissues.

  b., extension (free-end) A unit of a removable prosthesis that extends anteriorly or posteriorly, terminating without end support by a natural tooth.

  b., film A thin, flexible, transparent sheet of cellulose acetate or similar material.

  b., mandibular The body of the mandible, on which

the teeth and alveolar tissues are situated.

  b., material Any substance from which a denture base may be made (e.g., acrylic resin, vulcanite, polystyrene resin, metal).

  b., metal The basal surface of a denture constructed of metal (e.g., aluminum, gold, cobalt-chromium), to which the teeth are attached.

  b., plastic A denture base, baseplate, or record base made of a plastic material.

  b., record *See* baseplate.

  b., shellac Certain resinous materials adapted to maxillary or mandibular casts to form baseplates.

  b., sprue *See* crucible former.

  b., temporary *See* baseplate.

  b., trial *See* baseplate.

Basedow's disease (băs′ĕ-dōz) *See* goiter, exophthalmic.

baseplate (record base, temporary base, trial base) A temporary form representing the base of a denture and used for making maxillomandibular (jaw) relation records, arranging artificial teeth, or trial placement in the mouth.

  b., stabilized A baseplate lined with a plastic or other material to improve its adaptation and stability.

  b., wax *See* wax, baseplate.

basic metabolic rate *See* basal metabolic rate.

basic services Frequently insurance companies split dental procedures into basic and major categories. Basic services usually consist of the diagnostic, preventive, and routine restorative dental services. The plan may provide different deductibles, co-insurance, and maximums for basic vs. major services as an incentive to good dental care.

basion (bā′sē-ahn) The midline point at the anterior margin of the occipital foramen.

basis The principal active ingredient in a prescription

basophil (bā′sō-fĭl) *See* leukocyte.

basophilia (bā-sō-fĭl′ē-ah) (basophilic granular degeneration, basophilic stippling) An aggregate of bluestaining granules found in erythrocytes; seen in lead poisoning, leukemia, malaria, severe anemias, and certain toxemias.

basophilic line (bā-sō-fĭl′ĭk) *See* line, basophilic.

batch processing Data processing in which a number of similar input data items are grouped together and processed during a single machine run with the same program.

Battle's sign *See* sign, Battle's.

bayonet A binangled instrument, the nib or blade of which is generally parallel to the shaft; resembles a bayonet. *See also* angle former, bayonet; condenser, bayonet.

beading A term used to denote the scribing of a shallow groove (less than 0.5 mm in width or depth) on a cast that outlines the major connector. It is used to transfer the design to the investment cast and to ensure tissue contact of the major connector.

beam A stream or approximately unidirectional emission of electromagnetic radiation or particles.

   b., central The center of the beam of roentgen rays emitted from the tube.

   b., useful The part of the primary radiation that passes through the aperture, cone, or other collimator.

beaver-tail retractor *See* retractor, beaver-tail.

Bednar's aphtha *See* aphtha, Bednar's.

beeswax A low-melting wax that is an ingredient of many dental waxes.

Begg appliance *See* appliance, Begg.

behavior The manner in which a person acts or performs. Any or all of the activities of a person, including physical action learned and unlearned, deliberate or habitual.

   b. management Techniques used to control or modify an action or performance of a subject. In dentistry, usually associated with the management of oral hygiene behavior, dietary behavior, or patient behavior under stress.

   b. modification To alter, change or transfer an action from a socially unacceptable and destructive act to a socially acceptable nondestructive action. In dentistry, usually associated with oral habits, such as finger or thumb sucking, mouth breathing, nail biting, and smoking.

Behcet's syndrome *See* syndrome, Behcet's.

Beilby's layer *See* layer, Beilby's.

Bell's palsy, sign, palsy test *See under appropriate noun.*

Benadryl Trade name for diphedyramine hydrochloride, an antihistamine with anticholinergic (drying) and sedative side ef fects

Bence Jones protein *See* protein, Bence Jones.

Benedict's test *See* test, Benedict's.

beneficiary 1: A person eligible for benefits under a dental plan. Synonyms: eligible individual; enrollee; member. **2:** A person who receives benefits under a dental benefit contract. *See also* covered person; insured; member; subscriber).

benefit booklet A booklet or pamphlet provided to the subscriber that contains a general explanation of the benefits and related provisions of the dental benefits program. Also known as a "Summary Plan Description."

benefit plan summary The description or synopsis of employee benefits required by ERISA to be distributed to the employees.

benefits 1: The cash benefit paid for various procedures performed. **2:** The list of dental services or procedures covered by the insurance policy and referred to as the schedule of benefits. Synonym: coverage.

benign (bē-nīn′) The inability of a neoplasm to metastasize when describing it.

Bennett angle, movement *See under appropriate noun.*

benzathine penicillin G Penicillin G linked with dibenzylethylene diamine to form a slowly absorbable injectable antibiotic effective against penicillin-susceptible organisms.

benzocaine Ethyl 4-aminobenzoate, an ester-like anesthetic with low water solubility and low solubility; used topically in direct application to abraded, ulcerated, or lacerated tissues, including oral mucosa.

benzyol-arginine naphthylamide A bacterial enzyme that mimics the activity of trypsin. BANA is used as a marker of bacterial growth in dental plaque or as a marker for the diagnosis of periodontal disease involving *B. gingivalis, B. forsythus, and Treponema denticola.*

benzoyl peroxide A chemical incorporated into the polymer of resins to aid in the initiation of polymerization.

beriberi (asjike, athiaminosis, endemic multiple neuritis, endemic polyneuritis, hinchazon, inchacao, kakke, loempe, panneuritis endemica, perneiras) A nutritional disease resulting from a deficiency of thiamine. Classically it is characterized by multiple neuritis, muscular atrophy, weakness, cardiovascular changes, and progressive edema.

Besnier-Boeck-Schaumann disease (běz′nē-ā běk shaw-′măn) *See* sarcoidosis.

beta-hemihydrate (bā″tah-hĕm-ē-hī′drāt) The physical state of hemihydrate of calcium sulfate-plaster of paris.

betatron (bā′tah-trahn) A machine that produces high speed electrons through magnetic induction.

bevel The inclination that one surface makes with another when not at right angles; in cavity preparation, a cut that produces an angle of more than 90 degrees with a cavity wall.

   b., cavosurface The incline or slant of the cavosurface angle of a prepared cavity wall in relation to the plane of the enamel wall.

   b., contra (reverse bevel, internal bevel) Blade placement toward the base of the periodontal pocket that will separate the sulcular from the external epithelium.

   b., instrument The sloping keen edge of a cutting instrument.

   b., reverse *See* bevel, contra.

BHN *See* number, Brinell hardness; test, Brinell hardness.

bicarbonate A salt resulting from the incomplete neutralization of carbonic acid, such as from passing excess carbon dioxide into a base solution.

Bicillin Trade name. *See* benzathine penicillin G.

bicuspid (bĭ-kŭs′pĭd) *See* premolar.

b.i.d. Abbreviation for bis in die, a Latin phrase meaning twice a day.

Biermer's anemia (bēr′merz) *See* anemia, pernicious.

bifid tongue (bī′fĭd) *See* tongue, bifid.

bifid uvula *See* uvula, bifid.

bifurcation (bī-fer-kā′shŭn) The division into two parts or branches, such as any two roots of a tooth.

bilateral (bī-lăt′er-ŭl) Pertaining to both sides.

bilharziasis (bĭl″har-zī′ah-sĭs) *See* schistosomiasis.

bilirubinemia (bĭl″ē-roo″bĭ-nē′mē-ah) Presence of bilirubin in the blood. It may result from obstruction within or without the liver or to increased hemolysis. The total serum bilirubin in an adult is 0.2 to 0.7 mg/100 ml.

bilirubinuria (bĭl″ē-roo″bĭ-nū′rē-ah) Presence of bilirubin in the urine. More often, an excess of bilirubin in the urine resulting from excessive hemolysis.

billing The procedure of preparing a financial statement.

bimaxillary (bī-măx′ĭl-ăr-ē) Pertaining to the right and left maxillae; sometimes incorrectly used to refer to the maxillae and mandible.

    b., protrusion *See* protrusion, bimaxillary.

bimeter (bī′mē-tĕr) A gnathodynamometer with a central bearing point adjustable to varying heights. *See also* gnathodynamometer.

Bimler appliance *See* appliance, Bimler.

binangle (bĭn′ăngl) An instrument having two offsetting angles in its shank. The angles keep the cutting edge or the face of the nib within 3 mm of the axis of the shaft.

binder A substance, usually sticky, that holds the solid particles in a mixture together, thus aiding in the preservation of the physical form of the mixture.

binding Reversible combination of various drugs with body constituents such as plasma proteins.

binocular loupe *See* loupe, binocular.

biofeedback The instrumented process or technique of learning voluntary control over automatically regulated body functions; useful in the treatment of braxism, temporomandibular joint dysfunction, pain, and anxiety control in the dental setting.

    b., electromyographic (EMG) An instrumented process that helps patients learn control over muscle tension levels previously under automatic control; especially useful in treatment of dental disorders, such as bruxism, temporomandibular joint dysfunction, tension headaches, and other disorders involving the muscles of mastication. In addition to neuromuscular education, EMG biofeedback is useful in treating dental phobias, anxiety, and pain control by helping patients learn deep muscle relaxation techniques.

    b., temperature An instrumented learning process whereby a patient learns to control temperature of body parts. Training in self-controlled vasodilation (handwarming) technique has been found useful in

treating migraine headaches and anxiety in dental patients.

bioflavonoids Naturally occurring flavone or courmarin derivatives having the activity of so-called vitamin P. Its use in controlling gingival bleeding remains controversial.

bioglass A fused silic containing aluminum oxide that presents a surface-reactive glass film that is compatible with connective and epithelial tissues. Bioglass is a material used as a surface coating in blade and endosteal implants.

biologic Pertaining to biology.

biology The science of life or living matter, in all its forms and phenomena.

biomechanics (bī″ō-mē-kăn′ĭks) *See* biophysics.

biometrics (bī″ō-mĕt′rĭks) The science of the application of statistical methods to biologic facts.

bionator A removable orthodontic appliance designed to correct functional and skeletal anterior-posterior discrepancies between the maxilla and mandible.

biophysics (bī″ō-fĭz-ĭks) **(biomechanics)** The science that deals with the forces that act on living cells of the living body, the relationship between the biologic behavior of living structures and the physical influences to which they are subjected, and the physics of vital processes.

    b., dental The branch of biophysics that deals with the biologic behavior of oral structures as influenced by dental restorations.

biopsy (bī′ŏp-sē) The removal of a tissue specimen or other material from the living body for microscopic examination to aid in establishing a diagnosis.

    b., aspiration (needle biopsy) The procedure of obtaining a biopsy specimen by aspiration through a needle; used for bone or deep soft tissue lesions

    b., excisional The removal of an entire lesion, usually including a significant margin of contiguous normal tissue, for microscopic examination and diagnosis.

    b., exploratory Exploration combined with biopsy to determine method and degree of local extension, usually of bone or deep soft tissue lesions.

    b., incisional The surgical removal of a selected mass of a lesion and adjacent normal tissue for microscopic examination and diagnosis.

    b., needle *See* biopsy, aspiration.

    b., punch Biopsy material obtained by use of a punch.

biotin (bī′ō-tĭn) *See* vitamin, biotin.

biotransformation Chemical and physical changes produced in drugs after they enter the body (e.g., hydrolysis, conjugation).

bird-face *See* brachygnathia; retrognathism.

birth control pills Oral contraceptives, usually a mixture of a steroid having progestational activity and an estrogen.

birthday role Coordination of benefits regulation stipulating that the primary payer of benefits for dependent children is determined by the parent's birthdates. Regardless of which parent is older, the dental benefits program of the parent whose birthdate falls first in a calendar year is considered primary. (Does not apply to "self-funded" programs.)

bis Prefix meaning that two like or mirror-image moieties are joined together to form a chemical compound.

biscuit Firing bakes, or stages (referred to as low, medium, and high), during the fusing of dental porcelain preceding the final, or glaze, bake.

bisexual Engaged in or desiring sexual contact with persons of both sexes.

bismuth poisoning (bĭz'mŭth) *See* bismuthosis.

bismuthia (bĭz-mū'thē-ah) Discoloration of mucous membranes and skin from bismuth poisoning.

bismuthism *See* bismuthosis.

bismuthosis (bĭz"mŭth-ō'sĭs) (bismuth poisoning, bismuthism) Acute or chronic bismuth intoxication resulting from the ingestion or injection of bismuth salts. Possible manifestations include albuminuria, exfoliative dermatitis, gastrointestinal disturbances, and stomatitis. *See also* stomatitis, bismuth.

bite 1: The part of an artificial tooth on the lingual side between the shoulder and the incisal edge of the tooth. **2:** An interocclusal record or relationship. *See also* denture space; distance, interarch; record, interocclusal; record, maxillomandibular.

b. analysis *See* analysis, occlusal.

b., balanced *See* occlusion, balanced.

b. block 1: In intraoral radiography a film holder that the patient bites to provide stable retention of the film packet. **2:** Occlusion rim. *See also* rim, occlusion.

b., close *See* distance, small interarch.

b., closed 1: An abnormal overbite. **2:** A decrease in the occlusal vertical dimension produced by factors such as tooth abrasion and loss or failure of eruption of supportive posterior teeth. *See also* distance, reduced interarch.

b. closing *See* dimension, vertical decrease.

b., convenience *See* occlusion, acquired, eccentric.

b., edge-to-edge An occlusion in which the incisal edge of maxillary incisors meets the incisal edge of mandibular incisors. *See also* occlusion, edge-to-edge.

b. fork *See* fork, face-bow.

b. guard *See* guard, bite.

b. guard splint *See* splint, acrylic resin bite-guard.

b., locked *See* occlusion, locked.

b., marks Distinctive tooth patterns in a wound, which may have forensic or legal implications.

b., normal *See* occlusion, normal.

b., open A malformation in which the anterior teeth do not occlude in any mandibular position.

b. opening *See* dimension, vertical, increasing occlusal.

b. opening bends Bends made in maxillary and mandibular light round wires mesial to the molar tubes.

b. plate *See* plane, bite.

b. raising *See* dimension, vertical, increasing occlusal.

b. record *See* path, generated occlusal.

b., rest *See* position, rest, physiologic.

b. rim *See* rim, occlusion.

b., working *See* occlusion, working.

biteplane (bīt'plān) A removable appliance that covers the occlusal surfaces of the teeth to prevent their articulation.

bite-wing film *See* film, bite-wing.

bite-wing radiograph *See* radiograph, bite-wing.

biting, cheek *See* habit.

biting, lip *See* habit.

biting, nail *See* habit.

biting pressure *See* pressure, occlusal.

biting strength *See* strength, biting.

blade *See* instrument parts.

blanching, gingival *See* gingival, blanching.

Blandin and Nuhn's gland *See* gland, Blandin and Nuhn's.

blastomatoid lesion (blăs-tō'mah-toid) Overzealous reactive process, which, because of tumescence, has some features of neoplasia. A specific tissue element, such as fibroblasts, endothelial cells, osteoblasts, osteoclastic giant cells, or nerves, predominates in a specific lesion to form granuloma pyogenicum, giant cell reparative granuloma, traumatic fibroma, tori, or traumatic neuroma.

Blastomyces brasiliensis (blăs"tō-mī'sēz) A species of fungus causing South American blastomycosis, not found in the United States.

Blastomyces dermatitidis (blăs"tō-mī'sēz der"mah-tīt'ĭ-dĭs) A species of fungus causing North American blastomycosis.

blastomycosis (blăs"tō-mī-kō'sĭs) Infection resulting from the fungus *Blastomyces dermatitidis* (North American blastomycosis) or to *Blastomyces brasiliensis* (South American blastomycosis); characterized by chronic suppurative lesions. The disseminated form is usually fatal.

b., South American A fungous infection that often begins when organisms enter the body through the oral mucosa, producing local ulcers or through an extraction site, producing papillary lesions. Dissemination leads to granulomatous lesion of the lymph nodes, gastrointestinal tract, and liver and lungs and to microabscesses of the skin. The causative agent is *Blastomyces brasiliensis*.

bleaching The use of a chemical oxidizing agent (sometimes in combination with heat) to lighten tooth discolorations. *See also* agent, bleaching.

bleeding The flowing of blood.

b., gingival *See* gingival bleeding.

b., occult Hemorrhage of such small proportions that the blood can be detected only by chemical test, the microscope, or the spectroscope.

b. points A series of puncture points made through the gingival tissue; used as a guide for making the gingivectomy incision.

b. time The time required for blood to stop flowing from a tiny wound. Normal bleeding time is from 2 to 6 minutes. Bleeding time is increased in disorders of platelet count, uremia, and ingestion of aspirin and other antiinflammatory medications.

blindness, color (defective color vision) Decreased ability to detect differences in color. *See also* achromatopsia.

b., blue-yellow color Color disability in which the spectrum is seen in reds and greens; a form of protanopia.

b., red-green color The common form of color disability, in which the entire spectrum is constituted by yellows and blues; a form of protanopia.

Bloch-Sulzberger syndrome *See* syndrome, Bloch-Sulzberger.

block A mental obstacle that prohibits a patient from having favorable responses to the dentist and suggested treatment plans.

b., data A physical unit of data that can be conveniently stored by a computer on an input or output device. The block is normally composed of one or more logical records or a portion of logical record. Synonym: physical record.

b., field The reversible interruption of nerve conduction over terminal branches by infiltration of a suitable agent into the area.

b., nerve The reversible interruption of conduction along a nerve trunk or its branches because of the absorption of a suitable agent. Also, regional anesthesia secured by extraneural or paraneural injection in close proximity to the nerve whose conductivity is to be cut off.

blocking The process of obstructing or deadening, as a nerve.

b. agent *See* agent, blocking.

blockout (wax out) Elimination of undesirable undercut areas on a cast to be used in the fabrication of a removable denture.

blood The fluid circulating through the heart, arteries, capillaries, and veins; carries nutrients and oxygen to body tissues.

b., bad Lay term for syphilis.

b. calcium The level of calcium in the blood plasma, generally regulated by parathyroid gland activity in conjunction with the degree of calcium ingestion, absorption, use, and excretion. Normal value is 8.5 to 11.5 mg/100 ml of blood serum.

b. cell count An estimation of the number or types of circulating blood cells (e.g., red blood cell [erythrocytic], white blood cell, differential).

b. chemistry The determination of the chemical constituents of blood by assay in a clinical laboratory as part of a diagnostic protocol.

b. clot *See* clot, blood.

b., color index of A figure gained by dividing the hemoglobin percentage by the red blood cell percentage. In most anemias the result is below 1, but in pernicious anemia it is characteristically above 1.

b. disorders Hematologic dyscrasias that affect the component cells and plasma elements of the blood. Blood disorders are generally divided into two broad groups: those in which there is an increase in bulk (e.g., plethora, hydremia, polycythemia) and those in which there is a decrease in bulk (e.g., anhydremia, dehydration, anemia).

b. dyscrasias (disorders) Pathologic conditions in which any of the constituents of the blood are abnormal or are present in abnormal quantity, such as leukemia or hemophilia.

b. groups The division of blood into types on the basis of the compatibility of the erythrocytes and serum of one individual with the erythrocytes and serum of another individual. The groups are immunologically and genetically distinct.

b. pressure *See* pressure, blood.

b. products Constitutents of whole blood that are used in replacement therapy, such as plasma or platelets.

b. sugar The concentration of sugar (chiefly glucose— "true blood sugar") in the blood. It is usually kept within a narrow range by an interplay of many factors: glycogenolysis, glyconeogenesis, intestinal absorption, insulin, insulin "antagonists," and other hormones. In the testing of total reducing substances, the normal range of concentration of fasting blood sugar is 80 to 120 mg/ml; in the testing of "true blood sugar," the normal range of concentration is 70 to 100 mg/ml.

b. urea nitrogen (BUN) Nitrogen in the form of urea in whole blood or serum. Its concentration is a gross measure of renal function. The upper limit of the normal range is 25 mg/100 ml.

b., volume index of The volume of red blood cells/ total volume of blood times 100 = vol% of packed red blood cells (hematocrit index). A value greater than 1 indicates an abnormally large number or size of erythrocytes.

blower, chip *See* syringe, air, hand.

blowpipe A torch that employs gas-oxygen, or oxygen and acetylene, to melt metal in dental casting and soldering procedures.

blue, methylene (mĕth'ĭ-lēn) **1:** A dye used to color

bacteria for microscopic examination. **2:** An aniline dye often used as an antiseptic and topical analgesic in the treatment of lesions of the oral mucous membranes and skin.

blue nevus *See* nevus, blue.

blunderbuss apex *See* apex, blunderbuss.

BMR *See* basal metabolic rate.

board certification The examination program that establishes the clinical proficiency of a dental specialist according to the procedures established by the individual specialty certification board under the rules and authority of the Council on Dental Education of the American Dental Association.

board certified The status of a dental specialist, such as an orthodontist, who has become a Board Diplomate by successfully completing the certification program of the recognized certification board in that special area of practice.

board diplomate A dental specialist who has achieved certification by the recognized certifying board in that specialty, as attested by a diploma from the board.

board eligible The status of a dental specialist whose educational qualifications have been verified by acceptance of an application for certification by the recognized certifying board. Board eligibility depends on advanced education in the specialty and on timely progress toward completion of the certification procedure. Regular renewal is required to maintain eligibility until the examination is completed.

board qualified An unrecognized term used variously and inaccurately to identify any of the stages from educational qualification to certification.

bodily movement *See* movement, body.

body Any mass or collection of material.

b., Donovan An extracellular structure found in macrophages in lesions of granuloma inguinale.

b., foreign Any object or material that is not normal for the area in which it is located.

b., ketone The compounds acetoacetic acid, betahydroxybutyric acid and acetone, which are formed in the liver and released to the blood. Elevated levels occur during excessive fat use, such as in diabetes or starvation.

b., Lipschütz Any one of the eosinophilic oval structures see in the nuclei of cells found in herpes virus infection.

b., Schaumann (shaw′măn) A round to oval cytoplasmic inclusion composed of concentric deposits of an amorphous material. Seen in the giant cells of sarcoidosis, in beryllium lesions, and sometimes in other giant cells.

b., Verocay A component of Antoni type A tissue seen in neurilemoma. *See also* neurilemoma.

Boeck's disease (běks) *See* sarcoidosis.

Boeck's sarcoid (běks) *See* sarcoidosis.

Bogarad's syndrome *See* syndrome, auriculotemporal.

Bohn's nodules *See* nodules, Bohn's.

Boley gauge *See* gauge, Boley.

Bolton analysis A computation developed by Wayne Bolton for the evaluation of tooth size discrepancies between upper and lower arches.

Bolton plane *See* plane, Bolton-nasion.

Bolton point, triangle *See under appropriate noun.*

Bolton-nasion plane *See* plane, Bolton-nasion.

bolus (bō′lŭs) A mass of food ready to be swallowed or a mass passing through the intestines.

bond The force that holds two or more units of matter together.

b., primary or chemical A bond that requires some change in structure of matter. Primary bonds are ionic, covalent, or metallic.

b., secondary or physical (sometimes called *van der Waals' forces*) A bond that involves weak interatomic attractions such as variation in physical mass or location of electrical charge.

bonding Adhesion of orthodontic attachments to the teeth without use of an interposed band.

b., alveolar The specialized bone structure that contains the alveoli or sockets of the teeth and supports the teeth.

b., alveolar, architecture The structural pattern of the alveolar bone and its subjacent latticework of supporting bone. The alveolar bone is thin and compact adjacent to the periodontal membrane. The trabecular bone connects and reinforces the individual alveoli. The architecture of a bone is the result of functional stimuli to that bone, the stimuli varying as to type, intensity, and duration.

b., alveolar, metabolism The metabolic activity occurring within alveolar bone, which is generally slower than that occurring within metaphyseal bone but more rapid than that of diaphyseal bone.

b. apposition *See* bone deposition.

b., basal That part of the mandible and maxillae from which the alveolar process develops.

b., bundle The bone that forms the immediate bone attachment of the numerous bundles of collagen fibers of the periodontal ligament that have been incorporated into the bone.

b. bur A drill designed to cut into bone.

b. calcium content The amount of calcium stored in bone tissue. Plasma calcium is in constant exchange with the calcium of the extracellular fluid and bones. The parathyroid gland maintains the constancy of the calcium concentration in the plasma. The bones serve as a reservoir of calcium and phosphate to provide for the other needs of the body and to supply minerals for deposition in the skeleton.

b., cancellous (spongiosa, spongy bone, supporting

bone, trabecular bone) The bone that forms a trabecular network, surrounds marrow spaces that may contain either fatty or hematopoietic tissue, lies subjacent to the cortical bone, and makes up the main portion (bulk) of a bone.

b., cancellous, atrophy of disuse Wasting of bone tissue occurring with loss of function of a part (e.g., a tooth). The supporting bone assumes an osteoporotic nature, and the marrow remains fatty or hematopoietic.

b. cells Osteoblasts, osteocytes, osteoclasts, and osteoprogenerator cells.

b. changes, mechanical factors Pressure and tension forces play an important role in determining bone structure. Improperly controlled appliances can resorb bone faster than deposition can occur, causing mobile teeth and traumatic occlusion. Poor vascularity is a concomitant cause of undue pressure and tension and may inhibit repair and frequently may cause necrosis.

b. chips Small pieces of cancellous bone generally used to fill in bony defects and to precipitate recalcification.

b., compact Hard, dense bone comprising the outer cortical layer and consisting of an infinite variety of periosteal bone, endosteal bone, and haversian systems.

b. conduction See conduction, bone.

b. crest The most coronal portion of alveolar bone.

b. density The compactness of bone tissue. The demonstration of bone density by means of radiographs is directly dependent on the quantity of inorganic salts contained in the bone tissue.

b. deposition Apposition or formation of new bone as a normal physiologic process.

b. development See bone, endochondral, formation; bone formation; bone, membrane, formation.

b., direct Individual placement of attachments on the teeth at the time of adhesion.

b., effect of external radiation to Damage to the bones of adults is most often seen after heavy and localized x-ray treatment.

b., endochondral (ĕn″dō-kŏn′dral) A bone that is developed in relation to antecedent cartilages (e.g., long bones, mandible). See also bone, membrane.

b., endochondral, formation Primarily a replacement of previously formed embryonic cartilage with an adult bony structure; a more complex bone formation than membrane bone. The actual replacement of cartilage by bone is only part of the process, however, because much of the bone is laid down directly external to the embryonic cartilage. See also bone, membrane, formation.

b. formation The deposition of an organic mucopolysaccharide matrix (osteoid) that is subsequently mineralized with calcium salts. See also bone apposition; bone deposition.

b. graft, autogenous See graft, autogenous bone.

b. graft, donor site See donor site.

b. graft, onlay See graft, onlay bone.

b. graft, recipient site See recipient site.

b. groove Osteotomy into or near the crest of the alveolar ridge for placement of an endosteal blade type of implant.

b. groove, canted An osteotomy sloped to avoid the mandibular canal or to keep the implant infrastructure within the medullary confines.

b., indirect Positioning of attachments on a dental cast and transferring them to the teeth en masse for adhesion by means of a molded matrix bone. The material of the skeleton of most vertebrate animals; the tissue comprising bones.

b., internal reconstruction of The formation of bone on the tensional side of the periodontal ligament with concurrent resorption from the marrow space; contralaterally, resorption of alveolar bone with apposition from the endosteum in the marrow space.

b., interproximal The bone that forms the septa between the teeth; consists primarily of a spongiosa of supporting bone covered by a layer of cortical bone. See also septum, interdental.

b. involvement Changes in the alveolar and/or supporting bone occurring as a sequel to, or accompanying, inflammatory or dystrophic disease; usually of a resorptive nature.

b. lamella Bone having the appearance of layers of thin leaves or plates. This appearance is produced by the lines that represent periods of inactivity of bone formation.

b., malar (zygomatic bone) A quadrangular bone on each side of the face that unites the frontal and superior maxillary bones with the zygomatic process of the temporal bone. It forms the cheek prominence, a portion of the lateral wall and floor of the orbit, and parts of the temporal fossa and infratemporal fossa.

b., marble See osteopetrosis.

b. marrow The soft vascular tissue that fills bone cavities and cancellous bone spaces and consists primarily of fat cells, hematopoietic cells, and osteogenetic reticular cells.

b., membrane A bone developed within membrane but having no antecedent cartilage (e.g., parietal, frontal, bones of upper face). See also bone, endochondral.

b., membrane, formation The membrane bone forms directly from the mesenchyme, first as a thin, flattened, irregular bony plate or membrane in the dermis, gradually expanding at its margins and becoming thickened by the deposition of successive layers of additional bone on the inner and outer surfaces. *See also* bone, endochondral, formation.

b. membranes Membrane structures associated with the growth, development, and repair of bone: the periosteum, a connective tissue layer adjacent to bone surfaces; periodontal membrane, a modified periosteum associated with tooth structure; and endosteum, a thin layer of connective tissue lining the walls of the bone marrow spaces.

b., microscopic appearance of Composition of bone tissue as viewed under a microscope. Microscopically, bone is composed of osteocytes embedded within lacunae in a calcified intercellular matrix. Extending from the lacunae are minute canals called *canaliculi*, which communicate with canaliculi of adjacent lacunae. Through this system of canals, nutrient material reaches the osteocytes and provides avenues for the removal of waste products of metabolism. Bone is deposited in incremental layers (lamellae) around haversarian canals, the lamellae toward the surface of the bone being more or less parallel to it.

b. mineral content, chemistry of The hardness of bone results from its mineral content in the organic matrix. The minerals, (commonly designated as bone salts) and the organic matrix make up the interstitial substance of bone. The bone salts consist essentially of hydroxyapatite ($Ca_{10}[PO_4]_6[OH_2]$), carbon dioxide, and water, together with small amounts of other ions.

b., onlay *See* graft, onlay bone.

b., perichondrial Bone that is deposited in concentric layers around the long shaft of the bone in a manner similar to the growth of endochondral bone.

b., physical properties of Compact bone has the following physical characteristics: specific gravity, 1.92 to 1.99; tensile strength, 13,000 to 17,000 psi; compressive strength, 18,000 to 24,000 psi; compressive strength parallel to the long axis, 7150 psi; compressive strength at right angles to the long axis, 10,800 psi. These physical characteristics make bone particularly suitable for carrying out its functions of weight bearing, leverage, and protection of vulnerable viscera.

b. rarefaction A decreased density of bone, i.e., a decrease in the weight per unit of volume.

b. recession *See* recession, bone.

b., resorption and repair of An adaptive physiologic mechanism ocurring as long as the individual retains the natural dentition. *See also* resorption of bone.

b., resting lines in Lines created by alternating periods of bone formation and rest, giving a tierlike appearance to lamellar bone.

b., reversal lines in Irregular lines containing concavi-

ties directed away from the bundle bone and serving as a histologic indication that resorption has taken place up to that line from the marrow side.

b. sequestrum *See* sequestrum.

b., sphenoid An irregular, wedge-shaped bone located at the base of the skull in front of the temporal bone and the basilar portion of the occipital bone. It is composed of a body that is more or less cuboidal in shape and hollowed out interiorly to form the sphenoidal air sinuses. Extending from the body laterally are two great wings and two small wings. Projecting below the body are two pterygoid processes. The lateral surfaces of the pterygoid processes give origin to the external ptergoid muscles, whereas the medial surfaces give origin to the internal pterygoid muscles.

b., spongy *See* bone, cancellous.

b. support The amount of alveolar and trabecular bone adjacent to a tooth that can provide attachment, investment, and support for the tooth.

b., supporting *See* bone cancellous.

b., supporting, atrophy of disuse *See* bone, cancellous, atrophy of disuse.

b. surgery *See* surgery, osseous.

b., thickened margin of Widening of the crest of the alveolus, primarily on the buccal and/or lingual aspects, varying from a thick ledge to a "beading" of the bone margin; results in a more or less bulbous contour of the gingival tissue overlying it.

b., trabecular *See* bone, cancellous.

b. wax *See* wax, bone.

b., woven So termed because of the character and pattern resulting from the interweaving of broad bands of bone.

b., zygomatic *See* bone, malar.

Bonwill-Hawley chart *See* chart, Hawley.

Bonwill's triangle *See* triangle, Bonwill's.

bony crater A concave resorptive defect in the alveolar crest, usually occurring interdentally.

bony crepitus *See* crepitus, bony.

borax Often a principal ingredient in casting fluxes. Used in gypsum products as a retarder for the setting reaction and a strengthener for hydrocolloids.

border The circumferential margin or edge.

b., denture (denture edge, denture periphery) The limit, boundary, or circumferential margin of a denture base.

b., mandibular (mandibular plane) Tangent to the lower border of the mandible. A line joining point gonion to point gnathion.

b. molding Shaping of an impression material by the manipulation or action of the tissues to determine the denture border position.

b. movement *See* movement, border.

b. seal The contact of the denture border with the underlying or adjacent tissues to prevent the passage of air or other substances.

b. structures The oral structures that bound the borders of a denture.

b. tissues, movement. The action of the muscles and other structures adjacent to the borders of a denture.

boutons terminaux *See* end-feet.

Bowen's disease *See* carcinoma in situ.

box, light *See* illuminator.

boxing The building up of vertical walls, usually in wax, around an impression to produce the desired size and form of the base of the cast.

b. strip *See* strip boxing.

brachycephalic (brăk″ē-sĕ-făl′ĭk) Descriptive term applied to a broad, round head having a cephalic index of more than 80.

brachygnathia (brăk″ĭg-nā′thē-ah) (bird-face, micrognathia) Marked underdevelopment of the mandible. *See also* retrognathism.

bracing Resistance to the horizontal components of masticatory force.

bracket A small metal attachment fixed to a band that serves as a means of fastening the arch wire to the band.

bradycardia (brăd-ē-kar′dē-ah) Abnormal slowness of the heart as evidenced by a slowing of the pulse rate (under 50 beats/minute).

bradydiastole (brăd″ē-dī-ăs′tō-lē) Abnormal prolongation of the diastole.

bradykinin One of a number of plasma kinins, a potent vasodilator; one of the physiologic mediators of an anaphylaxis reaction.

brachydactyly Abnormal shortness of the fingers, usually associated with some congenital syndrome.

bradypnea (brăd″ē-nē′ah) Abnormal slowness of breathing.

bradythesia (brăd″ē-thē′zē-ah) Slowness or dullness of perception.

brain, electrical activity of Electrical energy that can be observed as waves with electroencephalographic equipment. These rhythms and patterns have been organized into a system that imputes values for the state of health and disease. Electrical evidence of brain activity of the cerebral cortex reveals that different potential patterns are produced by different states of mental activity (e.g., tension, mental work, sleep).

brainstem The part of the brain, presumably the oldest part phylogenetically, in which are located centers for many simple but basically important reactions within the nervous system. The brainstem includes the primitive forebrain, the midbrain, and the hindbrain.

branchial nerve *See* nerve, branchial.

Branemark technique *See* osseointegration.

breach of contract *See* contract, breach of.

break-even point The level of patient visits or net reve-nues at which the revenues for a period are equal to the expenses incurred in that period.

breath Air inhaled and exhaled in respiration.

b., bad (offensive) *See* halitosis.

breathing, mouth The process of inspiration and expiration of air primarily through the oral cavity. It is commonly seen in nasal conditions, such as deviated septum, hypertrophied adenoids, and allergies, and may produce excessive drying of the oral mucosa with a tendency to gingival hyperplasia.

bregma (brĕg′mah) The point at which sagittal and coronary sutures meet.

Breuer's reflex *See* reflex, Hering-Breuer.

bridge Colloquial expression for a fixed partial denture. *See* denture, partial, fixed.

b., cantilever *See* denture, partial, fixed, cantilever.

b., fixed *See* denture, partial, fixed.

b., removable A colloquial expression for a removable partial denture. *See also* denture, partial, removable.

b. splint *See* splint, fixed.

Brill-Symmers disease *See* lymphoma, giant follicular.

Brinell hardness number *See* number, Brinell hardness.

Brinell hardness test *See* test, Brinell hardness.

brittle Friable; technically, a brittle material is one in which the proportional limit and ultimate strength are close together in value. *See also* ductility.

broach An instrument with numerous protruding barbs from a metal shaft. It is generally used to engage the dental pulp for extirpation.

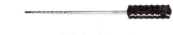

Endodontic broach

b., barbed *See* broach.

b. holder An instrument similar to a pin vise used to hold a broach.

b., pathfinder *See* broach, smooth.

b., smooth (pathfinder, pathfinder broach) An instrument used for locating the orifice of a root canal and exploring the canal to determine the accessibility of the root end.

Broders' classification *See* index, Broders'.

Broders' index *See* index, Broders'.

bromism (brō′mĭzm) The toxic state induced by excessive exposure to or ingestion of bromine or bromine-containing compounds.

bromopnea (brōm″ahp-nē′ah) *See* halitosis.

bronchia (brŏng′kē-ah) Bronchial tubes smaller than bronchi and larger than bronchioles.

bronchiarctia (brŏng′kē-ark′shē-ah) The stenosis of a bronchial tube.

bronchiectasis (brŏng″kē-ĕk′tah-sĭs) A chronic disease characterized by dilation of the bronchi and bronchioles, clinically recognizable by fetid breath and purulent matter; dilation of the bronchi, either local or general.

bronchiocele (brŏng′kē-ō-sēl″) A dilation or swelling of a branch smaller than a bronchus.

bronchiole (brŏng′kē-ōl) A terminal division of a bronchium.

bronchium (brŏng′kē-ŭm) One of the subdivisions of a bronchus.

bronchoconstriction (brŏng′kō-kahn-strĭk′shŭn) The reduction of the caliber of the bronchi.

bronchodilation (brŏng′kō-dī-lā′shŭn) The dilation of a bronchus; the operation of dilating a stenosed bronchus.

bronchodilator (brŏng′kō-dī-lā′tor) A drug that dilates, or expands, the size of the lumina of the air passages of the lungs by relaxing the muscular walls.

bronchospasm (brŏng′kō-spăzm) A spasmodic contraction of the muscular coat of the bronchial tubes, such as occurs in asthma.

bronchostenosis (brŏng′kō-stĕ-nō′sĭs) Stenosis of the bronchi; bronchiarctia.

Brooke's tumor *See* epithelioma adenoides cysticum.

brown pellicle *See* pellicle, brown.

bruise In medical jurisprudence a contusion; an injury made on the flesh of a person by an instrument without destroying its continuity, i.e., without breaking the skin.

bruit (brōōt) Extracardiac blowing sound heard at times over peripheral vessels; generally denotes cardiovascular disease.

brush, polishing An instrument consisting of natural, synthetic, or wire bristles, mounted on a mandrel or in a hub to fit on a lathe chuck; used to carry abrasive or polishing media to polish teeth, restorations, and prosthetic appliances.

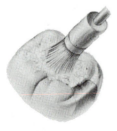

Brush used to polish groove

b., bristle polishing A polishing brush with natural or synthetic bristles.

b., wheel polishing A polishing brush with bristles mounted like spokes of a wheel.

b., wire polishing A polishing brush with bristles of wire, usually steel or brass.

brushing *See* abrasion, denture.

bruxism (brŭk′sĭzm) The involuntary gnashing, grinding, or clenching of teeth. It is usually unconscious, whether the individual is awake or asleep; often associated with fatigue, anxiety, emotional stress, or fear; and frequently triggered by occlusal irregularities, usually resulting in abnormal wear patterns on the teeth, periodontal breakdown, or joint or neuromuscular problems.

BSP *See* test, Bromsulphalein.

bubo (bū′bō) A lymph node that is enlarged secondary to an infection. The process may lead to suppuration; seen in primary syphilis, chancroid, plague, malaria, and other infectious processes.

buccal (bŭk′ŭl) Pertaining to or adjacent to the cheek.

b. aspect *See* aspect, buccal.

b. contour *See* contour, buccal.

b. flange *See* flange, buccal.

b. notch *See* notch, buccal.

b. shelf *See* shelf, buccal.

b. splint *See* splint, buccal.

b. surface *See* suface, buccal.

b. tube *See* tube, buccal.

b. vestibule *See* vestibule, buccal.

buccoclusion (bŭk″ō-kloo′zhŭn) An occlusion in which the dental arch or group of teeth is buccal to the normal position.

buccolingual relationship *See* relationship, buccolingual.

buccolingual stress *See* stress, buccolingual.

buccoversion (bŭk″ō-ver′zhŭn) Any deviation from the normal line of occlusion toward the cheeks.

buck knife *See* knife, buck.

buckling The crowding of anterior teeth in the dental arch.

budget plan A method of financing dental accounts in which arrangements are made for the patient to pay a series of small amounts on his account, usually over a period of 12 to 18 months.

buffer Any substance in a fluid that tends to lessen the change in hydrogen ion concentration, which otherwise would be produced by adding acids or alkalis.

bug An error in a computer program.

bulb, speech *See* aid, speech, prosthetic, pharyngeal section.

bulimia Repeated secretive bouts of excessive eating followed by self-induced vomiting, purging, and anorexia, usually accompanied by feelings of guilt, depression, and self-disgust. Oral signs may include decalcification of the lingual aspect of the teeth.

bulla (bŭl′ah) A circumscribed, elevated lesion of the

skin containing fluid and measuring over 5 mm in diameter.

BUN *See* blood urea nitrogen.

Bunnell test *See* test, Paul-Bunnell.

bur A rotary cutting instrument of steel or tungsten carbide; supplied with cutting heads of various shapes.

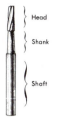

Head

Shank

Shaft

Parts of dental bur

b., carbide A bur made of tungsten carbide; used at high rotational speeds.

b., crosscut A bur with blades slotted perpendicularly to the axis of the bur.

b., end-cutting A bur that has cutting blades only on the end of its head.

b., excavating A bur used to remove dentin and debris from a cavity.

b., finishing A bur with numerous, fine-cutting blades placed close together; used to contour metallic restorations.

b., intramucosal insert base-preparing *See* insert, intramucosal.

b., inverted cone A bur with a head shaped like a truncated cone, the larger diameter being at the terminal (distal) end.

b., plug-finishing *See* bur, finishing.

b., round A bur with a sphere-shaped head.

b., straight fissure A bur without crosscuts that has a cylindrically shaped head.

b., tapered fissure A bur that has a long head with sides that converge from the shank to a blunt end.

burden of proof In a legal proceeding the duty to prove a fact or facts in dispute.

Burkitt's tumor (African lymphoma) A type of lymphosarcoma seen in African children. About half the patients have lesions in the jawbones. Recent evidence suggests a possible viral cause.

Burlew wheel A trade name for an abrasive-impregnated, knife-edged, rubber polishing wheel; used on a mandrel in the dental handpiece to smooth metallic restorations and tooth surfaces.

B. w., high luster Burlew wheel in which jeweler's rouge or iron peroxide is used as the abrasive agent.

B. w., midget (sulci Burlew wheel) A miniature form of Burlew wheel.

B. w., sulci *See* Burlew wheel, midget.

burn A lesion caused by contact of heat, radiation, friction, chemicals, etc., with tissue. Thermal burns are classified as follows: *first degree,* manifested by erythema; *second degree,* manifested by formation of vesicles; *third degree,* manifested by necrosis of the mucosa or dermis; *fourth degree,* manifested by charring into the submucous or subcutaneous layers of the body.

b., aspirin An irregularly shaped, whitish area on the mucosa caused by the topical application of acetylsalicylic acid.

burnisher An instrument shape with rounded edges used to burnish, polish, or work-harden metallic surfaces.

b., ball A burnisher with a working point in the form of a ball.

b., beaver-tail *See* burnisher, straight.

b., fishtail A burnisher that slightly resembles a fish's tail in shape.

b., straight A burnisher that resembles a beaver's tail in shape; the broad, flat blade is smoothly continuous with the shank, meeting it in a slight curve; the edges and the point′ are smoothly rounded.

burnishing A process related to polishing and abrading; the metal is moved by mechanically distorting the normal space lattice. Commonly accomplished during the polishing of soft golds.

burnout Elimination by heat of an invested pattern from a set investment to prepare the mold to receive casting metal.

b., high heat The use of temperature over 1100° F (593.5° C) to effect wax elimination.

b., inlay (wax) Elimination of wax from an invested inlay flask. *See also* wax elimination.

b., job The condition of having no energy left to care, resulting from chronic, unrelieved job-related stress and characterized by physical and emotional exhaustion and sometimes by physical illness.

b., radiographic Excessive penetration of the x-ray beam of an object or part of an object, producing a totally black overexposed area on the radiograph.

b., wax *See* burnout, inlay; wax elimination.

business area The area adjacent to the reception room in which the receptionist conducts the business affairs of the office and directly through which patients must pass both to enter and leave the dental office.

business hours (office hours) Those hours of the day during which professional, public, or other kinds of business are ordinarily conducted.

business office The room reserved for the dentist in which the business of the dental practice is conducted.

butt To place directly against the tissues covering the residual veolar ridge; to bring any two square-ended surfaces into contact, as a butt joint.

button The excess metal remaining from the casting and sprue; located at the end of the sprue, opposite the casting.

    b., implant *See* insert, intramucosal.

buttonhole approach A method of surgical treatment of a periodontal abscess in which, after an incision is made in the fluctuant abscess, an additional attempt is made to curet the area adjoining the root and the fundus of the abscess through the destroyed portion of the alveolar plate or bone.

cachexia (kah-kĕk′sē-ah) Weakness, loss of weight, atrophy, and emaciation caused by severe or chronic disease.

　c., hypophyseal *See* disease, Simmonds′.
　c., hypopituitary *See* disease, Simmonds′.

café-au-lait spots *See* spots, café-au-lait.

cafeteria plan Employee benefits plan in which employees select their medical insurance coverage and other nontaxable fringe benefits from a list of options provided by the employer. Cafeteria plan participants may receive additional, taxable cash compensation if they select less expensive benefits.

caffeine (kăf′ēn) A white, odorless, bitter compound isolated from tea and coffee that is used as a stimulant of the central nervous system. *See also* aspirin; phenacetin; caffeine.

Caffey′s disease *See* hyperostosis, infantile cortical.

calcific metamorphosis (of dental pulp) A frequently observed reaction to trauma; characterized by partial or complete obliteration of the pulp chamber and canal.

calcification (kăl″sĭ-fĭ-kā′shŭn) The process whereby calcium salts are deposited in an organic matrix. The condition may be normal as in bone and tooth formation or pathologic in nature.

　c., dystrophic Pathologic deposition of calcium salts in necrotic or degenerated tissues.
　c., metastatic Pathologic deposition of calcium salts in previously undamaged tissues. This process is due to an excessively high level of blood calcium, such as in hyperparathyroidism.

calcifying epithelial odontogenic tumor (Pindborg tumor) An uncommon tumor arising from odontogenic epithelium characterized by focal areas of calcification. It has the same age, sex, and site distribution as the ameloblastoma.

calcination (kăl′sĭ-nā′shŭn) A process of removing water by heat; used in the manufacture of plaster and stone from gypsum.

calcinosis (kăl-sĭ-nō′sĭs) **1:** Deposition of calcium salts in various tissues due to hypercalcemia and tissue degeneration. **2:** Presence of calcification in or under the skin. The condition may occur in a localized form (calcinosis circumscripta) or in a generalized form (calcinosis universalis).

calcium (kăl′sē-ŭm) A basic element, with an atomic weight of 40.07, found in nearly all organized tissues. Essential for mineralization of bone and teeth. The normal level of calcium in the bood is 9 to 11.5 mg/100 ml. A deficiency of calcium in the diet or in use may lead to rickets or osteoporosis. Overexcretion in hyperparathyroidism leads to osteoporotic manifestations. *See also* factor IV.

　c., blood *See* blood calcium.
　c. fluoride A compound that is used as a flux in the manufacture of some silicate cements.
　c., hydroxide A white powder that is mixed with water or another medium and used as a base material in cavity liners and for pulp capping.
　c., phosphate An odorless, tasteless white powder, the various forms of which are sometimes used as abrasives in dentifrices.
　c., salts Calcium present in salivary fluid as phosphates and carbonates. These salts are believed to form dental calculus on their precipitation from saliva.
　c., sulfate *See* alpha-hemihydrate; beta-hemihydrate; gypsum.
　c., tungstate A chemical substance used in crystal form to coat screens; the screens fluoresce when struck by roentgen rays.

calculus (calcareous deposit) A concretion composed of calcium phosphate, calcium carbonate, magnesium phosphate, and other elements within an organic matrix composed of desquamated epithelium, mucin, microorganisms, and other debris.

　c., dental A salivary deposit of calcium phosphate and carbonate with organic matter on the teeth or a dental prosthesis.
　c., serumal *See* calcium, subgingival.
　c., subgingival Calculus deposited on the tooth structure and found apical to the gingival margin within the confines of the gingival cervix, gingival pocket, or periodontal pocket. Usually darker, more pigmented, and denser than supragingival calculus.
　c., supragingival Calculus deposited on the teeth occlusal or incisal to the gingival crest.

calibrated probe *See* probe, periodontal.

calibration of x-ray unit *See* unit, x-ray calibration.

caliper, axis-orbital A caliper used to record facial measurements that is also capable of transferring them to an adjustable articulator. It consists of (1) a hinge-bow, (2) a bite fork covered with compound, (3) an indicator of the axis-orbital plane, (4) an upright rod to hold the orbital indicator in place, (5) a toggle to freeze the bow's base to the bite fork, and (6) a toggle to attach and allow adjustments for the support of the indicator. Synonym: hinge-bow transfer recorder.

Callahan's method *See* method, chloropercha.

callus (kăl′ŭs) The tissue near and about the broken fragments of a bone that becomes involved in the repair of the fracture through various stages of exudate, fibrosis, and new bone formation.

calorie The amount of heat required to raise one gram of water one degree Celsius at atmospheric pressure, also called gram calorie or small calorie. A great calorie or kilocalorie consists of 1000 small calories. The large calorie is the unit used to denote the heat expenditure of an organism and/or the fuel or energy value of food.

Camper's line *See* line, Camper's.

camphorated parachlorophenol (păr″ah-klō″rō-fē′nol) A mixture of 35% parachlorophenol and 65% camphor; used to treat root canals and periapical infections.

Campylobacter rectus A microorganism associated with progressive periodontal destruction and refractory forms of periodontitis.

canal(s) Portion of the root that contains the pulp tissue and is bounded by dentin.

  c., accessory root A lateral branching of the main root canal, usually occurring in the apical third of the root.

  c., branching *See* canal, collateral pulp.

  c., collateral pulp (branching canal) A dental pulp canal branch that emerges from the root at a place other than the apex.

  c., interdental (nutrient canal) The nutrient channels that pass upward through the body of the mandible. Seen as radiolucent lines on radiographs.

  c., mandibular A channel extending from the mandibular foramen on the medial surface of the ramus of the mandible to the mental foramen. It contains mandibular blood vessels (arteries and veins) and a portion of the mandibular branch of the trigeminal nerve.

  c., nutrient *See* canal, interdental.

  c., pulp The space in the radicular portion of the tooth occupied by the pulp.

  c., root *See* canal, pulp.

    c., root, measurements A technique employing the use of radiographs for determining the length of the root canal.

canaliculus (kăn-ah-lĭk′-ū-lŭs) A minute channel that extends from or to the lacunae of bone and cementum and contains filamentous processes of the cells that oc-cupy the lacunae; interconnects with canaliculi extending from neighboring lacunae.

cancer (kăn′sĕr) A malignant neoplasm. Term is sometimes incorrectly used to include all neoplasms, benign or malignant. *Carcinoma* and *sarcoma* are more limiting terms.

cancrum oris (kăng′krŭm aw′rĭs) *See* stomatitis, gangrenous.

Candida albicans (kăn′dĭ-dah ăl′bĭ-kănz) A budding, yeastlike fungus present in the normal flora of the mucous membrane of the female genital tract and respiratory and gastrointestinal (including the mouth) tracts that is capable of assuming a pathogenic role in the production of oral and systemic moniliasis (thrush, monilial infection, etc.).

candidiasis (kăn″dĭ-dī′ah-sĭs) Infection by *Candida albicans*. *See also* moniliasis; thrush.

  c., pseudomembranous Forms loosely adherent (wipeable), yellowish-white plaques on the oral mucosal surface.

  c., erythematous (atrophic) Forms smooth red patches on the hard or soft palate, the buccal mucosa, or the dorsal surface of the tongue.

  c., hyperplastic Forms white plaques that cannot be removed by wiping or scraping.

  c., angular cheilitis Forms fissures or ulcers radiating from the angles of the mouth often accompanied by white plaques. Usually observed in elderly patients, although when observed in a young person, it may be an indicator of HIV infection. Candidiasis of the esophagus, trachea, bronchi, or lungs are indicator diseases associated with group IV HIV infection. *See also* acquired immunodeficiency syndrome; AIDS; ARC.

canine (kā′nīn) (cuspid) One of the four pointed teeth in humans, situated one on each side of each jaw, distal to the lateral incisor; forms the keystone of the arch. The term *canine* is increasingly preferred to cuspid.

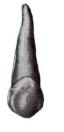 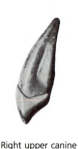 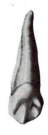

Labial surface | Right upper canine / Mesial surface | Lingual surface

c. fossa *See* fossa, canine.

c. guidance A concept of occlusal function in which

the canine teeth are assigned a major control role in the excursive movements of the mandible.

canker (kăng′ker) *See* herpes labialis.

c. sore *See* sore, canker.

cannula (kăn′ū-lah) A tube for insertion into the body; its caliber is usually occupied by a trocar during the act of insertion.

cantilever bridge *See* denture, partial, fixed, cantilever.

cantilever partial denture *See* denture, partial, fixed, cantilever.

cantle A fragment, piece, portion.

capacity Legal qualification, competency, power, or fitness.

c., functional residual (normal capacity) The volume of gas in the lungs at resting expiratory level.

c., iron-binding A measure of the binding capacity of iron in the serum; helps to differentiate the causes of hypoferremia. This capacity tends to increase in iron deficiency and diminishes in chronic diseases and during infection.

c., normal *See* capacity, functional residual.

c., total lung (TLC) The volume of air in the lungs at the end of maximal inspiration.

c., vital (VC) The maximal volume of air that can be expired after maximal inspiration.

capillarity (kăp″ĭ-lăr′ĭ-tē) The phenomenon by which a film of fluid is drawn and held between two closely approximating surfaces.

capillary(ies) (kăp′ĭ-lăr″ē) The terminal vessels uniting the arterial with the venous systems of the body. Capillaries are organized into extensive branching reticular beds to provide a maximum surface for exchange of fluids, electrolytes, and metabolites between tissues and the vascular system. The capillary bed has the largest cross-sectional area of the entire vascular system.

c., attraction The quality or state that, because of surface tension, causes elevation or depression of the surface of a liquid that is in contact with a solid. Considered to be one of the factors in retention of complete dentures.

capital budgeting The process of planning expenditures on assets whose returns are expected to extend beyond 1 year.

capitation 1: The practice of dentistry financed by a set fee per person per given period of time. A form of contracted dental care, usually by a corporation, institution, or other group. **2:** System by which the contracting dentist, assuming the financial risk, is compensated at a fixed per-capita rate, usually on specific, predetermined dental services as appropriate and necessary to eligible subscribers. **3:** A capitation dental benefits program is one in which a dentist or dentists contract with the program's sponsor or administrator to provide all or most of the dental services covered

under the program to subscribers in return for payment on a per-capita basis.

c., fee A predetermined per-person charge made by the carrier for benefits available under an insurance plan.

capitulum (kah-pĭt′ū-lŭm) A little head. Term used by some European writers instead of head or condyle.

c. mandibulae *See* process, condyloid.

capping, pulp The covering of an exposed dental pulp with a material that protects it from external influences.

c., direct pulp Application to the exposed pulp of a drug or material for the purpose of stimulating repair of the injured pulpal tissue.

c., indirect pulp A chemical (usually calcium hydroxide) placed over a layer of carious dentin remaining over the potentially exposed pulp to protect the pulp from external irritants.

capsule, joint A fibrous sac or ligament that encloses a joint and limits its motion. It is lined with synovial membrane.

c., temporomandibular joint *See* articulation, temporomandibular, capsule.

carat A standard of fineness of gold, 24 carats being taken as expressing absolute purity.

carbamazepine An anticonvulsant and specific analgesic for trigeminal neuralgia sometimes used in the treatment of herpes zoster under a physician's supervision.

carbenicillin A semisynthetic penicillin that is acid resistant and rapidly absorbed from the small intestine and thus suitable for oral administration.

carbide bur *See* bur, carbide.

carbohemia (kar″bō-hē′mē-ah) Imperfect oxygenation of the blood.

carbohemoglobin (kar″bō-hē″mō-glō′bĭn) Hemoglobin compounded with CO_2.

carbohydrates A group of organic compounds with the class name saccharides, which are the aldehydic or ketonic derivative of polyhydric alcohols. Carbohydrates that include sugar, starch, cellulose, and gum are generally synthesized by green plants. Carbohydrates constitute the main energy source in the diet and are classified as mono-, di-, tri-, and poly-saccharides.

carbohydrate tolerance *See* tolerance, carbohydrate.

carbon-coated A vitreous carbon coating to either an endosteal or blade implant to improve tissue compatability.

carbon markings The markings made on the teeth when, with articulating paper interposed, the mandibular teeth are brought in contact with the maxillary teeth.

carbonate hydroxyapatite (kr′ bon-āt hī-drok″sē-ăp′ ah-tīt) Term indicating the composition and crystal structure of hard tissues.

carcinoma (kar-sĭ-nō′mah)

c., adenoid cystic (cylindroma, adenocystic carci-

noma, adenocystic basal cell carcinoma, basaloid mixed tumor) A pseudoadenomatous basal cell carcinoma originating from salivary glands, the cells of which resemble basal cells and form duct-like or cystlike structures. It grows slowly but is malignant.

c., basal cell (basal cell epithelioma, rodent ulcer, turban tumor) An epithelial neoplasm with a basic structure resembling the basal cells of the epidermis. It develops from basal cells of the epidermis or from the outer cells of hair follicles or sebaceous glands, particularly the middle third of the face. It rarely, if ever, metastasizes but is locally invasive. It does not arise from oral mucosa.

c., basosquamous Carcinoma that histologically exhibits both basal and squamous elements. It may occasionally be seen in the oral cavity; considered to have a greater tendency to metastasize than basal cell carcinoma.

c., epidermoid (squamous cell carcinoma) A malignant epithelial neoplasm with cells resembling those of the epidermis. The term *squamous cell carcinoma* is used for intraoral lesions of this nature.

c., exophytic A malignant epithelial neoplasm with marked outward growth like a wart or papilloma.

c., in situ A dysplastic epithelial disease involving the skin and mucous membrane and considered to be precancerous. Dyskeratosis is evident, but there is no invasion.

c., intraepithelial *See* carcinoma, in situ.

c., mucoepidermoid A malignant epithelial tumor of the salivary gland; characterized by acini with mucus-producing cells.

c., squamous cell *See* carcinoma, epidermoid.

c., transitional cell A malignant tumor arising from a transitional type of stratified epithelium.

cardiac Relating to the heart.

c. arrest A stopping of heart action; a complete cessation of heart function.

c. massage *See* massage, cardiac.

c. pacemaker *See* pacemaker.

c. output The volume of blood put out by the heart per minute; the product of the stroke volume and the heart rate per minute.

cardioinhibitory (kar″dē-ō-ĭn-hĭb′ĭ-tor-ē) Restraining or inhibiting the movements of the heart.

cardiokinetic (kar″dē-ō-kĭ-nĕt′ĭk) Exciting the heart; a remedy that excites the heart.

cardiopulmonary Pertaining to the heart and lungs.

cardiovascular disease Any one of a number of abnormal conditions that involve dysfunction of the heart and blood vessels, including but not limited to systemic hypertension; atherosclerosis, including coronary heart disease; and rheumatic heart disease.

cardiovascular system The network of structures including the heart and blood vessels that convey the blood throughout the body.

care As a legal term, the opposite of negligence.

c., reasonable Such care as an ordinarily prudent person would exercise under the conditions existing at the time that person is called on to act.

caries (kā′rē-ēz) In general medicine, the decay or death of a bone.

c., dental An infectious disease with progressive destruction of tooth substance, beginning on the external surface by demineralization of enamel or exposed cementum.

c., arrested dental State existing when the progress of the decay process has halted.

c., healed dental *See* caries, dental, arrested.

c., incipient dental A decayed part of a tooth where the lesion is just coming into existence.

c., proximal dental Decay occurring in the mesial or distal surface of a tooth.

c., rampant dental A suddenly appearing, widespread, rapidly progressing type of caries.

c., recurrent dental Extension of the carious process beyond the margin of a restoration.

c., residual dental (residual carious dentin) Decayed material left in a prepared cavity and over which a restoration is placed.

c., senile dental (senile decay) Caries noted particularly in old age when supporting tissues have receded; occurs in cementum, usually on proximal surfaces of the teeth.

cariogenicity The ability of a substance to induce or potentiate the formation of dental caries.

cariostatic agents Agents that inhibit or arrest dental caries formation. *See* flourides, sealants.

carious (ka′rē-ŭs) Pertaining to caries or decay.

c., dentin *See* wax, carious.

carnauba wax *See* wax, carnauba.

Carnoy's solution *See* solution, Carnoy's.

carotene (kăr′ō-tēn) An orange pigment found in carrots, leafy vegetables, and other foods that may be converted to vitamin A in the body.

carotenemia (kăr″ō-tĕ-nē′mē-ah) Excess carotene in the blood, producing a pigmentation of the skin and mucous membranes that resembles jaundice.

carotid (ka-rot′ĭd) Either one of the two main right and left arteries of the neck.

carrier 1: A person harboring a specific infectious agent without clinical evidence of disease and who serves as a potential source or reservoir of infection for others. May be a healthy carrier or a convalescent carrier. **2:** The party of the dental plan contract who agrees to pay claims or provide service. Synonyms: insurer, underwriter, or administrative agent. *See also* third party.

c., amalgam An instrument used to carry plastic amal-

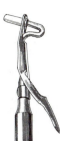

Amalgam carrier

gam to the prepared cavity or mold into which it is to be inserted.

c., foil *See* foil passer.

cartilage A derivative of connective tissue arising from the mesenchyme. Typical haline cartilage is a flexible, rather elastic material with a semitransparent, glasslike appearance. Its ground substance, or matrix, is a complex protein (chondromucoid) through which there is distributed a large network of connective tissue fibers. There are cartilage cells distributed throughout the matrix that are rounded and do not have the branching characteristics of bone cells. The cells are isolated in the matrix they have secreted and normally have no blood vessels. Therefore nutrients and metabolites are exchanged with the circulation by passage through the ground substance (matrix).

c., articular A thin layer of hyaline cartilage located on the joint surfaces of some bones. Not usually found on articular surfaces of temporomandibular joints, which are covered with an avascular fibrous tissue.

c., cricoid The lowest cartilage of the larynx.

caruncle, submaxillary The orifice of the sublingual (Wharton's) duct that opens into the mouth on a small papilla on either side of the lingual frenum.

carver (carving instrument) An instrument used to shape a plastic material, such as wax or amalgam.

c., amalgam An instrument used to shape plastic amalgam.

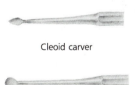

Cleoid carver

Discoid carver

carving Shaping and forming with instruments.

case Term often incorrectly used instead of the appropri-

ate noun (e.g., patient, flask, denture, or casting). "Case" is not synonymous with "patient" because the latter is the human being affected with the disease.

c., charting Recording of a patient's status of health or disease.

c., dismissal The technique of illustrating to the patient what has been accomplished, usually done during the last appointment of a series.

c., history *See* history, case.

c., management The monitoring and coordination of treatment rendered to patients with specific diagnoses or requiring high cost or extensive services.

c., presentation Explanation of dental needs to the patient.

c. summary Enumeration of all the services to be performed for an estimated amount of money.

cash budget A schedule showing cash flows (receipts, disbursements, net cash) for a firm over a specified period.

cash cycle The length of time between the purchase of raw materials and the collection of accounts receivable generated in the sale of the final product.

cash flow Reported net income of a corporation plus amounts charged off for depreciation, depletion, amortization, and extraordinary charges to reserves, which are bookkeeping deductions and not paid out in actual dollars and cents. A yardstick used in recent years to offer a better indication of the ability of a company to pay dividends and finance expansion from self-generated cash than the conventional reported net income figure.

cassette (kah-sĕt′) A lighttight container in which x-ray films are placed for exposure to x radiation; usually backed with lead to eliminate the effect of backscattered radiation.

c., cardboard (cardboard filmholder) A cardboard envelope of simple construction suitable for use in making radiographs on "direct exposure" or "no-screen" types of x-ray films.

c., screen-type A cassette usually made of metal, with the exposure side of low−atomic number material, such as Bakelite, aluminum, or magnesium, and containing intensifying screens between which a "screen type" of film or films may be placed for exposure to x radiation.

cast 1: *n.* An object formed by pouring plastic or liquid material into a mold where it hardens. **2:** *v.* To throw metal into an impression to form the casting.

c., bar splint *See* splint, cast bar.

c., dental A positive likeness of a part or parts of the oral cavity reproduced in a durable hard material.

c., diagnostic A positive likeness of dental structures for the purpose of study and treatment planning.

c., gnathostatic A cast of the teeth trimmed so that the occlusal plane is in its normal position in the mouth when the cast is set on a plane surface. Such casts are used in the gnathostatic technique of orthodontic diagnosis.

c., implant A positive reproduction of the exposed bony surfaces made in a surgical bone impression and on which an implant frame is designed and fabricated.

   c., diagnostic implant A cast made from a conventional mucosal impression on which the wax trial denture and surgical impression trays are made or selected.

c., investment *See* cast, refractory.

c., keying of The process of forming the base (or capital) of a cast so that it can be remounted accurately. Also referred to as the split-cast method of returning a cast to an articulator.

c., master An accurate replica of the prepared tooth surfaces, residual ridge areas, or other parts of the dental arch reproduced from an impression from which a prosthesis is to be fabricated.

c., corrected master A dental cast that has been modified by the correction of the edentulous ridge areas as registered in a supplemental, correctable impression.

c., preextraction A cast made before the extraction of teeth. *See also* cast, diagnostic.

c., preoperative *See* cast, diagnostic.

c., record A positive replica of the dentition and adjoining structures, used as a reference for conditions existing at a given time.

c., refractory A cast made of materials that will withstand high temperatures without disintegrating and that, when used in partial denture casting techniques, expands to compensate for metal shrinkage.

c., study *See* cast, diagnostic.

c., working An accurate reproduction of a master cast; used in preliminary fitting of a casting to avoid injury to the master cast.

casting 1: *n.* A metallic object formed in a mold. 2: *v.* Forming a casting in a mold.

   c., vacuum The casting of a metal in the presence of a vacuum. *See also* casting machine, vacuum.

casting flask *See* flask, refractory.

casting machine A mechanical device used for throwing or forcing a molten metal into a refractory mold.

   c.m., air pressure A casting machine that forces metal into the mold by compressed air.

   c.m., centrifugal A casting machine that forces the metal into the mold by centrifugal force.

   c.m., vacuum A casting machine in which the metal is cast by evacuation of gases from the mold. Atmospheric pressure actually forces metal into mold.

casting model *See* cast, refractory.

casting ring *See* flask, refractory.

casting temperature *See* temperature, casting.

casting wax *See* wax, casting.

Castle's intrinsic factor *See* factor, Castle's intrinsic.

catabolism (kah-tăb′ō-lĭzm) The destructive process (opposite of the anabolic-metabolic processes) by which complex substances are converted into more simple compounds. A proper relation between anabolism and catabolism is essential for the maintenance of bodily homeostasis and dynamic equilibrium.

   c. of energy Dissipation of energy in living tissues as work or heat (one phase of metabolism, the other being anabolism).

   c. of substance Destructive metabolism; the conversion of living tissues into a lower state of organization and ultimately into waste products.

catalase reaction (kăt′ah-lās) The response of bubbling in the presence of hydrogen peroxide given by blood exudates or transudates.

catalysis (kah-tăl′ĭ-sĭs) The increase in rate of a chemical reaction, induced by a substance called a *catalyst*, which takes no part in the reaction and remains unchanged.

catalyst (kăt′ah-lĭst) A substance that induces an increased rate of a chemical reaction without entering into the reaction or being changed by the reaction.

catamenia (kăt″ah-mē′nē-ah) Menstruation. Frequently used to designate age at onset of menses.

catatonia (kăt″ah-tō′nē-ah) A form of schizophrenia characterized by alternating stupor and excitement. A patient's arms often retain any position in which they are placed.

catgut Sheep's intestine prepared as a suture and used for ligating vessels and closing soft tissue wounds.

cathode A negative electrode from which electrons are emitted and to which positive ions will be attracted. In x-ray tubes, the cathode usually consists of a helical tungsten filament, behind which a molybdenum reflector cup is located to focus the electron emission toward the target of the anode.

cathode-ray tube A vacuum tube in which a beam of electrons is focused to a small point on a luminescent screen and can be varied in position to form a pattern.

cation (kăt′ī-ahn) A positively charged ion.

cationic detergent *See* detergent, cationic.

cat-scratch disease *See* fever, cat-scratch.

casualty insurance Insurance against loss due to accidents, usually applied to property but may apply to bodily injury or death due to accident.

causalgia (kaw-zăl′jē-ah) A postextraction localized pain phenomenon usually characterized by a continuous burning senation.

cause of action Generally, a ground or reason for a legal action; a wrong subject to legal redress.

   c., proximate *See* proximate cause.

caustic, *adj.* Destructive of living tissue by chemical burning action.

cavity A carious lesion or hole in a tooth.

c., access *See* access cavity.

c., axial surface A cavity occurring in a tooth surface where the general plane is parallel to the long axis of the tooth.

c. classification Carious lesions are classified according to the surfaces of a tooth on which they occur (labial, buccal, occlusal, etc.), type of surface (pit and fissure or smooth surface), and numerical grouping (G.V. Black's classification).

c., artificial classification (G.V. Black) Classification of cavities.

Class 1 Cavities beginning in structural defects of the teeth, as in pits and fissures.

Class 2 Cavities in proximal surfaces of premolars and molars.

Class 3 Cavities in proximal surfaces of canines and incisors that do not involve removal and restoration of the incisal angle.

Class 4 Cavities in proximal surfaces of canines and incisors that require removal and restoration of the incisal angle.

Class 5 Cavities in the gingival third (not pit cavities) of the labial, buccal, or lingual surfaces of the teeth.

Class 6 (not included in Black's classification) Cavities on incisal edges and cusp tips of the teeth.

c., complex A cavity that involves more than one surface of a tooth.

c. floor The base-enclosing side of a prepared cavity. *See also* cavity, prepared.

c., gingival (gingival third cavity) A cavity occurring in the gingival third of the clinical crown of the tooth (G.V. Black's Class 5)

c. lining Material applied to the prepared cavity before the restoration is inserted to seal the dentinal tubules for protection of the pulp.

c. medication Drug used to clean or treat a cavity before inserting a dressing, base, or restoration.

c., nasal (nasal fossa) Two irregular spaces that are situated on either side of the midline of the face, extend from the cranial base to the roof of the mouth, and are separated from each other by a thin vertical septum. In radiographs the nasal cavity appears over the roots of the upper incisors as a large, structureless, radiolucent area.

c., pit and fissure A cavity that begins in minute faults in the enamel caused by imperfect closure of the enamel.

c. preparation The orderly operating procedure required to remove diseased tissue and to establish in a tooth the biomechanically acceptable form necessary to receive and retain a restoration.

c., prepared The form developed in a tooth to receive and retain a restoration.

c., prepared, floor of The flat bottom or enclosing base wall of a prepared cavity; on an axial plane it is called the *axial wall*, and on the horizontal plane it is called the *pulpal wall*.

c., prepared, impression A negative likeness of a tapered type of prepared cavity.

c., proximal A cavity occurring on the mesial or distal surface of a tooth.

c., pulp The space in a tooth bounded by the dentin; contains the dental pulp. The part of the pulp cavity within the coronal portion of the tooth is the pulp chamber, and the part found within the root is the pulp canal, or root canal.

c., simple A cavity that involves only one surface of a tooth.

c., smooth surface A cavity formed by decay beginning in surfaces of teeth that are without pits, fissures, or enamel faults.

c. toilet G.V. Black's final step in cavity preparation. Consists of freeing all surfaces and angles of debris.

c. varnish *See* varnish, cavity.

c. wall *See* wall, cavity.

CBC Abbreviation for complete blood count in which all the blood cells are counted per cubic millimeter, including a differential counting of the white blood cells (leukocytes).

CDC Abbreviation for the Centers for Disease Control.

cavosurface angle *See* angle, cavosurface.

cavosurface bevel *See* bevel, cavosurface.

CD4 (T4) lymphocyte An immunologically important white cell that is responsible for cell-mediated immunity. It is the cell invaded by the retrovirus HIV in which the virus replicates itself.

cell(s) The basic unit of vital tissue. One of a large variety of microscopic protoplasmic masses that make up organized tissues. Each cell has a cell membrane, protoplasm, a nucleus, and a variety of inclusion bodies. Each type of cell is a living unit, with its own metabolic requirements, functions, permeability, ability to differentiate into other cells, reproducibility, life expectancy, etc.

c., connective tissue The fibroblast, which for purposes of clarity is characterized by such terms as *perivascular connective tissue cell* or *young connective tissue cell.*

c., defense A cell, mobilized within inflamed, irritated, or otherwise diseased tissue, that acts as a protective element to neutralize or wall off the foreign irritant. Defense cells include plasma cells, polymorphonuclear leukocytes, and the cells of the reticuloendothelial system.

c., differentiation The development of the cells into the various basic cell units of tissue: the epithelial cell and the nerve cell, which arise from the ectodermal tissue layer of the embryo; and the blood, muscle, bone, cartilage, and other connective tissue cells, which arise from the mesodermal tissue of the embryo. The mature tissue cell has many intermediary, transitional forms that are sequential in their development from the primitive, less differentiated anlage cell forms. These intermediary forms are evident clinically in disease in the blood dyscrasias, tumors, and inflammation, and in health in the normal processes of growth, development, healing, and repair.

c., endosteal A reticular cell that is modified and identified by its location; the endosteum is a condensation of the stroma of the bone marrow.

c., germ A cell of an organism whose function it is to reproduce an entity similar to the organism from which the germ cell originated. Germ cells are characteristically haploid.

c., giant A large cell frequently having several nuclei.

c., homeostasis *See* homeostasis, cell.

c., Langerhans' Star-shaped cells of unknown function that appear to be permanent residents of the epithelium.

c., mesenchymal An embryonic connective tissue cell with an outstanding capacity for proliferation. Capable of further differentiation into reticular cells or osteoblasts. When persisting in the adult organism, the cells are usually arranged in loose connective tissue along the small blood vessels or in reticular fibers. They are identified by their location and their capacity to differentiate into other cell types, such as smooth muscle cells in the formation of new arteries, phagocytes in inflammatory processes, and bone cells in the formation of new bone tissue.

c., plasma A cell of disputed origin (lymphatic vs. undifferentiated mesenchymal cell) that is seen in chronic inflammation and certain disease states and tumors but not normally in the circulating blood. The cell is larger than a lymphocyte and has an eccentric nucleus with basophilic nuclear chromatin peripherally located like figures on a clock face. Currently, the cells are believed to produce and carry antibodies.

c., reticular A cell of reticular connective tissue, such as in the stroma of the bone marrow, where it retains both osteogenic and hematopoietic potencies; it is identified by its location, morphology, potency, and direct origin from mesenchymal cells.

c., Sternberg-Reed A giant tumor cell believed to be derived from reticular cells; it contains from one to many nuclei and is seen in Hodgkin's disease.

c., Tzank A degenerated epithelial cell caused by acantholysis and found especially in pemphigus.

cellulitis (sĕl-ū-lī'tĭs) A diffuse inflammatory process that spreads along fascial planes and through tissue spaces without gross suppuration.

celluloid strip *See* strip, plastic.

cellulose, oxidized (sĕl'ū-lōs) Cellulose, in the form of cotton, gauze, or paper, that has been more or less completely oxidized.

cement A material that produces a mechanical interlocking effect on hardening.

c., dental Any one of the materials used in dentistry as luting agents, bases, and temporary restorations. *See also* cement, dental, acrylic resin; cement, dental, zinc oxide–eugenol; cement, silicate; cement, zinc phosphate.

c., acrylic resin dental A dental cement, dispensed as a powder and a liquid, that is mixed as any other cement. The powder contains polymethyl methacrylate, a filler, plasticizer, and polymerization initiator. The liquid monomer is methyl methacrylate with an inhibitor and an activator.

c., copper dental A zinc phosphate cement to the powder of which has been added a copper oxide.

c., dental base An insulating layer of cement placed in the deeper portion of a prepared cavity to insulate the pulp.

c., Kryptex dental *See* cement, silicophosphate.

c., silicious dental *See* cement, silicate.

c., zinc oxide-eugenol dental Least irritating of the cements. The powder is essentially zinc oxide with strengtheners and accelerators. The liquid is basically eugenol.

c. dressing Postoperative dressing applied after periodontal surgery.

c. dressing, dental, Kirkland *See* dressing, Kirkland cement.

c. line *See* line, cement.

c., polycarboxylate Dental cement used for dementation of cast restorations and orthodontic appliances and as bases. Prepared by mixing a zinc oxide powder with a liquid of polycarboxylic acid.

c., sealer A compound used in filling a root canal; it is inserted in a plastic condition, solidifies after placement, and fills any irregularities in the surface of the canal.

c., silicate A relatively hard, translucent, restorative material used primarily in anterior teeth. Prepared by mixing a liquid and a powder. The powder is an acid-soluble glass prepared by the fusion of CaO, SiO, Al_2O_3, and other ingredients with a fluoride flux. The liquid is a buffered phosphoric acid solution.

c., silicophosphate (Kryptex cement) A combination zinc phosphate and silicate cement. Less translucent, less irritating, and less soluble than silicate and stronger than zinc phosphate cement.

c., zinc phosphate A material used for cementation of inlays, crowns, bridges, and orthodontic appliances; occasionally used as a temporary restoration. Prepared by mixing a powder and a liquid. The powders are composed primarily of zinc oxide and magnesium oxides. The principal constituents of the liquid are phosphoric acid, water, and buffer agents.

cemental line *See* line, cemental.

cemental repair *See* repair, cemental.

cemental spicule (spĭk´ūl) *See* spicule, cemental.

cemental spike *See* spicule, cemental.

cemental tear A small portion of cementum forcibly separated, either partially or completely, from the underlying dentin of the root as a result of occlusal force; seen on the tension side in occlusal traumatism.

cementation (sē-mĕn-tā´shŭn) Attachment of an appliance or a restoration to natural teeth or attachment of parts by means of a cement.

cementicle (sē-mĕn´tĭ-cul) A calcified body sometimes found in the periodontal ligament of older individuals. It is presumed that degenerated epithelial cells form the nidus for this calcification.

cementifying fibroma *See* fibroma, cementifying.

cementing line *See* line, cemental.

cementoblast (sē-mĕn´tō-blăst) The cell that forms the organic matrix of cementum. Derived from the inner aspect of the cental sac during the initial formation of cementum or from the mesenchymal cell of the periodontal membrane after completion of primary cementogenesis. The cementoblast, trapped within cellular cementum, becomes a cementocyte.

cementoclasia (sē-mĕn˝tō-klā´zē-ah) Destruction of cementum by cementoclasts.

cementocyte (sē-mĕn´tō-sīt) The cell found within lacunae of cellular cementum, which possesses protoplasmic processes that course through the canaliculi of the cementum; derived from cementoblasts trapped within newly formed cementum.

cementoenamel junction *See* junction, cementoenamel.

cementoid The most recent layer covering the surface of cementum that is uncalcified.

cementoma (sē-mĕn-tō´mah) **(traumatic osteoclasia)** An endontogenic tumor associated with the apices of teeth. It may be present as a mass of fibrous connective tissue, as fibrous connective tissue with spicules of cementum, or as a calcified mass resembling cementum and having few cellular elements.

c., first-state *See* fibroma, periapical.

cementopathia (sē˝mĕn-tō-păth´ē-ah) The concept wherein necrotic, diseased cementum and lack of productivity of cementum are implicated in the causation of periodontitis and periodontosis.

cementoproximal Pertaining to the proximal surface apical to the cementoenamel junction of the clinical crown of a tooth.

cementum (sē-mĕn´tŭm) A specialized, calcified connective tissue that covers the anatomic root of a tooth, giving attachment to the periodontal ligament.

c., acellular Cementum that contains no cementocytes.

c., cellular Portion of the calcified substance covering the root surfaces of the teeth. It is bonelike in nature and contains cementocytes embedded within lacunae, with protoplasmic processes of the cementocytes coursing through canaliculi that anastomose with canaliculi of adjacent lacunae. The lacunae are dispersed through a calcified matrix arranged in lamellar form. Cellular cementum is localized primarily at the apical portion of the root but may deposit over the acellular cementum or serve to repair areas of cemental resorption.

c., collagen fibrils of Fibrils that penetrate the cementum surface and are continuous with the periodontal fibers necessary for tooth support.

c., lamellar Cementum in which layers of appositional cementum are arranged in a sheaflike pattern, the layers of cementum being more or less parallel to the cemental surface and demarcated by incremental lines that represent periods of inactivity of cementum formation.

c., necrotic Nonvital cementum that is situated coronal to the bottom of the periodontal pocket.

c., secondary Term used to imply all subsequent layers of cementum formed after the primary layer. It may be cellular or acellular.

center, rotation A point or line around which all other points in a body move.

central bearing Application of forces between the maxillae and mandible at a single point that is located as near as possible to the center of the supporting areas of the upper and lower jaws. The purpose is to distribute closing forces of the jaws evenly throughout the areas of the supporting structures during the registration and recording of maxillomandibular (jaw) relations and during the correction of occlusal errors.

c.-b. device A device that provides a central point of bearing or support between upper and lower occlusion rims. It consists of a contracting point that is attached to one occlusion rim and a plate on the other rim that provides the surface on which the bearing point rests or moves.

c.-b. point *See* point, central-bearing.

central occlusion *See* occlusion, centric.

central processing unit (CPU) The central processor of the computer system contains the internal memory unit (memory), arithmetic logic unit (ALU), and input/output control unit (I/O control).

central tendency The tendency of a group of scores to cluster around a central representative score. The statistics most frequently used for measures of central tendency are the mean, median, and mode.

centric (sĕn´trĭk) (objectionable as a noun) An adjective that should be used in conjunction with a noun to describe jaw and tooth relationships. *See* position, centric; relation, centric; occlusion, centric; occlusion, centric relation.

c. checkbite *See* record, occluding, centric relation.

c. occlusion *See* occlusion, centric.

c. position *See* position, centric.

c. relation *See* relation, centric.

centrifugal force (sĕn-trĭf′-ū-găl) *See* force, centrifugal.

cephalic index An anthropometric value based on the ratio between the width and length of the head.

$$\text{cephalic index} = \frac{\text{maximum head (or skull) width} \times 100}{\text{maximum head (or skull) length}}$$

cephalogram (sĕf′ah-lō-grăm) A cephalometric radiograph. On tracings of these films, anatomic points, planes, and angles are drawn that assist in the evaluation of the patient's facial growth and development.

cephalometer (sĕf′ah-lom′ĕ-ter) *See* cephalostat.

c., radiographic *See* cephalostat.

cephalometric analysis *See* analysis, cephalometric.

cephalometric landmark *See* landmark, cephalometric.

cephalometric radiograph A radiograph of the head made with precise reproducible relationships between x-ray source, subject, and film. The generally accepted distances between x-ray source and the center of the subject are 5 feet (152.4 cm) or 150 cm. The distance between subject and film is usually 12 cm but may be standardized at a different value or varied with patient size and recorded for each exposure. The two standard orientations are lateral (profile) and posteroanterior (PA).

cephalometric skeletal analysis Assessment of the facial type of skeleton; the relationship of the parts to each other, to the skull, and to an estimated "normal."

cephalometric tracing A tracing of selected structures from a cephalometric radiograph made on translucent drafting paper or film for purposes of measurement and evaluation.

cephalometrics (sĕf-ah-lō-mĕt′rĭks) Scientific study of the measurements of the head.

cephalometry (sĕf-ah-lom′ĕ-trē) Measurement of the bony structure of the head using reproducible lateral and anteroposterior radiograms.

cephalophore (sĕf′ah-lō-for) A cephalostat designed to take in-sequence–oriented facial photographs and gnathostatic models.

cephalosporins Semisynthetic derivatives of an antibiotic originally derived from the microorganism *Cephalosporium acremonium*. Cephalosporins are similar in structure to penicillins.

cephalostat (sĕf′ah-lō-stăt) A head-positioning device that assures reproducibility of the relations between an x-ray beam, a patient's head, and an x-ray film in radiography.

ceramics The art of making dental restorations, or parts of restorations, from fused porcelain.

c., orthoclase *See* feldspar.

cerebellum (sĕr-ĕ-bĕl′ŭm) A major division of the brain behind the cerebrum and above the pons and fourth ventricle, consisting of a median lobe, two lateral lobes, and major connections, through pairs of peduncles, to the cerebrum, pons, and medulla oblongata. The cerebellum is intimately connected with the auditory vestibular apparatus and the proprioceptive system of the body and hence is involved in maintenance of body equilibrium, orientation in space, and muscular coordination and tonus.

cerebral palsy *See* palsy, cerebral.

cerebrum (sĕr′ĕ-brŭm) The largest portion of the brain. Operating at the highest functional level and occupying the upper part of the cranium, the cerebrum consists of two hemispheres united at the bottom by commissures of large bundles of nerve fibers. As with all parts of the nervous system, each part of the cerebrum has highly specific functions (e.g., a specific outer cortical area controls voluntary chewing, whereas certain inner subcortical areas are involved in involuntary jaw posture).

certificate of eligibility An official identification card or similar document issued to program beneficiaries as evidence of entitlement to services.

certificate of insurance A statement issued to a group member describing in general terms the policy provisions for eligibility, deductibles, coinsurance, allowances, and maximums. Used in lieu of issuing copies of the group or master contract to each individual employee member of an insured group.

certificate holder 1: The person, usually the employee, who represents the family unit covered by the dental benefits program; other family members are referred to as "dependents." **2:** Generally refers to a subscriber of a traditional indemnity program. **3:** In reference to the program for dependents of active-duty military personnel, the certificate holder is called the *sponsor*. *See also* Subscriber. Synonyms: subscriber, enrollee.

certified dental assistant A person who has completed the Certification Board of the American Dental Assistant Association.

cervical (ser′vĭ-kal) Relating to the neck, or cervical line, of a tooth.

c. appliance *See* appliance, cervical.

c. convergence *See* convergence, cervical.

c. line *See* junction, cementoenamel.

c. fibers *See* nerve, fibers.

chalazion forceps (kah-lā′zē-ahn) *See* forceps, chalazion.

chamber An enclosed area.

c., ionization An instrument for measuring the quantity of ionizing radiation, in terms of the charge of electricity associated with ions produced within a defined volume of air.

c., air-equivalent ionization A chamber in which the materials of the wall and electrodes produce ionization essentially similar to that in a free-air ionization chamber.

c., air-wall ionization An ionization chamber with walls of material of low atomic number, having the same effective atomic number as atmospheric air.

c., extrapolation ionization An ionization chamber with electrodes whose spacing can be adjusted and accurately determined to permit extrapolation of its reading to zero chamber volume.

c., free-air ionization An ionization chamber in which a delimited beam of radiation passes between the electrodes without striking them or other internal parts of the equipment. The electric field is maintained perpendicular to the electrodes in the collecting region; as a result, the ionized volume can be accurately determined from the dimensions of the collecting electrode and limiting diaphragm. This is the basic standard instrument for dosimetry within the range of 5 to 400 kV.

c., monitor ionization An ionization chamber used for checking the constancy of performance of the roentgen-ray apparatus.

c., pocket ionization A small, pocket-sized ionization chamber used for monitoring radiation exposure of personnel. Before use it is given a charge, and the amount of discharge is a measure of the quantity of radiation received.

c., standard ionization *See* chamber, ionization, free-air.

c., thimble ionization A small cylindrical or spherical chamber, usually with walls of organic material.

c., thin-wall ionization An ionization chamber having walls so thin that nearly all secondary corpuscular rays reaching them from external materials can penetrate them easily.

c., tissue-equivalent ionization A chamber in which the walls, electrodes, and gas are selected to produce ionization essentially equivalent to the characteristics of the tissue under consideration.

c., pulp (pulp cavity) The space occupied by the pulp.

c., relief A recess in the impression surface of a denture, created to reduce or eliminate pressure from the corresponding area of the mouth.

c., suction *See* chamber, relief.

chamfer (shăm′fer) In extracoronal cavity preparations, a marginal finish that produces a curve from an axial wall to the cavosurface.

chancre (shăng′ker) (autochthonous ulcer) The primary lesion of syphilis, located at the site of entrance of the spirochete into the body, that occurs about 3 weeks after contact; begins as a papule and develops into a clean-based shallow ulcer. Secondary infection may produce suppuration. Has the appearance of a button-like mass because of the contiguous induration and rolled border. Weeping characteristics are also present.

c. of lip The primary lesion of syphilis that often appears as an ulcerated or crusted, indurated lesion with a brownish or copper-colored weeping base when located on the lip. The lesion is teeming with *Treponema pallidum*. **c., soft** *See* chancroid.

chancroid (shăng′kroid) **(soft chancre)** A venereal disease caused by *Haemophilus ducreyi*. It is characterized by a soft chancre that is a necrotic draining ulcer similar to a chancre but without characteristic induration. A regional bubo may occur.

channel A definite furrow, groove, or tubelike passage.

c., vascular A blood or lymph vessel through which inflammatory infiltrate and periodontitis can proceed from a localized superficial area to involve the deeper structures of the periodontium.

character One of a set of elementary symbols that may be arranged in groups to express information. They may include the decimal digits 0 to 9, the letters A to Z, punctuation marks, operation symbols, and any other single symbol that a computer may read, store, or write.

characteristics, sex Primary: those organs concerned with reproduction, such as the gonads and genitalia. Secondary: differences in voice range and timbre, muscularity, and distribution of hair and adipose tissue.

Charcot's joint *See* joint, Charcot's.

charges The financial obligation made to a patient account for services rendered, usually on a quoted fee for explicit services provided.

charlatan A quack, a person who pretends to have skills or knowledge that he or she does not possess.

Charles' law *See* law, Charles'.

chart A sheet of paper, pasteboard, etc., that presents a graphic representation of a condition or state.

c., Bonwill-Hawley *See* chart, Hawley.

c., dental A diagrammatic chart of the teeth on which the findings from the clinical and radiographic examinations are recorded.

c., Hawley (Bonwill-Hawley chart) Graded outlines of dental arch sizes based on the mesiodistal diameters of the six anterior teeth.

c., health *See* chart, history.

c., history Forms and records for obtaining a thorough medical and oral history combined with a complete record of findings that enables one to gather and have on hand the necessary records to render total patient care.

c., tooth *See* chart, dental.

Charters' method *See* method, Charters'.

charting Tabulation of the progress of a disease; the compilation of a clinical record.

Chayes' attachment (shaz) Believed to be the first internal precision attachment. *See also* attachment, intracoronal.

Cheadle's disease (chē′dĕlz) *See* scurvy, infantile.

checkbite *See* record, interocclusal.

    c., centric *See* record, interocclusal, centric; record, maxillomandibular, centric.

    c., eccentric *See* record, interocclusal, eccentric.

    c., lateral *See* record, interocclusal.

    c., protrusive *See* record, interocclusal, protrusive.

cheek biting Chewing of one's cheek (buccal mucosa) because of malocclusion, oral habit, or lack of coordination in the chewing cycle.

cheilion (kī′lē-ahn) The corner of the mouth.

cheilitis (kī-lī′tĭs) (perléche) Inflammation of the lip.

    c., actinic (solar cheilitis) Crusting, desquamation, ulceration, atrophy, and inflammation of the lips, more especially the lower lip, due to chronic exposure to the elements and actinic rays of sunlight.

    c., cigarette paper Focal areas of inflammation of the lips caused by cigarette paper sticking to the surface and injury produced by efforts to remove it.

    c., glandularis apostematosa Chronic diffuse nodular enlargement of the lower lip associated with purulent inflammatory hyperplasia of the mucous glands and ducts. Rare, unknown etiology.

    c., solar *See* cheilitis, actinic.

cheiloplasty (kī′lō-plăs″tē) Corrective surgery or restoration of the lips.

cheilorraphy (kī-lor′ah-fē) Surgical repair of a congenital cleft lip.

cheiloschisis (kī-los′kī-sĭs) *See* harelip.

cheilosis (kī-lō′sĭs) A noninflammatory condition of the lip usually characterized by chapping and fissuring. It is characteristic of vitamin B complex deficiency of the mouth orifice and/or monilial infection.

    c., angular Transverse fissuring at the angles of the mouth attributable to deficiences of the B complex group of vitamins, loss of the vertical dimension, drooling of saliva, and superimposed monilial infection.

cheilotomy (kī-lot′ō-mē) Incision into, or excision of, a part of the lip.

chelation (kē-lā′shŭn) Chemical reaction of a metallic ion (e.g., calcium ion) with a suitable reactive compound (e.g., ethylenediamine tetra-acetic acid) to form a compound in which the metal ion is tightly bound.

chemamnesia (kĕm-ăm-nē′zē-ah) Reversible amnesia produced by a chemical or drug.

Chemclave Brand name for chemical vapor sterilizer that uses a mixture of alcohols, ketones, formaldehyde, and water heated to approximately 127 degrees Centigrade under a pressure of at least 20 pounds per square inch. ADA accepted.

chemoreceptor (kē″mō-rē-sĕp′tor) A specialized sensory end organ adapted for excitation by chemical substances (e.g., olfactory and gustatory receptors) or specialized sense organs of the carotid body that are sensitive to chemical changes in the bloodstream.

chemotherapeutic agent *See* agent, chemotherapeutic.

cherubism (cher′ŭ-bĭzm) **(familial intraosseous swelling) 1:** A fibroosseous disease of the jaws of genetic nature. The swollen jaws and raised eyes give a cherubic appearance; multiple radiolucencies are evident on radiographic examination. **2:** A familial form of fibrous dysplasia that is characterized by unilateral or, more often, bilateral swelling of the jaws in children. *See also* dysplasia, fibrous.

chew-in technique The method by which the dentist records a patient's occlusal paths in the wax patterns to be used in making restorations. In making the grooves and ridges in the wax patterns directly, the dentist asks the patient to make right-and-left and fore-and-aft sliding occlusal strokes to generate the paths of the opposite prominences. *See also* path, generated occlusal.

chewing The movements of the mandible during mastication; controlled by neuromuscular action and limited by the anatomic structure of the temporomandibular joints.

    c. cycle *See* cycle, chewing.

    c. force *See* force, chewing.

Cheyne-Stokes reflex *See* respiration, Cheyne-Stokes.

Cheyne-Stokes respiration *See* respiration, Cheyne-Stokes.

chickenpox *See* varicella.

chi square (χ^2) A nonparametric statistic used with discrete data in the form of frequency count (nominal data) or percentages or proportions that can be reduced to frequencies. Highly used to determine differences between categories (e.g., yes-no; visits dentist every 6 months, 1 year, 2 years, 5 years); compares the observed results to the expected results to determine significant differences. May be used with many categories of response.

child In the law of negligence and in the laws for the protection of children, a term used as the opposite of adult (generally under the age of puberty), without reference to parentage and distinction of sex.

child abuse The physical, sexual, or emotional maltreatment of a person under 18 years of age. Child abuse occurs predominantly with children under the age of three. Symptoms include bruises and contusions, medical record of repeated trauma, radiographic evidence of fractures, emotional distress, and failure to thrive.

child neglect A form of child abuse in which proper care is denied or withheld.

chin cup *See* cup, chin.

chip A logic element, containing electronic circuit components, both active and passive, embedded in a cohesive material of any shape.

c. blower *See* syringe, air, hand.

chisel An instrument modeled after the carpenter's chisel; intended for cutting or cleaving hard tissue. The cutting edge is beveled on one side only; the shank may be straight or angled.

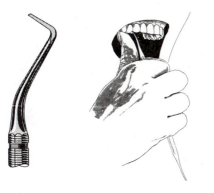

Binangle chisel

c., contra-angle (binangle chisel) A chisel-shaped, binangled, paired cutting instrument whose blade meets the shank at an angle greater than 12 degrees.

c., posterior *See* chisel, contra-angle.

c., Wedelstaedt A chisel with a blade that is continuous with the shank; has no constricting neck; curves rather than angles into the shank; is available in varying widths.

chiropractic A branch of the healing arts that deals with the nervous system and its relationship to the spinal column and its interrelationship with other body systems in health and disease. The primary spinal and paraspinal structural derangements chiropractors are concerned with are known as chiropractic subluxations. Treatment is referred to as chiropractic management or adjustment.

Chlamydia A genus of microorganisms that live as intercellular parasites having a number of properties in common with gram-negative bacteria. Two species of *Chlamydia* organisms have been identified; both are pathogenic to humans.

C. trachomatis An organism that lives in the conjunctive of the eye and the epithelium of the urethra and cervix and is responsible for conjunctivitis, lymphogranuloma venereum, and trachoma.

C. psittaci An organism that infests birds and causes a type of pneumonia in humans (psittacosis).

chloral hydrate A sedative and hypnotic.

chloramine solution *See* solution.

chloramphenicol A broad-spectrum antibacterial and an-

tirickettsial agent that should be reserved for serious infections in which other agents are ineffective.

chlordiazepoxide A psychopharmacologic compound used for the relief of anxiety. Brand name Librium.

chloride shift (klō'rīd) *See* phenomenon, Hamburger's.

chlorhexidine gluconate A antiseptic antimicrobial skin cleanser possessing bactericidal activities. Brand name Hibiclens.

Chlormycetin Brand name for chloramphenicol. *See also* chloramphenicol.

chloroformization (klō″rō-form″ĭ-zā′shŭn) The administration of chloroform.

chloropercha (klor″ō-per′chah) A solution obtained by mixing various amounts of chloroform with guttapercha.

c. method *See* method, chloropercha.

chlorophyllin (klor″ō-fĭl′ĭn) Any of a number of products resulting from the reaction of certain decomposition products of chlorophyll with copper and/or other metallic ions.

chlortetracycline (klor″tĕt-rah-sī′klēn) **(Aureomycin)** A broad-spectrum antibiotic possessing bacteriostatic properties of some value in the treatment of disease produced by large viruses (the psittacosis and lymphogranuloma inguinale groups).

choice of path of placement *See* placement, choice of path of.

cholagogue (kō′lah-gahg) A substance that stimulates emptying of the gallbladder and flow of bile.

choleretic (kō″ler-ĕt′ĭk) A substance that stimulates production of bile by the liver.

cholesterol (kō-lĕs′ter-ol) A lipid common to all animal, but not plant, cells. As a sterol, it contains the cyclopentenophenanthrene nucleus. High levels are found in nerve tissue, atheromas, gallstones, cysts, etc. Normally 140 to 220 mg are present in 100 ml of blood.

choline A lipotropic or transmethylation factor found in most animal tissue either free or in combination as lecithin, acetylcholine, or as cytidine diphosphate. Its acetate form (acetylcholine) is essential for synaptic transmission. Administration of choline appears to improve memory and has shown some beneficial use in Alzheimer's disease.

cholinergic (kō-lĭn-er′jĭk) **(parasympathomimetic)** Producing or simulating the effects of acetylcholine.

c. blocking agent *See* agent, blocking, cholinergic.

cholinesterase (kō-lĭn-ĕs′ter-ās) An esterase that hydrolyzes acetylcholine. It is an enzyme that is widely distributed throughout the muscles, glands, and nerves of the body and converts the acetylcholine into choline and acetic acid.

cholinolytic (kō″lĭn-ō-lĭt′ĭk) *See* anticholinergic.

chondrodystrophia fetalis (kŏn″drō-dĭs-trō′fē-ah fētăl′ĭs) *See* achondroplasia.

chondroectodermal dysplasia (kŏn″drō-ĕk-tō-dĕrm′al

dĭs-plā'zē-ah) **(Ellis-van Creveld syndrome)** A syndrome characterized by the following tetrad: (1) bilateral polydactyly; (2) chondrodysplasia of the long bones resulting in acromelic dwarfism; (3) anomaly of the teeth, nails, hair, and maxillary and mandibular region anteriorly; and (4) heart malformation.

chondroma (kahn-drō'mah) A benign tumor of cartilage. However, many chondrosarcomas arise in preexisting chondromas.

chondrotin A mucopolysaccharide present in the ground substance or matrix of connective tissue, particularly cartilage.

chondromyxosarcoma (kahn"drō-mĭk"sō-sar-kō'mah) Chondrosarcoma that exhibits an appreciable amount of myxomatous degeneration. *See also* chondrosarcoma.

chondrosarcoma (kahn"drō-sar-kō'mah) A malignant neoplasm composed of cartilage-like tissue.

chorea (kō-rē'ah) **(St. Vitus' dance)** A disorder of the central nervous system resulting in purposeless, involuntary athetoid (writhing) movements of the muscles of the face and extremities. It may be associated with or follow rheumatic fever (Sydenham's chorea), hysteria, senility, or infections, or it may be a hereditary disorder (Huntington's chorea).

Christian's disease *See* disease, Hand-Schuler-Christian.

Christmas disease *See* hemophilia B.

chromium-cobalt-molybdenum A stainless alloy used in interosseous implants for dental prosthesis.

chromosome (krō'mō-sōm) One of a number of small, dark-staining, and more or less rod-shaped bodies situated in the nucleus of a cell. At the time of cell division, chromosomes divide and distribute equally to the daughter cells. They contain genes arranged along their length. The number of chromosomes in the somatic cells of an individual is constant (diploid number), whereas just half this number (haploid number) appears in germ cells.

  c., aberration Any rearrangement of chromosome parts as a result of breakage and reunion of broken ends.

chronic Characterized by a long, slow course as opposed to acute.

cicatrix (sĭk'ah-trĭks, sĭ-kā'trĭks) **(scar)** The result of healing by second intention; characterized microscopically by excessive collagenation of the granulation tissue.

cicatrization (sĭk"ah-trĭ-zā'shŭn) Conversion of granulation tissue into scar tissue.

cineradiography (sĭn"ĕ-rā-dē-og'rah-fē) The making of motion pictures by means of roentgen rays and image intensification. Studies are used for diagnosis and research purposes. Speech patterns can be studied during the process of phonation; the action of the tongue, jaws, and palate can be studied during mastication and deglutition.

cingulum (sĭng'gū-lŭm) The portion of incisor teeth and canines, occurring on the lingual or palatal aspects, that forms a convex protuberance at the cervical third of the anatomic crown. Represents the lingual or palatal developmental lobe of these teeth.

  c. modification Alteration of the lingual form of an anterior tooth to provide a definite seat for the support of a rest unit of a removable partial denture.

ciprofloxacin A synthetic broad-spectrum antibacterial agent suitable for oral administration effective against some periodontal organisms.

circulation Movement of blood through blood vessels.

  c., coronary Circulation of blood within heart muscle.

  c., peripheral The passage of fluids, elctrolytes, and metabolites through the walls of terminal vessels of the vascular tree into and out of the tissue spaces.

  c., pulmonary Circulation of venous blood from the right ventricle of the heart, to the lungs, and back to the left atrium of the heart.

  c., systemic Circulation of oxygenated blood from the left ventricle of the heart to the various tissues and of venous blood back to the right atrium of the heart.

circulatory system System for circulation of blood, consisting of heart, arteries, arterioles, capillaries, venules, and veins.

circumferential wiring *See* wiring, circumferential.

cirrhosis A chronic degenerative disease of the liver in which blood flow is restricted and metabolic and detoxification functions are impaired or destroyed. Cirrhosis is most commonly the result of chronic alcohol abuse.

citric acid A white, crystalline, organic acid freely soluble in water and alcohol. It can be extracted from citrus fruits or through a fermentation of sugars. It is a key intermediary in metabolism. *See also* citric acid cycle.

citric acid cycle A sequence of enzymatic reactions involving the metabolism of carbon chains of sugars, fatty acids, and amino acids to yield carbon dioxide, water, and high-energy phosphate bonds. Also called *Krebs' citric acid cycle* or *tricarboxylic acid cycle.*

citrin (sĭt'rĭn) *See* factor, platelet 1.

civil action A noncriminal legal action.

civil law A statutory law as opposed to common law or judge-made law (such as case law). The dental practice act is a civil law.

claim 1: In a juridical sense, a demand of some type made by one person or another. **2:** A request for payment under a dental benefits plan. **3:** A statement listing services rendered, the dates of services, and itemization of costs. Includes a statement signed by the beneficiary and treating dentist that services have been rendered. The completed form serves as the basis for payment of benefit.

claimant Person who files a claim for benefits. May be the patient or the certificate holder.

claim form The form used to file for benefits under a dental benefits program, includes sections for the patient and the dentist to complete.

claims payment fraud The intentional manipulation or alteration of facts submitted by a treating dentist resulting in a lower payment to the beneficiary and/or the treating dentist than would have been paid if the manipulation had not occurred.

claims reporting fraud The intentional misrepresentation of material facts concerning treatment provided and charges made, in that this misrepresentation would cause a higher payment.

claims review 1: In dental prepayment, the routine examination by a carrier or intermediary of the claim submitted to it for payment or for predetermination of benefits; may include determination of eligibility, coverage of service, and plan liability. **2:** In quality assurance, examination by organizations of claims as part of a quality review or use review process.

clamp A device used to effect compression or retention.

  c., cervical *See* clamp, gingival.

  c., gingival (cervical clamp) A rubber dam clamp intended to retract gingival tissues.

    c., Ferrier 212 gingival A purposely unbalanced gingival rubber dam clamp for retracting gingival tissue from the field of operation. It must be stabilized to position with modeling compound. Developed by W.I. Ferrier.

    c., Hatch gingival An adjustable gingival rubber dam clamp.

  c., rubber dam (rubber dam retainer) A device made of spring metal and used to retain a rabber dam in place or to improve the operating field by isolating it from the oral environment.

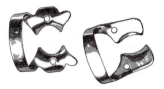

Rubber dam clamps

  c., root rubber dam A clamp whose jaws are designed to fit on the root surfaces of a tooth; usually used for the retention of a rubber dam.

Clarke-Fournier glossitis (foor-ne-a′) *See* glossitis, interstitial sclerous.

Clark's rule *See* rule, Clark's.

clasp An extracoronal direct retainer of a removable par-

tial denture, usually consisting of two arms, a retentive arm and a reciprocal arm, joined by a body that may connect with an occlusal rest.

  c., Adams A formed wire clasp, of modified arrowhead design, using the buccomesial and distoproximal undercuts of a tooth for retention.

  c., arm Clasp extensions, usually from minor connectors, that provide retention, reciprocation, or stabilization.

    c., arm, reciprocal An arm of a clasp, usually at or occlusal to the height of contour, located in such a manner as to reciprocate any force arising from an opposing clasp arm on the same tooth.

    c., arm, retentive (retention terminal) A clasp amn that is flexible and engages the infrabulge area at the terminal end of the arm.

    c., arm, fatigue of A situation in which the retentive arm of a clasp metal has undergone flexure at the same point repeatedly, and fracture has resulted. Tapering the clasp arm tend to distribute the flexure and to reduce such tendency to fracture.

  c., arrowhead A wire clasp, for retention of removable appliances, whose active elements are in the shape of an arrowhead and engage the mesioproximal and distoproximal undercuts on the buccal aspect of adjacent teeth.

  c., back-action A clasp that originates on one surface of a tooth and traverses the suprabulge area to another surface, where it is supported by an occlusal rest; it then continues to encircle the tooth on the third surface, where it terminates in the infrabulge area beyond the opposite angle of the tooth surface where it originated.

  c., bar A clasp whose arms are bar-type extensions from major connectors or from within the denture base; the arms pass adjacent to the soft tissues and approach the point of contact on the tooth in a cervico-occlusal direction.

    c., bar, arm A clasp arm that originates from the denture base or from a major or minor connector. It consists of the arm that traverses but does not contact the gingival structures and a terminal end that approaches its contact with the tooth in a cervico-occlusal direction.

  c., cast A clasp made of an alloy that has been cast into the desired form and retains its crystalline structure.

  c., circumferential A clasp that encircles more than 180 degrees of a tooth, including opposite angles, tent of the clasp, at least one terminal being in the infrabulge area (cervical convergence).

    c., circumferential arm A clasp arm that has its origin in a minor connector and follows the contour of the tooth approximately in a plane perpendicular to the path of placement of the removable partial denture.

c., reciprocal, circumferential arm An arm of a clasp located in such a manner as to reciprocate any force arising from an opposing clasp arm on the same tooth.

c., retentive circumferential arm (retention terminal) A circumferential clasp arm that is flexible and engages the infrabulge area at the terminal end of the arm.

c., stabilizing circumferential arm A circumferential clasp arm that is rigid and contacts the tooth at or occlusal to the surveyed height of contour.

c., combination A clasp that employs a wrought wire retentive arm and a cast reciprocal or stabilizing arm. A clasp that employs a bar type of retentive arm and a cast reciprocal or stabilizing arm.

c., continuous A secondary lingual bar.

c. design Determination of the shape and construction of a clasp with its position outlined on the cast.

c., embrasure (em-bra′zhur) A clasp used where no edentulous space exists. It passes through the embrasure, using two occlusal rests, and clasps the two teeth with circumferential clasps that have a common body.

c. flexibility The property of a clasp that enables it to be bent without breaking and to return to its original form. Factors that affect the flexibility of a retentive clasp arm are its length, diameter, crosssection form, structure, and the alloy of which it is made.

c. flexure *See* flexure, clasp.

c., formed *See* clasp, wrought.

c., mesiodistal A type of clasp that embraces the distolingual and mesial surfaces of a tooth and takes its retention in either or both mesial and distal undercuts.

c., retentive, flexibility of Ability of the retentive clasp to deform sufficiently to escape from a retentive undercut area without permanent deformation.

c., Roach *See* clasp, bar.

c., stress-breaking action of Relief for the abutment teeth from all or part of torquing occlusal forces; partially achieved by having a retentive arm of maximum flexibility that will provide adequate retention.

c., wrought (formed clasp) A clasp made of an alloy that has been drawn into various forms of wire.

classification Systematic arrangement according to characteristics of groups or classes.

c., Angle's *See* Angle's classification, modified.

c., Broders' *See* index, Broders'.

c., cavity *See* cavity, classification.

c. of habits Compilation of habits that may cause periodontal disease. Habit neuroses include lip biting, cheek biting, biting of foreign objects, and abnormal tongue pressure against the teeth. Occupational habits include thread biting, musician's habits, holding nails in the mouth, etc. Miscellaneous habits include thumb-sucking, pipe smoking, incorrect toothbrushing habits, cracking nuts with the teeth, and mouth breathing.

c., Kennedy *See* Kennedy classification.

c. of motion A classification system that identifies the extent of involvement of the body in completing a dental motor task.

Class 1 Motions of the fingers only.

Class 2 Motions of the fingers and wrist.

Class 3 Motions of the fingers, wrist, and elbow.

Class 4 Motions of the fingers, wrist, elbow, and upper arm.

Class 5 Motions of the fingers, wrist, elbow, upper arm, and body.

c. of partial dentures Grouping of partially edentulous situations based on various conditions (e.g., location of the edentulous space, location of remaining teeth, position of direct retainers, and ability of oral structures to support a partial denture).

c. of periodontal diseases Division of periodontal diseases into three classes: (1) inflammation—gingival abrasion, gingivitis, marginal periodontitis; (2) dystrophy—disuse atrophy, occlusal traumatism, periodontosis; and (3) combinations of inflammatory and dystrophic diseases—periodontosis and periodontitis, occlusal traumatism, and periodontitis.

c. of pockets Division of pockets into two classes: (1) suprabony-gingival and periodontal and (2) infrabony, according to number of osseous walls-three osseous walls, two osseous walls, one osseous wall.

cleansing, biomechanical The process of cleaning and shaping a root canal with endodontic instrumentation in conjunction with irrigating solutions.

cleansing solution *See* solution, cleansing.

clearance 1: A condition in which moving bodies may pass without hindrance. **2:** Removal from the blood by the kidneys (e.g., urea or insulin) or by the liver (e.g., certain dyes).

c., interocclusal The difference in the height of the face when the mandible is at rest and when the teeth are in occlusion. This is determined by measuring the amount of space between the upper and lower teeth when the mandible is in the position of physiologic rest. The difference between the rest vertical dimension and the occlusal vertical dimension of the face, as measured in the incisal area. *See also* distance, interocclusal.

c., occlusal A condition in which the lower teeth may pass the upper teeth horizontally without contact or interference.

cleat A fixed point of anchorage, usually in the form of a metal spur or loop embedded in the acrylic resin base of a Hawley retainer or soldered onto an arch wire, to which a rubber dam elastic or other device is attached during orthodontic tooth movement.

cleft(s) A longitudinal fissure of opening.

c., facial Fissures along the embryonal lines of the junction of the maxillary and lateral nasal processes; usually extend obliquely from the nasal ala to the outer border of the eye.

c., gingival A cleft of the marginal gingiva; may be caused by many factors, such as incorrect tooth-brushing, a breakthrough to the surface of pocket formation, or faulty tooth positions, and may resemble V-shaped notches.

c. lip A congenital anomaly of the face caused by the failure of fusion between embryonic maxillary and medial nasal processes.

c., occult *See* submucous cleft.

c., operated (postoperative cleft) A cleft that has been surgically repaired.

c. palate A congenital anomaly of the oral cavity caused by the failure of fusion between the embryonic palatal shelves.

c. palate prosthesis *See* prosthesis, cleft palate.

c., postoperative *See* cleft, operated.

c., Stillman's Small fissures extending apically from the midline of the gingival margin in teeth subjected to trauma. Although these clefts may be found in traumatism, they are not necessarily diagnostic of occlusal trauma.

c., submucous *See* submucous cleft.

c., unoperated A cleft of the palate that has not been surgically repaired.

cleidocranial dysostosis *See* dysostosis, cleidocranial.

clenching The nonfunctional forceful intermittent application of the mandibular teeth against the maxillary teeth.

cleoid (klē'oid) A carving instrument having a blade shaped like a pointed spade or claw, with cutting edges on both sides and the tip.

clicking A sound associated with dysfunction of the temporomandibular joint, also the sound made by poor fitting dentures.

climate, occlusal The new occlusal relationship and environment produced by occlusal adjustment, orthodontic tooth movement, or a periodontal prosthesis.

clindamycin A semisynthetic antibiotic effective against a broad range of aerobic gram-positive cocci, anaerobic gram-negative bacilli, and anerobic and microaerophilic gram-positive cocci. Brand name Cleocin HCL.

clinic, table A display or demonstration of a topic, limited to scope, for transmitting information to a small number of persons at a time.

clinical crown *See* crown, clinical.

clinical crown:clinical root ratio *See* ratio, clinical crown:clinical root.

clinical diagnosis *See* diagnosis, clinical.

clinoidale (klīn-oid'al) The most superior point on the contour of the anterior clinoid.

clioquinol An antifungal oinment or cream used topically to treat angular cheilitis. Brand name Vioform.

clonus (klō'nŭs) Alternating muscular spasm and relaxation in rapid succession.

closed bite *See* bite, closed.

closed panel 1: In a prepayment plan, a group of dentists sharing office facilities who provide stipulated services to an eligible group for a set premium. For beneficiaries of plans using closed panels, choice of dentists is limited to panel members. Dentists must accept any beneficiary as a patient. **2:** A closed panel dental benefits plan exists when patients eligible to receive benefits can receive them only if services are provided by dentists who have signed an agreement with the benefits plan to provide treatment to eligible patients. As a result of the dentist reimbursement methods characteristic of a closed panel plan, only a small percentage of practicing dentists in a given geographical area are typically contracted by the plan to provide dental services.

closed procedure Reduction of a fracture of the maw or placement of an implant without surgical flap retraction.

Clostridium A genus of spore-forming anaerobic bacteria of the Bacillaceae family.

C. bifermentans Causes gas gangrene.

C. botulinum Causes botulism.

C. perfringens Causes food poisoning, cellulitis and wound infections.

C. tentani Causes tetanus.

closure The act or condition of being brought together or closed up.

c., adjustive arcs of Arcs of jaw closure found in deflective malocclusion caused by an intercusping of the teeth that does not coincide with a centrically related jaw closure.

c., arcs of mandibular Circular or elliptic arcs created by closure of the mandible.

c., centric path of The path traversed by the mandible during closure when its associated neuromuscular mechanism is in a balanced state of tonus.

c., velopharyngeal Closure of nasal air escape by the knee-action elevation of the soft palate and contraction of the posterior pharyngeal wall.

c., voluntary arcs of A jaw closure direction consciously made by a patient.

clot Coagulated blood, plasma, or fibrin.

c., blood A coagulum formed of blood of a semisolidified nature.

clotrimazole A synthetic broad-spectrum antifungal agent that inhibits the growth of pathogenic yeasts including *Candida albicans* and other species of the genus *Candida*. Brand name Lotrimin.

clotting factors Chemical and cellular constituents of the blood responsible for the conversion of fibrinogen into a mesh of insoluble fibrin causing the blood to coagulate or clot.

clubbing (pulmonary osteoarthropathy) Deforming enlargement of the terminal phalanges of the fingers. It is usually acquired and may be associated with certain cardiac and pulmonary diseases.

clutch A device made for gripping the teeth in a dental arch, to which face-bows or tracing devices may be attached rigidly enough to behave in space relations during the movements as if they were jaw outgrowths.

CMV Abbreviation for cytomegalovirus. *See* cytomegalovirus.

coagulating current *See* current, coagulating.

coagulation time *See* time, coagulation.

coated tongue *See* tongue, coated.

coating, enteric (ĕn-ter′ĭk) A tablet covering that resists the action of the fluids and enzymes in the stomach but dissolves readily in the upper intestine.

coating material A biologically acceptable, usually porous, nonmetal applied over the surface of a metallic implant, with the expectation that tissue ingrowth will occur in the pores. Often a carbon polymer or ceramic substance.

cobalt-chromium alloy *See* alloy, cobalt-chromium.

coccidioidomycosis An infectious fungal disease caused by the inhalation of spores of the bacterium *Coccidioides immitis,* which is carried on windborne dust particles. Although endemic in the southeastern United States, coccidioidomycosis is considered among the opportunistic infections that are indicators of AIDS.

code A system of recording information by symbols so that only selected people will know the meaning. Used also to conserve space.

　c. of ethics A series of principles used as a guide in assisting a dentist to fulfill the moral obligations of professional dental practice.

codeine (kō′dēn) A crystalline alkaloid, morphine methyl ether that is used as an analgesic and antitussive.

coding Writing instructions for a computer either in machine language or nonmachine language.

Coecal (kō′kăl) Trade name for dental stone (Hydrocal).

coefficient, absorption *See* absorption coefficient.

coefficient, phenol The ratio of potency of a given germicide to that of phenol under standard conditions.

coefficient of thermal expansion *See* expansion, thermal coefficient.

cofactor V *See* factor VII.

cognition (kog-nĭsh′ŭn) The higher mental processes of understanding, reasoning, knowledge, intellectual capacity, etc.

cognitive (kog′nĭ-tĭv) Pertaining to the faculty of knowing, perceiving, or being aware; an expression of intellectual capacity.

cognovit note A note that confesses judgment and justice of the claim and to which the maker has no available legal defense.

cohere To stick together, to unite, to form a solid mass.

cohesion Ability of a material to adhere to itself.

cohesive Capable of cohering or sticking together so as to form a mass.

coinsurance 1: A means of sharing, dividing, or splitting the cost of dental services between the dental plan and the insured patient. A common division is 80%/20%. This means the insurance company will pay 80% of the cost of the dental service, and the patient will pay 20%. Percentages vary and may be applied to scheduled or usual, customary, and reasonable fee plans. **2:** A provision of a dental benefits program by which the beneficiary shares in the cost of covered services, generally on a percentage basis. The percentage of a covered dental expense that a beneficiary must pay (after the deductible is paid). A typical coinsurance arrangement is one in which the third party pays 80% of the allowed benefit of the covered dental service and the beneficiary pays the remainder of the charged fee. Percentages vary and may apply to table of allowance plans; usual, customary, and reasonable plans; and direct reimbursement programs.

　c. clause A provision in an insurance contract stipulating that the insurer will pay a specified share of dental expenses covered by the plan.

cold, clinical applications of Clinical uses of cold to treat cold injury (e.g., frostbite), relieve pain in burn injury, relieve pain in severe and acute inflammation (pulpitis), and relieve pain and swelling in contusions, abrasions, and sprains. *See also* heat and cold, applied.

cold , physiologic effects of In reference to application of cold to a local area, marked vasoconstriction followed by vasodilation and edema. In extreme exposure the effects include a significant drop in temperature on the surface and a lesser drop in deeper tissue layers, depending on the degree of cold and duration of application; decreased phagocytosis; a decrease in local metabolism; and analgesia to varying degrees of anesthesia of the part exposed to cold.

cold sore *See* sore, canker; herpes labialis.

cold welding *See* welding, cold.

cold work Deformation of the space lattice of metals by mechanical manipulation at room temperature. The process alters certain properties (e.g., ductility).

cold-curing resin *See* resin, autopolymer.

collagen An intercellular constituent of connective tissue and bone consisting of bundles of tiny reticular fibrils, most noticeable in the white glistening inelastic fibers of tendons, ligaments, and fascia.

collagenase An enzyme capable of depolymerizing collagen, found in some microorganisms and believed to contribute to periodontal disease.

collapse A state of extreme prostration and depression with failure of circulation; abnormal falling in of the walls of any part or organ; and, with reference to a lung, an airless or fatal state of all or part of the lung.

collar The small part of the root of a tooth that is a part of an artificial tooth (denture).

collective bargaining The negotiations between organized labor and employers on matters such as wages, hours, working conditions, and health and welfare programs.

collimation (kol″ĭ-mā′shŭn) Literally, making parallel. In radiology refers to the elimination of the peripheral (more divergent) portion of a useful x-ray beam, by means of metal tubes, cones, or diaphragms interposed in the path of the beam. *See also* diaphragm.

collimator (kol′ĭ-mă-ter) A diaphragm of system of diaphragms made of an absorbing material and designed to define the dimensions and direction of a beam of radiation.

collision tumor *See* tumor, collision.

colloid (kol′oid) A suspension of particles in a dispersion medium, the particles generally ranging in size from 1 to 100 mμ. Hydrocolloids and silicate cements are examples of dental colloids.

color blindness *See* blindness, color.

color, temper The color produced by the thickening of the oxide coating on carbon steel as temperature is increased. Used as an indication of the degree of tempering.

coloring, extrinsic Coloring from without, as in the application of color to the external surface of a prosthesis.

coloring, intrinsic Coloring from within. The incorporation of pigment within the material of a prosthesis.

coma (kō′mah) A state of unconsciousness from which the patient cannot be aroused, even by powerful stimulation. It is gradual in onset, prolonged, and not spontaneously reversible.

    c., diabetic Unconsciousness accompanying severe diabetic acidosis. It may develop from omission of insulin, surgical complications, or disregard of dietary restrictions. Premonitory symptoms include weakness, anorexia, dry skin and mouth, drowsiness, abdominal pain, and fruity breath odor. Late symptoms are coma, air hunger, low blood pressure, tachycardia, dehydration, soft and sunken eyeballs, glycosuria, hyperglycemia, and a high level of ecetoacetic acid. *See* shock, insulin.

combination clasp *See* clasp, combination.

command The portion of an instruction that specifies the operation to be performed. A term used with hardware operations.

comminution of food *See* food, comminution of.

common deductible A deductible amount that is common to the dental and another health insurance policy (usually a major medical policy). In a major medical policy with a $100 common deductible, once $100 of medical or dental expense has been incurred under either policy or both, no further deductible is required.

common law Judge-made law, as contrasted with statutory law. It is that body of law that originated in England and was in force at the time of the American Revolution; modified since that time on a case-by-case basis in the courts.

communicable period The period of time when the infectious agent that causes a communicable disease may be transmitted to a susceptible host, such as in diseases that intially involve the mucous membrane (i.e., diphtheria and scarlet fever). The period of communicability is from the time of exposure to the disease until termination of the carrier state, if one develops.

communication The technique of conveying thoughts or ideas between two people or groups of people.

    c., privileged Certain classes of communications between persons who stand in a confidential or fiduciary relationship to each other that the law will not permit to be divulged in court. Examples of confidential relationships are those of psychiatrist and patient and attorney and client. Confidentiality of communications depends on the law in each state.

community dentistry A branch, discipline, or specialty of dentistry that deals with the community and its aggregate dental or oral health rather than that of the individual patient. Formal recognition of dentists engaged in community dentistry is through the American Board of Public Health Dentistry.

compact To form by uniting or condensing particles with the application of pressure (e.g., the progressive insertion and welding of foil and the building up of plastic amalgam in a preparation.)

compacter A rotary instrument used in the McSpadden endodontic technique to condense the guttapercha cone into the root canal.

compaction The act of compacting or the state of being compact.

compensating curve *See* curve, compensating.

compensation The monetary reward for rendering a service; insurance providing financial return to employees in the event of an injury that occurs during the performance of their duties and that prohibits work. Compulsory in many states.

    c., unemployment Insurance covering the employee so that compensation may be provided for loss of income due to unemployment.

competence A measure of the degree of a person's ability to cope with all aspects of the environment.

competent Having legal capacity, ability, or authority.

compiler A computer program that translates a high-level language program into a corresponding machine instruction. The program that results from compiling is a translated and expanded version of the original program.

complaint The most troublesome of symptoms disclosed by the patient.

  c., chief The symptom or reason for which the patient seeks treatment. The most troublesome symptom.

complemental air *See* volume, inspiratory reserve.

complete blood count *See* count, blood, complete.

complete denture *See* denture, complete.

complex A combination of a number of things; the sum or total of various things.

  c., craniofacial The bones and surrounding soft structure of the cranium and face.

  c., dentofacial Referring to the dentition and surrounding structures.

component(s) A part or element.

  c., A *See* factor II.

  c. of force *See* force, component of.

  c. of partial denture *See* denture, partial, components of.

  c., salivary *See* lysozyme.

  c., thromboplastic cellular (TCC) *See* factor, platelet, 3.

composite odontoma *See* odontoma, composite.

composite resin *See* resin, composite.

composition, modeling *See* plastic; compound.

compound 1: A combination of elements held together in a well-defined pattern by chemical bonds. In pharmacy, a mixture of drugs. **2:** A thermoplastic substance used as a nonelastic impression material.

  c. A, B, E, F, S *See* corticoid, adrenal.

  c. cone A compound in the form of a cone or pyramid; used for impressions of individual preparations.

  c., impression (modeling compound) *See* compound.

  c., intermetallic A compound of two metals in which the metals are only partially soluble in one another; exhibits a homogeneous grain structure, but the atoms do not intermingle randomly in all proportions.

  c., modeling *See* compound, impression.

  c. tracing stick A compound dispensed in stick form.

  c., tray A compound similar to impression compound but with less flow and more viscosity when soft and more rigidity when chilled.

comprehensive orthodontic therapy A coordinated approach to improvement of the overall anatomic and functional relationships of the dentofacial complex, as opposed to partial correction with more limited objectives such as cosmetic improvement. Usually but not necessarily uses fixed orthodontic attachments as a part of the treatment appliance. Includes treatment and adjunctive procedures (such as extractions, maxillofacial surgery, other dental services, nasopharyngeal surgery, speech therapy) directed at malrelationships within the entire dentofacial complex. Optimal care requires periodic evaluation of patient needs, especially during the growing years. Treatment is most effective when begun in the deciduous or mixed dentition and accomplished in successive phases as the face matures. Active correction in the adult dentition can usually be accomplished in one phase.

compression Act of pressing together or forcing into less space.

  c. molding *See* molding, compression.

  c. of tissue *See* tissue, displaceability.

compressive strength *See* strength, compressive.

compromise (kahm′prō-mīz″) Arrangement arrived at, in or out of court, for settling a disagreement on terms considered by the parties to be fair.

compulsion (kahm-pŭl′shŭn) A repetitive, stereotyped, and often trivial motor action, whose performance is compelled even though the person does not wish to perform the act. Oral habits (bruxism, clenching, etc.) may be compulsions.

computed tomography A radiographic body scanning technique in which thin or narrow layer sections of the body can be imaged for diagnostic purposes. The technique uses a computer-linked x-ray machine to focus the x-rays on a particular section of the body to be viewed.

computer A device capable of accepting data in the form of facts and figures, manipulating them in a prescribed way, and supplying the results of these processes as meaningful information. This device usually consists of input and output devices, storage, arithmetic and logic units, and a control unit. Usually an automatic, stored-program machine is implied.

  c., digital A computer that operates on discrete data by performing arithmetic and logic processes on these data.

  c. language The vocabulary and syntax of a set of symbols that are used to instruct a computer what to do (e.g., COBOL, FORTRAN, BASIC, PASCAL).

  c. output microfilm (COM) A system that allows a computer user to produce microfilm copies of computer output. The COM unit operates independently of the CPU and is therefore called an *offline device*. Output from computer processing is recorded on magnetic tape, which is later removed from the computer's tape handler, mounted on the COM unit, and recorded on microfilm.

conceal To hide; secrete; withhold from the knowledge of others.

Concise Brand name for diacrylate resin adhesives used in composite restorations and for bonding orthodontic appliances to the enamel.

concrescence (kahn-krĕs′ĕns) **1:** The union of two teeth

63

after eruption by the fusion of their cementum surfaces. **2:** Fusion of teeth after their roots have formed. The union is effected by cementum. *See also* fusion.

condensation (kahn″dĕn-sā′shŭn) Commonly used term for the insertion and compression or compaction of dental materials into a prepared cavity. *Compaction* is a more accurate term than *condensation*. *See also* compaction.

condenser (kahn-dĕn′ser) (formerly called *plugger)* An instrument or device used to compact or condense a restorative material into a prepared cavity. Its working end is called the *nib* or *point*; the end of the nib is termed the *face*. The face may be smooth or serrated.

c., amalgam (amalgam plugger) An instrument used to condense plastic amalgam.

c., automatic *See* condenser, mechanical.

c., back-action A condenser with the shank bent into a Ushape so that the condensing force is a pulling motion rather than the usual pushing force.

c., bayonet A condenser in which the offset of the nib and the approximately right-angled bends in the shank permit a better line of force for condensation of direct filling gold. There are many variations in angles, length, and diameter of the nib.

c., electromallet (McShirley's electromallet) An electromechanical device for compacting direct filling gold. Frequency of blows may be varied from 200 to 3600 strokes/min; the intensity of the blow is controlled electronically.

c., foil A condenser used to compact direct filling gold.

c., long-handled foil A hand condenser of varied design for compacting gold foil.

c., foot A foil condenser with the nib shaped like a foot.

c., hand An instrument that compacts material, the force being applied by the muscular effort of the operator with or without supplementary force from a mallet in the hand of the assistant.

c., Hollenback *See* condenser, pneumatic.

c., mechanical (automatic mallet) A device to supply an automatically controlled blow for condensing restorative material. It may be spring-activated, penumatic, or electronically controlled.

c., parallelogram A condenser, the face of which is shaped like a rectangle or a parallelogram.

c., pneumatic (Hollenback condenser) A pneumatic mechanical device developed by George M. Hollenback to supply a compacting force. The force is delivered by controlled pneumatic pressure. Blows are variable in intensity, with speed variable up to 300 strokes/min.

c. point *See* point, condenser.

c., round A condenser, the face of which has a circular outline.

c., stepping The orderly movement of a condenser point over the surface of gold foil or amalgam during its placement and compaction.

condensing force *See* force, condensing.

condensing osteitis *See* osteitis, condensing.

condensor (spreader) An instrument used in filling a root canal to compress the filling material in a lateral direction.

conduct, dishonorable Conduct that mars the character and lessens the reputation; conduct that is shameful, disgraceful, base.

conduction The carrying of sound waves, heat, light, nerve impulses, or electricity.

c., air The process of transmitting sound waves to the cochlea by way of the outer and middle ear. In normal hearing, practically all sounds are transmitted in this way, except those of the hearer's own voice, which are transmitted partly by bone conduction.

c., bone The transmission of sound waves or vibrations to the cochlea by way of the bones of the cranium.

c., impulse Conduction of an impulse along the nerve fiber, which is accompanied by an alteration of the electrical potential of the fiber tissue and an exchange of electrolytes across the nerve fiber membrane.

conductivity Capacity for conduction; ability to convey.

c., electrical Ability of a material to conduct electricity. Metals are usually good conductors, and nonmetals are poor conductors.

c., thermal Ability of a material to transfer heat. It is of great importance in dentistry, where a low thermal conductivity is desirable in restorative material and a high thermal conductivity is desirable when soft tissue is covered.

condylar (kahn′dĭ-lar) Pertaining to the mandibular condyle.

c. axis *See* axis, condylar.

c. guide *See* guide, condylar.

c. guide inclination *See* guide, condylar, inclination.

condyle (kahn′dīl) The rounded surface at the articular end of a bone.

c. head Redundant term; the word *condyle* means head. *See* condyle.

c., mandibular The articular process of the mandible; the condyloid process of the mandible.

c., neck of *See* process, condyloid, neck of.

c., orbiting *See* orbiting condyle.

c. path The path traveled by the mandibular condyle in the temporomandibular joint during the various mandibular movements.

c., lateral, path The path of the condyle in the glenoid fossa when a lateral mandibular movement is made.

c., protrusive, path The path of the condyle when

the mandible is moved forward from its centric position.

c. rod *See* rod, condyle.

c., rotating The condyle on the side of the bolus formation, or the one that is braced and placed and rotated while the bolus is being chewed.

condylectomy (kahn″dĭl-ĕk′tō-mē) Surgical removal of a condyle.

condyloid process *See* process, condyloid.

condyloplasty A surgical procedure to alter the shape of the condyle to remove the effects of degenerative disease.

condylotomy (kahn″dĭ-lot′ō-mē) Surgical division through, without removal of, a condyle; or removal of a portion, usually the articular surface, of a condyle.

cone 1: A geometric shape with a circle for its base that tapers evenly to an apex. **2:** A solid substance, usually guttapercha or silver, having a tapered form similar in length and diameter to a root canal; used to fill the space once occupied by the pulp in the root of the tooth. **3:** An accessory device on a dental x-ray machine, designed to indicate the direction of the central axis of its x-ray beam and to serve as a guide in establishing a desired source-to-film distance.

c. distance The distance between the focal spot and the outer end of the cone; usually expressed in inches or centimeters. Modern dental roentgen-ray units usually have cone distances of from 5 to 20 inches (12.5 to 50 cm).

c., long A tubular ″cone″ designed to establish an extended anode-to-skin distance, usually within a range of from 12 to 20 inches (30 to 50 cm).

c., short A conical or tubular ″cone″ having as one of its functions the establishment of an anode-to-skin distance of up to 9 inches (22.5 cm).

confidential An express or implied agreement that the dentist will not disclose the information received from a patient to anyone not directly involved in the care and treatment or not legally capable of requiring disclosure; generally an ethical rather than legally enforceable consideration in dentistry.

congenital Present at birth and usually developed in utero.

congestion *See* hyperemia.

congestive heart failure An abnormal condition characterized by circulatory congestion (retention of fluids) caused by cardiac or kidney disorders. This condition usually develops chronically in association with the retention of sodium and water by the kidneys. Acute congestive heart failure may result from myocardial infarction of the left ventricle.

conjugate 1: *v.* To unite. **2:** *n.* The product of conjugation.

conjugation In biochemistry, the union of a drug or toxic substance with a normal constituent of the body, such as glucuronic acid, to form an inactive product that is then eliminated.

connective tissue *See* tissue, connective.

connector The part of a partial denture that unites its components.

c. bar *See* bar, connector.

c., cross arch bar splint A removable cross arch connector used to stabilize weakened abutments that support a fixed prosthesis by attachment to teeth on the opposite side of the dental arch. It can be removed by the dentist but not by the patient.

c., major A metal plate or bar (e.g., lingual bar, linguoplate, palatal bar) used to join the units of one side of a removable partial denture to those located on the opposite side of the dental arch.

c., anterior palatal major A major connector uniting bilateral units of a maxillary removable partial denture. It is a thin metal plate that is located in the anterior palatal region.

c., lingual bar major A type of connector used to unite the right and left components of a mandibular removable partial denture and occupy a position lingual to the alveolar ridge.

c., linguoplate major A major connector formed by the extension of a metal plate from the superior border of the regular lingual bar, across gingivae, and onto the cingulum of each anterior tooth.

c., posterior palatal major (posterior palatal bar) A major transpalatal connector located in the posterior palatal region. It is used when the anterior palatal bar alone is insufficient to provide the necessary rigidity.

c., secondary lingual bar major (Kennedy bar) Often called a *continuous clasp* or *Kennedy bar*. It rests on the cingulum area of the lower anterior teeth and serves principally as an indirect retainer and/or stabilizer for weakened anterior lower teeth.

c., minor The connecting link between the major connector or base of a removable partial denture and other units of the restoration, such as direct and indirect retainers, rests.

c., nonrigid A connector used where retainers or pontics are united by a joint permitting limited movement. It may be a precision or a nonprecision type of connector.

c., rigid A connector used where retainers or pontics are united by a soldered, cast, or welded joint.

c., saddle *See* connector, major.

c., subocclusal A nonrigid connector positioned gingival to the occlusal plane.

consciousness A state in which the individual is capable of rational response to questioning and has all protective reflexes intact, including the ability to maintain a patent airway.

consent Concurrence of wills; permission.

c., express Consent directly given by voice or in writing.

c., implied Consent made evident by signs, actions, or facts, or by inaction or silence.

consideration Inducement to make a contract. It may be a benefit to the promisor or a loss or detriment to the promisee. To be consideration it must be regarded as such by both parties.

Consolidated Omnibus Budget Reconciliation Act (COBRA) Legislation relative to mandated benefits for all types of employee benefits plans. The most significant aspects within this context are the requirements for continued coverage for employees and/or their dependents for 18 months who would otherwise lose coverage (30 months for dependents in the event of the employee's death).

consonant A conventional speech sound produced, with or without laryngeal vibration, by certain successive contractions of the articulatory muscles that modify, interrupt, or obstruct the expired airstream to the extent that its pressure is raised.

c., semivowel (1,t) Consonants that are like vowels both perceptually and physiologically.

constitution General makeup of the body as determined by genetic, physiologic, and biochemical factors. It may be markedly influenced by environment.

construction, single denture The making of one upper or lower denture as distinguished from a set of two complete dentures.

consultant A professional or nonprofessional person who, by virtue of special knowledge of professional or nonprofessional aspects of a dental practice, is sought out for advice and training.

consultation A meeting of persons to discuss or decide something.

c., professional Joint deliberation by two or more dentists and/or physicians to determine the diagnosis, treatment, or prognosis for a particular patient.

c., patient A meeting between the dentist, patient, and other interested persons for the purpose of discussing the patient' s dental needs, proposing treatment, and making business arrangements.

consumer One who may receive or is receiving dental service; the term is also used in health legislation and programs as someone who is never a practitioner or is not associated in any direct or indirect way with the supplying or provision of dental services.

contact The act of touching or meeting.

c., balancing The contact established between the upper and lower dentures at the side opposite the working side (anteroposteriorly or laterally) for the purpose of stabilizing the dentures.

c., deflective occlusal (cuspal interference) A condition of tooth contacts that diverts the mandible from a normal path of closure to centric jaw relation or causes a denture to slide or rotate on its basal seat. *See also* contact, interceptive occlusal.

c., faulty Imperfections in the contact between adjacent teeth. Often leads to food impaction between the teeth, with subsequent initiation or perpetuation of periodontal lesions.

c., initial The first meeting of opposing teeth on elevation of the mandible toward the maxillae.

c., interceptive occlusal An initial contact of teeth that interferes with the normal movement of the mandible. *See also* contact, deflective occlusal.

c., premature *See* deflective occlusal; contact, interceptive occlusal.

c., working A contact of the teeth made on the side of the dental arch toward which the mandible has been moved.

contaminated Made radioactive by the addition of minute quantities of radioactive material.

contamination, radioactive Deposition of radioactive material in any place where it is not desired, and particularly where its presence may be harmful or may constitute a radiation hazard.

contingent (kahn-tǐn′jĕnt) Dependent for effect on something that may or may not occur.

continuant A speech sound in which the speech organs are held relatively fixed during the period of production.

continuing education Postgraduate study offered either in institution of higher learning by groups with an organized dental program or by individuals who are especially qualified in certain areas. Required by some state licensing boards for license renewal. Credit accumulated for special qualifications to join special interest groups.

continuous bar retainer *See* retainer, continuous bar.

continuous clasp *See* retainer, continuous bar.

continuous loop wiring *See* wiring, continuous loop.

contour, *n.* The external shape, form, or surface configuration of an object.

c., buccal The shape of the buccal aspect of a posterior tooth. It normally has occlusocervical convexity, with its greatest prominence at the gingival third of the clinical buccal surface.

c., gingival The shape of the natural or artificial gingiva as it approximates the natural or artificial tooth.

c., height of The greatest convexity of a tooth viewed from a predetermined position.

c., anatomic height of A line encircling a tooth to designate its greatest convexity.

c., surveyed height of A line scribed or marked on a cast, that designates the greatest convexity with respect to a selected path of denture placement and removal.

c., proximal The form of the mesial or distal surface of a tooth.

c., restoration The restoration of a proper contour where surfaces of teeth have been destroyed because of disease processes or excessive wear.

c., tooth A shape of a tooth that is essential to a healthy gingival unit because it enables the bolus of food to be deflected from gingival margins during mastication.

contouring, occlusal Correction, by grinding, of gross disharmonies of the occlusal tooth form (e.g., uneven marginal ridges, plunger cusps, extruded teeth, malpositioned teeth) to establish a harmonious occlusion and protect the periodontium of the tooth.

contouring pliers *See* pliers, contouring.

contra-angle (kahn″trah-ang′gl) More than one angle. An instrument having two or more offsetting angles of such degree that the end of the instrument is kept within 3 mm of the axis of the shaft.

contract **1:** An agreement based on sufficient consideration between two or more competent parties to do or not to do something that is legal. **2:** A legally enforceable agreement between two or more individuals or entities that confers rights and duties on the parties. Common types of contracts include: **3:** Contracts between a dental benefits organization and an individual dentist to provide dental treatment to members of an alternative benefits plan. These contracts define the dentist's duties both to beneficiaries of the dental benefits plan and the dental benefits organization, and usually define the manner in which the dentist will be reimbursed; and **4:** Contracts between a dental benefits organization and a group plan sponsor. These contracts typically describe the benefits of the group plan and the rates to be charged for those benefits.

c., breach of The failure, without legal excuse, to perform an obligation or duty in a contract.

c. dentist A practitioner that contractually agrees to provide services under special terms, conditions and financial reimbursement arrangements.

c. dentistry **1:** Providing dental care under a specific set of guidelines and for a specific set of individuals under an accepted written agreement by the patient, dentist, and employer. **2:** The practice of dentistry whereby the dentist enters into a written agreement with either patients or an employer to provide dental care for a set group of people.

c., express A contract that is an actual agreement between the parties, with the terms declared at the time of making, being stated in explicit language either orally or in writing.

c. fee schedule plan A dental benefits plan in which participating dentists agree to accept a list of specific fees as the total fees for dental treatment provided.

c., implied A contract not evidenced by explicit agreement of the parties but inferred by the law from the acts and circumstances surrounding the transactions.

c., open-end **1:** A contract that permits periodic reevaluation of the dental plan during the contract year. If indicated by the reevaluation, dental services may be deleted or added to achieve a balance between the premium and cost of service provided. **2:** A contract that sets no dollar limits on the total services to be provided to beneficiaries but does list the particular services that will be included in the plan.

c. practice Dental practice in which an employer or third-party administrator contracts directly with a dentist or group of dentists to provide dental services for beneficiaries of a plan. *See also* closed panel.

c. contract term The period of time, usually 12 months, for which a contract is written.

contraception A process or technique for the prevention of pregnancy by means of a medication, device, or method that blocks or alters one or more of the processes of reproduction in such a way that sexual union can occur without impregnation.

contraction **1:** Shortening, shrinkage, or reduction in length or size. **2:** A condition in which teeth or other maxillary and mandibular structures (e.g., the dental arch) are nearer than normal to the median plane.

c., metal Shrinkage associated with the congealing of a metal from its molten state to a solid after having been cast. *See also* expansion, thermal.

c., muscle Development of tension in a muscle in response to a nerve stimulus.

c., muscle, changes in striation bands Alterations in bands of striated muscle during contraction. Striated muscle is composed of a darker A band and a lighter 1 band. Both of these alternating bands develop tension during contraction but not to the same degree. In isometric contraction (clenched teeth), the sarcomere muscle unit remains unchanged in length, whereas the A band (the darker band) actually shortens and the I band (the lighter band) lengthens. When a muscle is passively stretched (as when the mandible is opened by gravity), the A band lengthens relatively more than the I band, and during isotonic contraction practically all the shortening is in the A segment. It is thus concluded that the contractile properties are not the same throughout the sarcomere—the unit of contractility. It is suggested that the darker A band has a greater concentration of contractile substance than the I band and that, in addition to contractile elements, the I band contains elastic noncontractile elements that constitute a series of elastic components throughout the fibril. Thus there is, throughout a fiber, an arrangement of dark, contractile components alternating with lighter, elastic components.

c., muscle, chemical factors in The chemical constituents and action involved in the contraction of muscle fibers. Muscle is a structure whose working units are built up largely from two proteins, actin and myosin, which appear to be organized into separate filaments running longitudinally through the muscle fibers. Neither type of filament runs continuously along the length of the fiber, although the effect is that of a continuous structure. The filaments are organized into a succession of groupings of one type of fiber. Each group is arranged in a regular palisade to overlap the next group of fibers, which are similarly arranged in palisades. This gives a banded appearance to the fiber. The thicker filaments contain myosin and are restricted to the A bands, where they give rise to a higher density and birefringence. The thinner filaments contain actin and extend to either side of the Z band, which is at the center of the I band. When the muscle contracts or is stretched, the two groups of filaments slide past each other like the alternating units of a sliding gate. The controlled sliding motion is presumably brought about through the mediation of oblique cross links between the filaments. These cross links are the structural expression of the biochemical interaction between actin and myosin. The chemical substance that initiates the interaction between these fibrils is adenosine triphosphate (ATP). The final effect of the interaction between ATP, myosin, and actin is to enable the two types of filaments to crawl past each other to create the shortened state of the muscle.

c., concentric muscle Unresisted ordinary shortening of muscle.

c., eccentric muscle Increase in muscle tonus during lengthening of the muscle. Eccentric contraction occurs when muscles are used to oppose movement but not to stop it (e.g., the action of the biceps in lowering the forearm gradually and in a controlled manner). Eccentric contractions are called *isotonic* because the muscle changes length.

c., isometric muscle Increase in muscular tension without a change in muscle length, as in clenching the teeth.

c., isotonic muscle Increase in muscular tension during movement without resistance (either lengthening or shortening), as in free opening and closing of the jaws.

c., postural muscle Maintenance of muscular tension (usually isometric muscular contraction) sufficient to maintain posture.

c., smooth muscle, mechanism of The mechanisms that regulate the functions of smooth muscle fibers. These regulatory mechanisms vary and are affected principally by two methods. First, the parasympathetic and sympathetic nerve fiber endings of the autonomic nervous system form a reticulum around the muscle cells before entering them. The action of these fibers is antagonistic; they act directly on the muscle cell—not on each other. Examples of the structures principally under the control of the autonomic nerve mechanism are the blood vessels and the pilomotor fibers. Second, the selection response to rhythmic activity associated with the automaticity of a viscus or other organ depends on local or hormonal factors. An example of this mechanism is the function of the uterus under the control of the estrogenic hormone.

c., static muscle Contraction in which opposing muscles contract against each other and prevent movement. Fixation action of a muscle in a static contraction is termed *isometric* because it develops tension without changing length.

contractor, independent One who, exercising an independent employment, contracts to do a piece of work according to the conditions of the contract and without being subject to control except as to the result of the work.

contracture A permanent shortening (contraction) of a muscle.

contraindication (kahn″trah-ĭn″dĭ-ka′shŭn) Any symptom or circumstance indicating the inappropriateness of a form of treatment otherwise advisable.

contrast, radiographic (radiographic image) The differences in photographic or film density produced on a radiograph by structural composition of the object radiographed or by varying amounts of radiation.

c., radiographic, long-scale An increased number of grays between the blacks and whites on a radiograph. Higher kilovoltages increase the scale of contrast.

c., radiographic, short-scale A minimum number of grays between the blacks and whites on a radiograph. Lower kilovoltages decrease the scale of contrast.

contributory negligence *See* negligence, contributory.

contributory plan A method of payment for group insurance coverage in which part of the premium is paid by the employee and part is paid by the employer or union.

contributory program A dental benefits program in which the enrollee shares in the monthly premium of the program with the program sponsor (usually the employer). Generally done through payroll deduction.

controlled-release therapeutic systems A drug or hormone delivery system that releases a predetermined amount of drug or hormone into the body over a specified period of time.

control, stress Any method used to diminish or remove the stress load generated by occlusal contact, whether the contact is functional in origin or the result of a habit cycle.

contusion (kahn-tū′zhŭn) A bruise that is usually produced by an impact from a blunt object and that does not cause a break in the skin.

convenience form *See* form, convenience.

convergence, cervical The angle formed between the cervicoaxial inclination of a tooth surface on the one side and a diagnostic stylus of a dental cast surveyor in contact with the tooth at its height of contour.

conversational mode A method of using a computer from an on-line terminal. Transactions originating at a remote point require a response from the central computer's files.

conversion privilege The right of an individual covered by a group dental insurance policy to continue having coverage on a direct payment basis when association with the insured group is terminated.

converter, rotary A motor generator set or unit that when operated by one type of current, produces another (e.g., the conversion of alternating to direct current).

convertin *See* thromboplastin, extrinsic.

coolant (koo′lănt) Air or liquid directed onto a tooth, tissue, or restoration to neutralize the heating effect of a rotary instrument.

Cooley's anemia *See* thalassemia major.

Cooley's trait *See* thalassemia minor.

Coolidge filament transformer, tube *See under appropriate noun.*

coordination Harmonious functioning, such as muscles.
  c. of benefits clause 1: A provision in an insurance contract that when a patient is covered under more than one group dental plan, benefits paid by all plans will be limited to 100% of the actual charges after each deductible has been satisfied. **2:** COB: A method of integrating benefits payable under more than one plan. Benefits from all sources should not exceed 100% of the total charges.

Copal resin A mixed resin of diverse plant origin used in cavity varnishes. The effectiveness is questioned in protecting the pulp from the phosphoric acid in dental cements.

copayment Beneficiary's share of the dentist's fee after the benefits plan has paid.

cope The upper half of a flask in the casting art; hence also the upper, or cavity, side of a denture flask.

coping (thimble) A thin metal covering or cap over a prepared tooth.
  c., paralleling A casting placed over an implant abutment to make it parallel to other natural or implant abutments.
  c., transfer A covering or cap, made of metal, acrylic resin, or other material, and used to position a die in an impression.

copolymer (kō-pahl′ĭ-mer) Polymerization of two or more monomers that have slightly different chemical formulas. Used in dentistry to impart certain desirable physical properties (e.g., flow).

copolymerization (kō-pahl-ĭ-mer-ĭ-ză′shūn) Formation of a copolymer.

coproporphyrinuria (kahp″rō-por″fĭ-rĭ-nū′rē-ah) Presence of an abnormal concentration of coproporphyrin in the urine. Normal values range from 70 to 250μg/day. An increased amount of coproporphyrin III occurs in the urine in clinical lead poisoning, exposure to lead without clinically apparent symptoms, infections, malignant disease, and alcoholic cirrhosis, after ingestion of small amounts of ethanol, or normally in some individuals.

cord(s) A long organ or body that is rounded.
  c., spinal The central nervous system cord contained in the vertebral column. The spinal cord is essential to the regulation and administration of various motor, sensory, and autonomic nerve activities of the body. Through its pathways it conducts impulses from the extremities, trunk, and neck to and from the higher centers and to consciousness. It thus provides for simple reflexes, has control over visceral activities, and participates in the conscious activities of the body.
  c., vocal Membranous structures in the throat that produce sound; the thyroarytenoid ligaments of the larynx. The inferior cords are called the *true vocal cords,* and the superior cords are called the *false vocal cords.*

core The central part. A section of a mold, usually of plaster, made over assembled parts of a dental restoration or construction to record and maintain the relationships of the parts so that the parts can be reassembled in their original positions.
  c., amalgam Foundational replacement of the badly mutilated crown of a tooth whose purpose is to provide a rigid base for retention of a cast crown restoration. The core may be retained by undercuts, slots, pins, or the pulp chamber of an endodontically treated tooth.
  c., cast A metal casting, usually with a post in the canal or a root, designed to retain an artificial crown.
  c., composite Composite resin buildup to provide retention for a cast crown restoration.
  c., laboratory A section of a mold, usually of plaster, made over assembled parts of a dental restoration or construction to record and maintain the relationships of the parts so that the parts can be reassembled in their original positions.

core-vent implant system An ADA provisionally accepted endosseous implant system using the criteria of osseous integration constructed of medical grade titanium alloy after the design of Branemark in which the submergible apical portion is of a hollow-vented design. The superior part is machined to receive a variety of prosthodontic abutments.

corium, gingival (kō′rē-ŭm) The most stable, inert, and mature phase of connective tissue elements of the gingiva lying between the periosteum and the lamina propria mucosae.

cornea The transparent anterior part of the eye.

cornification Conversion of epithelium to a hornlike substance. *Keratinization* is a more specific term implying the formation of true keratin.

coronal Pertaining to the crown portion of teeth.

coronoid process *See* process, coronoid.

coronoidectomy (kor″ō-noid-ĕk′tō-mē) Surgical removal of the coronoid process of the mandible.

corporate dentistry 1: Dental care provided for a specific group of employees within a single business under a contract arrangement or on a salaried basis, with costs borne by the corporation. **2:** A company-owned and operated dental care facility that provides services to employees and sometimes dependents.

corpuscle(s) Any small body, mass, or organ.

c., blood A formed element in the blood. *See also* erythrocyte, leukocyte, lymphocyte, monocyte.

c., Golgi's Small spindle-shaped proprioceptive endorgan located in tendons and activated by stretch.

c., Krause's Bulboid encapsulated nerve endings located in mucous membranes and activated by cold.

c., Meissner's Medium encapsulated nerve endings found in the skin and activated by light touch.

c., Merkel's Specialized sensory nerve endings located in the submucosa of the mouth and activated by light touch.

c., Pacini's Large sensory nerve endings, scattered widely in subcutaneous tissues, joints, tendons, etc., and activated by deep pressure.

c., Ruffini's Specialized sensory nerve organs in the skin and mucous membranes for perceiving heat. Temperatare variations of less than 5° C are not readily received by these end organs.

corrected master cast *See* cast, master, corrected.

correction, occlusal Correction of malocclusion, by whatever means is employed, including the elimination of disharmony of occlusal contacts.

corrective A prescription ingredient designed to compensate for or nullify specific undesirable effects of the principal pharmaceutical agent and the adjuvent.

correlation A statistical procedure used to determine the degree to which two (or more) variables vary together. Correlation does not suggest a cause-effect relationship but only the degree of parallelism or concomitance between the variables; the cause of which may be unknown. The Pearson product-moment correlation (r) is the most frequently used, and this coefficient is used unless another is specified.

c. coefficient number The result of statistical computation, that indicates the strength of the tendency of two or more variables to vary concomitantly. The coefficient is expressed in fractions (i.e., r = 80), ranging from 1 to + 1 that indicates the magnitude of the relationship between the variables. Perfect direct correspondence is expressed by + 1; perfect inverse correspondence by −1; complete lack of correspondence by 0. Fractional values are not read as percents.

c., linear A correlation in which the regression line, that line which best describes the relationship between the two variables, is a straight line, so that for any increase in the magnitude of one variable, there will be a proportional change in the magnitude of the other variable.

c., multiple A complex correlation procedure in which scores on two or more variables are combined to predict scores on another variable called the *dependent variable*.

correspondence Written or typed communication between two individuals or groups of individuals.

corrosion Electrolytic or chemical attack of a surface. Usually refers to the attack of a metal surface.

cortex The outer layer of an organ or other structure.

c., adrenal The outer layer of the adrenal gland, the site of secretion of the adrenocortical hormones.

c., cerebral The outer gray matter of cerebrum, where many of the higher functions—volition, consciousness, conceptualization, sensation, etc.—are carried out.

corticalosteotomy (kor″tĭ-kahl-ŏs′tō-mē) An osteotomy through the cortex at the base of the dentoalveolar segment, which serves to weaken the resistance of the bone to the application of orthodontic forces.

corticoid, adrenal (kor′tē-koid) An adrenal corticosteroid hormone (e.g., 11-dehydrocorticosterone [compound A], corticosterone [compound B], 11-deoxycorticosterone [cortexone, DOC], cortisone [compound E], cortisol [compound F], 11-desoxycortisol [substance S], aldosterone, androgen, progesterone, estrogen, and many other inactive steroids). *See also* aldosterone, androgen, corticosterone, cortisone, estrogens, hydrocortisone, progesterone.

corticosteroid (kor″tĭ-kō-ster′oid) *See* steroid, adrenocortical.

corticosterone (Kendall's compound B) (kor″tĭ-kōster′ōn; kor″tĭ-kos′ter-ōn) An adrenal corticosteroid hormone that is necessary for the maintenance of life in adrenalectomized animals; protects against stress, influences muscular efficiency, and influences carbohydrate and electolyte metabolism.

corticotropin (kor″tĭ-kō-trō′pĭn) A purified preparation of adrenocorticotropic hormone derived from the pituitary gland of animals. *See also* ACTH.

cortin General term for the hormonal secretions of the adrenal cortex.

cortisol *See* hydrocortisone.

cortisone (17-hydroxy-11-dehydrocorticosterone, Kendall's compound E) A hormone produced by the adrenal cortex; a glucocorticoid, 17-hydroxy-11-dehydrocorticosterone; useful in the treatment of rheumatoid arthritis, lupus erythematosus, some allergic conditions, etc. Has marked antiinflammatory properties. Excess production or administration produces signs of hyperadrenocorticalism (Cushing's syndrome) with hyperlipemia and obesity hyperglycemia, edema, etc.

cosmetic orthodontics Limited orthodontic therapy for the purpose of improving appearance, such as the closing of an unsightly diastema between central incisors that presents no other handicap.

cost containment Features of a dental benefits program or of the administration the program designed to reduce or eliminate certain charges to the plan.

cost-effective, *n.* The minimal expenditure of dollars, time, and other elements necessary to achieve the health care result deemed necessary and appropriate.

cost sharing The share of health expenses that a beneficiary must pay, including the deductibles, copayments, coinsurance, and charges over the amount reimbursed by the dental benefits plan.

Costen's syndrome *See* syndrome, Costen's.

cothromboplastin (kŏ-thrahm″bō-plăs′tĭn) *See* thromboplastin, extrinsic.

cotton, absorbent Fibers or hairs of the seed of cultivated varieties of Gossypium herbaceum, so prepared that the cotton readily absorbs liquid.

cotton pliers *See* pliers, cotton.

cotton roll rubber dam clamp. *See* clamp, rubber dam, cotton roll.

Council on Dental Therapeutics An appointed Council within the Division of Scientific Affairs of the American Dental Association directed to study, evaluate, and disseminate information with regard to dental therapeutic agents, their adjuncts, and dental cosmetic agents that are offered to the public or profession.

cough A sudden noisy expulsion of air from the lungs.

   c., gander The characteristic clanging, brassy cough of tracheal obstruction.

count, blood, complete Determination of the number of red blood cells (erythrocytes), white blood cells, and platelets in an accurately measured volume of blood. It usually includes the quantity of hemoglobin per cubic millimeter of blood. A normal red blood count is 4 to 5.5 million cells per cubic millimeter of blood.

count, platelet Determination of the number of platelets in a cubic millimeter of blood. The normal count is 200,000 to 500,000.

count, reticulocyte (rē-tĭk′ū-lō-sīt″) The number of reticulocytes in the circulating blood, giving some indication of bone marrow activity. The number is increased after acute blood loss and after recovery from anemia. The number is decreased in anemias associated with defective red cell or hemoglobin production (nutritional, endocrine, toxic, or displacement anemias). he normal range is 0.5% to 1.5% of the erythrocytes.

count, white blood cell Determination of the number of white blood cells in an accurately measured volume of blood. The normal value is from 4000 to 9000 per cubic millimeter of blood.

   c., differential white blood cell Determination of the number of each type of white blood cell in the peripheral blood. The relative count is obtained by counting the number of each type of cell in every 100 cells. The results are expressed in percentages. The normal figure for neutrophils is 60% to 70%, lymphocytes 20% to 35%, monocytes 2% to 8%, basophils 0% to 1%, and eosinophils 2% to 4%.

counter A device for enumerating ionizing events.

   c., Geiger-Müller (G-M counter, Geiger counter) A highly sensitive gas-filled radiation-measuring device.

   c., proportional A gas-filled radiation detection tube in which the pulse produced is proportional to the number of ions formed in the gas by the primary ionizing particle.

   c., scintillation The combination of phosphor, photomultiplier tube, and associated circuits for counting light emissions produced in the phosphor.

counterdie The reverse image of a die, usually made of a softer and lower fusing metal than the die. It is used to swage metal, wax, or other material over a die. *See also* die.

counterirritant An irritant that blocks perception of pain by diverting attention to the sensation that it produces.

coverage Benefits available to an individual covered under a dental benefits plan.

coverage *See* denture coverage.

covered charges Charges for services rendered or supplies furnished by a dentist that qualify as covered services and are paid for in whole or in part by the dental benefits program. May be subject to deductibles, copayments, coinsurance, annual or lifetime maximums, or table of allowances, as specified by the terms of the contract.

covered person An individual who is eligible for benefits under a dental benefits program.

covered services Services for which payment is provided under the terms of the dental benefits contract.

coverage year The 12-month period over which deductibles and maximum benefits apply for each person.

Coxsackie A disease. *See also* herpangina.

cracked tooth syndrome Transient acute pain experienced occasionally while chewing, which is difficult to locate and to reproduce. Likely to occur among nut crackers, ice crushers, and popcorn eaters. Usually a vertical crack or split in the tooth extending across a marginal ridge through the crown and into the root involving the pulp. Visible by transilluminated light or with the use of disclosing dyes.

Crane-Kaplan pocket marker *See* pocket marker, Crane-Kaplan.

cranial base The bones forming the base of the skull. In cephalometric analysis defined by the angle formed by a line drawn basion to point S (sella turcica) and from point S to point N (fronto-nasal suture).

cranial nerves The twelve pair of nerves emerging from the cranial cavity through various openings in the base of the skull, which are as follows: olfactory, optic, oculomotor, trochlear, trigeminal, abducens, facial, acoustic, glossopharyngeal, vagus, accessory, and hypoglossal.

cranial prosthesis An artificial replacement for a portion of the skull.

craniofacial anomalies Congenital malformations of the skull and face, frequently associated with genetically transmitted syndromes.

craniofacial dysostosis (krā″nē-ō-fā′shŭl dĭs″os-tō′sĭs) *See* dysostosis, craniofacial.

craniosynostosis Premature fusion of the cranial sutures resulting in a malformed head, which may lead to an increase in intracranial pressure and consequential brain damage.

craniofacial templates A series of cephalometric tracings of normal faces by age, sex, and race by which variations in the facial form of a patient can be determined and a treatment objective arranged.

craniometry (krā″nĕ-ahm′ĕ-trē) Study of the measurements of the skull.

craniopharyngioma (krā″nē-o-fah-rĭn″jē-ō′mah) A tumor histologically identical to ameloblastoma that arises from remnants of the craniopharyngeal duct.

craniotabes (krā″nē-ō-tā′bēz) A soft, yielding skull; shallow pitting and thinning of skull bones of infants due to congenital syphilis or rickets.

crater formation Formation of interdental depressions in the gingival tissues and/or subjacent bone; often associated with the destructive effects of necrotizing ulcerative gingivitis.

crazing Formation of small cracks on the surface of structures induced by release on internal stress.

c. of plastic teeth Minute cracks appearing on the surface of plastic teeth.

creosote *See* creosote, N.F. XI.

credit rating Evaluation of any person's responsibility toward meeting financial obligations.

creditor A person to whom a debt is owed by another person.

crenation (krē-nā′shŭn) Wrinkling of the surface of cells as a result of shrinkage in their volume.

c. of tongue Scalloping along the lingual periphery of the tongue caused by the tongue's lying against the lingual surface of the mandibular teeth.

creosote, N.F.XI (wood creosote) A mixture of phenols obtained from wood tar and occasionally used to treat root canals.

crepitus (krĕp′ĭ-tŭs) A crackling sound such as that produced by the rubbing together of fragments of a fractured bone or by air moving in a tissue space.

c., bony The crackling sound noted during auscultation; also the sensation noted during palpation when the fragments of a fractured bone are rubbed together.

crescent, sublingual The crescent-shaped area on the floor of the mouth formed by the lingual wall of the mandible and the adjacent part of the floor of the mouth.

crest A projecting ridge or structure.

c., alveolar *See* bone crest.

c., gingival The coronal margin of the gingival tissue.

crestal resorption Bone resorption at the border or crest of the dental alveolus. This bone loss follows tooth extraction and may result from periodontal infection or through the use of heavy orthodontic forces.

cretin A thyroid-deficient dwarfed individual with mental subnormality.

cretinism (krē′tĭ-rĭzm) **(congenital hypothyroidism) 1:** Marked retardation of physical and mental development caused by congenital lack of secretion of thyrotropic hormone by the pituitary gland. Slow tooth eruption is one of the results. **2:** A thyroid deficiency that results in retardation of physical and mental development.

crevice A narrow opening due to a fissure or a crack.

c., gingival The fissure between the free gingiva and enamel.

crib, Jackson A removable orthodontic appliance retained in position by crib-shaped wires.

crib, lingual An orthodontic appliance consisting of a wire framework suspended lingually to the maxillary incisor teeth; used to obstruct thumb and tongue habits.

crib splint *See* splint, crib.

cribriform Perforated (like a sieve).

c. plate The aveolar bone that forms the tooth socket and to which the periodontal ligament is attached (radiographically the lamina dura).

cricoid cartilage (krī′koid) *See* cartilage, cricoid.

cricoidynia (krī″koi-dĭn′ē-ah) Pain in the cricoid cartilage.

cricothyrotomy (krī″kō-thī-rot′ō-mē) An incision between the cricoid and thyroid cartilages for the purpose of maintaining a patent airway.

cri-du-chat syndrome (krē-doo-shăt') *See* syndrome, cri-du-chat.

crisis, adrenal Acute adrenocortical insufficiency, with clinical manifestations of headache, nausea, vomiting, diarrhea, confusion, costovertebral angle pain, circulatory collapse, and coma. May occur in relation to stress of dental or medical procedures in patients with latent adrenal disease or in patients who have undergone prior ACTH or cortisone therapy, especially without control or termination of therapy.

crisis, thyroid A complication occurring after thyroidectomy, or before or during other surgical procedures where even mild hyperthyroidism is present. It is characterized by tachycardia, a high temperature, nervousness, and occasionally delirium.

cristobalite (krĭs-tō'bah-līt) A form of crystalline silica used in dental casting investments because of its relatively high capacity for thermal expansion and resistance to breaking down by heat.

criteria Predetermined rules or guidelines for dental care, developed by dentists relying on professional expertise, prior experience, and the professional literature, with which aspects of actual instances of dental care may be compared. Explicit criteria are predetermined, specific, and measurable; implicit criteria are implied or understood but not directly expressed.

Crooke's tube *See* x-ray tube, Crooke's.

cross arch bar splint *See* connector.

cross arch bar splint connector *See* connector, cross arch bar splint.

cross arch fulcrum line *See* line, fulcrum, cross arch.

cross arch splinting *See* splinting, cross arch.

cross linkage *See* polymerization, cross.

cross polymerization *See* polymerization, cross.

cross-bite An occlusion with the line of occlusion of the mandibular teeth anterior and/or buccal to the maxillary teeth. *See also* occlusion, cross-bite.

c.-b., anterior Primary or permanent maxillary incisors locked lingual to mandibular incisors.

c.-b., posterior Primary permanent maxillary posterior teeth in lingual position in relation to the mandibular teeth.

cross-examination Questioning of a witness by the party against whom he has been called and examined.

cross-infection The transmission of a communicable disease from one person to another due to poor barrier protection.

cross-resistance *See* resistance, cross-.

cross-section form *See* clasp, flexibility of.

cross-tolerance *See* tolerance, cross-.

Crouzon's disease (kroo-zahnz') *See* dysostosis, craniofacial.

Crouzon's syndrome *See* dysostosis, craniofacial.

crowding A malocclusion characterized by inadequate arch circumference to accommodate the teeth in proper alignment.

crown That portion of a human too.h covered by enamel.

c., anatomic That portion of dentin covered by enamel.

c., artificial A dental prosthesis restoring the anatomy, function, and esthetics of part or all of the coronal portion of the natural tooth.

c., clinical 1: That portion of enamel visibly present in the oral cavity. **2:** The portion of a tooth that is occlusal to the deepest part of the gingival crevice.

c., extra-alveolar clinical The portion of a tooth that extends occlusally or incisally from the junction of the tooth root and the supporting bone.

c., complete A restoration that reproduces the entire surface anatomy of the clinical crown and fits over a prepared tooth stump.

c., complete veneer A restoration that reproduces the total clinical coronal surface contour of the tooth.

c., dowel A restoration that replaces the entire coronal portion of a tooth and derives its retention from a dowel extending into a treated (filled) root canal.

c., faced *See* crown, veneered metal.

c., full, restoration An individual tooth prosthesis encompassing the entire prepared clinical crown. *See also* crown, complete veneer.

c., jacket *See* crown, complete.

c., partial A restoration that covers three or more, but not all, surfaces of a tooth.

c., porcelain-faced An artificial crown that makes use of porcelain inlayed in or veneered onto the labial or buccal surface.

c.-root ratio Relation of the clinical crown to the clinical roots of the teeth—an important consideration in diagnosis, prognosis, and treatment planning.

c., stainless steel A preformed steel crown used for the restoration of badly broken-down primary teeth and first permanent molars. Also used as a temporary restoration of fractured permanent incisors.

c., three-quarter Term frequently used to designate a partial veneer crown.

c., veneered metal A complete crown that has one or more surfaces prepared for and covered by a tooth-colored substance such as porcelain or resin.

c. and bridge prosthodontics The division of prosthodontics that deals with crown restorations and the fixed type of tooth-borne partial denture prosthesis. *See also* prosthodontics, fixed.

Crozat appliance *See* appliance, Crozat.

CRT Abbreviation for cathode-ray tube.

crucible (kroo'sĭ-bl) A vessel or container that will withstand high heat and is used for melting or holding material.

c. former (sprue base) The stand or base into which a

sprued pattern is placed. It establishes the shape or form of the hollowed-out end of the investment in the casting ring, which will receive the molten metal on its course through the sprue hole. *See also* sprue former.

crushing strength *See* strength, compressive.

crust A hard coating surface layer composed of coagulated tissue fluid and blood products mixed with ephithelial and inflammatory cells covering a lesion formed by the rupture of a bulla, vesicle, or pustule.

cryolite (krī'ō-līt) (**sodium aluminum fluoride [Na₃AlF₆]**) A fluoride often used as a flux in the manufacture of silicate cements.

crystal(s) A naturally produced solid. The ultimate units of the substance from which it was formed are arranged systematically.

   c. gold *See* gold, mat.

   c., platinocyanide A chemical substance used in the manufacture of fluorescent screens. Barium platinocyanide was first used by Roentgen for this purpose.

   c., silver halide Silver compounds, usually silver bromide and silver iodide, that are impregnated in the photographic emulsion of film. These compounds, when acted on by actinic rays, are disintegrated, with the formation of metallic silver in a finely divided state. The photographic image results when the film is subjected to processing.

cubic centimeter (cc) Unit of volume sometimes used in prescription writing. For that purpose it may be considered identical with the milliliter (ml). *See also* milliliter.

cubital (kū'bĭ-tal) Pertaining to the forearm.

cubitus (kū'bĭ-tŭs) The forearm.

cuboid (kū'boid) (cuboidal) Resembling a cube in form.

cuboidal *See* cuboid.

culture Growth of microorganisms or other living cells on artificial media.

   c., bacterial Bacterial growth on or in an artificial medium. The medium used may be selective for a given type or genus of organism (e.g., tomato juice agar for lactobacilli).

   c., endodontic Growth of microorganisms obtained from root canals or periapical tissues.

   c. medium A substance, liquid or solid, used for cultivating bacteria.

   c., endodontic medium A specific medium used for endodontic cultures.

cumulative Increasing in effect.

cup, chin 1: An orthopedic device that directs a posterior and/or vertical force to the mandible, through the attachment of a cup fitting over the chin to a headcap. **2:** A drug used to cause muscle relaxation during anesthesia by blocking acetylcholine at the neuromuscular and synaptic junctions.

cure 1: Successful treatment of a disease or wound. **2:** A procedure or reaction that changes a plastic material to a hard material (e.g., vulcanization or polymerization. *See also* process).

curet, curette (kū-rĕt') A periodontal or surgical instrument having a sharp, spoon-shaped working blade; used for debridement. The periodontal curet, available in many sizes and shapes, is used for root and gingival curettage.

curettage (kū"rĕ-tahzh') Scraping or cleaning with a curet.

   c., apical (apoxesis) Curettement of diseased periapical tissue without excision of the root tip. *See also* curettage, subgingival.

   c., infrabony pocket Enucleation, by means of suitable instrumentation, of the inflammatory soft tissue elements lying within and surrounding the crest of an infrabony resorptive defect; also includes the débridement and planing of the root surface of the pocket.

   c., root Débridement and planning to smoothness of the root surface of a tooth in order to eliminate accretions on the root and to provide a suitable environment for the return of the gingival tissues to a state of health.

   c., subgingival The process of debridement of the epithelial attachment, the ulcerated and entire (pocket) epithelium, and subjacent inflamed and altered gingival corium; usually results in resolution of the inflammatory process and desirable shrinkage and repair of the edematous tissue.

Curette *See* curet.

curie (kū'rē) A measurement of radioactivity produced by the disintegration of unstable elements. The curie is that quantity of a radioactive nuclide in which the number of disintegrations per second is 3.700×10^{10}. Since the curie is a relatively large unit, the millicurie (0.00 curie) and the microcurie (one millionth of a curie) are more often used. It is important to note that the curie is based on the number of nuclear disintegrations and not on the number or amount of radiations emitted.

curing The act of polyimerization.

   c., denture, *See* denture curing.

cursor The pointer on the video screen that indicates the current position on the screen of the terminal.

current A measure of the number of electrons per second that pass a given point on a conductor.

   c., alternating A current that alternately changes its direction of flow. It usually consists of 60 complete cycles/sec.

   c., coagulating An electrical current, delivered by a needle, ball, or other variously shaped points, that coagulates tissue.

   c., direct An electrical current in which the electron

flow is in only one direction.

c., galvanic A direct current created by a battery. An electromotive force of 500 mV may exist in the mouth.

c., saturation The maximum current in a roentgen-ray tube that fully uses all electrons that are available at the cathode for the production of roentgen rays.

current dental terminology (CDT) A listing of descriptive terms and identifying codes developed by the American Dental Associatlon (ADA) for reporting dental services and procedures to dental benefits plans.

current procedural terminology (CPT) A listing of descriptive terms and identifying codes developed by the American Medical Association (AMA) for reporting practitioner services and procedures to medical plans and medicare.

curvature, occlusal *See* curve of occlusion.

curve Nonangular deviation from a straight line or surface.

c., alignment *See* alignment.

c., anti-Monson *See* curve, reverse.

c., compensating The curvature of alignment of the occlusal surfaces of the teeth that is developed to compensate for the paths of the condyles as the mandible moves from centric to eccentric positions. A means of maintaining posterior tooth contacts on the molar teeth and providing balancing contacts on dentures when the mandible is protruded. Corresponds to the curve of Spee of natural teeth.

c., dose-effect A curve relating the dose of radiation with the effect produced.

c., milled-in *See* path, milled-in.

c., Monson The curve of occlusion, described by Monson, in which each cusp and incisal edge touch or conform to a segment of the surface of a sphere 8 inches (20 cm) in diameter, with its center in the region of the glabella. *See also* curve, compensating.

c. of occlusion (occlusal curvature) 1: A curved occlusal surface that makes simultaneous contact with the major portion of the incisal and occlusal prominences of the existing teeth. **2:** The curve of a dentition on which the occlusal surfaces of the teeth lie. *See also* curve, reverse.

c., reverse A curve of occlusion that is convex upward when viewed in the frontal plane.

c., sine The wave form of an altemating current, characterized by a rise from zero to maximum positive potential, then descending below zero to its maximum negative value, and then rising to its maximum positive potential, to fall to zero again.

c. of Spee 1: Anatomic curvature of the occlusal alignment of teeth, beginning at the tip of the lower canine, following the buccal cusps of the natural premolars and molars, and continuing to the anterior border of the ramus, as described by von Spee. **2:**

The curve of the occlusal surfaces of the arches in vertical dimension, brought about by a dipping downward of the mandibular premolars, with a corresponding adjustment of the upper premolars.

c., survival A curve obtained by plotting the number or percentage of organisms surviving at a given time against a given dose of radiation. A curve showing the percentage of individuals surviving at different intervals after a particular dosage of radiation.

c. of Wilson By-product term of the thinking that supported the theory that occlusion should be spherical. The curve in the lower arch is concave, whereas the one in the upper arch is convex.

Cushing's syndrome *See* syndrome, Cushing's.

cusp A notably pointed or rounded eminence on or near the masticating surface of a tooth.

c. angle *See* angle, cusp.

c. height The shortest distance between the deepest part of the central fossa of a posterior tooth and a line connecting the points of the cusps of the tooth.

c., shoeing *See* restoration of cusps.

cusp-fossa relations Organic relations between a stamp cusp and its fossa.

cuspal interference *See* contact, deflective occlusal.

cuspid *See* canine.

cuspidor A fixture provided on some dental operating units into which patients can expectorate. In current practice, most operating fields are kept clear of saliva by high volume suction saliva ejectors.

customary fee The fee level determined by the administrator of a dental benefits plan from actual submitted fees for a specific dental procedure to establish the maximum benefit payable under a given plan for that specific procedure. *See also* fee, usual; fee reasonable.

cuticle The outer layer of the skin. Also, a layer that covers the free surface of an epithelial cell.

c., primary 1: The transitory remnants of the enamel organ and oral epithelium covering the enamel of a tooth after eruption. Synonym: Nasmyth's membrane. **2:** Believed to be the last substance formed by ameloblasts, mediating the attachment of ameloblasts to the enamel.

c., secondary 1: The second cuticle formed when the ameloblasts are replaced by the oral epithelium. It then covers the primary cuticle on the enamel and is the only cuticle on the cementum. **2:** A keratinized pedicle found between the gingival epithelium and the surface of a tooth.

cuticula dentis (ku-tik'u-lah den'tis) *See* cuticle, primary.

cutting instrument *See* instrument, cutting.

CVA See accident, cerebrovascular.

cyanocobalamin (sī″ah-nō-kō-băl′ah-mĭn) *See* vitamin B complex.

cyanosis (sī-ah-nō′sĭs) Characteristic bluish tinge or color of the skin and mucous membranes associated with reduction in hemoglobin brought about by inadequate respiratory change (5 gm/100 ml are necessary for color to be perceptible).

cyclamate A noncaloric artificial sweetening agent used in conjunction with saccharin presently banned by the FDA because of its carcinogenic potential.

cycle A succession of events.

  c., chewing A complete course of movement of the mandible during a single masticatory stroke.

  c., masticating Three-dimensional patterns of mandibular movements formed during the chewing of food.

cyclothymia (sī″klō-thī′mē-ah) *See* psychosis, manicdepressive.

cyclotron (sī′klō-trahn) A device for accelerating charged particles to high energies by means of an alternating electrical field between electrodes placed in a constant magnetic field.

cylindroma (sĭl-ĭn-drō′mah) An adenocystic basal cell carcinoma of the salivary glands. A malignant tumor that may occur in the sublingual, submandibular, parotid, or labial salivary glands. *See also* carcinoma, adenocystic.

cyclophosphamide An alkylating agent with antitumor properties, that also acts as a suppressor of B-cell activity and antibody formation, used to treat autoimmune diseases.

cyst (sĭst) A pathologic space in bone or soft tissue containing fluid or semifluid material and, in the oral regions, almost always lined by epithelium.

  c., branchial (branchial cleft cyst) Soft tissue cyst usually Seen on the lateral side of the neck, arising from epithelial illusions within the cervical lymph nodes. Microscopic examination shows the epithelial lining of stratified squamous epithelium surrounded by lymphoid tissue.

  c., calcifying and keratinizing odontogenic A cyst arising from odontogenic epithelium, with abundant production of keratin-containing ghost cells and areas of dystrophic calcification. This lesion has no age or sex distribution.

  c., dental *See* cyst, periodontal.

  c., dentigerous An epithelium-lined sac filled with fluid or semifluid material that surrounds the crown of an unerupted tooth or odontoma.

  c., dentoalveolar *See* cyst, periodontal.

  c., dermoid An epithelium-lined sac with one or more skin appendages (hair follicles, sweat glands, sebaceous glands) in its wall. It may be found in the floor of the mouth. This lesion should not be confused with the teratomatous dermoid cyst of the ovary.

  c., epidermoid An epithelium-lined sac containing fluid; possesses characteristics of the epidermis but does not have the skin appendages seen in dermoid cysts.

  c., eruption A dentigerous cyst that causes a clinically evident bulging of the overlying alveolar ridge.

  c., extravasation *See* cyst, traumatic.

  c., fissural A cyst that arises from the enslaved epithelium in maxillary suture lines due to fusion of the embryonic processes of the facial bones.

  c., follicular An odontogenic cyst that arises from the epithelium of the tooth bud and dental lamina. Follicular cysts include dentigerous, primordial, and multilocular cysts.

  c., lateral follicular A follicular cyst occurring on the lateral surface of a tooth, usually near the cementodentinoenamel junction. *See also* cyst, follicular.

  c., globulomaxillary An epithelium-lined sac formed at the junction point of the globular (median nasal) and maxillary processes. It is seen as a pear-shaped radiolucency between the maxillary lateral incisor and canine, and it separates their roots.

  c., hemorrhagic An extravasation cyst or lesion; traumatic bone cyst or lesion. This is not a true cyst but is probably a defect in the bone produced by traumia and repair. It appears as a definite radiolucent area with a sharply marked radiopaque border. It contains air and is lined by a thin endosteum. *See also* cyst, solitary bone.

  c., incisive canal *See* cyst, nasopalatine.

  c., indefinite bone *See* cyst, traumatic.

  c., lateral *See* cyst, periodontal.

  c., median palatal An epithelium-lined sac containing fluid; appears as a radiolucency in the midline of the palate. It is of developmental origin.

  c., mucous (mucocele) An epithelium-lined sac containing mucus. Mucous cysts in the sinus may appear as spherical, radiopaque areas.

  c., multilocular A follicular cyst containing many loculi, or spaces, and not associated with a tooth.

  c., nasoalveolar A fluid-containing sac lined by epithelium and located at the ala of the nose. A developmental cyst, it may simulate a nasal or periapical abscess.

  c., nasopalatine (nasopalatine duct) A cyst arising within the nasopalatine canal. Radiographically it may appear as a heart-shaped radiolucency between the maxillary central incisors. Histologically it may show mucous cells and nerve bundles in addition to a lining of stratified squamous or respiratory epithelium. The incisive canal cyst and the cyst of the papilla incisiva are the recognized subtypes.

  c., odontogenic An epithelium-lined sac produced from the tooth-forming tissues (e.g., primordial, dentigerous, and periodontal cysts).

  c., periapical *See* cyst, radicular.

  c., periodontal (dental root cyst, dentoalveolar cyst, lateral cyst, periapical cyst) An epitheliumlined sac containing fluid. Usually found at the apex of a pulp-involved tooth. Lateral types occur less frequently along the side of the root.

c., primordial An epithelium-lined sac containing fluid and appearing as a radiolucency in the jaws. It is derived from an enamel organ before any hard tissue is formed.

c., radicular (periapical cyst, root end cyst) A cyst that has a fibrous connective tissue wall and a lining of stratified squamous epithelium and that is attached to the apex of the root of a tooth with a nonvital pulp or a defective root canal filling.

c., residual An odontogenic cyst that remains within the jaw after the removal of the tooth with which it was associated. May be radicular or follicular.

c., root end *See* cyst, radicular.

c., solitary bone A pathologic bone space of disputed origin that may be either empty or filled with fluid. It may have a delicate connective tissue lining.

c., thyroglossal duct An epithelium-lined sac containing fluid formed in portions of the incompletely involuted thyroglossal duct, which connects the primitive pharynx with the tongue in embryonic life. These cysts may appear in the midline at any region from the subhyoid to the base of the tongue.

c., traumatic (extravasation cyst, extravasation lesion, traumatic bone lesion) A radiolucent lesion appearing chiefly in the mandible as a well-defined area with a radiopaque border; clinically it appears as a cavity lined by extremely thin periosteum and filled with air. Assumed to be caused by injury to young spongy bone, hemorrhage resorption, and then walling off by cortical bone. *See also* cyst, solitary bone.

cystadenoma (sĭs-tăd″ĕ-nō′mah) An adenoma with the development of cystic spaces due to dilation of acinar or ductal structures.

c., papillary, lymphomatosum (Warthin's tumor) A benign salivary gland tumor that consists of numerous cystic spaces lined by a double layer of epithelium. A dense aggregate of lymphocytes containing germinal centers surrounds the cystic spaces.

cytology The study of the anatomy, physiology, pathology, and chemistry of a cell.

cy., exfoliative (sĭ-tahl′ō jē) Study of desquamated cells.

cytomegalic inclusion disease *See* disease, salivary gland.

cytomegalovirus (CMV) A visceral disease virus, a member of the group of herpetoviruses having special affinity for the salivary glands. Considered one of the indicator infections of AIDS.

cytozyme (sī′tō-zīm) *See* thromboplastin.

D

Dalton's law *See* law, Dalton's.

dam A barrier to the passage of moisture or saliva.

   d., post- *See* seal, posterior palatal.

   d., rubber A thin sheet of latex rubber used to isolate a tooth or teeth and keep them dry during a dental procedure.

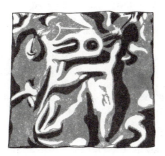

Rubber dam

   d., rubber punch A hand-punch instrument with progressively larger openings, used to make a hole(s) in the rubber dam.

damages Compensation or indemnity that may be recovered at law by any person who has suffered loss, detriment, or injury to person, property, or rights through the unlawful act or negligence of another.

   d., compensatory A sum that compensates the injured party for injury only.

   d., exemplary (punitive damages) Damages awarded to the plaintiff over those that will barely compensate for property loss. Such compensation may be awarded when the wrong done to the plaintiff involved violence, malice, or fraud by the defendant. The object is to provide compensation for mental suffering or loss of pride. It may be employed as punishment of the defendant.

   d., nominal A trifling sum awarded to a plaintiff in an action in which there is no substantial loss or injury to be compensated but in which the law still recognizes a technical invasion of rights or a breach of the defendant's duty. Also awarded in cases in which, although there has been a real injury, the plaintiff's evidence is not sufficient to show its amount.

   d., punitive *See* damages, exemplary.

Darier's disease *See* disease, Darier's.

darkroom A completely lightproof room or cubicle that is used in the processing of photographic, medical, and dental films. *See also* safe-light.

Darvon Brand name for porpoxyphene hydrochloride, a mild centrally acting narcotic analgesic agent.

data A collection of facts and figures, often called *raw data* to emphasize that they are unprocessed. Data are processed and interpreted to yield information.

   d. base An organized collection of data. A medical data base is all the information that exists in the practice at any time.

   d. processing The collection of data, processing of the data to obtain usable information, and communication of this usable information.

   d. set A hardware device that converts digital pulses (square waveform) into modulated frequencies (sinusoidal wave) for transmission, a process called *modulation*. It also converts modulated frequencies into voltage pulses, a process called *demodulation*. Synonym: modem.

daughter (decay product) A nuclide formed from the radioactive decay of another nuclide called the *parent*.

day sheet A form that permits systematic record keeping of treatment of patients and of monies received and spent.

Day's syndrome *See* syndrome, Riley-Day.

DDC Abbreviation for dideoxycytidine. *See* dideoxycytidine.

DDI Abbreviation for dideoxyinosine. *See* dideoxyinosine.

dead Without life; destitute of life.

   d. space *See* space; physiologic dead space; anatomic dead space.

deaf Without usable hearing.

deafen To make deaf; to cause the loss of all usable hearing.

deafness (dĕf'nĕss) Impaired hearing.

   d., central Impaired hearing due to interference with cerebral auditory pathways or in the auditory centers in the brain (e.g., cerebrovascular accidents and other degenerative brain diseases). Hearing aids are of little benefit.

d., conduction *See* deafness, transmission.

d., nerve Impaired hearing due to pathologic conditions in the auditory nerve or the hair cells of the organ of Corti in the inner ear (e.g., high-tone deafness, which comes with age, damage to the organ of Corti by noise, or a tumor of an auditory nerve). Hearing aids are usually of little benefit.

d., transmission (conduction deafness) Impaired hearing due to interference with passage of sound waves through the external ear (e.g., wax) or middle ear (e.g., otitis media, aerotitis media, or otosclerosis). May be characterized by greater interference with hearing of low tones. Hearing aids that amplify may help.

deanesthesiant (dē″an-ĕs-thē′zē-ănt) Anything that will arouse a patient from a state of anesthesia.

death (deth) **1:** Cessation of life; the stoppage of life beyond the possibility of resuscitation. **2:** The cause or occasion of loss of life.

d., brain In addition to the generally accepted definition of death, some states, either by statute or court decision, have added a ″brain death″ definition to the law, applicable where there has been an irreversible cessation of brain function.

debility (dē-bĭl′ĭ-tē) Weakness; lack of strength; asthenia.

debridement (dā-brēd-maw′) Removal of foreign material and or devitalized tissue from the vicinity of a wound.

d., epithelial (de-epithelization) *See* curettage, subgingival.

debris (dĕ-brē′) Foreign material or particles loosely attached to a surface.

d. of Malassez (măl-ah-sā′) Remnants of Hertwig's epithelial root sheath within the periodontal ligament.

debt A sum of money due by agreement; the contract may or may not be express and does not necessarily fix the precise amount to be paid.

debug To locate and correct any errors in a computer program.

decalcification (dē-kăl″sĭ-fĭ-kā′shŭn) Loss or removal of calcium salts from calcified tissues.

decay To deteriorate, putrefy.

d., dental *See* caries, dental.

d. product *See* daughter.

d., radioactive Disintegration of the nucleus of an unstable nuclide by the spontaneous emission of charged particles and/or photons.

d., senile *See* caries, dental, senile.

decibel (dĕs′ĭ-bĕl) A logarithmic ratio unit that indicates by what proportion one intensity level differs from another.

deciduous (dē-sĭd′ū-ŭs) That which will be shed. Pertaining specifically to the first dentition of humans or animals.

d. dentition Teeth that will be shed.

d. teeth The teeth constituting the first dentition.

declaration and provision for affairs A systematic statement of the affairs and estate of a person, in which all assets and property are listed.

decompression, nerve Release of pressure on a nerve trunk by surgical widening of the bony canal.

deductible 1: A stipulated sum the covered person must pay toward the cost of dental treatment before the benefits of the program go into effect. The deductible may be annual or payable only once and may vary in amount from program to program. **2:** The amount of dental expense for which the beneficiary is responsible before a third party will assume any liability for payment of benefits. Deductible may be an annual or one-time charge. and may vary in amount from program to program. (*See* family deductible.)

d. amount That portion of dental care expense the insured must pay before the plan's benefits begin.

d. clause A provision in an insurance contract stipulating that the insurer will pay only that amount that is in excess of a specified amount.

deep bite *See* overbite.

deep sensibility *See* sensibility, deep.

de-epithelization (dē-ĕp″ĭ-thē″lĭ-zā′shŭn) *See* debridement, epithelial.

DEF rate *See* rate, DEF.

defamation (dĕf-ah-mā′shŭn) The act of detracting from the reputation of another. The offense of injuring a person's reputation by false and malicious statements.

default An omission of that which should be done; failure to fulfill an obligation or a promise.

defect Absence of some legal requisite; an imperfection.

d., operative Incomplete repair of bone after root resection or periapical curettage.

d., osseous A concavity in the bone surrounding one or more teeth, resulting from periodontal disease.

d., speech Any deviation of speech that is outside the range of acceptable variation in a given environment.

defective, mental A mentally subnormal individual. A person in whom a basic nervous system defect may be assumed because of social and intellectual deficiencies (e.g., persons afflicted with microcephaly, hydrocephalus, mongolism).

defendant The party against whom relief or recovery is sought in a lawsuit.

defense The reasons, in law or fact, offered by the defendant in a legal proceeding as to why the plaintiff should not prevail.

   d. cell *See* cell, defense.

defibrillation (dē-fĭ″brĭ-lā′shŭn) The arrest of fibrillation, usually that of the cardiac ventricles. An intense alternating current is briefly passed through the heart muscle, throwing it into a refractory state.

defibrillator (dē-fĭ′brĭ-lā″tor) An apparatus for defibrillating the ventricles of the heart.

deficiency A lack or defect.

   d., ac-globulin *See* parahemophilia.

   d., dietary An inadequate amount of food intake or an insufficiency of any of the food elements necessary for proper nutrition.

   d., gingival hyperplasia in vitamin A Hyperplastic and hyperkeratotic gingival changes occurring with decreased ingestion, diminished absorption, faulty use, or overexcretion of vitamin A. For example, in diabetes the liver often cannot effectively convert carotene to vitamin A.

   d., mineral A form of nutritional deficiency produced by the inadequate ingestion, absorption, use, and/or overexcretion of essential inorganic elements such as calcium, magnesium, or phosphorus.

   d., nicotinic acid Deficiency of nicotinic acid in the diet, resulting in acute erythematous stomatitis, papiilary atrophy of the tongue, and ulcerative gingivitis.

   d., plasma thromboplastic antecedent *See* hemophilia C.

   d., protein A malnutritive state produced by inadequate ingestion, absorption, use, or overexcretion of essential protein elements. Degenerative lesions produced in the periodontium include osteoporosis of the alveolar and supporting bone and disappearance of fibroblasts and connective tissue fibers of the periodontal membrane.

   d., PTA *See* hemophilia C.

definition (image) The property of projected images relating to their sharpness, distinctness, or clarity of outline. Penumbra width is a measure of definition. *See also* resolution.

deflective occlusal contact *See* contact, deflective occlusal.

deformation (dē″for-mă′shŭn) Distortion; disfigurement.

   d., elastic Term applied when the alteration in shape of a material disappears as the causative load is removed.

   d., inelastic Deformation occurring when a material is stressed beyond its elastic limit.

   d., permanent Deformation occurring beyond the yield point so that the structure will not return to its original dimensions after removal of the applied force.

deformity Distortion or disfigurement of a portion of the body; may be congenital, familial, hereditary, acquired, pathologic, or surgical.

   d., gingival Deviation from the normal gingival topographic and architectural pattern.

degeneration, ballooning A condition seen in vesicles of viral origin, in which epithelial cells are washed from the vesicle wall. The cells swell and their nuclei undergo amitotic division, resulting in multinucleated giant cells that may be seen floating in vesicular fluid.

degeneration , basophilic granular (ba″so-til′ik) *See* basophilia.

degenerative joint disease A term to describe osteoarthritis. Osteoarthritis is a noninflammatory process as opposed to rheumatoid arthritis. Osteoarthritis occurs more frequently in women after the age of 40.

degloving Intraoral surgical exposure of the bony mandibular anterior region. This procedure can be performed in the posterior region if necessary.

deglutition (dĕg″loo-tĭsh′ŭn) **(swallowing)** A succession of muscular contractions from above downward or from the front backward; propels food from the mouth toward the stomach. The action is generally initiated at the lips; it proceeds back through the oral cavity, and the food is moved automatically along the dorsum of the tongue. When the food is ready for swallowing, it is passed back through the fauces. Once the food is beyond the fauces and in the pharynx, the soft palate closes off the nasopharynx, and the hyoid bone and larynx are elevated upward and forward. This action keeps food out of the larynx and dilates the esophageal opening so that the food may be passed quickly toward the stomach by peristaltic contractions. The separation between the voluntary and the involuntary characteristics of this wave of contractions is not sharply defined. At birth the process is already well established as a highly coordinated activity, i.e., the swallowing reflex.

degradation (dĕg-rah-dā′shŭn) Reduction of a chemical compound to a less complex compound.

degrees of freedom (df) A statistic, based on the number of observations and groups in a study, that is necessary to determine statistical significance. One looks up the degrees of freedom and the significance level in a table of significance values to determine if the magnitude of the value obtained is significant. Used with the t-test, chi square, analysis of variance, and correlation.

dehiscence (dē-hĭs′ĕns) A fissural defect in the facial alveolar plate extending from the free margin apically.

dehiscent (dē-hĭs′ ĕnt) Opened wide; fissured.

   d. mandibular canal A condition caused by bone resorption that leaves the mandibular canal without a covering or roof of bone.

dehydration (dē″hĭ-drā′shŭn) **1:** Removal of water (e.g., from the body or tissue). **2:** Decrease in serum fluid coupled with the loss of interstitial fluid from the body. Dehydration is associated with disturbances in fluid and electrolyte balance.

d. of gingivae The drying of gingival tissue, leading to a lowered tissue resistance, which can result in gingival inflammation; Seen in mouth breathing.

delayed expansion *See* expansion, delayed.

delict (dē-lĭkt′) A wrong or an injury; an offense; a violation of public or private obligation.

delinquent, *adj.* (dē-lĭng′kwĕnt) Pertaining to a debt or claim that is due and unpaid at the time due.

delirium (de-lir′ĭ-ŭm) A condition of mental excitement, confusion, and clouded sensorium, usually with hallucinations, illusions, and delusions; precipitated by toxic factors in diseases or drugs.

d. tremens A delirious state marked by distressing delusions, illusions, and hallucinations, constant tremor, fumbling movements of the hands, insomnia, and great exhaustion.

delivery Transfer of the possession of personal property from one person to another.

delta dental plan An active member organization of the Delta Dental Plans Association, formed and guided by state dental societies to provide prepaid dental care to the public on a group basis.

demand In economics, refers to the buying of services or goods; in dental care, generally denotes the active request for and purchase of dental care services.

dementia A progressive, organic mental disorder characterized by chronic personality disintegration, confusion, disorientation, stupor, deterioration of intellectual capacity and function, and impairment or control of memory, judgment, and impulses (e.g., senile psychosis, also associated with AIDS).

Demerol (dĕm′er-ahl) Trade name for meperidine hydrochloride.

demurrer (dē-mĕr′ĕr) An admission of the facts charged by the opponent while maintaining that those facts are legally insufficient to establish liability.

denasality (dē-nā-săl′ĭ-tē) The quality of the voice when the nasal passages are obstructed, preventing adequate nasal resonance during speech.

dendrite (dĕn′drīt) **1:** Fingerlike projections formed during the solidification of crystalline materials. **2:** A branched, treelike protoplasmic process of a neuron that carries nerve impulses toward the cell body. *See also* axon.

denervation (dē″ner-vā′shŭn) Sectioning or removal of a nerve to interrupt the nerve supply to a part.

dens in dente (dĕnz ĭn dĕn′tā) (dens invaginatus, gestant odontoma) Anomaly of the tooth found chiefly in upper lateral incisors; characterized by invagination of the enamel, giving a radiographic appearance that suggests a ″tooth within a tooth.″

dens invaginatus (dĕnz ĭn-văj-ĭn-ā′tŭs) *See* dens in dente.

Densite (dĕn′sīt) Trade name for a form of alpha-hemihydrate with a low setting expansion and greater hardness; used for dies, models, and casts; sometimes referred to as a Class II stone.

densitometer (dĕn″sĭ-tŏm′ĕ-ter) An instrument for determining the degree of darkening of developed photographic or x-ray film, based on the use of a photocell to measure the light transmission through a given area of the film.

density Concentration of matter, measured by mass per unit volume.

d., radiographic The degree of darkening of exposed and processed photographic or x-ray film, expressed as the logarithm of the opacity of a given area of the film.

dental Relating to the teeth.

d. arch *See* arch, dental.

d. assistant *See* assistant, dental.

d. benefits organization Any organization offering a dental benefits plan. Also known as dental plan organization.

d. benefits plan Entitles covered individuals to specified dental services in return for a fixed, periodic payment made in advance of treatment. Such plans often include the use of deductibles, coinsurance, and/or maximums to control the cost of the program to the purchaser.

d. benefits program The specific dental benefits plan being offered to enrollees by the sponsor.

d. care Treatment of the teeth and their supporting structures.

d. caries *See* caries, dental.

d. cement *See* cement, dental.

d. chart *See* chart, dental.

d. cooperative A dental facility organized to provide dental services for the benefit of subscribers and not for profit. There is no discrimination as to who may subscribe, and each subscriber has equal rights and voice in the control of the cooperative. The operation of the cooperative usually rests with a lay board of directors elected by subscribers.

d. dysfunction *See* dysfunction, dental.

d. engine *See* engine, dental.

d. floss Waxed or plain thread of nylon or silk used to clean the interdental areas; an aid in oral physiotherapy.

d. geriatrics *See* geriatrics.

d. granuloma *See* granuloma, dental.

d. handpiece *See* handpiece.

d. history *See* history.

d. hygienist *See* hygienist, dental.

d. implant *See* implant.

d. insurance A policy that insures against the expense of treatment and care of dental disease and accident to teeth.

d. jurisprudence *See* jurisprudence, dental.

d. laboratory technician *See* technician, dental laboratory.

d. material *See* material, dental.

d. plan Any organized method for the financing of dental care.

d. porcelain *See* porcelain, dental.

d. prepayment A system for budgeting the cost of dental services in advance of their receipt.

d. prosthetic restoration *See* prosthesis, dental.

d., public health Preferably called *public health dentistry*, this is a specialty of dentistry that deals with dental health on a community, regional, or national basis rather than on a provider-to-patient basis. However, some programs sponsored by public health dental agencies do provide for direct patient care for otherwise underserved populations. *See also* community dentistry.

d. records Confidential documents containing the clinical and financial data of the dental patient.

d. review committee A group of dentists and administrative personnel that reviews questionable dental claims and can suggest policy decisions regarding dental care.

d. senescence *See* senescence, dental.

d. service corporation A legally constituted, not-for-profit organization that negotiates and administers contracts for dental care. Delta Dental Plans and Blue Cross/Blue Shield Plans are such plans.

d. staff The personnel employed or engaged by the dentist or his/her agent to conduct the assignable professional and management functions of the dental clinic, office, or practice.

d. stone *See* stone, dental.

d. tape *See* tape, dental.

d. unit *See* unit, dental.

dentate (den'tāt) Having teeth.

denticle (den'tĭ-kl) **(endolith, pulp nodule, pulpstone)** A calcified body found in the pulp chamber of a tooth; it may be composed either of irregular dentin (true denticle) or an ectopic calcification of pulp tissue (false denticle).

dentifrice A pharmaceutical compound used in conjunction with the toothbrush to clean and polish the teeth. Contains a mild abrasive, a detergent, flavoring agent, binder, and occasionally deodorants and various medicaments designed as caries preventives, (e.g., antiseptics).

d. abrasion *See* abrasion, dentifrice.

dentin (den'tĭn) **(dentine)** The portion of the tooth that lies subjacent to the enamel and cementum. Consists of an organic matrix on which mineral (calcific) salts are deposited; pierced by tubules containing filamentous protoplasmic processes of the odontoblasts that line the pulpal chamber and canal. It is of mesodermal origin.

d., carious Dentin that is involved in or affected by the carious process.

d., residual carious *See* caries, dental, residual.

d. dysplasia *See* dysplasia, dentinal.

d. eburnation (ē-bŭr-nā'shŭn) A change in carious teeth in which the softened and decalcified dentin assumes a hard, brown, polished appearance.

d., hereditary opalescent *See* dentinogenesis imperfecta.

d., hyperesthesia of Excessive sensibility of dentin.

d. irritation (tertiary dentin, reparative dentin) Formed in response to an injury or irritant.

d., sclerotic *See* dentin, transparent.

d., secondary Dentin formed or deposited on the walls of pulp chambers and canals subsequent to the complete formation of the tooth; due to certain metabolic disturbances that result in irritation and stimulation of the odontoblasts to renewed activity.

d., transparent (sclerotic dentin) Dentin formed as a defense mechanism in reaction to various stimuli. Dental tubules are obliterated by deposits of calcium salts that are harder and denser than normal dentin. This dentin appears transparent in ground sections.

d. wall The portion of the wall of a prepared cavity that consists of dentin.

dentine *See* dentin.

dentinocemental junction (den-te″nō-sē-men'tal) *See* junction, dentinocemental.

dentinoenamel junction *See* junction, dentinoenamel.

dentinogenesis imperfecta (den″tĭ-nō-jen'ĕ-sĭs ĭm-per fĕk'tah) **(hereditary opalescent dentin) 1:** Disturbance of the dentin of genetic origin; characterized by early calcification of the pulp chambers and root canals, marked attrition, and an opalescent hue to the teeth. **2:** A localized form of mesodermal dysplasia affecting the dentin of the tooth. It may be hereditary and may be associated with osteogenesis imperfecta. **3:** A hereditary condition associated with a defect in dentin formation; the enamel remains normal.

dentinoma (den″tĭ-nō'mah) An odontogenic tumor composed of regular or irregular dentin.

dentist One whose profession is to treat diseases and injuries of the teeth and oral cavity and to construct and insert restorations of and for the teeth, jaws, and mouth.

dentistry The science and art of preventing, diagnosing, and treating diseases, injuries, and malformations of the teeth, jaws, and mouth and of replacing lost or absent teeth and associated structures.

d., forensic *See* jurisprudence, dental.

d., four-handed The technique of chairside operating in which four hands are kept busy working in the oral cavity simultaneously.

d., operative The branch of oral health service concerned with operations to restore or reform the hard dental tissues (e.g., operations necessitated by caries, trauma, impaired function and for improvement of appearance).

d., prosthetic *See* prosthodontics.

d., psychosomatic Dentistry that concerns itself with the mind-body relationship.

d., washed-field Constant flushing of the operative field with an irrigant (usually water) and the evacuation of the washing (debris, etc.) from the mouth by vacuum airstream. *See also* technique, hydroflow.

dentition (děn-tǐsh'ŭn) The natural teeth in position in the dental arches.

d., artificial Artificial substitutes for the natural dentition. *See also* denture.

d., deciduous *See* dentition, primary.

d., mixed The complement of teeth in the jaws after the eruption of some of the permanent teeth but before all the deciduous teeth are absent.

d., natural The natural teeth, as considered collectively, in the dental arches.

d., permanent (secondary dentition, permanent teeth) The 32 teeth of adulthood that either replace or are added to the complement of deciduous teeth.

d., primary The teeth that erupt first and are usually replaced by the permanent teeth.

d., prognosis of Evaluation by the dentist of the prospect of recovery from dental disease, combined with a forecast of the probability of maintaining the dentition and associated structures in function and health.

d., secondary *See* dentition, permanent.

d., transitional More commonly referred to as the mixed dentition. The transitional period usually begins with the eruption of the first permanent molars and ends with the exfoliation of the last primary tooth. In time span about 6 years from age 6 to 12.

dentode (děn-tōd) An exact reproduction of a tooth on a gnathographically mounted cast.

dentoenamel junction *See* junction, dentinoenamel.

dentofacial deformity Malformation of the dentofacial complex with resultant disabling disharmony in size and/or form, as well as function. Includes malocclusion, cleft lip and palate, other skeletal deformities, and muscular dysfunctions.

dentofacial orthopedics A more descriptive synonym for orthodontics; the adjustment of relationships between and among teeth and facial bones by the application of outside forces and/or the stimulation and redirection of functional forces within the craniofacial complex.

dentoform A mock-up of the dentition and alveolar structures; used as a teaching aid or for display purposes.

dentulous (děnt'ū-lŭs) **(dentulism)** Having the natural teeth present in the mouth.

denture An artificial substitute for missing natural teeth and adjacent tissues.

d., acrylic resin A denture made of acrylic resin.

d., artificial *See* denture.

d., basal surface of (impression surface of denture, foundation surface of denture) The part of a denture base that is shaped to conform to the basal seat for the denture.

d. brush A brush designed especially for cleaning dentures.

d. characterization Modification of the form and color of the denture base and teeth to produce a more lifelike appearance.

d., complete (complete dental prosthesis) A dental prosthesis that replaces all of the natural dentition and associated structures of the maxillae or mandible.

d. coverage The extent to which the oral tissue is covered by the denture base.

d. curing The process by which the denture-base materials are hardened in a denture mold to the form of a denture. *See also* process.

d. design A planned visualization of the form and extent of a denture.

d. dislodging force *See* force, denture dislodging.

d., duplicate A second denture intended to be a copy of the first denture.

d. edge *See* border, denture.

d. esthetics *See* esthetics, denture.

d., finish of The final perfection of the form of the polished surfaces of a denture.

d. flange *See* flange.

d. foundation The portion of the oral structures that supports the complete or partial denture base under occlusal load. *See also* area, basal seat.

d. foundation, surface of *See* denture, basal surface of.

d., full Improper term. *See* denture, complete.

d., heel of *See* distal end.

d., immediate (immediate-insertion denture) A removable dental prothesis constructed for placement immediately after removal of the remaining natural teeth.

d., implant A denture that gains its support, stability, and retention from a substructure that is implanted under the soft tissues of the basal seat of the denture and is in contact with bone.

d., implant, substructure *See* substructure, implant.

d., implant, superstructure *See* superstructure, implant.

d., impression surface of *See* denture, basal surface of.

d., interim A dental prosthesis to be used for a short

interval of time.

d., maintenance of An important part of prosthodontic treatment and a major factor in the longevity of the service that the restoration can be expected to give.

d., metal base A denture with a base of gold, chrome-cobalt alloy, aluminum, or other metal.

d., model, wax *See* denture, trial.

d. packing *See* packing, denture.

d., partial (partial dental prosthesis) A prosthesis that replaces one or more, but less than all, of the natural teeth and associated structures.

  d., bilateral partial A dental prosthesis that supplies teeth and associated structures on both sides of a semiedentulous arch.

  d., cantilever partial *See* denture, partial, fixed, cantilever.

  d., components of partial The units that compose a removable partial denture (e.g., the base, the artificial teeth, direct and indirect retainers,major and minor connectors).

  d., construction of partial The science and technique of designing and constructing partial dentures.

  d., extension partial A removable partial denture that is retained by natural teeth at one end of the denture base segments only; a portion of the functional load is carried by the residual ridge.

d., fixed partial A tooth-borne partial denture that is intended to be permanently attached to the teeth or roots that furnish support to the restoration.

  d., cantilever fixed partial A fixed dental prosthesis that has one or more abutments at one end of the fixed partial denture supporting pontic(s) at its other end.

d., removable partial A partial denture that can be readily placed in the mouth and removed by the wearer.

d., temporary partial *See* denture, partial, treatment.

d., tissue-borne partial A removable partial denture that is not supported entirely by the natural teeth.

d., tooth-borne partial A partial denture that is supported entirely by the teeth that bound the edentulous area covered by the base.

d., tooth-borne/tissue-borne partial A partial denture that gains support from both an abutment tooth or teeth and from the structures of an edentulous area covered by the base.

d., treatment partial (temporary partial denture) A dental prosthesis used for the purpose of treating or conditioning the tissues that are called on to support and retain a denture base.

d., unilateral partial A dental prosthesis that restores lost or missing teeth on one side of the arch only.

d. overlay A complete denture that is supported by both tooth and muscosa. Remaining teeth are used

to provide additional stability to the denture.

d. periphery *See* border, denture.

d., polished surface of The portion of the surface of a denture that extends in an occlusal direction from the border of the denture and includes the palatal surface. It is the part of the denture base that is usually polished and includes the buccal and lingual surfaces of the teeth.

d. processing *See* processing, denture.

d. provisional A prosthetic appliance to be used for a short period of time for reasons of esthetics, function, or occlusal support; more commonly referred to as a temporary, interim, or transitional denture. A provisional denture is usually an immediate denture and is most often employed in the maxillary arch.

d. retention *See* retention, denture.

d. space The space between the residual ridges and between the cheeks and the tongue that is available for dentures. *See also* distance, interarch.

d. stability *See* stability, denture.

d., temporary A denture intended to serve for a very short time in a temporary or emergency situation.

d., transitional A removable partial denture that serves as a temporary prosthesis to which teeth will be added as more teeth are lost and that will be replaced after postextraction tissue changes have occurred. A transitional denture may become an interim denture when all the teeth have been removed from the dental arch.

d., trial (wax model denture) A temporary denture, usually made of wax on a baseplate, that is used for checking jaw relation records, occlusion, and the arrangement and observation of teeth for esthetics.

denture-bearing area *See* area, basal seat.

denture-sore mouth *See* mouth, denture-sore.

denture-supporting area *See* area, basal seat.

denture-supporting structure *See* structure, denture supporting.

deoxyribonucleic acid probes A nucleic acid fragment labeled with a radioisotope that is complementary to a sequence in another nucleic acid fragment that will bind to it and thus identify it. It is used as a diagnostic tool to identity the species of microbe involved in an infectious process such as refractory periodontal disease.

dependency State of being dependent.

d., drug Psychic craving for, habituation to, or addiction to a chemical substance; the term replaces *drug addiction*, which emphasizes physiologic craving.

d., emotional An emotional need manifested by a marked and habitual inclination to rely on another for comfort, support, guidance, and decision; the tendency to seek help of others in making decisions or in carrying out difficult actions; the need to be mothered, loved, taken care of, emotionally supported. In extreme cases such persons lose their ability to function independently.

dependents Generally the spouse and children of a subscriber, as defined in a contract. Under some contracts, parents or other members of the family may be beneficiaries.

depletion, salt (dē-plē'shŭn) A condition resulting from inadequate water intake, low intake of sodium and chlorides in the alimentary tract, and secretion of sweat and urine. The most significant of these losses are the gastrointestinal fluid losses resulting from vomiting, diarrhea, and fistulas.

depolarization (dē-pō″lar-ĭ-zā'shŭn) Neutralization of polarity; the breaking down of polarized semipermeable membranes, as in nerve or muscle cells in the induction of impulses.

deponent One who gives under oath testimony that is reduced to writing.

deposit, bismuth *See* stomatitis, bismuth.

deposit, calcareous *See* calculus.

deposition (dĕp-ō-zĭ'shŭn) Evidence given by a witness under interrogatories, oral or written, and usually written down by an official person and intended to be used on the trial of an action in court.

depot (dē'pō) In physiology, the site of accumulation, deposit, or storage of body products not immediately or actively involved in metabolic processes (e.g., a fat depot).

depreciation Normally, charges against earnings to write off the cost, less salvage value, of an asset over its estimated useful life. It is a bookkeeping entry and does not represent any cash outlay, nor are any funds earmarked for the purpose. Following are three classic methods of applying depreciation: straight line, sum of the year's digits, and double declining balance.

depressant (dē-prĕs'ănt) A medicine that diminishes functional activity.

depression (dē-prĕsh'ŭn) Decrease of functional activity.

  d., psychologic A clinical syndrome of neurotic or psychotic proportions, consisting of lowering of mood tone (feelings of painful dejection), difficulty in thinking, and psychomotor retardation. As used by the layman, depression ordinarily refers only to the mood element, which would be more appropriately labeled dejection, sadness, gloominess, despair, or despondency. Many such patients lack motivation and concern for their oral health or dental needs.

derivative (dē-rĭv'ah-tĭv) A chemical substance that is the result of a chemical reaction.

dermatalgia (der-mah-tăl'jē-ah) Pain, burning, and other sensations of the skin unaccompanied by any structural change; probably caused by some nervous disease or reflex influence.

dermataneuria (der″mat-ah-nū'rē-ah) Derangement of the nerve supply of the skin, causing disturbance of sensation.

dermatitis (der-mah-tī'tĭs) Inflammation of the skin.

  d. herpetiformis Dermatitis characterized by grouped, erythematous, papular, vesicular, pustular, or bullous lesions occurring in various combinations, often accompanied by vesicobullous and ulcerative lesions of the oral mucous membranes.

  d. infectiosa eczematoids (Engman's disease) A pustular eczematous eruption that frequently follows or occurs coincidentally with some pyogenic process.

  d., radiation Inflammation of the skin resulting from a high dose of radiation. The reaction varies with the quality and quantity of radiation used and is usually transitory.

dermatoma A circumscribed thickening or hypertrophy of the skin.

dermatome A instrument for cutting thin slices or layers of skin for grafting or for sequentially removing small lesions.

dermatomyositis (der″mah-tō-mī″ō-sī'tĭs) **(polymyositis, dermatomucosomyositis)** A form of collagen disease related to scleroderma and lupus erythematosus. The skin lesions are diffuse erythematous desquamations or rashlike lesions. The skin symptoms are related to a variety of patterns of myositis.

dermatosclerosis (der″mah-tō-sklĕ-rō'sĭs) *See* scleroderma.

dermatosis (der″mah-tō'sĭs) Any disease of the skin.

desaturation (dē-săt″ŭr-ā'shŭn) Conversion of a saturated compound (e.g., stearin) into an unsaturated compound (e.g., olein) by the removal of hydrogen.

desensitization (dē-sĕn″sĭ-tĭ-zā'shŭn) A condition of insusceptibility to infection or an allergen; established in experimental animals by the injection of an antigen that produces sensitization or an anaphylactic reaction. After recovery, a second injection of the antigen is made, bringing about no reaction and thus producing desensitization.

desiccate (dĕs'-ĭ-kāt) To dry by chemical or physical means; for example, electrocoagulation can produce desiccation in tissues.

desiccation (dĕs″ĭ-kā'shŭn) Excessive loss of moisture; the process of drying up. *See also* electrocoagulation.

design, *v.* To plan and/or delineate by drawing the outline of a proposed prosthesis.

desmolysis (dĕs-mol'ĭ-sĭs) Destruction and disintegration of connective tissue. Some authorities associate this desmolytic process with the destruction of connective tissue lying between the enamel and oral epithelium, which thus permits proliferation of the oral epithelium and fusion of enamel and oral epithelium.

desmosomes *See* epithelium, desmosomes of.

detector, radiation *See* radiation detector.

detention Restraint; custody; confinement.

detergent (dē-tĕr′jĕnt) A cleanser. Also applied in a more specific sense to chemicals that possess surface-active properties in water and whose solutions are therefore able to wet surfaces that are normally water repellent and thereby assist in the mechanical dispersion and emulsification of fatty or oily material and other substances that soil the surface.

    d., anionic A detergent in which the cleansing action resides in the anion. Soaps and many synthetic detergents are anionic.

    d., cationic A detergent in which the cleansing action resides in the cation. Many such detergents are strong germicides (e.g., those that contain quaternary ammonium compounds).

    d., nonionic A cleanser that acts by depressing the surface tension of water but does not ionize.

    d., synthetic A cleanser, other than soap, that exerts its effect by lowering the surface tension of an aqueous cleansing mixture.

detoxicate (dē-tok′sĭ-kāt) *See* detoxify.

detoxify (detoxicate) To remove the toxic quality of a substance.

developer A chemical solution that converts the invisible (latent) image on a film into a visible one composed of minute grains of metallic silver.

developing, time-temperature method Procedure of developing dental films; a solution of fixed temperature is used, and the films are immersed in the solution for a specific length of time.

developing, visual method Procedure of developing dental films in which the films are placed in the developing solution and watched by holding them from time to time before a safelight. Correct development has occurred when the film becomes so dark that it is difficult to distinguish between tooth and bone structure.

development The process by which the individual reaches maturity.

    d. of film *See* film, processing.

developmental disabilities Pathologic conditions that start developing before the age of 18 and that limit normal physiologic or mental function and usually persist throughout life.

developmental disturbances Interruptions in the normal growth and development of a child.

deviation (dē″vē-ā′shŭn) Turning from a regular course; deflection.

devital tooth *See* tooth, pulpless.

dextran (dĕk′străn) **(C$_6$H$_{12}$O$_6$ • H$_2$O)** A water-soluble polymer of glucose of high molecular weight. A purified form, having an average molecular weight of 75,000, is used in 6% concentration in isotonic sodium chloride solution to expand plasma volume and maintain blood pressure in emergency treatment of hemorrhagic and traumatic shock.

dextro- Prefix designating that an aqueous solution of a substance rotates the plane of polarized light to the right. *See also* isomers, optical.

dextrorotatory (dĕk″strō-rō′tah-tor″ē) Turning the plane of polarization, or rays of polarized light, to the right.

dextrose (dĕks′trōs) Dextrorotatory glucose, a monosaccharide occurring as a white, crystalline powder; colorless and sweet.

diabetes (dī-ah-bē′tēz) A deficiency condition involving carbohydrate metabolism and characterized by the habitual discharge of an excessive amount of urine.

    d., bronzed The combination of hemochromatosis and diabetes mellitus. The skin takes on a bronzed appearance due to the deposition of an iron-containing pigment in the skin.

    d. insipidus 1: A metabolic disturbance characterized by marked urinary excretion and great thirst but no elevation of sugar in the blood or urine. **2:** A pituitary dysfunction characterized by an insufficient output of the antidiuretic hormone and leading to polyuria and polydipsia.

    d., juvenile Diabetes mellitus occurring in children and adolescents, usually of a more severe and rampant nature than diabetes mellitus in adults, with consequent difficulty of regulation.

    d. mellitus A metabolic disorder, due primarily to a defect in the production of insulin by the islet cells of the pancreas, with resultant inability to use carbohydrates. Characterized by hyperglycemia, glycosuria, polyuria, hyperlipemia (due to imperfect catabolism of fats), acidosis, ketonuria, a lowered resistance to infection, etc. Periodontal manifestations may include recurrent and multiple periodontal abscesses, osteoporotic changes in alveolar bone, fungating masses of granulation tissue protruding from periodontal pockets, a lowered resistance to infection, and delay in healing after periodontal therapy.

    d., phlorizin Glycosuria due to inhibition of phosphorylation of phlorizin. It is not related to an endocrine disturbance.

diadochokinesia (dī″ah-dō″kō-kĭ-nē′zē-ah) The act or process of repeating at maximum speed some simple cyclical reciprocating movement such as raising and lowering of the mandible or protrusion and retraction of the tongue.

diagnosis Translation of data gathered by clinical and radiographic examination into an organized, classified definition of the conditions present.

    d., clinical Determination of the specific disease or diseases involved in producing symptoms and signs by examination of the patient and use of analogy.

    d., differential The process of identifying a condition by differentiating all pathologic processes that may produce similar lesions.

d., final The diagnosis arrived at after all the data have been collected, analyzed, and subjected to logical thought. Treatment may be necessary in some instances before the final diagnosis is made.

d., radiographic Limited term used to indicate those radiologic interpretations which cannot be verified or disproved by clinical examination.

diagnosis-related group A system of classifying hospital patients on the basis of diagnosis consisting of distinct groupings. A DRG assignment to a case is based on the patient's principal diagnosis, treatment procedures performed, age, gender, and discharge status.

diagnostic cast *See* cast, diagnostic.

diagnostic equilibration A measuring method of determining and recording on dentodes the amount and the direction that interfering cusps deflect the closure direction of the mandible, as can be seen in mountings.

dialysis (dī-ăl′ĭ-sĭs) Diffusion through a membrane.

diamond A crystalline carbon substance, the hardest natural substance known, used industrially and in dentistry for cutting and grinding.

diaphragm (dī′ah-frăm) **1:** A musculotendinous partition that separates the thorax and abdomen. **2:** A metal barrier plate, often of lead, pierced with a central aperture so arranged as to limit the emerging, or useful, beam of roentgen rays to the smallest practical diameter for making radiographic exposures. *See also* collimation; collimator; distance, cone, long; source-collimator distance.

d., Potter-Bucky *See* grid, Potter-Bucky.

diaphysis (dī-ăf′ĭ-sĭs) Shaft of a long bone.

diarthrosis (dī″ăr-thrō′sĭs) A freely movable joint enclosed in a fluid-filled cavity and limited variously by muscles, ligaments, and bone.

diastema (dī″ah-stē′mah) An abnormal space between two adjacent teeth in the same dental arch.

diastole (dī-ăs′tō-lē) **1:** The rhythmic period of relaxation and dilation of a chamber of the heart during which it fills with blood. **2:** The period after the contraction of the heart muscle, during which the aorta releases the potential energy stored in its elastic tissue. The energy is converted into kinetic energy and sustains the pressure necessary for steady flow of blood in the vessels. The pressure measured at this period is the lowest attained during the cardiac pumping cycle and is called the *diastolic pressure*. The normal pressure in the adult is approximately 120/80 mm Hg (systolic/diastolic) and increases with age from 128/85 at 45 years of age to 135/89 at 60 years of age.

diathermy (di′ah-ther″mē) A generalized rise in tissue temperature produced by a high-frequency alternating current between two electrodes. The temperature rise is produced without causing tissue damage.

diathesis (dī-ăth′ĕ-sĭs) A tendency, based on body makeup; constitutional, hereditary, or acquired states of the body that cause a predisposition or susceptibility to diseases.

d., hemorrhagic A condition that may be due to defects in the coagulation mechanism, defects in the blood vessel wall, or both.

diazepam A generic central nervous system drug that acts on parts of the limbic system, the thalamus and hypothalamus, inducing a calming effect. Used in the management of short-term anxiety disorders, the relief of the symptoms of anxiety, and for the short-term relief of skeletal muscle spasm. Brand name Valium.

Dick's test *See* test, Dick's.

dideoxycytidine A dideoxynucleoside under study as an antiviral in the treatment of AIDS.

dideoxyinosine A dideoxynucleoside under study as an antiviral in the treatment of AIDS.

die The positive reproduction of the form of a prepared tooth in any suitable hard substance, usually in metal or specially prepared (improved) artificial stone.

d. lubricant A material applied to a die to serve as a separating medium so that the wax pattern will not adhere to the die but may be withdrawn from it without sticking.

d., stone A positive likeness in artificial (dental) stone; used in the fabrication of a dental restoration.

d., waxing A mold into which wax is forced for the production of standardized wax patterns.

diet The food and drink consumed by a given person from day to day. Not all the diet is necessarily used by the body. For this reason diet and nutrition must be differentiated.

d., alkaline A diet that is basic in reaction; produced by the addition of alkaline salts, including sodium bicarbonate.

d., lysine-poor A diet deficient in lysine, an essential amino acid. It is necessary that all the essential amino acids be present in the diet; should one or more be absent, proper use of the others cannot occur. Periodontal changes described in experimental animals with lysine deficiency include osteoporosis of supporting bone, disintegration and failure of replacement of periodontal fibers, etc.

dietary analysis *See* analysis, dietary.

dietary consistency The physical character of the diet. It may tend to produce or modify periodontal disease.

diethylstilbestrol (dī-ĕth′ĭl-stĭl-bĕs′trol) An estrogenic substance, $C_{18}H_{20}O_2$, that has an estrogenic activity considered to be greater than that of estrone. Useful in treating menopausal symptoms and occasionally used in the therapy of chronic desquamative gingivitis associated with artificial or natural menopause.

differential force A term sometimes used to describe the design and application of an orthodontic appliance to distribute the reciprocal forces of the appliance over significantly different root areas with the objective of eliciting a differential response.

difficult eruption *See* teething.

diffusibility (dĭ-fūz″ĭ-bĭl′ĭ-tē) Capable of being diffused.

diffusion (dĭ-fū′zhun) A property of ions or molecules of a solute that permits them to pass through a membrane or to intermingle by rapid or gradual permeation with the molecules of a solvent.

digit A single symbol or character representing a quantity.

digit-sucking An oral habit, usually referred to as finger or thumb sucking, that is not unusual in preschool children. Prolonged, persistent, or vigorous sucking into the transition dentition period can cause tooth displacement malocclusions.

digitalization (dĭj″ĭ-tăl-ĭ-zā′shŭn) Administration of digitalis in sufficient amount by any of several types of dosage schedules to build up the concentration of digitalis glycosides in the body of a patient.

dilaceration (dĭ-lăs″er-ā′shŭn) Severe angular distortion in the root of a tooth or at the junction of the root and crown. It results from trauma during tooth development.

Dilantin enlargement *See* hyperplasia, gingival, Dilantin.

Dilantin gingival hyperplasia *See* hyperplasia, gingival, Dilantin.

Dilantin sodium (dĭ-lăn′tĭn sō′dē-ŭm) Trade name for diphenylhydantoin sodium.

dilation (dĭ-lā′shŭn) The act of stretching or dilating.

diluent (dĭl′ū-ĕnt) An agent that dilutes the strength of a solution or mixture; medication that dilutes any one of the body fluids.

dilute (dĭ-lūt′) To make weaker the strength of a solution or mixture.

dimension, vertical 1: A vertical measurement of the face between any two arbitrarily selected points that are conveniently located one above and one below the mouth, usually in the midline.   **2:** The vertical height of the face with the teeth in occlusion or acting as stops. *See also* relation, vertical.

   v. d., decrease Decrease of the vertical distance between the mandible and the maxillae by modifications of teeth or of the positions of teeth or occlusion rims, or through alveolar or residual ridge resorption.

   v. d., increase Increase of the vertical distance between the mandible and the maxillae by modifications of teeth and the positions of teeth or occlusion rims.

   v. d., occlusal The vertical dimension of the face when the teeth or occlusion rims are in contact in centric occlusion.

   v. d., rest The vertical dimension of the face with the jaws in the rest relation.

   v. d., rest, decrease May or may not accompany a decrease in occlusal vertical dimension. It may occur without a decrease in occlusal vertical dimension in patients with a preponderant activity of the jaw-closing musculature, as in chronic gum chewers or patients with muscular hypertension.

   v. d., rest, increase May or may not accompany an increase in occlusal dimension. It sometimes occurs after the removal of remaining occlusal contacts, perhaps as a result of the removal of noxious reflex stimuli.

dimensional stability *See* stability, dimensional.

dimethylbenzene (dī-mĕth″ĭl-bĕn′zēn) *See* xylene.

Dimitri's disease (dē-mē′trēz) *See* disease, Sturge-Weber-Dimitri.

diphenhydramine hydrochloride A generic antihistamine with anticholinergic (drying) and sedative side effects used for the amelioration of allergic reactions. Brand name Benadryl.

diphenylhydantoin sodium (dī-fĕn″ĭl-hī-dăn′tō-ĭn) **(Dilantin sodium)** A drug used for the control of convulsive grand mal and petit mal epileptic seizures; often associated with the production of a profuse gingival hyperplasia.

diphtheria (dĭf-thē′rē-ah) An acute disease caused by *Corynebacterium diphtheriae* and resulting in swelling of the pharynx and larynx with fever.

diplomate A dental specialist who has achieved certification by the recognized certification board in that specialty, as attested by a diploma from the board.

diplopia (dĭ-plō′pē-ah) Seeing a single object as two images. May occur after fracture of the bony orbital cavity as a result of displacement of the globe of the eye inferiorly.

direct (di-rekt′) Relating to any restorative procedure performed directly on a tooth without the use of a die (e.g., a wax pattern formed in the prepared cavity), silver amalgam, or one of the powdered, granular, or foil golds compacted into a prepared cavity.

   d. access storage device A device used for storage of direct access files. It could be magnetic disk or diskette units.

   d. billing A process whereby the dentist bills a patient directly for his or her fees.

   d. gold Any of the forms of pure gold that may be compacted directly into a prepared cavity to form a restoration.

   d. pulp capping *See* capping, pulp, direct.

   d. reimbursement A self-funded program in which the individual is reimbursed based on a percentage of dollars spent for dental care provided, and which allows beneficiaries to seek treatment from the dentist of their choice.

   d. retainer *See* retainer, direct.

   d. retention *See* retention, direct.

director Person elected by shareholders at the annual

meeting to establish company policies. The directors appoint the president, vice presidents, and all other operating officers. Directors decide, among other matters, if and when dividends shall be paid.

disability 1: Want of legal qualification to do a thing; legal incompetency. **2:** Inability to function in the normal or usual manner; examples of an outcome measure are days missing from work or lessened productivity.

d., denial of A symptom in which patients deny the existence of a disease or disability. A patient who is edentulous may insist he eats better, looks better, and speaks better than if he had teeth. Another may insist that filthy, carious, periodontally involved teeth are beautiful and healthy and enhance his appearance. Denial by these patients is a nonrealistic attempt to maintain their predisease status. These patients regard ill health and disability as an imperfection, a weakness, and even a disgrace.

disarticulation (dĭs″ăr-tĭk″ū-lā′shŭn) Amputation or separation of joint parts, as in hemimandibulectomy, with inclusion of the condyloid process of the mandible.

disc *See* disk.

discharge To release; liberate; annul; unburden. To cancel a contract; to make an agreement or contract null and void.

discharge summary The clinical notes written by the discharging physician or dentist at the time of releasing a patient from the hospital or clinic, outlining the course of treatment, the status at release, and the postdischarge expectations and instructions.

d., purulent *See* pus.

disclosing solution A material, usually some form of dye, applied to the teeth to stain bacterial and mucinous plaque on the tooth surface.

disclusion (dĭs-klū′zhŭn) Separation of the occlusal surfaces of the teeth directly and simply by opening the jaws, or indirectly in excursions by the anterior teeth.

discoid (dĭs′koid) A carving instrument with a blade of circular form that has a cutting edge around the entire periphery.

discoloration, enamel *See* tetracycline.

discoloration, gingival *See* gingival discoloration.

discoplasty The surgical shaping or contouring of the meniscus of the temporomandibular joint.

discount 1: An allowance or deduction made from a gross sum. **2:** The procedure of reducing the amount of a professional fee.

discrimination, legal To treat unequally or unfairly on the basis of race, gender, national origin, religion, or handicap.

discrimination, tactile The ability to perceive two simultaneous touch stimuli; two-point discrimination. When the distance between the two stimuli is diminished to the amount that only one stimulus is perceived, a value is determined for the two-point discrimination

capacity of a special part. Thus correspondence is noted between the mobility of a structure and its discriminatory ability. A person's manual dexterity is also concomitant with the high specific activity of the lips and tongue and the facial and masticatory musculture. Thus the hands and the orofacial complex of structures complement each other, particularly in the masticatory function. When patients are anesthetized by local agents, they have diminished tactile sense and frequently bite their lips rather severely without being aware of it.

disease(s) (dĭ-sēz′) A definite deviation from the normal state; characterized by a series of symptoms. Disease may be caused by developmental disturbances, genetic factors, metabolic factors, living agents, and physical, chemical, or radiant energy, or the cause may be unknown.

d., Adams-Stokes (Adams-Stokes syndrome) A disease characterized by a slow and perhaps irregular pulse, vertigo, syncope, occasional pseudoepileptic convulsions, and Cheyne-Stokes respiration.

d., adaptation (adaptation syndrome) Metabolic disorders occurring as the result of adaptation or resistance to severe physical or psychologic stress. *See also* syndrome, general adaptation.

d., Addison's Chronic adrenocortical insufficiency due to bilateral tuberculosis, aplasia, atrophy, or degeneration of the adrenal glands. Symptoms include severe weakness, weight loss, low blood pressure, digestive disturbances, hypoglycemia, lowered resistance to infection, and abnormal pigmentation (bronze color of the skin, with associated melanotic pigmentation of the oral mucous membranes, particularly of the gingival tissues.

d., adrenocortical Disorders of adrenocortical function, giving rise to Addison's disease, Cushing's syndrome, adrenogenital syndrome, and primary aldosteronism.

d., Albers-Schonberg *See* osteopetrosis.

d., autoallergic *See* disease, autoimmune.

d., autoimmune (autoallergic disease, autoimmunization syndrome, chronic hypersensitivity disease, hypersensitivity disease) Any one of the diseases that are believed to be caused in part by reactions of hypersensitivity of the host tissue (antigens). Includes various hemolytic anemias, idiopathic thrombocytopenias, rheumatoid arthritis, systemic lupus erythematosus, glomerulonephritis, scleroderma, Hashimoto's thyroiditis, and Sjögren's syndrome.

d., Barlow's *See* scurvy, infantile.

d., Basedow's *See* goiter, exophthalmic.

d., Behçet's *See* syndrome, Behçet's.

d., Besnier-Boeck-Schaumann *See* sarcoidosis.

d., bleeder's *See* hemophilia.

d., blood A disease affecting the hematologic system

(e.g., anemia, leukemia, agranulocytosis purpura, infectious mononucleosis). Such a disease often results in lesions of the oral structures, particularly of the mucosal surfaces.

d., Bowen's *See* carcinoma in situ.

d., Brill-Symmers *See* lymphoblastoma, giant follicular.

d., brittle bone *See* osteogenesis imperfecta.

d., Caffey's *See* hyperostosis, infantile cortical.

d., cardiac A disease affecting the heart.

d., cat-scratch *See* fever, cat-scratch.

d., Cheadle's *See* scurvy, infantile.

d., Christmas *See* hemophilia B.

d., collagen (group disease, visceral angiitis) Collectively, a group of diseases affecting the collagenous connective tissue of several organs and systems. These diseases have in common similar biochemical structural alterations and include rheumatic fever, scleroderma, rheumatoid arthritis, systemic lupus erythematosus, periarteritis, and serum sickness.

d., combined system Pernicious anemia in which there is central nervous system damage associated with the hematologic findings.

d., communicable Any disease that may be transmitted directly or indirectly to a well person or animal from an infected person or animal. Any disease with the capacity for maintenance by natural modes of spread (e.g., by contact, by airborne routes, through drinking water or food, by arthropod vectors).

d., congenital Any disease present at birth. More specifically, one that is acquired in utero.

d., Coxsackie A *See* herpangina.

d., Crouzon's *See* dysostosis, craniofacial.

d., Cushing's *See* syndrome, Cushing's.

d., cytomegalic inclusion, generalized *See* disease, salivary gland.

d., Darier's (keratosis follicularis) An apparently genetic dermatologic disease that also involves mucous membranes. The oral lesions are whitish papdules of the gingiva, tongue, or palate. It is characterized histologically by the presence of corps ronds.

d., deficiency Disturbance produced by lack of nutritional or metabolic factors. Used chiefly in reference to avitaminosis.

d., degenerative joint *See* osteoarthritis.

d., demyelinating The diseases that have in common a loss of myelin sheath, with preservation of the axis cylinders (e.g., multiple sclerosis, Schilder's disease).

d., dental, hereditary Heritable defects of the dentition without generalized disease: amelogenesis imperfecta, dentinogenesis imperfecta, dentinal dysplasia, localized and generalized hypoplasia of enamel, peg-shaped lateral incisors, familial dentigerous cysts, missing teeth, giantism, and fused primary mandibular incisors. Dental defects occurring with generalized disease include dentinogenesis imperfecta with osteogenesis imperfecta, missing teeth with ectodermal dysplasia, enamel hypoplasia with epidermolysis bullosa dystrophia, retarded eruption with cleidocranial dysostosis, missing lateral incisors with ptosis of the eyelids, missing premolars with premature whitening of the hair, and enamel hypoplasia in vitamin D-resistant rickets.

d., dermatologic Any one of the diseases affecting the skin; often accompanied by pathologic manifestations of various mucosal surfaces of the body (e.g., the oral mucosa, genital mucosa, conjunctiva).

d., Engman's *See* dermatitis infectiosa eczematoides.

d., exanthematous Any one of a group of diseases caused by a number of viruses but having as a prominent feature a skin rash (e.g., smallpox, chickenpox, cowpox, measles, rubella).

d., familial A disease occurring in several members of the same family. Often used to mean members of the same generation and is occasionally used synonymously with hereditary disease.

d., Feer's *See* erythredema polyneuropathy; acrodynia.

d., fibrocystic (mucoviscidosis) A hereditary defect of most of the exocrine glands in the body, including the salivary glands. The secretion of the affected mucous glands is abnormally viscous.

d., foot-and-mouth (aphthous fever, epidemic stomatitis, epizootic stomatitis) Primarily a disease of animals caused by a filtrable virus that may be transmitted to humans and that occasionally produces symptoms. Human form is characterized by fever, nausea, vomiting, malaise, and ulcerative stomatitis. Skin lesions consisting of vesicles may appear, usually on the palms of the hands and soles of the feet. Spontaneous regression usually occurs within 2 weeks.

d., Fordyce's *See* spots, Fordyce's.

d., functional A disease that has no observable or demonstrable cause.

d., Gaucher's A constitutional defect in the metabolism of the cerebroside kerasin. This glycoprotein accumulates in the reticuloendothelial system and leads to splenomegaly, hepatomegaly, lymph node enlargement, and bone defects.

d., Graves' *See* goiter, exophthalmic.

d., group *See* disease, collagen.

d., Hand-Schüller-Christian (chronic disseminated histiocytosis X) A type of cholesterol lipoidosis characterized clinically by defects in membranous bones, exophthalmos, and diabetes insipidus.

d., Hansen's *See* leprosy.

d., heart Any abnormal condition of the heart (organic, mechanical, or functional) that causes difficulty.

d., arteriosclerotic heart A variety of functional changes of the myocardium that result from arteriosclerosis.

d., congenital heart Defective formation of the heart or of the major vessels of the heart.

d., rheumatic heart Scarring of the endocardium resulting from involvement in acute rheumatic fever. The process most often involves the mitral valve.

d., thyrotoxic heart Cardiac failure occurring as the result of hyperthyroidism or its superimposition on existing organic heart disease. Thyrotoxicosis is an important cause of auricular fibrillation.

d., hemoglobin C A disease due to an abnormal hemoglobin (hemoglobin C); occurs primarily in blacks and causes a mild normochromic anemia, target cells, and vague, intermittent arthralgia.

d., hemolytic, of newborn Hemolysis due to isoimmune reactions associated with Rh incompatibility or with blood transfusions in which there is an incompatibility of the ABO blood system. Several forms of the disease occur: erythroblastosis fetalis, congenital hemolytic disease, icterus gravis neonatorum, and hydrops fetalis.

d., hemophilioid Hemophilic states (conditions) that clinically resemble hemophilia (e.g., parahemophila, hemophilia B [Christmas disease]).

d., hemorrhagic, of newborn A hemorrhagic tendency in newborn infants occurring usually on the third or fourth day of life; believed to be due to defects of prothrombin and factor VII, resulting from a deficiency of vitamin K.

d., hereditary A disease transmitted from parent to offspring through genes. Three main types of mendelian heredity are recognized: dominant, recessive, and sex linked.

d., hidebound See scleroderma.

d., Hodgkin's A generally fatal lymphomatous disorder of unknown etiology that has neoplastic and granulomatous characteristics. Chiefly involves the lymph nodes, but sometimes the spleen, liver, bone marrow, and other organs are involved. Three variants include Hodgkin''s paragranuloma, Hodgkin's granuloma (classical or common type), and Hodgkin's sarcoma. All have in common the presence of Sternberg-Reed, or Dorothy Reed, cells and lymph node enlargement. Cervical lymph nodes are often the first to be affected. *See also* cell, Sternberg-Reed.

d., hypersensitivity See disease, autoimmune.

d., chronic hypersensitivity See disease, autoimmune.

d., iatrogenic A disease arising as a result of the actions or words of a physician or dentist (e.g., an ob-

session of having heart disease or bruxism as a result of a misunderstanding on the part of a patient).

d., idiopathic (ĭd″ē-ō-păth′ĭk) A disease in which the cause is not recognized or determined.

d., infectious Pathologic alterations induced in the tissues by the action of microorganisms and/or their toxins. Some of the infectious diseases involving the oral tissues are herpes zoster, herpetic gingivostomatitis, moniliasis, syphilis, and tuberculosis.

d., kissing See mononucleosis, infectious.

d., Letterer-Siwe (sē′veh) **(acute disseminated histiocytosis X, nonlipid histiocytosis, nonlipid reticuloendotheliosis)** A fatal febrile disease of unknown cause occurring in infants and children; characterized by focal granulomatous lesions of the lymph nodes, spleen, and bone marrow. Results in enlargement of the lymph nodes, spleen, and liver, defects of the flat and long bones, anemia, and sometimes purpura.

d., lipoid storage (lipoidosis, reticuloendothelial granuloma) Any one of a group of diseases in which lipid substances accumulate in the fixed cells of the reticuloendothelial system. Included are Gaucher's disease, Niemann-Pick disease, and the Hand-Schüller-Christian complex. Other storage diseases include lipochondrodystrophy (gargoylism) and cerebral sphingolipidosis.

d., Lobstein's See osteogenesis imperfecta.

d., Marie's See acromegaly.

d., Mediterranean See thalassemia major.

d., Mikulicz' (mĭk′ū-lĭch) A benign hyperplasia of the lymph nodes of the parotid or other salivary glands and/or the lacrimal glands.

d., Moeller's See scurvy, infantile.

d., molecule A disease associated with genetically determined abnormalities of protein synthesis at the molecular level.

d., muscle Pathologic muscle tissue changes. Such changes reveal few structural alterations, and the highly differentiated contents of muscle fibers tend to react as a whole. The pathologic features that distinguish one muscle disease from another are the age and character of changes within a muscle, distribution of those changes within one or several muscles, presence of inflammatory cells and parasites, and coexistence of pathologic changes in other organs. Muscles undergo a number of degenerative changes. There are alterations in the striation in certain pathologic states, caused by cloudy swelling, granular degeneration, waxy or hyaline degeneration, and other cellular modifications, such as multiplication of the sarcolemmic nuclei and phagocytosis of muscle fibers.

d., neuromuscular A condition in which various areas of the central nervous system are affected; results in dysfunction or degeneration of the musculature and disabilities of the organ.

d., Niemann-Pick (nē'măn) A congenital, familial disorder occurring chiefly in Jewish female infants, terminating fatally before the third year, and characterized by the accumulation of the phospholipid sphingomyelin in the cells of the reticuloendothelial system.

d., oral, hereditary Heritable defects of oral and paraoral structures (excluding the dentition) without generalized defects; includes ankyloglossia, hereditary gingivofibromatosis, and possible cleft lip and cleft palate. Many oral and paraoral defects are associated with generalized defects (e.g., Peutz-Jeghers, Franceschetti, Ehlers-Danlos, Pierre Robin, Sturge-Weber syndromes; hemorrhagic telangiectasia; Crouzon's disease; sickle cell disease; acatalasemia; white spongy nevus; xeroderma pigmentosum; gargoylism; neurofibromatosis; familial amyloidosis; and achondroplasia).

d., organic A disease in which actual structural changes have occurred in the organs or tissues.

d., Osler's *See* erythremia.

d., Owren's *See* parahemophilia.

d., paget's *See* osteitis deformans.

d., periodic *See* disorders, periodic.

d., periodontal Any disturbance of the periodontium or supporting structures of the teeth. Diseases affecting the periodontium include periodontitis, periodontosis, gingivitis, gingival enlargement, atrophy, and traumatism and may be loosely divided into two types: inflammatory and dystrophic. Etiological factors may be local or systemic or may involve an interplay between the two.

　d., etiological factors of periodontal The local and systemic factors, singly or in combination, that initiate periodontal lesions.

　d., local factors of periodontal The environmental conditions within the oral cavity that initiate, perpetuate, or alter the course of diseases of the periodontium (e.g., calculus, diastemata between teeth, food impaction, prematurities in the centric path of closure, tongue habits).

d., peripheral vascular A disease of arteries, veins, and/or lymphatic vessels.

d., pink *See* acrodynia.

d., Pott's Spinal curvature (kyphosis) resulting from tuberculosis.

d., psychosomatic A disease that appears to have been precipitated or prolonged by emotional stress; manifested largely through the autonomic nervous system. Various conditions may be included (e.g., certain forms of asthma, dermatoses, migraine headache, hypertension, peptic ulcer, rheumatoid arthritis, ulcerative colitis). Occlusal trauma associated with bruxism is often considered to be a disease of this type. *See also* disorder, psychophysiologic, autonomic, and visceral.

d., Quincke's *See* edema, angioneurotic.

d., Recklinghausen's (von Recklinghausen's disease) *See* hyperparathyroidism; osteitis; generalized fibrosa cystica; neurofibromatosis.

d., Rendu-Osler-Weber (ron'dū) *See* telangiectasia, hereditary hemorrhagic.

d., rheumatic *See* rheumatism.

d., rickettsial A disease caused by microorganisms of the family Rickettsiaceae (e.g., Rocky Mountain spotted fever, rickettsialpox, typhus, Q fever).

d., Riga-Fede (rē'gah-fā'dā) Ulceration of the lingual frenum of infants due to abrasion by natal or neonatal teeth.

d., Sainton's *See* dysostosis, cleidocranial.

d., salivary gland (generalized cytomegalic inclusion) A generalized infection in infants caused by intrauterine or postnatal infection with a cytomegalovirus of the group of herpesviruses. Manifestations include jaundice, purpura, hemolytic anemia, vomiting, diarrhea, chronic eczema, and failure to gain weight.

d., Schüller's (shĭl'erz) *See* osteoporosis.

d., Selter's *See* acrodynia

d., sex-linked A hereditary disorder transmitted by the gene that also determines sex (e.g., hemophilia).

d., sickle cell A hematologic disorder due to the presence of an abnormal hemoglobin (hemoglobin S) that permits the formation or results in the formation of sickle-shaped red blood cells. Two forms of the disease occur: sickle cell trait and sickle cell anemia. *See also* anemia, sickle cell; trait, sickle cell.

d., Simmonds' (pituitary cachexia, hypophyseal cachexia, hypopituitary cachexia) Panhypopituitarism due to destruction of the pituitary gland, usually from hemorrhage or infarction.

d., students' *See* mononucleosis, infectious.

d., Sturge-Weber-Dimitri (encephalotrigeminal angiomatosis) A congenital condition characterized by venous angioma of the meninges and cerebral cortex and ipsilateral angiomatous lesions of the face and jaws.

d., subclinical A latent, incipient, or mild form of a disease that does not produce known, clinically detectable manifestations. Abuse of the term occurs by including diseases deduced to be present only on the basis of borderline laboratory values.

d., Sutton's *See* periadenitis mucosa necrotica recurrens.

d., Swift's *See* acrodynia.

d., systemic Any disease involving the whole body.

　d., oral manifestations of systemic The lesions occurring within the stomatologic system in association with systemic diseases, often influenced by the local environmental factors within the oral cavity

d., Takahara's (tah″kah-hăr′ahz) A form of rare progressive oral gangrene occurring in childhood and seen only in Japan. Apparently related to a congenital lack of enzyme catalase (acatalasemia). Characterized by a mild to severe form of a peculiar type of oral gangrene that may develop at the roots of the teeth or the tonsils. Loss of teeth occurs, with necrosis of the alveolar bone. Patients become symptom free after puberty.

d., transmissible Any disease capable of being transmitted from one individual to another; any disease capable of being maintained in successive passages through a susceptible host, usually under experimental conditions (e.g., by injection). *See also* disease, communicable.

d., Vaquez' (vah-kāz′) *See* erythremia.

d., von Recklinghausen's, of bone *See* hyperparathyroidism; osteitis fibrosa cystica, generalized.

d., von Recklinghausen's, of skin *See* neurofibromatosis.

d., Weil's (vīlz) (epidemic jaundice) An acute febrile disease caused by *Leptospira icterohaemorrhagiae or L. canicola*. Manifestations include fever, petechial hemorrhage, myalgia, renal insufficiency, hepatic failure, and jaundice.

d., Werlhof's (verl′hofs) *See* purpura, thrombocytopenic.

disharmony, occlusal A phenomenon in which contacts of opposing occlusal surfaces of teeth are not in harmony with other tooth contacts and with the anatomical and physiological controls of the mandible. *See also* contact, deflective occlusal; contact, interceptive occlusal; malocclusion.

disinfect (dĭs″in-fĕkt′) To destroy pathogenic microorganisms.

disinfectant (dĭs″ĭn-fĕk′tănt) A chemical especially for use on instruments to destroy most pathogenic microorganisms.

disinfection The process of destroying of pathogenic organisms or of rendering them inert.

disintegration, nuclear A spontaneous nuclear transformation (radioactivity) characterized by the emission of energy and/or mass from the nucleus. When numbers of nuclei are involved, the process is characterized by a definite half-life.

d., induced nuclear Disintegration resulting from artificial bombardment of a material with high-energy particles such as alpha particles, deuterons, protons, neutrons, or gamma rays.

disk (disc) A thin, flat, circular object.

d., abrasive A disk with abrasive particles attached to one or both of its surfaces or its edge.

Disks

d., diamond A disk of steel with diamond chips bonded to its surface.

d., garnet A disk with particles of garnet as the abrading medium.

d., Jo-dandy Trade name for a separating disk. *See also* disk, separating.

d., lightning A steel separating disk.

d., Merkel's *See* corpuscle, Merkel's.

d. pack A set of circular magnetic surfaces mounted coaxially on a shaft for computer storage of files. Can be used for storage of serial or direct access files.

d., polishing A disk with an extremely fine abrasive; used to finish and polish a surface.

d., safe-side A separating disk with abrasive on one side only; the other side is smooth.

d., sandpaper An abrasive disk with sandpaper as the abrading medium.

d., separating A disk of steel or hard rubber.

d. storage A storage device that uses magnetic recording on flat, rotating disks.

d. of temporomandibular joint A plate of fibrous tissue that divides the temporomandibular joint into an upper and a lower cavity. The disk is attached to the articular capsule and moves forward with the condyle in free opening and protrusion.

dislocation Displacement of any part, especially a bone or bony articulation.

dislodgment Movement or removal of a prosthesis from its established position.

disorder(s) Derangement of function.

d., coagulation Any one of the hemorrhagic diseases caused by a deficiency of plasma thromboplastin formation (deficiency of antihemophilic factor, plasma thromboplastic antecedent, Hageman factor, Stuart factor), deficiency of thrombin formation (deficiency of prothrombin, factor V, factor VH, Stuart factor), and deficiency of fibrin formation (afibrinogenemia, fibrinogenopenia).

d., periodic A variety of disorders of unknown cause that have in common periodic recurrence of manifestations. Such disorders are usually benign, resist treatment, often begin in infancy, and occasionally have a hereditary pattern. Included are periodic sialorrhea, neutropenia, arthralgia, fever, purpura (anaphylactoid purpura), edema (angioneurotic edema), abdominalgia, and periodic parotitis (recurrent parotitis).

d., platelet Hemorrhagic disease due to an abnormality of the blood platelets (e.g., thrombocytopenia, thrombasthenia).

d., psychophysiologic, autonomic, and visceral Standard psychiatric nomenclature for what are commonly known as psychomotor disorders. The disorders are disturbances of visceral function, secondary to chronic attitude and long continued reaction to stress. These disorders may occur in any organ innervated by the autonomic nervous system, since overactivity or underactivity of that system due to stress appears to trigger the disorder. *See also* disease, psychosomatic.

d., visual Disorders that may result from injury or disease to the eyeball and its adnexa, the retina, or the cornea (e.g., contusions of the orbit and eyelids, opacities of the lens, corneal scars, vascular changes to the retina). These peripheral disorders are effective in causing partial or total loss of vision in one or both eyes. They are simple, concrete, and fundamental. One sees or one does not see, and gray visions are generally quantitative differences that affect the perception of light and shadow and color and form. Visual disorders may also result from injury or disease to the optic tract fibers, optic chiasma, cerebral pathways, and visual cortex in the occipital region of the cerebrum. These disorders are qualitative deviations from normal, and the symptoms include visual field defects such as tubular vision found in hysteria, complete blindness in one or both eyes due to optic nerve injury, and hemianopsia, in which vision may be lost in one half of the visual field of one or both eyes. Other visual disorders include night and day blindness, color blindness, and the serious visual agnosia that results from trauma, tumor, or vascular disorders in the visual cortex of the cerebrum.

displaceability of tissue *See* tissue, displaceability.

disprove To refute or to prove to be false by affirmative evidence to the contrary.

dissection, neck Removal of the lymph nodes and contiguous tissues from a primary site in the mandibular and/or maxillofacial area as treatment of neoplastic cells that have involved the regional cervical lymphatic system.

dissolve To terminate, cancel, annul, disintegrate. To release the obligation of anything, as to dissolve a partnership.

distal Away from the median sagittal plane of the face and following the curvature of the dental arch.

d. end The most posterior part of a removable dental restoration or denture flange.

distance The measure of space intervening between two objects or two points of reference.

d., anode-film *See* distance, target-film.

d., cone The distance between the focal spot and the outer end of the cone; usually expressed in inches or centimeters. Modern dental roentgen-ray units usually have cone distances of from 5 to 20 inches (12.5 to 50 cm).

d., long cone Long (extended) cone distance is usually 14 to 20 inches (35 to 50 cm). *See also* cone, long.

d., short cone A focal-skin distance of 9 inches (22.5 cm) or less; usually refers to the distance as determined by the cone supplied by the manufacturer in the basic x-ray unit.

d., focal-film *See* distance, target-film.

d., interarch (interridge distance) The vertical distance between the maxillary and mandibular arches under conditions of vertical relations that must be specified.

d., large interarch A large distance between the maxillary and mandibular arches.

d., small interarch A small distance between the maxillary and mandibular arches.

d., interocclusal (interocclusal gap, free-way space) The distance between the occluding surfaces of the maxillary and mandibular teeth when the mandible is in its physiological rest position. This can be determined by calculating the difference between the rest vertical dimension and the occlusal vertical dimension of the face.

d., interridge *See* distance, interarch.

d., object-film The distance, usually expressed in centimeters or inches, between the object being radiographed and the cassette or film.

d., target-film (anode-film distance, focal-film distance) The distance between the focal spot of the tube and the film; usually expressed in inches or centimeters.

distention A state of dilation.

distoclusion Lower teeth occluding distal to their normal relationship to the uppers, as in an Angle Class II malocclusion.

d., bilateral Distoclusion on both sides.

d., unilateral Distoclusion on one side.

distomolar A supernumerary (fourth) molar located posterior to the third molar.

distortion 1: Deviation from the normal shape or condition. **2:** Modification of the speech sound in some way so that the acoustic result only approximates the standard sound and is not accurate. **3:** Twisting or deformation. Loss of accuracy in reproduction of cavity form.

d., film-fault Imperfection in the size or shape of a film image by either magnification, elongation, or foreshortening.

d., horizontal Disproportional change in size and shape of the image in the horizontal plane due to oblique horizontal angulation of the x-ray beam.

d., magnification Proportional enlargement of a radiographic image. It is always present to some degree in oral radiography but is minimized with extended focal-film distances.

d., vertical (foreshortening) Disproportional change in size, either elongation or foreshortening, due to incorrect vertical angulation or improper film placement.

distoversion Placement of a tooth farther than normal from the median plane or midline.

distraction Placement of teeth or other maxillary or mandibular structures farther than normal from the median plane.

disturbances, occlusal Derangements in the patterns of occlusion.

ditch (ditching) Undesirable loss of tooth substance in the region of a restoration margin (usually gingival).

ditching *See* ditch.

diuretic (dī″ū-rĕt′ĭk) **1:** *n.* A drug that increases the formation of urine. **2:** *adj.* Pertaining to the increased formation of urine.

dizziness An unpleasant sensation of disturbed relations to surrounding objects in space.

DMF index rate *See* rate, DMF index.

DNA probe *See* deoxyribonucleic acid probes.

DO cavity A cavity on the distal and occlusal surfaces of a tooth. *See also* cavity, Class 2.

doctor A learned person; one qualified in a science or art; one who has received the highest academic degree in a particular field.

dolichocephalic (dol′ĭ-kō-sĕ-făl′ĭk) Pertaining to a long and narrow head (with a cephalic index below 75).

dolor (dō′lor) Pain.

donor site The portion of the body from which an organ or tissue is removed for transplant or grafting.

donor tissue Tissue contributed by the donor to be used in tissue or organ transplant.

Donovan body *See* body, Donovan.

dope Slang term denoting any drug taken temporarily or habitually without medical cause and that is intended to alter mood.

dorsal (dor′săl) Pertaining to the back or to the posterior part of an organ.

dorsum sella (dŏr′sŭm sĕl′ah) Most posterior point on the internal contour of sella turcica.

dosage (dō′sĭj) The amount of a medicine or other agent administered for a given case or condition.

dose (dōs) **1:** The quantity of drug necessary to produce a desired effect. **2:** The total radiation delivered to a specified area or volume or to the whole body. *See also* also dose, radiation absorbed.

d., absorbed (D) The amount of energy imparted by ionizing particles to unit mass of irradiated material at a place of interest. The unit of absorbed dose is the rad (100 ergs/Gm).

d., air X-ray dose delivered at a point in free air; expressed in roentgens. It consists only of the radiation of the primary beam and the radiation scattered from surrounding air; does not include backscatter from radiated matter (e.g., tissue).

d., booster Portion of an immunizing agent given at a later time to stimulate the effects of a previous dose of the same agent.

d., cumulative The total accumulated dose resulting from a single or repeated exposure to radiation of the same region or of the whole body. If used in area monitoring, it represents the accumulated radiation exposure over a given period of time.

d., depth The absorbed dose of radiation imparted to matter at a particular depth below the surface, usually expressed as percentage depth dose. *See also* dose, percentage depth.

d. distribution A representation of the variation of dose with position in any region of an irradiated object. The dose distribution may be measured using detectors small enough to avoid disturbing the distribution; or it may be calculated and expressed in mathematical form.

d., doubling The amount of ionizing radiation, absorbed by the gonads of the average person in a population over a period of several generations, that will result in a doubling of the current rate of spontaneous mutations.

d. equivalent (DE) The product of absorbed dose and modifying factors, namely the quality factor (QF), distribution factor (DF), and any other necessary factors. The unit of dose equivalent is the rem (rads × qualifying factors).

d., erythema The dose of radiation necessary to produce a temporary redness of the skin. This dose varies with the quality of radiation.

d., exit The absorbed dose delivered by a beam of radiation at the surface through which the beam emerges from a phantom or patient.

d., exposure *See* exposure.

d., fractionation A dose given by a number of shorter exposures over a longer period than would be required if the dose was given by a continuous exposure in one session at the same dose rate.

d., gonadal The dose of radiation absorbed by the gonads.

d., integral (integral absorbed dose, volume dose) The total energy absorbed by a part or object during exposure to radiation. The unit of integral dose is the gram rad (100 ergs).

d., lethal 1: The amount of a drug that would prove fatal to the majority of persons. **2:** The amount of radiation that will be or may be sufficient to cause the death of an organism.

d., median lethal (LD$_{50}$) The amount of ionizing radiation required to kill, within a specified period, 50% of the individuals in a large group or population of animals or organisms.

d., minimum lethal (MLD) The minimal amount of a drug that will kill an experimental animal.

d., maintenance The quantity of drug necessary to sustain a normal physiologic state or a desired blood or tissue level of drug.

d., maximum permissible (MPD) The maximum relative biologic effect dose that the body of a person or specific parts thereof shall be permitted to receive in a stated period of time. In most instances, for the x radiation used in dental radiography, it is satisfactory to consider the RBE dose in rems numerically equal to the absorbed dose in rads and the absorbed dose in rads numerically equal to the exposure dose in roentgens. *See also* dose, weekly permissible.

d., median effective (ED$_{50}$) A dose that, under standard conditions, is effective in 50% of a randomly selected group of subjects.

d., percentage depth The ratio (expressed as a percentage) of the absorbed dose at a given depth in an irradiated body, to the absorbed dose at a fixed reference point on the central ray, usually the surface-absorbed dose.

d., priming A quantity several times larger than the maintenance dose; used at the initiation of therapy to establish rapidly the desired blood and tissue levels of the drug.

d. protraction A method of radiation administration delivered continuously over a relatively long period at a relatively low dosage rate.

d., radiation The amount of energy absorbed per unit mass of tissue at a site of interest. NOTE: This definition limits the use of "dose" to conform with the 1962 recommendations of the International Commission on Radiological Units and Measurements (ICRUM). The following terms therefore become obsolete. They will be found in this glossary under the general heading of *exposure: air dose, cumulative dose, exposure dose,* and *threshold dose.*

d., radiation-absorbed (rad) The unit of absorbed dose, with a value of 100 ergs per gram.

d. rate The time rate at which radiation dose is applied, expressed in either roentgens per unit time or rads per unit time.

d., skin *See* dose, surface-absorbed.

d., surface-absorbed The absorbed dose delivered by a radiation beam at the point where the central ray passes through the superficial layer of the phantom or patient.

d., therapeutic A quantity several times larger than the maintenance dose; used in vitamin therapy in which a marked deficiency exists.

d., threshold The minimum dose that will produce a detectable degree of any given effect.

d., tissue The dose absorbed by a tissue or the tissues in a region of interest.

d., tolerance *See* dose, maximum permissible.

d., toxic The amount of a drug that causes untoward symptoms in the majority of persons.

d., transit A measure of the primary radiation transmitted through the patient and measured at a point on the central ray at some point beyond the patient.

d., U.S.P. *See* dose, median effective (ED$_{50}$); dose, lethal, median (LD$_{50}$); dose, lethal, minimum (MLD); drug, official.

d., volume *See* dose, integral.

d., weekly permissible A dose of ionizing radiation accumulated in 1 week and of such magnitude that, in view of present knowledge, exposure at this weekly rate for an indefinite period of time is not expected to cause appreciable bodily injury during a person's lifetime.

dose-effect curve *See* curve, dose-effect.

dosimetry (dō-sĭm′ĕ-trē) The accurate and systematic determination of the amount of radiation to which an animal or person has been exposed during a given period of time.

dovetail A widened or fanned-out portion of a prepared cavity, usually established deliberately to increase the retention and resistance form.

d., lingual A dovetail established as a step portion, with lingual approach, in some Class 3 and Class 4 preparations; used to supplement the retentions and resistance form.

d., occlusal A dovetail established at the terminal of the occlusal step of a proximal cavity.

dowel A post or pin, usually made of metal, fitted into a prepared root canal of a natural tooth to improve retention of a restoration.

downcoding A practice of third-party payers in which the benefits code has been changed to a less complex and/or lower cost procedure than was reported.

Down syndrome A congenital condition characterized by varying degrees of mental retardation and multiple developmental defects. It is most commonly caused by the presence of an extra chromosome 21. It is also called *trisomy 21* or *trisomy G syndrome. Mongolism* is an archaic and discredited term.

downtime The time interval during which a device is malfunctioning or inoperative.

doxycycline A tetracycline used in the treatment of refractory forms of periodontal disease.

drachm (drăm) *See* dram.

draft *See* draw.

drag The lower, or cast, side of a denture mold or flask, to which the cope is fitted. The base of the cast is embedded in plaster or stone, with the remainder of the denture pattern exposed to be engaged by the plaster or stone in the cope (the upper part of the flask).

drain Any substance that provides a channel for release or discharge from a wound.

　d., cigarette *See* drain, Penrose.

　d., Penrose (cigarette) A thin-walled rubber tube through which a piece of gauze has been pulled.

dram (drachm) A unit of weight that equals the eighth part of the apothecaries' ounce. Symbol ʒ.

draught (drăft) *See* draw.

draw (draft, draught) The taper or divergence of the walls of a preparation for insertion of a cemented restoration.

drepanocythemia (drĕp″ah-nō-sī-thē′mē-ah) *See* anemia, sickle cell.

dressing, Kirkland cement A surgical dressing applied to the tissues after periodontal surgery; consists of zinc oxide, tannic acid, and powdered rosin, admixed with a liquid composed of lump rosin, sweet almond oil, and eugenol.

dressing, postoperative surgical A surgical cement dressing applied to the teeth and tissues after surgical periodontal therapy. Possesses supportive, protective, hemostatic, analgesic, and other properties.

DRG Abbreviation for diagnosis-related group.

drift *See* tooth, drifting.

drill A cutting instrument for boring holes by rotary motion.

　d., bibevel A drill with two flattened sides and the end cut in two beveled planes.

　d., spear-point A drill with a tribeveled, or threeplaned, point.

　d., twist A drill with one or more deep spiral grooves that extend from the point to the smooth part of the shaft.

drilling Boring a hole with a rotary cutting instrument; used in reference to pinholes. (Objectionable as a term describing the general preparation of cavities with rotary instruments.)

drip The continuous slow intravenous introduction of fluid containing nutrients or drugs.

droplet spread Transmission of an infection through the projection of oral and nasal secretions by coughing, sneezing, or talking.

dropsy (drahp′sē) *See* anasarca.

drug(s) A substance used in the prevention, cure, or alleviation of disease or pain or as an aid in some diagnostic procedures.

　d. abuse Excessive or improper use of drugs, especially through self-administration for nonmedical purposes. This term has increased significance because of the enactment of the Comprehensive Drug Abuse Prevention and Control Act of 1970, which replaces the Harrison Narcotic Act.

　d., antibiotic Chemical compounds obtained from certain living cells of lower plant forms, such as bacteria, yeasts, and molds, and from synthesis. They are antagonistic to certain pathogenic organisms and have a lethal effect on them.

　d., antiseptic A chemical compound used to reduce the number of microorganisms in the oral cavity.

　d., autonomic A drug that mimics or blocks the effects of stimulation of the autonomic nervous system.

　d., desensitizing A pharmaceutical used to diminish or eliminate sensitivity of teeth to physical, chemical, thermal, or other irritants (e.g., strontium chloride, silver nitrate [ammoniacal], sodium fluoride, formalin, zinc chloride).

　d., endodontic Any one of the drugs used in treating the dental pulp and dental periapical tissues.

　d., nonofficial A drug that is not listed in the *United States Pharmacopeia (U.S.P.)* or the *National Formulary (N.F.)*.

　d., official A drug that is listed in the *U.S.P.* or *N.F.*

　d., officinal (of-ĭs′ĭn-al) Drugs that may be purchased without a prescription. More commonly called *over-the-counter (OTC) drugs*.

　d., over-the-counter (OTC) A drug that may be purchased without a prescription. Sometimes called a *nonlegend drug* because its label does not bear the prescription legend required on all drugs that may be dispensed only on prescription.

　d., parasympathetic Belladonna alkaloids that inhibit glandular secretions of the nose, mouth, pharynx, and bronchi. This is the chief reason for using atropine and scopolamine for preanesthetic medication.

　d., parasympatholytic (par″ah-sĭm″pah-thō-lĭt′ĭk) A drug that blocks nerve impulses passing from parasympathetic nerve fibers to postganglionic neuroeffectors.

　d., parasympathomimetic (par″ah-sĭm″pah-thō-mĭ-met′ĭk) A drug that has an effect similar to that produced when the parasympathetic nerves are stimulated.

　d., proprietary A drug that is patented or controlled by a private organization or manufacturer.

dry field The isolation of a surgical or operating field from body fluids such as saliva and blood. A dry field is essential in the placement of some sealants and restorative fillings.

dry heat A method of sterilization of suitable instruments using a well-calibrated and time-controlled convection oven.

dry socket *See* socket, dry.

Dry-foil Trade name for tinfoil that is supplied with an adhesive powder or coating on one side.

dual choice (dual option) Federal legislation that requires employers to give their employees the option to enroll in a local health maintenance organization rather than in the conventional employer-sponsored health program.

dual impression technique *See* technique, impression, dual.

duct A small passage.

    d., nasopalatine *See* cyst, nasopalatine.

    d., Stensen's The excretory duct of the parotid gland; it passes lateral to the masseter muscle and enters the oral cavity through the buccal tissues adjacent to the maxillary first and second molars.

    d., Wharton's The excretory duct of the submaxillary glands; opens into the oral cavity at the sublingual papillae of the mucous membrane of the floor of the mouth behind the lower incisor teeth.

ductility (dŭk-tĭl′ĭ-tē) The property of a material that allows permanent deformation under tension without rupture. It is measured as percentage increase in length on rupture compared with original length and is termed *percentage elongation* or *elongation.*

Duke's test *See* test, Duke's.

Dunlop file *See* file, Hirschfeld-Dunlop.

duplication The procedure of accurately reproducing a cast or other object.

    d. impression *See* duplication.

duty That which is due from a person; that which a person owes to another; an obligation.

dwarf, pituitary (pĭ-tū′ĭ-tār″ē) An individual who is of small stature as a result of a deficiency of growth hormones. Such dwarfs usually are well proportioned.

dwarfism Deficient growth and development leading to small stature and often skeletal deformity. It may be associated with ovarian agenesis, pituitary insufficiency, mongolism, progeria, rickets, renal disease, dietary deficiency, achondroplasia, cleidocranial dysostosis, osteogenesis imperfecta, microcephaly, hydrocephaly, sexual precocity, delayed adolescence.

dye, occlusal registration A water-soluble dye used as an aid in locating occlusal contacts. A valuable aid in effecting the fine adjustments in the final phases of the selective grinding procedure.

dyes, treatment The dyes used in medicine and dentistry in the treatment of diseased states, the most useful of which are the rosanilin dyes (e.g., gentian violet, crystal violet) and the fluorescein dyes (e.g., Mercurochrome), which possess antiseptic and protective properties.

dynamic relation *See* relation, dynamic.

dysautonomia, familial (dĭs″aw-tō-nō′me-ah) *See* syndrome, Riley-Day.

dyscrasia (dĭs-krā′zē-ah) **1:** A morbid condition, especially one that involves an imbalance of component elements. **2:** Abnormal composition of the blood (e.g., in leukemias, anemias).

dysdiadochokinesia (dĭs″dī-ah-dō″kō-kĭ-nē′zē-ah) Disturbance of musculoskeletal function. There is a disorganization in the reciprocal innervation of agonists and antagonists and a loss of the ability to stop one act in terms of rate, magnitude, and the direction of movement and immediately to follow it with another act diametrically opposite (e.g., alternately elevating and depressing the mandible). Another example is observed in the inappropriate use of the tongue during mastication when it is necessary to change, reverse, and modify the energy and direction of movement.

dysesthesia (dĭs″ĕs-thē′zē-ah) Impairment of the senses, especially of the sense of touch. Painfulness of any sensation not normally painful.

dysfunction (dĭs-fŭnk′shŭn) **(malfunction)** Any abnormality or impairment of function or the inability of a body, organ, or organ system to perform normally.

    d., dental Abnormal functioning or impairment of the functioning of the dental organ.

    d., endocrine Abnormality in the function of an endocrine gland, either by hypofunction or hyperfunction of the secretory elements of the gland.

dysgnathia (dĭs-nā′thē-ah) Those abnormalities that extend beyond the teeth and include the maxillae, the mandible, or both. *See also* anomaly, dysgnathic.

dyskeratosis (dĭs′ker-ah-tō′sis) An irreversible alteration in the maturation of stratified squamous epithelium. Refers to an increase of abnormal mitosis, individual cell keratinization, epithelial pearls within the spinous layer, loss of polarity of the cells, hyperchromatism, nuclear atypia, and basilar hyperplasia.

dysmenorrhea (dĭs″mĕn-ō-rē′ah) Painful menstruation.

dysmetria (dĭs-mē′trē-ah) Loss of ability to gauge distance, speed, or power of movement associated with muscle function; for example, the patient is unable to control the force of closure and strikes the opposite occluding teeth with greater vigor than necessary.

dysostosis (dĭs-ōs-tō′sis) Defective ossification.

    d., cleidocranial (klī″dō-krā′nē-al) **(Sainton's disease)** A familial disease or congenital disorder characterized by failure to form, or retarded formation of, the clavicles; delayed closure of the sutures and fontanels; and delayed eruption of teeth, with formation of supernumerary teeth. It is characterized by underdevelopment of the maxillae; agnesis or aplasia of the clavicle; abnormalities in other skeletal bones and muscles; and irregularities of the dentition. The syndrome may be mutational or transmitted on an autosomal dominant basis.

    d., craniofacial (Crouzon's disease, Crouzon's syndrome) A condition of unknown etiology that is similar to cleidocranial dysostosis but differs in that the clavicles are not affected. *See also* dysostosis, cleidocranial.

d., faciomandibular Developmental disturbance of the cranial bones and hypoplasias of the upper part of the face. The mandibular body is underdeveloped, but the ramus is hyperplastic. The teeth are crowded and malposed.

d. multiplex *See* syndrome, Hurler's.

dysphagia (dĭs-fā'jē-ah) Difficulty in swallowing. It may be due to lesions in the mouth, pharynx, or larynx, neuromuscular disturbances, or mechanical obstruction of the esophagus (e.g., dysphagia of Plummer-Vinson syndrome [sideropenic dysphagia], peritonsillar abscess, Ludwig's angina, carcinoma of the tongue, pharynx, larynx).

dysphoria (dĭs-for'ē-ah) A feeling of discomfort or restlessness. *See also* euphoria.

dysplasia (dĭs-plā'zē-ah) **1:** Developmental abnormality. *See also* dysplasia, dentinal. **2:** Reversible, regressive alteration in adult cells, seen as alterations in their size, shape, orientation, and functions; leads to change in tissue architecture and is related to chronic inflammation or protracted irritation. Abnormality of development. **3:** Disharmony between component parts.

d., anteroposterior (anteroposterior facial dysplasia) An abnormal anteroposterior relationship of the maxillae and mandible to each other or to the cranial base.

d., craniofacial Disharmony between the cranium and the face.

d., dentinal A genetic disturbance of the dentin characterized by early calcification of the pulp chambers and root canals and by root resorption. It is differentiated from dentinogenesis imperfecta by the latter's characteristics of attrition and relative freedom from root resorption.

d., dentofacial Disharmony between teeth and bones of the face (e.g., crowding, spacing).

d., ectodermal A disease of genetic origin characterized by failure to form ectodermal derivatives. Sweat glands and teeth may be missing (anhidrosis and anodontia, respectively), and there may be scant hair, faulty fingernails, and malformation of the iris.

d., fibroosseous *See* dysplasia, fibrous.

d., fibrous (fibro-osseous dysplasia) A metabolic disturbance characterized by replacement of the bone marrow with fibrous tissue and slow, progressive remolding and enlargement of the bone. It may be monostotic (limited to one bone) or polyostotic (present in many bones). Albright's syndrome shows polyostotic fibrous dysplasia and other symptoms. The monostotic lesions may be identical with ossifying fibroma or with osseous dysplasia. *See also* osteofibroma; syndrome, Albright's.

d., polyostotic fibrous Fibrous dysplasia occurring in more than one bone. *See also* dysplasia, fibrous; osteofibroma; syndrome, Albright's.

d., maxillomandibular Disharmony between one jaw and the other.

d., osseous A chronic reaction of the bone to injury characterized by replacement of the bone marrow with fibrous connective tissue, unilateral enlargement of the maxillae or mandible, and characteristic radiographic findings. It is similar to or identical with monostotic fibrous dysplasia and ossifying fibroma.

d., focal osseous *See* fibroma, periapical.

dyspnea (dĭsp nē'ah) Difficult, labored, or gasping breathing; inspiration, expiration, or both may be involved.

dysrhythmia (dĭs-rĭth'mē-ah) Disordered rhythm.

dystonia (dĭs-tō'nē-ah) Disorder or lack of tonicity.

dystrophy (dĭs'trō-fē) Faulty nutrition. Often used to refer to the results of faulty nutrition, i.e., wasting away.

d., muscular A chronic, degenerative, noncontagious, progressive disorder of unknown etiology manifested by weakness and wasting away of the voluntary muscles.

Eames' technique (mēz) *See* technique, Eames'.

earnings report A statement issued by a company showing its earnings or losses over a given period. The earnings report lists the income earned, expenses, and net result. Synonym: income statement.

EBIT Abbreviation for earnings before interest and taxes.

eburnation (ē″ber-nā′shŭn) Increase in bony density into an ivory-like mass. *See also* osteitis, condensing; dentin eburnation.

eccentric (ĕk-sĕn′trĭk)   **1:** Deviation from the normal or conventional.   **2:** Away from the central or reference position.

  e. checkbite *See* record, interocclusal, eccentric.

  e. jaw relation *See* relation, jaw, eccentric.

  e. occlusion *See* occlusion, eccentric.

  e. position *See* position, eccentric.

ecchymosis (ĕk′ ĭ-mō′sĭs) Discoloration of mucous membranes caused by a diffuse extravasation of blood. Frequently called a *bruise*.

echoviruses (ECHO) An enteric pathogen associated with fever and mild respiratory disease; sometimes may produce an aseptic menigitis.

econonics In dentistry, a broad term that covers all the business aspects of dental practice.

ectodermal dysplasia A developmental disturbance of tissues derived from the ectoderm (e.g., hair, nails, sweat glands, teeth). Dental findings are partial anodontia and microdontia.

ectomorph (ĕk′tō-morf) A constitutional body type (Sheldon's classification) characterized by long, fragile bones and a highly developed nervous system.

ectopic eruption *See* eruption, ectopic.

ectropion (ĕk-trŏ′pē-on) Eversion, or rolling outward, of the eyelid margin.

eczema (ĕk′zē-mah) An inflammatory skin disease characterized by vesiculation, inflammation, watery discharge, and the development of scales and crusts. The large variety of types can be distinguished according to location and etiology.

ED₅₀ *See* dose, median effective.

edema (ĕ-dē′mah) Accumulation of fluid in the tissues or in the peritoneal or pleural cavities. Primary factors favoring edema are increased capillary hydrostatic pressure (increased venous pressure), decreased osmotic pressure of plasma (hypoproteinemia), decreased tissue tension and lymphatic drainage, increased osmotic pressure of tissue fluids, and increased capillary permeability. Additional renal and hormonal factors are important. Clinical manifestations may consist of a steady weight gain or localized or generalized swelling.

  e., angioneurotic (angioedema, giant urticaria, Quincke's disease) Spontaneous swelling of the lips, cheeks, eyelids, tongue, soft palate, pharynx, and glottis, frequently associated with allergy to foods or drugs and lasting from several hours to several days. Involvement of the glottis results in obstruction of the airway.

  e., cardiac Edema due to venous congestion in association with congestive heart failure; tends to appear first in such dependent parts as the legs.

  e., dependent Edema that changes its position with the posture of dependent parts (e.g., edema of the legs in progressive heart failure).

  e., periorbital Edematous swelling of the eyelids in association with local injury, allergic reactions, hypoproteinemia, trichinosis, myxedema, etc.

  e., pitting Persistent indentation of the skin when pressure is applied to an edematous area.

edentate (ē-dĕn′tāt) Without teeth.

edentulate (ē-dĕn′tū-lāt) *See* edentulous.

edentulism (ĕ-dĕn′tū-lĭzm) The condition of being edentulous, without teeth.

edentulous (ē-dĕn′tū-lŭs) Without teeth; lacking teeth.

edge strength *See* strength, edge.

edge-to-edge bite *See* occlusion, edge-to-edge.

edge-to-edge occlusion *See* occlusion, edge-to-edge.

edgewise appliance *See* appliance, edgewise.

EDP Abbreviation for electronic data processing.

Edtac Trade name for a chelating agent used to soften calcified tissue.

education of patient Effective communication between the dentist (and/or auxiliaries) and the patient concerning dentistry and the principles of treatment and prevention. The procedure of increasing the patient's knowledge of the oral cavity and its care to the point where the reasons for proposed dental services are understood.

effect The result of an action.

  e. of external radiation on bone *See* osteoradionecrosis.

  e. of function on bone *See* law, Wolff's.

  e., heel (anode heel effect) Variation of intensity over the cross section of a useful x-ray beam, due to the angle at which x-rays emerge from beneath the surface of the focal spot, which causes a differential attenuation of photons comprising the useful beam.

  e., lysing The disintegrating action on tissue components produced by the toxic and compressive products of inflammation. In gingival inflammation, lysis of the gingival fibers must occur before apical migration of the epithelial attachment can occur. In microbiology, the presence of complement in the antigen-antibody complex is necessary for bacterial lysis. Hemolysis occurs with coexistence of erythrocyte, antibody, and complement.

  e., wedging An effect produced by food impaction that forces the teeth apart.

effective half-life *See* life, radioactive.

effectiveness The degree to which action(s) achieve the intended health result under normal or usual circumstances.

effector (ĕ-fĕk′tor) **1:** A motor or secretory nerve ending in an organ, gland, or muscle; consequently called an *effector organ*. **2:** An on-the-job organ of the body that responds to stimulations asking for corrections. Antonym: receptor.

efferent (ĕf′er-ĕnt) Conveying away from a center toward the periphery.

efficiency Operation of a dental practice in such a way that both business and professional services are performed in a minimum amount of time without sacrificing quality of work, sympathetic attitude, and kindliness.

eH Symbol for oxidation-reduction potential, which is regarded as a significant factor in the protection of the body against anaerobic bacteria. The eH of living tissue of pH level 7.4 is about 0.12 volt.

Ehlers-Danlos syndrome (ā′lerz dăn′lōs) *See* syndrome, Ehlers-Danlos.

EIA Abbreviation for enzyme immunoassay; better known as ELISA for enzyme-linked immunosorbent assay used to detect the presence of HIV antibody to HIV in the blood.

Eikenella corrodens A gram-negative rod-shaped facultatively anaerobic bacteria that is part of the normal flora of the oral cavity but may become an opportunistic pathogen in immunocompromised patients.

ejector By common usage, a device used to remove debris and fluids by negative pressure. Correct term for such a device, however, is *aspirator*. *See also* aspirator.

  e., saliva A device (containing a removable tip) that is

attached to a vacuum supply to remove saliva from a dental field of operation.

  e., saliva, tip A removable tip, made of metal, glass, rubber, plastic, or a combination of these, that is attached to a saliva ejector and bent to fit over lower teeth and reach the floor of the oral cavity.

elastic, *adj.* Referring to property of a solid substance that permits recovery of its shape after a deformation resulting from force application.

  e. deformation *See* deformation, elastic.

  e. impression *See* impression, elastic.

  e., intermaxillary *See* elastic, maxillomandibular.

  e., intramaxillary An elastic band used within either the maxillary or mandibular arch.

  e. limit *See* limit, elastic.

  e., maxillomandibular An elastic band used between the maxillary and mandibular dentitions.

  e. memory 1: The property of a material (e.g., wax), enabling it, after being warmed, bent, and cooled, to return to its original form on rewarming. **2:** A rubber plastic band used to apply force to the teeth.

elasticity The quality or condition of being elastic.

  e., modulus of (Young's modulus) A measurement of elasticity obtained by dividing stress below the proportional limit by its corresponding strain value. A measure of stiffness.

elastomer (ē-lăs′tō-mer) A soft, rubberlike material; synthetic rubber. A rubber base impression material (e.g., silicone, mercaptan).

elastosis (e″lăs-tō′sĭs) Degeneration of the elastic tissues; found particularly in the lips and associated with senile or actinic cheilitis.

  e., senile A dermatologic disease, which is the result of degeneration of the elastic connective tissue.

elderly An adjective used to describe a person who is beyond middle age and approaching old age. It is politically correct to refer to those over 65 as senior citizens. *See also* geriatric dentistry.

electroanesthesia (ē-lĕk″trō-ăn-es-thē′zē-ah) Local or general anesthesia induced by electric current.

electrocoagulation (ē-lĕk″trō-kō-ăg″ū-lā′shŭn) The use of electrically generated heat to destroy tissue by coagulation necrosis. Usually a platinum wire electrode or loop is used.

electrocortin (ē-lĕk″trō-kor′tĭn) *See* aldosterone.

electrode (ē-lĕk′trōd) An instrument with a point or a surface from which a current can be discharged into or received from the body of a patient or a solution.

electroencephalograph **(EEG)** (ē-lĕk″trō-ĕn-sĕf′ah-lō-grăf) An instrument for recording the electrical activity of the brain.

electrogalvanism (ē-lĕk-trō-găl′văn-ĭzm) **(galvanism)** The flow of electric current between two different metals in an electrolyte solution. Dissimilar metals used in different intraoral restorations.

electrolyte (ē-lĕk′trō-līt) A solution that conducts electricity by means of its ions.

　e. affinity The attraction of the electrolytes in the body to the different fluid compartments of the intracellular and extracellular environments. Sodium is the predominant cation in the extracellular fluid; potassium is the predominant cation within the cells; chlorine and bicarbonate are the predominant anions in the plasma and interstitial fluids; and phosphates and proteins are the chief anions in the cells.

　e. balance, fluid and *See* fluid and electrolyte balance.

electrolyzer (ē-lĕk′trō-lī″zer) **(ionizer)** An electric apparatus designed for use in a root canal to break down a treatment chemical into its various ions by direct current. *See also* electrosterilizer.

electromallet, McShirley's *See* condenser, electromallet.

electromedication *See* electrosterilization.

electrometer (ē″lĕk-trom′ĕ-ter) An electrostatic instrument for measuring the potential difference between two points. In radiology, electrometers are used to measure changes in the potential of charged electrodes due to ionization occasioned by radiation.

electromyography (ē-lĕk″trō-mī-ŏg′rah-fē) Detection, recording, and interpretation of electric voltage generated by the skeletal muscles.

electron (ē-lĕk′tron) **(e)** A negatively charged elementary particle constituent in every neutral atom, with a mass of 0.000549 amu or 9.1×10^{-28} g. (Particles with an equal but opposite charge are called *positrons*.)

　e. beam *See* electron stream.

　e. stream (electron beam, cathode ray, cathode stream) A stream of electrons emitted from the negative electrode (cathode) in a roentgen-ray tube; their bombardment of the anode gives rise to the roentgen rays.

electronic Pertaining to the application of that branch of science that deals with the motion, emission, and behavior of currents of free electrons, especially in vacuum, gas, or phototubes and special conductors or semiconductors. Contrasted with electric, which pertains to the flow of large currents in wires only.

　e. knife *See* knife, electronic.

electroplating Plating by electrolysis. Impressions are plated in dentistry to form metalized working dies.

electropolishing Removal of a minute layer of metal by electrolysis to produce a bright surface.

electrosection An incision created by electrosurgery, ideally by using a fully rectified, alternating high-frequency current and producing minimal cellular injury.

electrosterilization Medication of a prepared root canal by use of electrolysis of the medicament.

electrosterilizer An electric apparatus designed for use in

root canal treatment for the electrolysis of a halide, such as sodium iodide, to release iodine in the cleaned root canal for the purpose of destroying residual organisms. *See also* electrolyzer.

electrosurgery The use of electrically generated energy from high-frequency alternating currents to cut or alter tissue within definite limits.

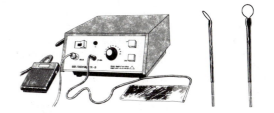

Electrosurgical unit. *Left,* Control box and foot or hand control, and two terminals. *Right,* Probe tips.

element A simple substance that cannot be decomposed by chemical means and is made up of atoms that are alike in their peripheral electronic configuration and chemical properties but differ in their nuclei, atomic weights, and radioactive properties.

elephantiasis (ĕl″ĕ-făn-tī′ah-sĭs) A chronic disease caused by filariasis of the lymph channels with resultant inflammation and blockage. The term is also used for hypertrophy of tissues from other causes (e.g., gingival elephantiasis).

　e. gingivae *See* fibromatosis gingivae.

elevator An instrument used to raise or lift something.

　e., dental One of a variety of blades used for engaging teeth and/or roots to remove them from their alveoli.

　e., malar An instrument used to elevate or reposition the zygomatic bone.

　e., periosteal A thin blade used to lift periosteum from bone.

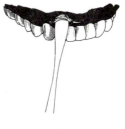

Periosteal elevator

eligibility date The date an individual and/or dependents become eligible for benefits under a dental benefits contract. Often referred to as effective date.

eligible person *See* beneficiary.

eligibility rules Conditions that define who may be entitled to dental benefits, when persons first become entitled to such benefits, and any provisions that determine how long an individual remains entitled to benefits.

ELISA Acronym for enzyme-linked immunosorbent assay used to detect the presence of HIV antibody to HIV in the blood.

elixir (ē-lĭk′ser) A pleasantly flavored sweetened hydroalcoholic solution of a drug intended for oral administration.

elliptocytosis (ē-lĭp″tō-sī-tō′sĭs) **(ovalcytosis, oval cell anemia)** A hereditary anomaly in which the red blood cells are elliptical, or oval shaped, and are predisposed to hemolysis.

elongation (ē″long-gā′shŭn) The process or condition of increasing in length before breaking; indicates ductility (e.g., a metal).

  e., % 1: The increase in length of a material after fracture in tension.   **2:** A mechanical test usually employed to measure ductility.

embedded Referring to a tooth, root tip, or foreign body that is covered in bone.

embolism (ĕm′bō-lĭzm) The clogging of a vessel by matter (e.g., a clot, air, oil) that is carried by the bloodstream to some point where the lumen of the vessel narrows (opposite of thrombosis, in which the clotting mechanism is organized in situ).

  e., air *See* aeroembolism.

embolus (ĕm′bō-lŭs) A blood clot or other material that travels in the bloodstream and then lodges in a vessel and obstructs circulation.

embrasure An opening, as in a wall. The space between the curved proximal surfaces of the teeth.

  e., buccal An embrasure that opens toward the cheeks.

  e. clasp *See* clasp, embrasure.

  e. hook An extension of a removable partial denture into the embrasure above the contact area between two adjacent teeth, which resists movement in a cervical direction.

  e., interdental The spaces formed by the interproximal contours of adjoining teeth, beginning at the contact area and extending lingually, facially, occlusally, and apically.

  e., labial An embrasure that opens toward the lips.

  e., lingual An embrasure that opens toward the tongue.

  e., occlusal An embrasure that opens toward the occlusal surface or plane.

emergency An unforeseen occurrence or combination of circumstances that calls for immediate action or remedy; pressing necessity; exigency.

  e. treatment Treatment that must be rendered to the patient immediately because of acute infection or pain.

emesis (ĕm′ĕ-sĭs) The sudden expulsion of gastric contents through the esophagus into the pharynx. The act is partly voluntary and partly involuntary.

emetic (ē-mĕt′ĭk) A drug that induces vomiting.

emetine hydrochloride (ĕm′ĕ-tēn) An alkaloid, $C_{29}H_{40}N_2O_4$•2HC1, regarded as a protozoacide and formerly used in the treatment of periodontitis as well as in the treatment of amebic dysentery.

EMF Abbreviation for erythrocyte-maturing factor.

eminence, retromylohyoid (ĕm′ĭ-nĕns, ret″-rō-mī-lō-hī′oid) The distal end of the lingual flange of a lower denture. It occupies the retromylohyoid space.

eminenectomy (ĕm″ ĭ-nĕn-ĕk′tō-mē) Operative removal of the anterior articular surface of the glenoid fossa.

emollient (ē-mol′yĕnt) An agent that is soothing to the skin or mucous membrane; makes the skin softer or smoother.

emotiometabolic (ē-mō″shē-ō-mĕt″ah-bol′ĭk) Modifying metabolism as a result of emotion.

emotion A complex feeling-state (affect) accompanied by characteristic motor and glandular activities; feelings; mood.

emotional Characterizing a person experiencing an emotion; manifesting emotional behavior, rather than logical, rational behavior; a person who is easily or excessively given to emotion.

empathy Putting oneself into the psychologic frame of reference of another, so that the other person's feeling, thinking, and acting are understood and to some extent predictable. A desirable trust-building characteristic of a helping profession. It is embodied in the sincere statement, ″I understand how you feel.″ Empathy is different from sympathy in that to be empathetic one understands how the person feels rather than actually experiencing those feelings as in sympathy.

emphysema (ĕm″fĭ-sē′mah) **1:** A swelling due to air in the tissue spaces. In the oral and facial regions it may be caused either by air introduced into a tooth socket or gingival crevice with the air syringe or by blowing of the nose.   **2:** Permanent dilation of the respiratory alveoli.

employee A person who, under the direction and control of the employer, performs services for remuneration.

Employee Retirement Income Security Act (ERISA): A federal act, passed in 1974, that established new standards and reporting/disclosure requirements for employer-funded pension and health benefits programs. To date, self-funded health benefit plans operating under ERISA have been held to be exempt from state insurance laws. This exemption is currently under review.

employer-sponsored plan A program supported totally or in part by an employer or group of employers to provide dental benefits for employees. The plan may be administered directly by the employer or another person or group under a contractual arrangement. Part of the cost may be borne by the employee.

empyema (ĕm″pī-ē′mah) The presence of pus in a cavity, hollow organ, or space (e.g., the pleural cavity).

emulsifiers An agent such as gum arabic or egg yolk used to suspend droplets of oil in a water-based solution. An agent to maintain any element or particle in suspension within a fluid medium.

emulsion (ē-mul′shŭn) A colloidal dispersion of one liquid in another. *See also* suspension.

   e., double A suspension of sensitive silver halide salts impregnated in gelatin and coated on both sides of a radiographic film base.

   e., silver A suspension of sensitive silver halide salts impregnated in gelatin and used for coating photographic plates, radiographic films, etc.

   e., single A suspension of sensitive silver halide salts impregnated in gelatin and coated on only one side of a radiographic film base.

enamel 1: The hard, glistening tissue covering the anatomic crown of the tooth. It is composed chiefly of hexagonal rods of hydroxyapatite, sheathed in an organic matrix (approximately 0. 15%), and oriented with their long axis approximately at right angles to the surface. **2:** The outermost layer or covering of the coronal portion of the tooth that overlies and protects the dentin.

   e., mottled *See* fluorosis, chronic endemic dental.

   e. pearl *See* pearl, enamel.

enameloma *See* pearl, enamel.

enanthem (ĕn-ăn′thĕm) *See* enanthema.

enanthema (ĕn″ăn-thē′mah) (enanthem) Lesions involving the mucous membrane.

encounter form A document or record used to collect data about given elements of a patient visit to a dental office or similar site that can become part of a patient record or be used for management purposes or for quality review activities.

end organ The expanded termination of a nerve fiber in muscle, skin, mucous membrane, or other structure.

   e. o., proprioceptor Sensory end organs, located chiefly in the muscles, tendons, and labyrinth, that provide information on the movements and position of the body. Four specific end organs are the muscle spindles; Golgi corpuscles, stimulated by tension; Pacini's corpuscles, stimulated by pressure; and bare nerve endings, stimulated by pain.

   e. o., sensory Sensory nerve fibers that end peripherally as either unmyelinated fibers or special structures called *receptors*. Receptors are situated in the skin, mucous membranes, muscles, tendons, joints, and other structures and also in such special sense organs as those for vision, hearing, smell, and taste.

The receptors are organized into a system that relates them to the environment: exteroceptors, interoceptors, and proprioceptors.

end section The distal portion of a twin-wire labial arch wire, consisting of a tube in which the anterior section of the labial arch is engaged.

end-bulb *See* end-feet.

end-feet (boutons terminaux, end-bulb) Small, terminal enlargements of nerve fibers that are in contact with the dendrites or cell bodies of other nerve cells; the synaptic ending of a nerve fiber.

ending A termination; the point at which something is concluded.

   e., annulospiral A nerve ending, associated with an intrafusal muscle fiber, that is stimulated by a stretch impulse resulting from the extension of a muscle. The ending is in the form of a gradual spiral around the length of the intrafusal muscle fiber in the muscle spindle and is connected to the coarse myelinated fibers.

   e., flower spray A sensory nerve ending that is attached to the distal end of an intrafusal muscle fiber and that is stimulated when the muscle fiber contracts, pulling on the nerve ending.

   e., free nerve The peripheral terminal of the sensory nerve.

endocarditis, subacute bacterial (ĕn″dō-kar-dī′tĭs) **(SBE)** Bacterial infection involving the endocardium that occurs primarily after bacteremia and the establishment of bacterial vegetation on an area of defective endocardium such as is found in patients with rheumatic or congenital heart disease.

endochondral bone *See* bone, endochondral.

endocrine Refers to either the gland that secretes directly into the systemic circulation or the substance secreted.

   e. diseases An abnormal condition caused by some malfunction of an endocrine gland.

   e. system The interrelated nature of the physiological function of endocrine glands.

endodontally involved (ĕn″dō-dŏn′tah-lē) Pertaining to disease of the dental pulp and dental periapical tissues.

endodontia (ĕn″dō-don′shē-ah) *See* endodontology.

endodontic implant A metallic implant extending through the root canal into the periapical bone structure to increase support and retention of the tooth.

endodontic techniques Procedures used in pulpless teeth or teeth that are to be made pulpless.

endodontics (ĕn″dō-don′tĭks) The branch of dental practice that applies the knowledge of endodontology.

endodontist (ĕn″dō-don′tĭst) A dentist who practices endodontics as a specialty.

endodontology (ĕn″dō-don-tahl′ō-jē) **(endodontia, pulp canal therapy, root canal therapy)** The division of dental science that deals with the etiology, diagnosis, prevention, and treatment of diseases of the dental pulp and their sequelae.

endolith (ĕn'dō-lĭth) *See* denticle.

endosteal implants *See* implants endosteal.

endosteum (ĕn-dŏs'tē-ŭm) A thin layer of connective tissue that lines the walls of the bone marrow cavities and haversian canals of compact bone and covers the trabeculae of cancellous bone. It has both osteogenic and hematopoietic potencies and, like the periosteum, takes an active part in the healing of fractures.

endothelioma (ĕn″dō-thē″lē-ō'mah) *See* tumor, Ewing's.

endotoxin (ĕn'dō-tahk'sĭn) A nondiffusible lipid polysaccharide-polypeptide complex formed within bacteria (some gram-negative bacilli and others); when released from the destroyed bacterial cells, it is capable of producing a toxic manifestation within the host.

end-plate A complex hypolemmal terminal arborization of a motor nerve fiber in a bed of specialized sarcoplasm; it transmits nerve impulses to muscle.

    e.-p., motor The end-plate by which impulses from nerves are transmitted to the muscle fibers. It is a modification of the sarcolemma and is continuous with it. The end-plate potential generated by the nerve impulse activates the muscle impulse.

end-to-end bite *See* occlusion, edge-to-edge.

end-to-end occlusion *See* occlusion, edge-to-edge.

Endur Brand name for a two-paste diacrylate resin adhesive used as a bonding agent in orthodontics.

energy Capacity for doing work.

    e., atomic Energy that can be liberated by changes in the nucleus of an atom.

    e., binding Energy represented by the difference in mass between the sum of the component parts and the actual mass of the nucleus of an atom.

    e. dependence The characteristic response of a radiation detector to a given range of radiation energies or wavelengths as compared with the response of a standard free-air chamber. Emulsions also show energy dependence.

    e., excitation Energy required to change a system from its ground state to an excited state. With each excited state there is associated a different excitation energy. *See also* excitation.

    e., ionizing The average energy lost by ionizing radiation in producing an ion pair in a gas. (For air it is about 33 eV.)

    e., kinetic Energy possessed by a mass because of its motion.

    e., nuclear *See* energy, atomic.

    e., photon (hv) Electromagnetic energy in the form of photons, with a value in ergs equal to the product of their frequency in cycles per second and Planck's constant (E = hv).

    e., potential Energy inherent in a mass because of its position with reference to other masses.

    e., radiant The energy of electromagnetic waves, such as radio waves, visible light, x-rays, and gamma rays.

engine, dental An electric motor that, by means of a continuous-cord drive over pulleys, activates a handpiece that holds a rotary instrument.

engineering, dental The application of physical, mechanical, and mathematical principles to dentistry.

Engman's disease *See* dermatitis, infectiosa eczematoides.

enlargement Increase in size.

    e., Dilantin *See* hyperplasia, gingival, Dilantin.

    e., idiopathic Gingival enlargement, of unknown causation, clinically characterized by a firm, rounded thickening of the gingival tissues and histologically characterized by connective tissue hyperplasia of the gingival corium.

enostosis (ĕn″os-tō'sĭs) A bony growth located within a bone cavity or centrally from the cortical plate. *See also* osteoma.

enrollee Individual covered by a benefit plan *see* beneficiary).

Entamoeba gingivalis (ĕn″tah-mē'bah) A genus of protozoan amoeba found in the mouth; repeatedly, but not conclusively, associated with the initiation and/ or perpetuation of periodontitis.

enteric coating (ĕn-ter'ĭk) *See* coating, enertic.

entropion (ĕn-trō'pē-on) Inversion, or infolding, of the eyelid margin.

enucleate (ĕ-noo'klē-āt) To remove a lesion in its entirety.

enunciation An auxiliary function of teeth, particularly those in the anterior sector of the dental arch; the formation of sounds as in speech.

enuresis (ĕn-ū-rē'sĭs) Involunatry urination (e.g., during general anesthesia, at night).

environment (ĕn-vī'ron-mĕnt) The aggregate of all the external conditions and influences affecting the life and development of an organism.

    e., extracellular External, or interstitial, environment provided and maintained for the tissue cells.

    e., oral The aggregate of all oral conditions and influences.

Environmental Protection Agency (EPA) A federal agency charged with the approval and overseeing of the use and disposal of hazardous materials. Workplace management of hazardous materials falls under the jurisdiction of the Occupational Safety and Health Administration (OSHA).

enzyme (ĕn'zīm) A protein substance that acts as a catalyst to speed up metabolic and other processes involving organic materials. Some enzymes function within cells; others function in the extracellular fluids and tissue spaces and organs. They are active in all major tissue functions, such as cellular respiration muscle contraction, digestive processes, and energy consumption, and are produced intracellularly.

eosinophil (ē″ō-sĭn′ō-fĭl) *See* leukocyte, eosinophilic.

eosinophilia (ē″ō-sĭn″ō-fĭl′ē-ah) An absolute or relative increase in the normal number of eosinophils in the circulating blood. Various limits are given (e.g., absolute eosinophilia if the total number exceeds 500/mm^3 and relative if greater than 3% but total less than 500 mm^3. It may be associated with skin diseases, infestations, hay fever, asthma, angioneurotic edema, adrenocortical insufficiency, and Hodgkin's disease.

eosinophilic granuloma *See* granuloma, eosinophilic.

EPA *See* Environmental Protection Agency

ephelis (ĕh-fē′lĭs) (freckle) Circumscribed macular collection of pigment in the epidermis or oral mucosa. Increased amount of melanin pigment is seen in the region of the basal layer of cells.

epidemiology (ĕp′ĭ-dĕm″ē-ol′ō jē) The science of epidemics and epidemic diseases, which involve the total population rather than the individual. Its aim is to determine those factors in the group environment that make the group more or less susceptible to disease.

epidermolysis bullosa (ĕp″ĭ-dermahl′ĭ-sĭs) A disease of the skin characterized by bullae, vesicles, cysts, and, often, associated mandibular enlargement. *See also* syndrome, Goldscheider's; syndrome, Weber-Cockayne.

epiglottis (ĕp″ĭ-glot′ĭs) An elastic cartilage, covered by mucous membrane, that forms the superior part of the larynx and guards the glottis during swallowing.

epilepsy (ĕp′ĭ-lĕp″sĕ) General term for a variety of disorders characterized by abnormalities of consciousness and convulsions due to brain damage. Drugs used in the treatment of symptoms (e.g., hydantoin sodium, diphenylhydantoin sodium) promote gingival hyperplasia.

epiloia (ĕp-ĭ-loi′yah) *See* syndrome, BournevillePringle.

epinephrine (ĕp″ĭ-nĕf′rĭn) A hormone secreted by the adrenal medulla that stimulates hepatic glycogenolysis, causing an elevation in the blood sugar, vasodilation of blood vessels of the skeletal muscles, vasoconstriction of the arterioles of the skin and mucous membranes, relaxation of bronchiolar smooth muscles, and stimulation of heart action. Used in local anesthetics for its vasoconstrictive action.

epiphysis (ē-pĭf′ĭ-sĭs) Terminal portion of a long bone. It is separated from the diaphysis during growth by a cartilaginous zone that serves as a growth center. Once ossification unites the epiphysis with the diaphysis, growth is completed.

epispinal (ĕp-ĭ-spī′nal) Located on the spinal column.

epistaxis (ĕp″ĭ-stăk′ sĭs) (nosebleed) Bleeding from the nose.

epithelial (ĕp-ĭ-thē′lē-al) Pertaining to the epithelium.

e. attachment *See* attachment, epithelial.

e. cuff, attached The attachment of the gingival epithelium to the enamel, including the close approximation of the free gingiva to the tooth.

e. cuff, implant The band of tissue that is constricted around an implant abutment post.

e. inclusion Bits of epithelial tissue introduced into bone crypts during perforation osteotomies. *See also* osteotomy, perforation.

epithelioma (ĕp″ĭ-thē″lē-ō′mah) An epithelial cancer.

e. adenoides cysticum (Brooke's tumor, trichoepithelioma) A form of basal cell carcinoma believed to arise from the epithelium of hair follicles. Regarded as a less invasive form of basal cell carcinoma.

e., basal cell *See* carcinoma, basal cell.

epithelium (ĕp″ĭ-thē′lē-ŭm) The structural arrangement of the various cellular components of epithelium characterized by two basic forms: medium suprapapillary width with medium-length rete pegs, and narrow suprapapapillary width with long rete pegs.

e., basement membrane of *See* membrane, basement.

e., desmosomes of An electromicroscopic finding of intercellular bridges that serve to attach adjacent epithelial cells to each other.

e., enamel, inner The innermost layer of cells (ameloblasts) of the enamel organ that deposit the organic matrix of the enamel on the crown of the developing tooth. Also the innermost layer of Hertwig's epithelial root sheath.

e., enamel, outer The outermost layer of cells of the enamel organ. It is separated from the inner enamel epithelium in the area of the developing crown by the stratum intermedium and stellate reticulum and lies immediately adjacent to the inner enamel epithelium in the area of the developing root.

e., enamel, reduced Combined enamel epithelium; the remains of the enamel organ after enamel formation is complete. After eruption of the tip of the crown, that part of the combined epithelium remaining on the enamel surface is called the *epithelial attachment*.

e., gingival A stratified squamous epithelium consisting of a basal layer; it is keratinized or parakeratinized when comprising the attached gingiva.

e., hyperplastic Increase in thickness, with alterations in structure, produced by proliferation of cellular elements of epithelium. The stratum spinosum epidermidis is usually the layer of cells that become thickened, resulting in acanthosis.

e., oral The epithelial covering of the oral mucous membranes. Composed of stratified squamous epithelium of varying thickness and varying degrees of keratinization.

e., pocket The epithelium that lines the gingival or periodontal pocket. Its most prominent characteristics are the presence of hyperplasia and ulceration, with exposure to the corium of the gingiva.

e., squamous Epithelium consisting of flat, scalelike cells.

e., stratified squamous The variety of epithelium prevalent as the covering of the oral mucous membrane and of dermal surfaces; composed of layers of cells oriented parallel to the surface. The various layers of cells in order of ascent from basement membrane to surface are stratum germinativum, stratum spongiosum, stratum granulosum, stratum lucidum (in dermal epithelium), and stratum corneum. The gingival epithelium generally exhibits some degree of keratinization, variable from parakeratosis to hyperkeratosis.

e., sulcal The stratified squamous epithelium forming the covering of the soft tissue wall of the gingival sulcus, or crevice. Extends from the gingival margin to the line of attachment of the epithelium to the tooth surface.

epithelization (ĕp′ ĭ-thē″lē-zā′shŭn) The natural act of healing by secondary intention; the proliferation of new epithelium into an area devoid of it but which naturally is covered by it.

epizootic fever Another name for foot and mouth disease in cloven-footed animals; also known as aphthous fever; caused by a type of coxsackievirus, uncommon in the United States. The disease in man is characterized by malaise, fever, headache, itchy skin, and a sensation of dry mouth despite heavy salivation. Vesicles appear in the mouth, around the lips, and on the hands and feet. Vesicles and ulcers of the mouth disappear within about 10 days.

epoxy resin (ē-pahk′sē) *See* resin, epoxy.

Epstein-Barr virus A herpetovirus associated with Burkitt's lymphoma and reported in cases of infectious mononucleosis; more recently reported associated with AIDS.

Epstein's pearls *See* nodules, Bohn's.

epulis (ĕp′ū-lĭs) A tumor (tumescence) of the gingiva. **e., congenital** of newborn A raised or pedunculated lesion located on the anterior gingivae of the newborn. It is histologically similar to granular cell myoblastoma. *See also* myoblastoma, granularcell.

e. fissurata (inflammatory fibrous hyperplasia, redundant tissue) A curtainlike fold of excess tissue associated with the flange of a denture.

e., giant cell *See* granuloma, giant cell reparative, peripheral.

e. granulomatosa A tumorlike mass of red, easily bleeding, infected granulation tissue that occurs due to exuberant reparative phenomena. Seen arising from tooth sockets or is associated with exfoliating necrotic bone.

equilibration (ē″kwĭ-lĭ-brā′shŭn) The act of placing a body in a state of equilibrium.

e., diagnostic *See* diagnostic equilibration.

e., mandibular The act or acts performed to place the mandible in a state of equilibrium.

e. of mounted casts Equilibration of the occlusion of mounted casts made of a patient for the purpose of observing and recording what must be done to adjust the natural occlusion.

e., occlusal Modification of occlusal forms of teeth by grinding, with the intent of equalizing occlusal stress and of harmonizing cuspal relations in function.

equilibrator (ē″kwĭ-lĭ-brā′tor) An instrument or device used in achieving or maintaining a state of equilibrium.

equilibrium (e″kwi-lib′re-um) A state of balance between two opposing forces or processes.

e., functional The state of homeostasis within the oral cavity existing when biologic processes and local environmental factors, including the forces of mastication, are in a state of balance.

equipment The nonexpendable items used by the dentist in the performance of professional duties.

equity A free and reasonable claim or right; fairness; impartiality. The money value of a property or of an interest in a property in excess of claims or liens against it; a risk interest or ownership right in property.

equivalent Equal in force, value, measure, or effect; corresponding in function.

e., aluminum The thickness of pure aluminum affording the same radiation attenuation, under specified conditions, as the material or materials being considered.

e., concrete The thickness of concrete having a density of 2.35 g/cm^3 that would afford the same radiation attenuation, under specified conditions, as the material or materials being considered.

e., lead The thickness of pure lead that would afford the same radiation attenuation, under specified conditions, as the material or materials under consideration.

erg A unit of energy (equal to a force of 1 dyne acting through a distance of 1 cm) equal to 2.4×10^{-8} calories, or 6.24×10^6 eV.

ergotoxine (ĕr″gō-tŏx′ĭn) A potent alkaloid that paralyzes the motor and secretory nerves of the sympathetic system but has no effect on the inhibitory or parasympathetic nerves.

ERISA Acronym for the Employee Retirement Income Security Act of 1974. *See* Employee Retirement Income Security Act.

erosion (ē-rō′zhŭn) Chemical or mechanicochemical destruction of tooth substance, the mechanism of which is incompletely known, that leads to the creation of concavities of many shapes at the cementoenamel junction of teeth. The surface of the cavity, unlike dental caries, is hard and smooth.

error Violation of duty; fault; a mistake in the proceedings of a court in matters of law or of fact.

e., legal A mistaken judgment or incorrect belief as to the existence or effect of matters of fact or a false or mistaken conception or application of the law.

e. of measurement The deviation of an individual score or observation from its true value that is due to the unreliability of the instrument and of the individual who is measuring.

e., numerical The amount of loss or precision in a quantity; the difference between an accurate quantity and its calculated approximation. Errors occur in numerical methods; mistakes occur in programming, coding, data transcription, and operating; malfunctions occur in computers and are due to physical limitations of the properties of materials.

e., sampling Any mistake in drawing a sample that keeps it from being unrepresentative; selection procedures that are biased; error introduced when a group is described on the basis of an unrepresentative sample.

e., variance That part of the total variance due to anything irrelevant to a study that cannot be experimentally controlled.

eruption (ē-rŭp′shun) The migration of a tooth from within its follicle in the alveolar process of the maxilla or mandible into the oral cavity.

e., continuous The normal occlusal progression of teeth noted throughout a lifetime.

e. cyst A dentigerous cyst that causes a clinically evident bulging of the overlying alveolar ridge. *See also* cysts, eruption

e., ectopic Abnormal direction of tooth eruption, most common to mandibular first and third molars, which sometimes leads to abnormal resorption of the adjacent tooth.

eruption hematoma An eruption cyst that is blood filled, visualized as a bluish purple area of elevated tissue of the overlying alveolar ridge.

e., passive Increasing length of the clinical crown often seen with aging and in the absence of clinical evidence of inflammation. The stages of passive eruption are as follows: (1) the most apical limit of the epithelial attachment is at the cementoenamel junction; (2) the most apical limit of the attachment is on the cementum, with the base of the gingival sulcus still on the enamel surface; (3) the most apical limit of the epithelial attachment is on the cementum, with the base of the sulcus at the cementoenamel junction; and (4) both the base of the sulcus and the epithelial attachment are on the surface of the cementum.

e., surgical Surgical removal of tissues covering an ab-

normally unerupted tooth to allow its natural progress into position.

eruptive gingivitis *See* gingivitis, eruptive.

erythema (ĕr″ĭ-thē′mah) Patchy, circumscribed, or marginated macular redness of the skin or mucous membranes due to hyperemia or inflammation.

e. multiforme complex An acute, inflammatory dermatologic disease of uncertain etiology (although occasionally related to drug administration), characterized by erythematous macules, papules, vesicles, and bullae that appear on the skin and not infrequently on the oral mucosa. *See also* syndrome, Stevens-Johnson.

erythredema polyneuropathy (ĕ-rĭth″rĕ-dē′mah pol′ĭ-noo-rop′ah-thē **(acrodynia, Feer's disease, pink disease, Selter's disease, Swift's disease)** A disease of infancy believed to be due to mercury poisoning. It is manifested by itching of the hands and feet, profuse sweating, hypertension, vasomotor disturbances, bruxism, and precocious shedding of the teeth.

erythremia (er″ĭ-thrē′mĕ-ah) **(Osler's disease, polycythemia rubra, polycythemia vera, primary polycythemia, Vaquez' disease)** A myeloproliferative disease characterized by a marked increase in the circulating red blood cell mass. It may represent a neoplastic growth of erythropoietic tissue. Neutrophilia, thrombocytopenia, and splenomegaly are common. Manifestations include plethora, vertigo, headache, and thrombosis.

erythroblastosis fetalis (ĕ-rĭth″rō-blăs-tō′sĭs fē-tăl′ĭs) Excessive destruction of red blood cells begun before or shortly after birth. It may be due to an Rh factor reaction. The skin is yellow, and the teeth may be markedly discolored.

Erythrocin Brand name for erythromycin.

erythrocyte (ĕ-rĭth′rō-sīt) Red blood cell; a nonnucleated, circular, biconcave, discoid, hemoglobincontaining, oxygen-carrying formed element circulating in the blood.

erythrocyte count The number of red blood cells per cubic millimeter of blood.

erythrocyte indices Standard values of red blood cell numbers, morphologic characteristics, and behavior in comprehensive hematologic laboratory testing.

erythrocyte sedimentation rate (ESR) The rate at which red blood cells settle in a pipette of unclotted blood, measured in millimeters per hour. It is used as an index of inflammation.

erythrocyte-maturing factor (EMF) *See* vitamin, cyanocobalamin.

erythrocytosis (ĕ-rĭth″rō-sī-tō′sĭs) **(secondary polycythemia)** An increased circulating red blood cell mass due to compensatory effort to meet reduced oxygen content. May be seen in persons living at high altitudes, as well as in emphysema, pulmonary insufficiency, and heart failure.

erythromycin An antibiotic produced by a strain of Streptomyces erythroeus, effective against beta-hemolytic streptococci (viridans group) upper and lower respiratory tract, skin, and soft tissue infections of mild to moderate severity. Recommended by the American Heart Association and the American Dental Association for use in a regimen for prophylaxis against bacterial endocarditis in patients hypersensitive to pencillin.

erythroplasia of Queyrat (ĕ-rĭth″rō-plā′zē-ah of kuhrat′) A form of intraepithelial carcinoma. The oral lesions are usually Seen as plaques with a bright, velvety surface.

escharotic (ĕs-kah-rot′ĭk) A caustic or corrosive agent that has the strength to burn tissue.

E space The net difference between the combined mesiodistal width of the primary canine, primary first molar, and the primary second molar and that of the permanent canine, first premolar, and second premolar. In the mandible the mean leeway space is 3.4 mm and in the maxilla it is 1.9 mm. Synonym: leeway space.

essence (ĕs′ĕns) An alcoholic solution of an essential oil.

essential oil *See* oil, essential.

Essig-type splinting *See* splinting, Essig-type.

estate One's interest in land or other property.

    e. planning A detailed, written-out plan (usually arrived at with the advice of estate counselors), in which all the financial affairs of the dentist are clearly stated and provisions are made for alterations when changing conditions warrant it.

ester (ĕs′tĕr) Any compound formed from alcohol and an acid.

esterase (ĕs′ter-ās) An enzyme that catalyzes the hydrolysis of an ester into its alcohol and acid.

esthetics (ĕs-thĕt′ĭks) (**aesthetics**) The branch of philosophy dealing with beauty, especially with the components thereof, i.e., color and form.

    e. dentistry Refers to those skills and techniques used to improve the art and symmetry of the teeth and face to improve the appearance as well as the function of the teeth, mouth, and face.

    e., denture The cosmetic effect, produced by a denture, that affects the desirable beauty, charm, character, and dignity of the individual.

        e., denture base (gingival tissue esthetics) The esthetically proper tinting, contouring, and festooning of the gingival tissue portion of a denture base.

    e., gingival tissue *See* esthetics, denture base.

estimate The anticipated fee for dental services to be performed.

Estlander's operation *See* operation, Abbé-Estlander.

estoppel (ĕ-stop′ĕl) A preclusion, in law, that prevents a person from alleging or denying a fact because of his/her own previous act or allegation.

estradiol benzoate (ĕs″trah-dī′ol bĕn′zō-āt) A topical steroid (B-estradiol-3-benzoate) with estrogenic activity, useful in the treatment of lesions produced by diminution of bodily production of estrogens. Experimental administration to aged laboratory mice has resulted in an increased downgrowth of epithelial attachment along the root surface of teeth and subsequent production of periodontal disease.

estrin (ĕs′trĭn) Generic term for the *ovarian estrogens: estriol, estrone,* and *estradiol.*

estrogens (ĕs′trō-jĕnz) Collective term for substances capable of producing estrus. It is also applied to the estrogenic hormones in women. Estriol is the principal estrogen found in the urine of pregnant women and in the placenta. Synthetic estrogens include diethylstilbestrol, hexestrol, and ethynyl estradiol.

etch, acid *See* acid etching.

etching A process used to decalcify the superficial layers of enamel as a step in the application of sealants or bonding agents in preventive dentistry and orthodontics. The agent of choice is phosphoric acid in concentrations of 30% to 40%.

ether, diethyl (ē′thĕr, dī-ĕth′ĭl) (**ethyl ether, ether** $[C_2H_5]_2O$) A volatile ether used as an anesthetic that causes excellent muscle relaxation with minimal effect on blood pressure, pulse rate, and respiration. It is irritating to the respiratory passages and produces nausea.

ether, divinyl (ē′ther, di-vi′nil) (**divinyl oxide** $[CH_2:CH]_2O$) Highly volatile, unsaturated ether that is a rapid-acting anesthetic without the aftereffect of nausea produced by diethyl ether.

etherization (ē″ther-ĭ-zā′shŭn) Administration of ether to produce anesthesia.

ethics (ĕth′ĭks) **1:** The science of moral obligation; a system of moral principles, quality, or practice. **2:** The moral obligation to render to the patient the best possible quality of dental service and to maintain an honest relationship with other members of the profession and mankind in general.

ethyl chloride (ĕth′ĭl klō′rīd) (**C_2H_5Cl**) A colorless liquid that boils between 12° and 13° C. It acts as a local anesthetic of short duration through the superficial freezing produced by its rapid vaporization from the skin. It is used occasionally in inhalation therapy as a rapid fleeting general anesthetic, comparable to nitrous oxide but somewhat more dangerous.

ethylene (ĕth′ĭ-lēn) (**olefiant gas, CH_2CH_2**) A colorless gas of slightly sweet odor and taste; used as an inhalation anesthetic.

ethylene oxide sterilization A gas used to sterilize instruments, equipment and materials that would otherwise be damaged by heat, or liquid chemicals. Effective at room temperature. Requires between 10 and 16 hours to be effective. Gas must penetrate the material.

The gas is highly toxic and must be vented before opening the sealed sterilizing unit. Sterilized materials must also be well aerated before using.

etiology (ē″tē-ol′ō-jē) **1:** Causative factors. **2:** The factors implicated in the causation of disease. **3:** The study of the factors causing disease.

  e., local factors The environmental influences that may be implicated in the causation and/or perpetuation of a disease process.

  e., systemic factors Generalized biologic factors that are implicated in the causation, modification, and/ or perpetuation of a disease entity. Within the oral cavity, the actions of the systemic factors are modified by interaction with local factors.

eudaemonic (ū-dē-mon′ĭk) Pertaining to a drug that brings about a feeling of normal well-being in a previously depressed patient.

eugenol (ū′jĕ-nol) **1:** An allyl guaiacol obtainable from oil of cloves. Used with zinc oxide in a paste for temporary restorations, bases under restorations, and impression materials. Believed to have a palliative effect on dental pulp and possibly a limited germicidal effect. **2:** Colorless or pale yellow liquid obtained from clove oil; has a clove odor and pungent, spicy taste. Used as the liquid portion of zinc oxide and eugenol cements and in toothache medications.

eugnathia (ū-nā′thē-ah) The normal or proper relationship of the jaws to each other.

euphoria (ū-for′ē-ah) A sense of well-being or normalcy. Pleasantly mild excitement.

euphoric (ū-for′ĭk) A substance that produces an exaggerated sense of well-being.

eupnea (ūp-nē′ah) Easy or normal respiration.

eutaxia (ū-tăk′sē-ah) Muscular coordination in good order. Opposite of ataxia.

euthyroidism (ū-thī′roid-ĭzm) A state of normal thyroid function.

evacuation system A centralized vacuum system connected to each dental operating unit used to keep the oral cavity clear of water, saliva, blood, and debris, generally operating at a high volume, high velocity, and low pressure.

evaluation To make a judgment or appraisal of a condition or situation. In dentristry used to describe the clinical judgment of a patient's dental health or an appraisal of staff performance.

evidence Proof presented at a trial by the parties through witnesses, records, documents, concrete objects, etc., for the purpose of inducing the court or jury to believe their contentions.

  e., radiographic The shadow images depicted in radiographs.

Evipal (ē′vĭ-pahl) Trade name for hexobarbital, a rapid-acting barbiturate.

  e. sodium Trade name for hexobarbital sodium. An ul-

trashort-acting barbiturate of the *N*-methyl type whose pharmacologic actions, from a clinical standpoint, are essentially similar to thiopental (Pentothal).

evulsed tooth *See* tooth, evulsed.

evulsion (avulsion) The sudden tearing out, or away, of tissue due to a traumatic episode.

  e., tooth Displacement of a tooth from its alveolar housing; may be partial or complete.

  e., nerve The operation of tearing a nerve from its central origin by traction.

Ewing's sarcoma *See* tumor, Ewing's.

Ewing's tumor *See* tumor, Ewing's.

examination **1:** Inspection; search; investigation; inquiry; scrutiny; testing. **2:** Inspection and/or investigation of part or all of the body to measure and evaluate the state of health or disease. The examination may include visual inspection, percussion, palpation, auscultation, and measurement of mobility, as well as various laboratory and radiographic procedures.

  e., clinical Visual and tactile scrutiny of the tissues of and surrounding the oral cavity.

  e., gingival Observation of the primary visual symptoms of periodontal disease, including color changes; changes in surface texture; deviations from normal contour and structure, tissue tone, and vitality; presence or absence of clefts; and the position of attachment.

  e., intraoral Examination of all the structures contained within the oral cavity.

  e., radiographic 1: Production of the number of radiographs necessary for the radiologic interpretation of the part or parts in question. **2:** Study and interpretation of radiographs of the mouth and associated structures.

  e., extraoral radiographic Examination of the oral and paraoral structures by exposing films placed extraorally, in contrast to intraorally.

  e., anteroposterior extraoral radiographic Examination in which the film is placed at the posterior with the rays passing from the anterior to the posterior direction to record images.

  e., body section extraoral radiographic (tomogram) A radiographic procedure of various internal layers of the head and body accomplished by the synchronized movement of the roentgen-ray tube and film in parallel planes but in opposite directions from each other. Also known as tomography, laminagraphy, planigraphy, and stratigraphy.

  e., bregma-mentum extraoral radiographic Radiography in which the film is placed beneath the chin, with the rays directed downward through the junction of the coronal and sagittal sutures (bregma) to the chin (meritum).

e., cephalometric extraoral radiographic *See* cephalometric radiography.

e., lateral facial extraoral radiographic Examination by means of a lateral head film.

e., lateral head extraoral radiographic Examination in which the film is placed parallel to the sagittal plane of the head.

e., lateral jaw extraoral radiographic Examination in which the film is placed adjacent to the mandible.

e., mental extraoral radiographic Examination in which the film is placed beneath the chin and the radiation is directed through the long axis of the lower central incisors while the mouth is open. An examination for viewing the mental process.

e., panoramic extraoral radiographic Curved single film radiography in which the beam source and film rotate in a synchronized manner about the head, exposing oral structures sequentially with simultaneous exposure of corresponding areas of the film.

e., posteroanterior extraoral radiographic Examination in which the film is placed anteriorly, with the rays passing from the posterior to the anterior direction.

e., profile extraoral radiographic Lateral head examination to show the profile of bone and soft tissue outline. It uses a decrease in milliampere seconds or an increase in target-film distance for recording the soft tissue image.

e., stereoscopic extraoral radiographic Radiographic examination used in conjunction with a stereoscope for localization. Exposures of two films are made, with identical placement of each film adjacent to the part in question and with a different angulation for each exposure.

e., temporomandibular extraoral radiographic Examination in which the film is placed adjacent to the area to be examined, with the rays directed through a point 2 ½ inches (6.25 cm) above the tragus of the opposite external ear with a vertical angulation of 15 degrees and a horizontal angulation of 5 degrees downward. Various other techniques and angulations are used (including laminagraphy) in examining this area.

e., Waters extraoral radiographic Posteroanterior examination of the paranasal sinuses. The film is placed in contact with the nose and chin, with the rays directed at right angles to the plane of the film.

e., intraoral radiographic Radiography of the teeth and facial bones by placing films within the oral cavity and directing roentgen rays at various angles through the area of interest.

e., bite-wing intraoral radiographic Radiography in which an intraoral radiograph records on a single film the shadow images of the outline, position, and mesiodistal extent of the crowns, necks, and coronal third of the roots of both the maxillary and mandibular teeth and alveolar crests.

e., extradental intraoral radiographic Examination in which the film is placed between the teeth and the tissue of the cheek or lip for the exploration or localization of the internal structures of these tissues.

e., oblique occlusal intraoral radiographic Exploratory examination of the maxillae or mandible using an occlusal type of film placed between the teeth. The rays are directed obliquely downward or upward (usually 60 to 75 degrees in the vertical plane) and parallel to the sagittal plane.

e., periapical intraoral radiographic The basic intraoral examination, showing all of a tooth and the surrounding periodontium.

e., true occlusal topographic intraoral radiographic Radiography of the maxillae or mandible using an occlusal type of film placed between the teeth, with the rays directed at right angles to the plane of the film or through the long axis of the teeth adjacent to the part in question.

excavator, spoon (ĕks′kah-vā″tor) A paired hand instrument intended primarily to remove carious material from a cavity.

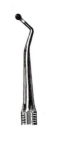

Spoon excavator

excess More than is necessary, useful, or specified.

e. marginal A condition in which the restorative material extends beyond the prepared cavity margin.

e. overhang Gingival margin excess.

excipient (ĕk-sĭp′ē-ĕnt) An ingredient included in a pharmaceutical preparation for the purpose of improving its physical qualities. *See also* binder; filler; vehicle.

excision (ĕk-sĭzh′ŭn) The act of cutting away or taking out.

e., local An excision limited to the immediate area of the lesion in question.

e., radical An excision involving not only the lesion in question but also anatomic parts remote from the site.

e., wide An excision involving the lesion in question and immediately adjacent anatomic structures.

excitant (ĕk-sīt′ănt) An agent that stimulates the activity of an organ.

excitation (ĕk-sī-tā′shŭn) The addition of energy to a system, thereby transferring it from its ground state to an excited state.

excursion A trip; movement from a mean position.

e., lateral Movement of the mandible from the centric position to a lateral or protusive position.

exclusions Dental services not covered under a dental benefits program.

exclusive provider organization (EPO) A dental benefits plan that provides benefits only if care is rendered by institutional and professional providers with whom the plan contracts (with some exceptions for emergency and out-of-area services).

execute To finish; accomplish; fulfill. To carry out according to its terms.

exercise prosthesis See prosthesis, exercise.

exercises, myotherapeutic See therapy, myofunctional.

exfoliation (ĕks-fō″lē-ā′shŭn) **(shedding)** Physiologic loss of the primary dentition.

exhalation (ĕks-hah-lā′shŭn) Giving off or sending forth in the form of vapor; expiration.

exhaustion (ĕg-zawst′yŭn) Loss of vital and nervous power from fatigue or protracted disease.

exhibit (ĕg-zīb′ĭt) A paper, document, or object presented to a court during a trial or hearing as proof of facts, or as otherwise connected with the subject matter, and which, on being accepted, is marked for identification and considered a part of the case.

exocytosis The appearance of migrating inflammatory cells in the epidermis.

exodontics (ĕk″sō-don′tĭks) The science and practice of removing teeth from the oral cavity as performed by dentists.

exolever (ĕks′ō-lē″ver) An instrument that uses the principles of leverage for extracting and removing teeth or roots of teeth from the oral cavity.

exophthalmos (ĕk″sof-thăl′mos) Abnormal protrusion of the eyeball. It is characteristic of toxic (exophthalmic) goiter.

exostosis (ĕk″sŏs-tō′sĭs) **(hyperostosis)** A bony growth projecting from a bony surface.

exotoxin (ĕk″sō-tok′sīn) The toxic material formed by microorganisms and subsequently released into their surrounding environments.

expanded duty auxiliary A person trained to carry out dental procedures more complex than the responsibilities usually delegated to dental auxiliaries.

expansile infrastructure endosteal implant An intraosseous implant device designed to enlarge or open after its insertion into the bone to provide retention.

expansion Increase in extent, size, volume, or scope.

e., delayed (secondary expansion) 1: Expansion occurring in amalgam restorations due to moisture contamination. **2:** Expansion exhibited by amalgam that has been contaminated by moisture during trituration or insertion.

e., dental arch Therapeutic increase in circumference of the dental arch by buccal and/or labial movement of the teeth.

e., hygroscopic Expansion, caused by absorption of water during setting of an investment, used to compensate for the shrinkage of mental from the molten to the solid state.

e., secondary See expansion, delayed.

e., setting Expansion that occurs during the setting or hardening of a material such as amalgam and gypsum products.

e., thermal Expansion due to heat. Thermal expansion of the mold is one of the important factors in achieving adequate compensation for the contraction of cast metal when it solidifies.

e., thermal coefficient A number indicating the amount of expansion caused by each degree of temperature change. The rate of change in restorative materials and tooth substance should be relatively the same.

experience rating A determination of the premium rate for a particular group partially or wholly on the basis of that group's own experience. Age, sex, use, and costs of services provided determine the premium.

experiment A trial or special observation made to confirm or disprove something doubtful; an act or operation undertaken to discover some unknown principle or effect or to test, establish, or illustrate some suggested or known truth.

expert One who has special skill or knowledge in a particular subject, such as a science or art, whether acquired by experience or study; a specialist.

expiration 1: Act of breathing forth or expelling air from the lungs. **2:** Cessation; termination; the expiration of a lease.

expiration date 1: Date on which the dental benefits contract expires. **2:** Date an individual ceases to be eligible for benefits.

explanation of benefits A written statement to a beneficiary, from a third-party payer, after a claim has been reported, indicating the benefits/charges covered or not covered by the dental benefits plan.

exploration 1: Examination by touch, either with or without instruments. For example, a carious lesion is explored with a special explorer, but the mucobuccal fold may be explored with the finger. **2:** The process of examination of a surface, with or without the use of instruments, to determine the condition or the surface depth of a defect or other similar diagnostic parameters.

explore To investigate.

explorer A dental instrument with a slender head honed to a fine point used to conduct a tactile examination and appraisal of pits and fissures, carious lesions, root surfaces, and margins of restoration.

explosion A violent, noisy outbreak due to a sudden release of energy.

exposure Uncovering; subjection to viewing or radiation.

e., air Radiation exposure measured in a small mass of air under conditions of electronic equilibrium with the surrounding air, that is, excluding backscatter from irradiated parts or objects.

e., chronic Radiation exposure of long duration, either continuous (protraction exposure) or intermittent (fractionation exposure); usually referring to exposure of relatively low intensity.

e., cumulative The total accumulated exposure resulting from repeated radiation exposures of the whole body or of a particular region.

e., double Two superimposed exposures on the same radiographic or photographic film.

e., entrance Exposure measured at the surface of an irradiated body, part, or object. It includes both primary radiation and backscatter from the irradiated underlying tissue or material.

e., erythema The radiation exposure necessary to produce a temporary redness of the skin. The exposure required will vary with the quality of the radiation to which the skin is exposed.

e., protraction Exposure to radiation continuously over a relatively long period at a low exposure rate.

e., pulp An opening through the wall of the pulp chamber uncovering the dental pulp.

e., accidental pulp Pulp exposure unintentionally created during instrumentation.

e., carious pulp Pulp exposure occasioned by extension of the carious process to the pulp chamber wall.

e., mechanical pulp *See* exposure, pulp, surgical.

e., surgical pulp (mechanical pulp exposure) Pulp exposure created intentionally or unintentionally during instrumentation.

e., radiographic A measure of the x or gamma radiation to which a person or object, or part of either, is exposed at a certain place, this measure being based on its ability to produce ionization. The unit of x or gamma radiation exposure is the roentgen (R).

e. rate, output Exposure to radiation at a specified point per unit of time, usually expressed in roentgens per minute.

e., surface *See* exposure, entrance.

e., threshold The minimum exposure that will produce a detectable degree of any given effect.

e. time The time during which a person or object is exposed to radiation, expressed in one of the conventional units of time.

express Stated distinctly and explicitly and not left to inference; set forth in words.

exsufflation (ĕk″sŭf-flā′shŭn) Forced discharge of the breath.

extension **1:** Enlargement in boundary, breadth, or depth. **2:** The process of increasing the angle between two skeletal levers having end-to-end articulation with each other; the opposite of flexion.

e. base *See* base, extension.

e. of benefits Extension of eligibility for benefits for covered services, usually designed to ensure completion of treatment commenced prior to the expiration date. Duration is generally expressed in terms of days.

e., gingiva, attached Gingival extension operation; a surgical technique designed to broaden the zone of attached gingiva by repositioning the mucogingival junction apically.

e., groove Enlargement of a cavity preparation outline to include a developmental groove.

e. for prevention A principle of cavity preparation enunciated by G.V. Black in 1891. To prevent the recurrence of decay, he advocated extension of the preparation subgingivally and axially and occlusally into an area that is readily polished and cleaned.

e., ridge An intraoral surgical operation for deepening the labial, buccal, and/or lingual sulci.

extenuate To lessen; to mitigate.

external oblique line (ō-blēk′) *See* line, external oblique.

external pin fixation *See* appliance, fracture.

external traction *See* traction, external.

exteroceptors (ek″ster-ō-sĕp′tors) Sensory nerve end receptors that respond to external stimuli; located in the skin, mouth, eyes, ears, and nose.

extirpation, pulp (ĕk″ster-pā′shŭn) *See* pulpectomy.

extracoronal (ĕk″strah-kor′ō-năl) Pertaining to that which is outside, or external to, the body of the coronal portion of a natural tooth.

e. retainer *See* retainer, extracoronal.

extract A concentrate obtained by treating a crude material, such as plant or animal tissue, with a solvent, evaporating part or all of the solvent from the resulting solution, and standardizing the resulting product.

extraction Removal of a tooth from the oral cavity by means of elevators and/or forceps.

e., serial Extraction of selected primary teeth over a period of years (often ending with removal of the first premolar teeth) to relieve crowding of the dental arches during eruption of the lateral incisors, canines, and premolars.

extrahazardous In the law of insurance, an action attended by circumstances or conditions of unusual danger.

extraoral Literally, outside of the mouth. Generally refers to an orthodontic appliance that extends outside the mouth to secure a firm base for force application within the mouth. *See* anchorage, extral oral.

extraoral anchorage Orthodontic force applied from a base outside the mouth. *See* anchorage.

extrapolate (ĕk-străp′ō-lāt) To infer values beyond the observable range from an observed trend of variables; to project by inference into the unexplored.

extrasystole (ĕk″strah-sĭs′tō-lē) A heartbeat occurring before its normal time in the rhythm of the heart and followed by a compensatory pause.

extravasation (ĕk-străv″ah-zā′shŭn) The escape of a body fluid out of its proper place (e.g., blood into surrounding tissues after rupture of a vessel, urine into surrounding tissues after rupture of the bladder).

extrinsic coloring Coloring from without (e.g., coloring of the external surface of a prosthesis).

extroversion A tendency of the teeth or other maxillary structures to become situated too far from the median plane.

extrude To elevate; to move a tooth coronally.

extrusion Movement of teeth beyond the natural occlusal plane that may be accompanied by a similar movement of investing tissues. *See also* eruption, continuous.

extubate (ĕks′tū-bāt) To remove a tube, usually an endotracheal anesthesia tube or a Levin gastric suction tube.

extubation (ĕks″tū-bā′shŭn) Removal of a tube used for intubation.

exudate (ĕks′ū-dāt) The outpouring of a fluid substance, such as exudated pus or tissue fluid.

  e., gingival The outpouring of an inflammatory exudate from the gingival tissues.

exudation (ĕks″ū-dā′shŭn) *See* exudate.

eye-ear plane *See* plane, Frankfort horizontal.

F-ratio (F-test) A value used in determining whether the difference between two variables is statistically significant or stable. A larger variance is divided by a smaller variance, both the results of analysis of variance procedures. The value for F is looked up in a table that shows the probability of occurrence of a ratio of this size.

fabrication (făb″rĭ-kā′shŭn) Construction or making of a restoration.

face, changeable area of The part of the face from the nose to the chin.

face form *See* form, face.

face-bow A caliper-like device that is used to record the relationship of the maxillae to the temporomandibular joints (or opening axis of the mandible) and to orient the casts in this same relationship to the opening axis of an articulator.

  f.-b., adjustable axis *See* face-bow, kinematic.

  f.-b., kinematic (hinge-bow) A face-bow attached to the mandible whose caliper ends (condyle rods) can be adjusted to permit the accurate location of the axis of rotation of the mandible.

facet (făs′ĕt) A flattened, highly polished wear pattern as noted on a tooth.

facial cleft *See* cleft, facial.

facial profile *See* profile, facial.

facies (fā′shē-ēz) The features, general appearance, and expression of a face.

facilitation Reinforcement of a lower level nerve stimulus by a higher level nerve stimulus. Thus a reflex that cannot be elicited by a subliminal impulse may be reinforced by an additional stimulus from a higher center. The combined effect of the two stimuli may cause a reflex response.

facsimile (făk-sĭm′ĭ-lē) A true copy that preserves all the markings and contents of the original.

fact A thing done; an event or a circumstance; an actual occurrence.

factor(s) A constituent, element, cause, or agent that influences a process or system; a gene; a dietary substance.

  f. I (fibrinogen, profibrin) *See* fibrinogen.

  f. II (prothrombin, component A, prothrombase, prothrombin B, thrombogen, thrombozyme) Considered to be the only essential precursor of thrombin.

  f. III (thromboplastin [tissue], thrombokinase, cytozyme [platelet], thrombokinin [blood], thromboplastic protein) *See* thromboplastin.

  f. IV (calcium, Ca + +) Ionized and/or bound calcium, which is generally required for the coagulation of blood, although some early phases of coagulation and the thrombin-fibrinogen reaction can take place without calcium.

  f. V (labile factor, proaccelerin, accelerin, acceleration factor, cofactor of thromboplastin, component A of prothrombin, plasma ac-globulin, plasma prothrombin conversion factor [PPCF], prothrombinase, prothrombin accelerator, prothrombin conversion accelerator I, thrombogen, thrombogene, proaccelerin-accelerin system) A factor apparently necessary for the formation of a prothrombin converting substance in blood and tissue extracts, i.e., intrinsic and extrinsic prothrombin activators. A deficiency results in parahemophilia (hypoproaccelerinemia).

  f. VI Term formerly used as indicating an intermediate product in the formation of thromboplastin and also used synonymously with accelerin and activated factor V. It has no designation at the present time.

  f. VII (stable factor, serum prothrombin conversion accelerator [SPCA], proconvertin, autoprothrombin I, cofactor V, component B of prothrombin, cothromboplastin, kappa factor, precursor of serum prothrombin conversion accelerator [pro-SPCA], prothrombin conversion factor, prothrombin converting factor, prothrombin conversion accelerator II, proconvertin-convertin system, prothrombinogen, serozyme, stable factor) A factor that accelerates the conversion of prothrombin to thrombin in the presence of factors III, IV, and V; a serum factor necessary for the formation of extrinsic prothrombin activator. A deficiency may be congenital, or it may be acquired in liver disease, vitamin K deficiency, or from prothrombinopenic agents used in anticoagulation therapy; it results in a prolonged (quantitative) one-stage prothrombin time test.

  f. VIII (antihemophilic factor [AHF], antihemophilic globulin, antihemophilic globulin A, antihemo-

philic factor A, plasma thromboplastin factor A [PTF-A], plasma thromboplastin factor [PTF], plasmokinin, platelet cofactor I, prothrombokinase, thrombocatalysin, thrombocytolysin, thrombokatilysin, thromboplastic plasma component [TPC], thromboplastinogen) A factor essential for the formation of blood thromboplastin. A deficiency results in classic hemophilia (hemophilia A); the clotting time is prolonged, and thromboplastin and prothrombin conversion is diminished.

f. IX (Christmas factor, plasma thromboplastin component [PTC], antihemophilic factor B, antihemophilic globulin B, autoprothrombin II, beta prothromboplastin, plasma factor X, plasma thromboplastin factor B [PTF-B], platelet cofactor II) A factor that is active in the formation of intrinsic blood thromboplastin. A deficiency results in Christmas disease (hemophilia B), which is caused by a decrease in the amount of thromboplastin formed.

f. X (Stuart-Prower factor, Stuart factor, Prower factor) A factor influencing the yield of intrinsic (plasma) thromboplastin. A deficiency results in a prolonged one-stage prothrombin time—brain tissue or Russell's viper venom are used to test for thromboplastin deficiency.

f. XI (plasma thromboplastin antecedent [PTA], antihemophilic factor C, PTA factor, plasma thromboplastin factor C [PTF-C]) A factor related to intrinsic (plasma) thromboplastin activation, which occurs when blood is exposed to a foreign surface. A deficiency results in hemophilioid states due to poor use of prothrombin. *See also* hemophilia C.

f. XII (Hageman factor, antihemophilic factor D, clot-promoting factor, fifth plasma thromboplastin precursor, glass factor) A factor whose absence results in a long clotting time and abnormal prothrombin consumption and thromboplastin generation tests when the tests are carried out in glass tubes. No abnormal bleeding tendency occurs with a deficiency of the factor.

f., acceleration *See* factor V.

f., antihemophilic (AHF) *See* factor VIII.

f., antihemophilic A *See* factor VIII.

f., antihemophilic B *See* factor IX.

f., antihemophilic C *See* factor XI.

f., antihemophilic D *See* factor XII.

f., antipernicious *See* vitamin B$_{12}$.

f. C (contact factor, contact activation product, third thromboplastic factor) A coagulation accelerator product formed by the interaction of active factor XII and factor XI.

f., Castle's intrinsic (intrinsic factor) A factor produced by the gastric mucosa, and possibly the duodenal mucosa, and considered to be responsible for the

absorption of vitamin B$_{12}$. *See also* anemia, pernicious.

f., Christmas *See* factor IX.

f., clot-promoting *See* factor XII.

f., clotting "Trace" proteins (excluding calcium) present in normal blood in such small amounts (except fibrinogen) that their presence is usually established by deductive reasoning and by genetic and biochemical characteristics. They are associated with thromboplastic activity and the conversion of prothrombin to thrombin.

f., contact *See* factor C.

f., environmental Local conditions that modify tissue response (e.g., narrow interdental spaces, saddle areas, attachment of frenula, oblique ridges).

f., erythrocyte-maturation (EMF) *See* vitamin B complex.

f., etiologic The element or influence that can be assigned as the cause or reason for a disease or lesion.

f., extrinsic *See* vitamin B complex.

f., familial A characteristic derived through heredity.

f., glass *See* factor XII.

f., glucocorticoid *See* hormone, "S".

f., Hageman *See* factor XII.

f., Hr Blood factors that are reciprocally related to the Rh factors. They are present in agglutinogens when the corresponding Rh factor is absent from the gene.

f., hyperglycemic *See* glucagon.

f., hyperglycemic-glycogenolytic *See* glucagon.

f., intrinsic *See* factor, Castle's intrinsic.

f., kappa *See* factor VII.

f., labile *See* factor V.

f., local Includes dental and bacterial plaques, bacterial toxins and irritants, calculus, food impaction, and other surface and locally placed irritants that are capable of injuring the periodontium.

f., pellagra-preventive *See* acid, nicotinic.

f., plasma, X *See* factor IX.

f., plasma prothrombin conversion (PPCF) *See* factor V.

f., plasma thromboplastin (PTF) Substances with thromboplastic activity contributed by the plasma. Included are the antihemophilic factor, Christmas factor, plasma thromboplastin antecedent, and Hageman factor. *See also* factor VIII.

> **f., plasma thromboplastin, A (PTF-A)** *See* factor VIII.
>
> **f., plasma thromboplastin, B (PTF-B)** *See* factor IX.
>
> **f., plasma thromboplastin, C (PTF-C)** *See* factor XI.
>
> **f., plasma thromboplastin, D (PTF-D)** Considered by some to be a fourth plasma substance with thromboplastic activity; not well characterized.

f., plasma X *See* factor IX.

f., platelet A substance on or in the surface of blood platelet necessary for coagulation in the absence of extravascular thromboplastic substances.

f., platelet, 1 (platelet ac-globulin, citrin) Either factor V or a factor with factor V activity; absorbed on platelets and accelerates conversion of prothrombin to thrombin.

f., platelet, 2 (platelet thrombin accelerator, platelet thromboplastic activity) A substance that accelerates the conversion of fibrinogen to fibrin.

f., platelet, 3 (thromboplastic cellular component [TCC], thromboplastinogenase, platelet activator) A substance associated with thromboplastin-generation activity.

f., platelet, 4 An antiheparin factor.

f., P.-P. (pellagra-preventive factor) *See* acid, nicotinic.

f., prothrombin conversion *See* factor VII.

f., prothrombin-converting *See* factor VII.

f., Prower *See* factor X.

f., psychosomatic Psychic, mental, or emotional factors that play a role in determining the initiation, course, and extent of a physical process; either directly or indirectly. Psychosomatic factors have been implicated in necrotizing ulcerative gingivitis (NUG), bruxism, clenching, oral habits, etc.

f., PTA (plasma thromboplastin antecedent factor) *See* factor XI.

f., reparative The ability of the tissues to heal or regenerate when they have been subjected to injury, disease, etc.

f., Rh Agglutinogens of red blood cells responsible for isoimmune reactions such as occur in erythroblastosis fetalis and incompatible blood transfusions.

f., spreading An enzyme that increases the permeability of ground substance.

f., stabile *See* factor VII.

f., stable *See* factor VII.

f., Stuart *See* factor X.

f., Stuart-Prower *See* factor X.

f., third thromboplastic *See* factor C.

failure Deficiency; inefficiency as measured by some legal standard; an unsuccessful attempt.

faint A state of syncope, or swooning.

falsify To forge; to give a false appearance to anything, as to falsify a record.

family 1: A body of persons who live in one house and under one head; a father, mother, and children; a husband and wife living together. **2:** The legal definition varies, depending on the jurisdiction and purpose for which the term is defined.

f. deductible A deductible that is satisfied by combined expenses of all covered family members. A plan with a $25 deductible may limit its application to a maxium of three deductibles, or $75, for the family, regardless of the number of family members.

f. membership A membership that includes spouses and/or dependents.

f. unit An insured group member and dependents who are eligible for benefits under a dental care contract; an accounting unit.

fascitis (fah-sī'tĭs) A tumorlike growth occurring in subcutaneous tissues in the mouth, usually in the cheek. A benign lesion sometimes mistaken for fibrosarcoma, it consists of young fibroblasts and numerous capillaries. It grows rapidly and may regress spontaneously.

fate Synonym for the more modern term *biotransformation*. *See also* biotransformation.

fatigue A condition of cells or organs under stress resulting in a diminution or loss of an individual's capacity to respond to stimulation.

f., muscle A peripheral phenomenon due to the failure of the muscle to contract when stimuli from the nervous system reach it. Occurs when muscle activity exceeds tissue substrate and oxygenation capacity.

fauces (faw'sēz) The archway between the pharyngeal and oral cavities; formed by the tongue, anterior tonsillar pillars, and soft palate.

FDA Abbreviation for the Food and Drug Administration. *See* Food and Drug Administration.

fear An emotion, generally considered negative and unpleasant, that is a reaction to a real or threatened danger; fright. Fear is distinguished from anxiety, which is a reaction to an unreal or imagined danger.

Fede's disease *See* disease, Riga-Fede.

fee Compensation for services rendered or to be rendered; payment for professional services.

f., customary A fee is customary if it is in the range of the usual fees charged by dentists of similar training and experience for the same service within the specific and limited geographic area (socioeconomic area of a metropolitan area or of a county).

f.-for-service plan A plan providing for payment to the dentist for each service performed rather than on the basis of salary or capitation fee.

f. schedule 1: A listing of maximum dollar allowances for dental procedures that apply under a specific contract. **2:** A list of the charges established or agreed to by a dentist for specific dental services.

f., reasonable A fee is considered reasonable if in the opinion of a responsible dental association's review committee it is the usual and customary fee charged for services rendered, considering the special circumstances of the case in question.

f., usual The fee customarily charged for a given service by an individual dentist to a private patient.

feedback The constant flow of sensory information back to the brain. When feedback mechanisms are deficient because of sensory deprivation, motor function becomes distorted, aberrant, and uncoordinated.

Feer's disease (fairz) *See* erythredema polyneuropathy.

feldspar (fĕld′spahr) A crystalline mineral of aluminum silicate with potassium, sodium, barium, or calcium— $NaAlSi_3O_8$ or $KAlSi_3O_8$. Feldspar melts over a range of 1100° to 2000° F (593.5° to 1093.5° C). An important constituent of dental porcelain.

f., orthoclase ceramic A clay found in large quantity in the solid crust of the earth. It acts as a filler and imparts body to the fused dental porcelaln.

fenestration (fĕn-ĕs-trā′shŭn) Opening, window, interstice.

f. in alveolar plate A round or oval defect or opening in the alveolar cortical plate of bone over the root surface.

Ferrier's separator (fer′ē-erz) *See* separator, Ferrier's.

festoon(s) (fĕs-toon′) A carving in the base material of a denture that simulates the contours of the natural tissues being replaced by the denture.

f., gingival The distinct rounding and enlargement of the margins of the gingival tissue found in early gingival involvement.

f., McCall's Enlargements of the gingival margins that may be associated with occlusal trauma.

festooning (fĕs-toon′ĭng) The process of carving the base material of a denture or denture pattern to simulate the contours of the natural tissues to be replaced by the denture.

fetor ex ore (fē′tor ĕks ō′rē) *See* halitosis.

fetor oris (fē′tor ō′rĭs) Bad breath, a common characteristic of ANUG. The degree of seriousness may be correlated with the amount of destruction present.

fever (pyrexia) Elevation of the body temperature.

f., acute necrotizing ulcerative gingivitis (ANUG) and acute primary keratotic gingivostomatitis (APKG) A moderate-to-high elevation of temperature is not a symptom of ANUG; however, the presence of a significantly elevated temperature might suggest the presence of APKG, a viral disease accompanied by a bleeding and tender gingiva, marked fetor oris, and lymphadenopathy.

f., aphthous *See* disease, foot-and-mouth.

f., cat-scratch (benign inoculation lymphoreticulosis, cat-scratch disease) A granulomatous process that occurs at the site of a scratch or bite of a house cat. Local lesions occur at the site of injury, with a regional adenitis that is out of proportion to the primary lesion occurring within 1 to 3 weeks. Systemic symptoms of infection may occur. Diagnosis is confirmed by reaction to cat-scratch antigen or the antigen of lymphogranuloma venereum, which is a related form of disease.

f., hay Rhinitis and conjunctivitis resulting from allergy; frequently caused by allergy to pollens.

f., rheumatic (roo-m̆at′ĭk) An apparently infectious disease produced by hemolytic streptococci or associated with their presence in the body; characterized by upper respiratory tract inflammation, cervical lymphadenopathy and lymphadenitis, polyarthritis, cardiac involvement, subcutaneous nodules, etc. The disease may be produced by an autoantibody reaction. A severe disease, apparently related to hypersensitive reaction to the hemolytic streptococci and characterized by polyarthritis, cardiac involvement, cervical lymphadenopathy, subcutaneous nodules, and low-grade fever.

f., scarlet (scarlatina) An acute disease caused by a specific type of streptococcus and characterized by a rash and a strawberry tongue.

f., uveoparotid (Heerfordt's syndrome, uveoparotitis) **1:** A disease characterized by inflammation of the parotid gland and of the uveal regions of the eye. **2:** Firm, nodular enlargement of the parotid glands, uveitis, and cutaneous lesions may be present. Considered to be a form of sarcoidosis. **3:** A syndrome consisting of sarcoidosis affecting the parotid glands, inflammation of the lacrimal glands, and inflammation of uveal tract of the eye.

fiber(s) An elongated, threadlike structure of organic tissue.

f., adrenergic Those nerve fibers, including most of the postganglionic sympathetic fibers, which transmit their impulses across synapses or neuroeffector junctions through the local release of the neurohormone more recently identified as norepinephrine and formerly designated sympathin.

f., alveolar White collagenous fibers of the peridontal membrane (ligament) that extend from the alveolar bone to the intermediate plexus, where their terminations are interspersed with the terminations of the cemental group of fibers.

f., alveolar crest Collagenous fibers of the peridontal membrane that extend from the cervical area of the tooth to the alveolar crest.

f., apical Fibers of the peridontal ligament radiating apically from tooth to bone.

f., association Extensions of nerve cells that are neither efferent nor afferent neurons but that furnish a pathway of connection between them.

f., bundle The gathering together of collagen fibers in a group, particularly the collagen fiber bundles of the periodontal membrane.

f., cemental Fibers of the periodontal membrane extending from the cementum to the zone of the intermediate plexus, where their terminations are interspersed with the terminations of the alveolar group of periodontal fibers.

f., circular Fibers in the free gingiva that encircle the tooth in a ringlike fashion.

f., collagen White fibers composed of collagen. The most conspicuous part of connective tissue, including the gingivae and periodontal membrane. Some fibers are distributed haphazardly throughout the connective tissue ground substance, and others are arranged in coarse bundles that exhibit a distinct orientation. Characterized by its hydroxyproline and hydroxylysine content.

f., crestal One group of periodontal ligament fibers extending from the cervical area of the tooth to the alveolar crest.

f., dentogingival Part of a fan-shaped fiber system that emerges from the supra-alveolar connective tissue and composed of circular, dentogingival, dentoperiosteal, and transseptal fiber groups.

f., dentoperisteal A fiber system emerging from the supra-alveolar part of the cementum of the tooth and passing outward beynd the alvelar crest in an apical direction into the mucoperiosteum f the attached gingiva.

f., gingival The group of fiber systems belonging to the gingival and supra-alveolar connective tissue and composed of circular, dentogingival, dentoperiosteal, and transseptal fiber groups.

f., horizontal Collagen fibers of the periodontal membrane that extend horizontally from the cementum to the alveolar bone.

f., nerve *See* fiber, nerve, mylinated; fiber, nerve, nonmedullated.

f., A-alpha nerve Large-diameter nerve fibers that connect into the substantia gelatinosa of the doral horns of the spinal cord before synapsing with the central transmission of the dorsal horn. A-alpha fibers are associated with the "gate-control" theory of pain.

f., A-beta nerve Large-diameter nerve fibers that are mechanoreceptors for pressure occurring in both the pulp and periodontal ligament, which are necessary to operate the gate mechanism.

f., A-delta nerve Small diameter nerve fibers that are mechanoreceptors for pain occurring in both the pulp and the periodontal ligament which are necessary to operate the gate mechanism.

f., C nerve Small-diameter nerve fibers that are mechanoreceptors for pain occurring in both the pulp and the periodontal ligament, which are necessary to operate the gate mechanism.

f., myelinated nerve A nerve fiber inside or outside the brain that is covered with an insulating medullary sheath along which are located nodes of Ranvier that facilitate as relay points the speed of nerve impulses over that of an equivalent nonmedulated fiber.

f., nonmedullated nerve A nerve fiber not covered by an insulating medullary sheath that is thus exposed to other tissue fluids and their respective electric potentials. In nonmedullated fibers, the impulse is relayed from point to continguous

point. Most of the nonmedullated fibers are within the substance of the central nervous system, and the distances between the cells are short.

f., oblique The group of collagen fibers in bundle arrangement in the periodontal ligament that are obliquely situated, with insertions in the cementum, and that extend more occlusally in the alveolus (approximately two thirds of the peridontal fibers fall into this group).

f., periodontal *See* ligament, periodontal.

f., principal The numerous bundles of collagenous tissue fibers arranged in groups that function as the mode of attachment of the tooth to the alveolus.

f., Sharpey's Collagenous fibers that become incorporated into the cementum.

f., transseptal A part of the gingival fiber system that extends from the supra-alveolar cementum of one tooth horizontally through the interdental attached gingiva above the septum of the alveolar bone to the cementum of the adjacent tooth.

fiberoptic lights A miniaturized light source that uses the property of flexible fiberglass strands to conduct light long distances with little or no distortion; used in intraoral application such as a light attached directly to the dental handpiece.

fibrillation (fĭ″brĭ-lā′shŭn) A local quivering of muscle fibers.

f., atrial Cardiac arrhythmia due to disturbed spread of excitation through atrial musculature.

f., auricular (aw-rĭk′ū-lar) An uncoordinated, independent contraction of the heart that results in marked irregularity of heart action.

f., ventricular Uncoordinated, independent contraction of the ventricular musculature resulting in cessation of cardiac output.

fibrinogen (fī-brĭn′-ō-jĕn) **(factor I, profibrin)** A soluble plasma protein (globulin) that is acted on by thrombin to form fibrin. The normal level is 200 to 400 mg/100 ml in plasma. Coagulation is impaired if the concentration is less than 100 mg/100 ml. Another form of fibrinogen called *tissue fibrinogen,* which has the power of clotting the blood without the presence of thrombin, occurs in body tissues.

fibrinokinase (fī″brĭ-nō-kī′nās) **(fibrinolysokinase, lysokinase)** An activator of plasminogen found in many animal tissues.

fibrinolysin (fī″brĭ-nol′ĭ-sĭn) *See* plasmin.

fibrinolysokinase *See* fibrinokinase.

fibroblast (fī′brō-blăst) A cell found within fibrous connective tissue, varying in shape from stellate (young) to fusiform and spindle shaped. Associated with the formation of collagen fibers and ground substance of connective tissue.

fibroblastoma (fī″brō-blăs-tō′mah) A tumor arising from

an ordinary connective tissue cell or fibroblast. The tumor may be a fibroma or a fibrosarcoma.

f., neurogenic See neurofibroma.

f., perineural See neurilemoma; neurofibroma.

fibrocystic disease See disease, fibrocystic.

fibroma (fī-brō′mah) A benign mesenchymal tumor composed primarily of fibrous connective tissue.

f., ameloblastic A mixed tumor of odontogenic origin characterized by the simultaneous proliferation of both the epithelial and mesenchymal components of the tooth germ without the production of hard structure.

f., calcifying See osteofibroma.

f., cementifying An intrabony lesion not associated with teeth, composed of a fibrous connective tissue stroma containing foci of calcified material resembling cementum; a rare odontogenic tumor composed of varying amounts of fibrous connective tissue with calcified material resembling cementum. Central lesion of the jaws.

f., irritation A localized peripheral, tumorlike enlargement of connective tissue due to prolonged local irritation and usuallly seen on the gingiva or buccal mucosa.

f. with myxomatous degeneration See fibromyxoma.

f., neurogenic See neurilemoma; neurofibroma.

f., odontogenic Central odontogenic tumor of the jaws, consisting of connective tissue in which small islands and strands of odontogenic epithelium are dispersed. A mesodermal odontogenic tumor composed of active dense or loose fibrous connective tissue; contains inactive islands of epithelium.

f., peripheral odontogenic A fibrous connective tissue tumor associated with the gingival margin and believed to originate from the periodontium. Often contains areas of calcification. Localized form of fibromatosis gingivae.

f., ossifying See osteofibroma.

f., periapical (benign periapical fibroma, fibrous dysplasia, first-state cementoma, focal osseous dysplasia, traumatic osteoclasia) A benign connective tissue mass formed at the apex of a tooth with a normal pulp.

fibromatosis (fī″brō-mah-tō′ sĭs) Gingival enlargement believed to be a hereditary condition that is manifested in the permanent dentition and characterized by a firm hyperplastic tissue that covers the teeth. Differentiation between this and diphenylhydantoin (Dilantin) hyperplasia is based on a history of drug ingestion.

f. gingivae (elephantiasis gingivae, idiopathic fibromatosis, idiopathic gingival hyperplasia) Generalized enlargement of the gingivae due to fibrous hyperplasia. Idiopathic in nature and similar in appearance to Dilantin hyperplasia.

f., hereditary gingival A condition possessing a familial attribute of distribution, in which there is gingival enlargement due to marked fibroplasia.

f., idiopathic See fibromatosis, gingivae.

fibromyxoma (fī″brō-mĭk-sō′mah) **(fibroma with myxomatous degeneration)** A fibroma that has certain characteristics of a myxoma; a fibroma that has undergone myxomatous degeneration. Combination of both fibrous and myxomatous elements.

fibro-osteoma (fī″brō-ahs″tē-ō′mah) See osteofibroma.

fibropapilloma (fī″brō-păp″ĭ-lō′mah) A lesion that resembles a benign neoplasm and shows fibroblastic and epithelial proliferation. Such lesions occur in regions of cheek chewing or other trauma. Since they are not true neoplasms, they may be better designated as irritation fibroses or fibrous hyperplasias.

fibrosarcoma (fī″brō-săr-kō′mah) Malignant mesenchymal tumor, the basic cell type being a fibroblast. Most fibrosarcomas are locally infiltrative and persistent but do not metastasize.

f., odontogenic An extremely rare malignant form of odontogenic fibroma.

fibrosis (fī-brō′sĭs) The process of forming fibrous tissue, usually by degeneration (e.g., fibrosis of the pulp).

f., hereditary gingival An uncommon form of severe gingival hyperplasia that may begin with the eruption of the deciduous or permanent teeth and is characterized by a firm, dense, pink gingival tissue with little tendency toward bleeding.

f., diffuse hereditary gingival An uncommon form of severe gingival hyperplasia considered to be of genetic origin. The tissue is pink, firm, dense, and insensitive and has little tendency to bleed.

fiduciary (fī-doo′shē-ăr′ē) A person who has a duty to act primarily for another's benefit, as a trustee. Also, pertaining to the good faith and confidence involved in such a relationship.

field An area, region, or space.

f. block See block, field.

f., operating The area immediately surrounding and directly involved in a treatment procedure (e.g., all the teeth included in a rubber dam application for the restoration of a single tooth or portions thereof).

f., radiation The region in which radiant energy is being propagated.

file, *n.* **1:** A metal tool of varying size and form with numerous ridges or teeth on its cutting surfaces; may be push-cut or pull-cut; used for smoothing or dressing down metals and other substances. **2:** A collection of records; an organized collection of information directed toward some purpose such as patient demographic data. The records in a file may or may not be sequenced according to a key contained in each record. **3:** *v.* To reduce by means of a file.

f.-access safeguards Methods of limiting certain users' access to particular data.

f., gold A file designed for removing surplus gold from gold restorations; may be pull-cut or push-cut.

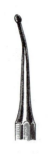

Gold file

f., Hirschfeld-Dunlop A variety of periodontal file used with a pull stroke for the removal of calculus; available in various angulations for approach to different surfaces of teeth.

f., root canal A small metal hand instrument with tightly spiraled blades used to clean and shape the canal.

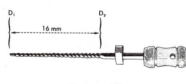

Root canal file

filled resin *See* resin, composite

filling A material used to fill a space. (Objectionable as a synonym for restoration.) *See also* restoration.

f., dental A lay term for restoration. *See* restoration, dental.

f.,"ditched" Refers to the marginal failure of amalgam restorations due to fracture of either the material or the tooth structure itself in that area.

f. material *See* material, filling.

f., postresection *See* filling, retrograde.

f., retrograde (postresection filling, retrograde obturation) A filling placed in the apical portion of a tooth root to seal the apical portion of the root canal.

f., root canal Material placed in the root canal system to seal the space previously occupied by the dental pulp.

f. technique *See* technique, filling.

f., treatment A temporary filling, usually of a sedative nature, used to allay sensitive dentin prior to the final restoration of the cavity.

film A thin, flexible, transparent sheet of cellulose acetate or similar material coated with a light-sensitive emulsion.

f. badge A pack of x-ray—sensitive film used for the detection and approximate measurement of radiation exposure for personnel-monitoring purposes; the badge may contain two or three films of differing sensitivity, and it may contain a filter that shields part of the film from certain types of radiation.

f. base *See* base, film.

f., bite-wing (interproximal film) A type of dental x-ray film that has a central tab or wing on which the teeth close to hold the film in position. *See also* examination, radiographic.

f. emulsion *See* emulsion, silver.

f. fault A defective result in a radiograph; usually caused by a chemical, physical, or electrical error in its production.

f. fault, black spots Spots caused by dust particles or developer on the films before development; also caused by outdated (expired) film.

f. fault, blurred A fault caused by film movement during exposure, bent film during exposure, double exposures, or flowing of emulsion during processing in excessively warm solution.

f. fault, dark A fault caused by overexposure of the film to radiation, film fog from extended development, accidental exposure to light (light leaks in film packet or dark room), or an unsafe darkroom light.

f. fault, distorted *See* distortion, film-fault.

f. fault, dyschroic fog A fogging of the radiograph, characterized by the appearance of a pink surface when the film is viewed by transmitted light and a green surface when the film is seen by reflected light. It usually is caused by an exhaustion of the acid content of the fixing solution (incomplete fixation).

f. fault, fogged A fault caused by stray radiation, use of expired film, or an unsafe darkroom light.

f. fault, light A fault caused by underexposure, underdevelopment (expired or diluted developing solution), development in temperatures that are too cold, or accidental use of a wrong film speed.

f. fault, reticulation A network of corrugations produced because of an excessive difference in temperature between any two of the three darkroom solutions.

f. fault, stained A fault caused by contaminated solutions, improper rinsing, exhausted solutions, improper washing, contamination by improper handling of the emulsions during or after processing, or film hangers containing dried fixer on the clips.

f. fault, static electricity Image in the emulsion that

has the appearance of lightning. Caused by rapid opening of the film pocket or transfer of static electricity from the technician to the film.

f. fault, white spots A fault caused by air bubbles clinging to the emulsion during development or by fixing solution spotted on the emulsion before development.

f. hanger An instrument or device for holding x-ray film during processing procedures.

f. holder, cardboard *See* cassette, cardboard.

f. image The shadow of a structure as depicted on a radiographic or photographic emulsion.

f., interproximal *See* film, bite-wing.

f. mounting Placement of radiographs in an orderly sequence on a suitable carrier for illumination and study.

f. packet A small, lightproof, moisture-resistant, sealed paper or plastic envelope containing an xray film (or two x-ray films) and a lead-foil backing designed for use in the making of intraoral radiographs.

f. placement Positioning of the x-ray film to receive the image cast by the roentgen rays.

f. processing Chemical transformation of the latent image, produced in a film emulsion by exposure to radiation, into a stable image visible by transmitted light. The usual procedure is basically a selective reduction of affected silver halide salts to metallic silver grains (development), followed by the selective removal of unaffected silver halide (fixation), washing to remove the processing chemicals, and drying.

    f. processing, rapid The use of high-speed chemicals or elevated temperatures to reduce processing time.

f. speed (film sensitivity) The amount of exposure to light or roentgen rays required to produce a given image density. It is expressed as the reciprocal of the exposure in roentgens necessary to produce a density of 1 above base and fog; films are classified on this basis in six speed groups, between each of which is a twofold increase in film speed.

f. on teeth Mucinous deposits on teeth, containing microorganisms, desquamated tissue elements, blood cellular elements, etc.; usually thin and adherent.

f. thickness Refers to thickness of a layer of material, particularly in reference to dental cements. In standardization tests it is the minimal thickness or layer obtained under a specific load.

f., x-ray *See* survey, radiographic.

filter A material placed in the useful beam to absorb preferentially the less energetic (less penetrating) radiations. *See also* filtration.

f., added Filter added to the inherent filter.

f., compensating A filter designed to shield less dense areas so that a more uniform image quality will be produced.

f., inherent Filtration introduced by the glass wall of the x-ray tube, any oil used for tube immersion, or any permanent tube enclosure in the path of useful beam.

f., total Sum of inherent and added filters.

filtration The use of absorbers for the selective attenuation of radiation of certain wavelengths from a useful primary beam of x radiation.

f., built-in Filtration effected by nonremovable absorbers deliberately built into the tube-head assembly to increase the inherent beam filtration.

f., external The action of absorbers external to the tube-head assembly, consisting of added filtration *(see above)* plus the attenuating effect of materials of which any closed-end cone such as a pointer cone may be made.

findings, radiographic (roentgenographic findings) The recorded radiographic evidence of normal and deviated anatomic structures.

fineness A means of grading alloys with regard to gold content. The fineness of an alloy is designated in parts per thousand of pure gold, pure gold being 1000 fine.

finger Any one of the five digits of the hand.

f., clubbed A condition seen in hypertrophic osteoarthropathy where the base angle between the base of the fingernail and adjacent dorsal surface of the terminal phalanx is obliterated and becomes 180 degrees or greater. The base of the nail projects downward, and the area of nail is increased.

f. positions The positions of the fingers when operating; refers not only to the fingers grasping the instrument but also to the fingers used for rests, support, and holding the tissues out of the way.

f. rest An integral part of instrumentation, in which the fingers of the working hand rest on the teeth, adjacent tissues, fingers of the opposing hand, etc., to improve control of the working stroke of an instrument by providing a fulcrum for movement of the working fingers and instruments.

f. strut A bar or similar component of the infrastructure of a subperiosteal or endosteal implant that projects from it, being attached only at one side.

finish line *See* line, finish.

finger sucking The habit of sucking the finger (or thumb) for oral gratification. It is normal in infants and young children as a comforting device, especially when tired or hungry. If the habit persists beyond the eruption of the permanent teeth, it may cause a malocclusion of the anterior teeth.

finish, satin The degree of finish of a polished surface that has been made very smooth but is without a high sheen.

finishing and polishing Removal of excess restoration

material from the margins and contours of a restoration, and polishing of the restoration.

firmware A special type of permanent program that takes the place of or accomplishes the function of traditional hardware components. Firmware is loaded into the equipment, either at the time it is manufactured or later, by the person installing the equipment or the person using the equipment.

first surgical stage (subperiosteal) The operation performed to obtain a direct bone impression.

fission (fĭsh'ŭn) The splitting of a nucleus into two fragments. Fission may occur spontaneously or may be induced artificially. In addition to the fission fragments, particulate radiation energy and gamma rays are usually produced during fission.

f., nuclear, products Elements (nuclides) or compounds resulting from nuclear fission.

f. products The nuclides produced by the fission of a heavy-element nuclide.

fissure A deep groove or cleft; commonly the result of the imperfect fusion of the enamel or adjoining dental lobes.

f., gingival See cleft, gingival.

f., pterygomaxillary The most posterior point in the anterior contour of the maxillary tuberosity.

fissured tongue See tongue, fissured.

fistula (fĭs'tū-lah) An abnormal tract connecting two body surfaces or organs or leading from a pathologic or natural internal cavity to the surface. The tract may be lined with epithelium.

f., alveolar A fistula communicating with the cavity of an alveolar abscess. More properly called *alveolar sinus*. See also sinus, alveolar.

f., arteriovenous See shunt, arteriovenous.

f., branchial A fistula associated with a branchial cyst; usually seen on the lateral surface of the neck.

f., dental See fistula, alveolar.

f. of lip Congenital malformation in which there is a deep pit or fistula on the mucosa of the lip; often bilateral and usually found on the lower lip.

f., oroantral An opening between the maxillary sinus and the oral cavity, most often through a tooth socket. See also fistula.

f., orofacial An opening between the cutaneous surface of the face and the oral cavity.

f., oronasal An opening between the nasal cavity and the oral cavity.

f., salivary An opening between a salivary duct and/ or gland and the cutaneous surface or into the oral cavity through other than the normal anatomic pathway.

fit Adaptation of any dental restoration. Adaptation of a denture to its basal seat, a clasp to a tooth, an inlay to a cavity preparation, etc.

fix To make firm, stable, immovable; to place in a de-

sired position and hold there. In dentistry, to secure in position, usually by means of cementation, a prosthesis such as a crown or a fixed partial denture.

fixation Act or result of fixing. In dentistry, the act of securing in position, usually by means of cementation, some treatment appliance such as a crown or fixed partial denture when willful removal of the restoration by the patient is not intended.

f., biphase pin See appliance, fracture.

f., elastic band Stabilization of fractured segments of the jaws by means of intermaxillary or maxillomandibular elastic bands applied to splints or appliances.

f. of elements by the skeleton Fixation of many elements for long periods of time in the bone matrix due to a special affinity of the elements for the matrix. Recent work with radioactive isotopes has firmly established the concept of the skeleton as a dynamic system. In addition to the changes in structure and in distribution of the bone mineral mediated by cellular activity, every ionic grouping in the mineral is capable of replacement.

f., external pin See appliance, fracture.

f., intermaxillary See fixation, maxillomandibular.

f., intraosseous Reduction and stabilization of fractured bony parts by direct fixation to one another with surgical wires, screws, pins, and/or plates.

f., mandibulomaxillary See fixation, maxillomandibular.

f., maxillomandibular (mandibulomaxillary fixation) Retention of fractures of the maxillae or mandible in the functional relations with the opposing dental arch through the use of elastic wire ligatures and interdental wiring and/or splints.

f., nasomandibular Mandibular immobilization, especially for edentulous jaws, using mandibulomaxillary splints, circummandibular wiring, and intraoral interosseous wiring through the nasal process of the maxillae.

f., osseous Immobilization of fractured bony segments.

f., radiographic In film processing, the chemical removal of all the undeveloped salts of the film emulsion, so that only the developed (reduced) silver will remain as a permanent image.

f., restorative The act of securing in position, usually by means of cementation, some treatment appliance, such as a crown or fixed partial denture, when willful removal of the restoration by the patient is not intended.

f., Roger-Anderson pin An appliance used in extraoral fixation of mandibular fractures and prognathisms. See also appliance, fracture.

fixed costs Costs that do not change to meet fluctuations in enrollment or in use of services (e.g., salaries, rent, business license fees, depreciation).

fixed fee schedule A list of specified fees for services that will be paid to dentists participating in a dental plan.

fixed partial denture *See* denture, partial, fixed.

fixed premium A specified amount charged for insurance that is not changed by such factors as size of family or initial year versus maintenance year of dental care coverage. Synonym: set premium.

flabby tissue *See* tissue, hyperplastic.

flaccid (flăk′sĭd) A relaxed or flabby state, as in a flail-like condition or paralysis of a muscle.

flag Any of various types of indicators used for identification. Also a character that signals the occurrence of some condition, such as the end of a word.

flange (flanj) The part of the denture base that extends from the cervical ends of the teeth to the border of the denture.

f.-(guide appliance) An appliance (prosthesis) with a lateral vertical extension designed to direct a re-sected mandible into centric occlusion.

f., buccal The portion of the flange of a denture that occupies the buccal vestibule of the mouth and that extends distally from the buccal notch.

f., contour of The topographic design of the flange of a denture.

f., labial The portion of the flange of a denture that occupies the labial vestibule of the mouth.

f., lingual The portion of the flange of a mandibular denture that occupies the space adjacent to the residual ridge and next to the tongue.

flap A sheet of soft tissue partially or totally detached to gain access to structures underneath or to be used in repairing defects in an adjacent or a remote part of the body.

f., envelope Mucoperiosteal tissue retracted from a horizontal linear incision (as along the free gingival margin), with no vertical component of the incision.

f., lingual tongue A flap used to repair a fistula of the hard palate, which combines the raising of a palatal flap to form the floor of the nose with a flap taken from the back or edge of the tongue to form the palatal surface.

f., mucoperiosteal A flap of mucosal tissue, including the periosteum, reflected from a bone.

f., pedicle A stalk-shaped flap.

f., sliding A flap that is advanced from its original location in a direction away from its base, to close a defect.

f., V-Y A flap in which the incision is shaped like a V and after closure like a Y, to lengthen a localized area of tissue. *See also* flap, Y-V.

f., Y-V A flap in which the incision is shaped like a Y

and after closure like a V, to shorten a localized area of tissue. *See also* flap, V-Y.

flash Excess material that is squeezed out of the mold (e.g., during packing of a denture by compression technique).

flask A metal case or tube used in investing procedures.

f., casting *See* flask, refractory.

f. closure The procedure of bringing the parts of a flask together to form a complete mold.

f., final, closure The last closure of a flask before curing and after trial packing of the mold with a denture base material.

f., trial, closure Preliminary closures made for the purpose of eliminating excess denture base or other plastic material and of ensuring that the mold is completely filled.

f., crown A small, sectional, metal boxlike case in which a sectional mold of plaster of paris or artificial stone is made for the purpose of compressing and curing plastics on small dental restorations.

f., denture A sectional, metal boxlike case in which a sectional mold of plaster of paris or artificial stone is made for the purpose of compressing and curing dentures or other resinous restorations.

f., injection A special flask designed to permit the filling of the mold after the flask is closed or to permit the addition of denture base material to that in the flask after the flask is closed.

f., refractory (casting flask, casting ring) A metal tube in which a refractory mold is made for casting metal dental restorations or appliances.

flasking The act of investing a pattern in a flask. The process of investing the cast and a wax denture in a flask preparatory to molding the denture base material into the form of the denture.

flavonoids A group of substances containing the plant pigment flavone. There is no known human requirement for them. They have a constrictor effect on the capillary bed and decrease permeability of blood vessels. Some beneficial effects of flavonoids have been described in the treatment of bruises, contusions, and sprains. Synonyms: bioflavonoids, vitamin P.

flexible benefits A benefits program in which an employee has a choice of credits or dollars for distribution among various benefit options (e.g., health and disability insurance, dental benefits, child care, pension benefits). *See also* cafeteria plans; flexible spending account.

flexible spending account Employee reimbursement account primarily funded with employee-designated salary reductions Funds are reimbursed to employee for health care (medical and/or dental), dependent care, and/or legal expenses, and are considered a nontaxable benefit.

flexibility The property of elastic deformation under loading.

flexion (flĕk'shŭn) The bending of a joint between two skeletal members to decrease the angle between the members; opposite of extension.

f.-extension reflex See reflex, flexion-extension.

flexure (flĕk'shĕr) The quality or state of being flexed.

f., clasp The flexure of a retentive clasp arm to permit passage over the surveyed height of contour, thus permitting the seating or removal of the clasp.

floor of cavity See cavity, floor.

floppy disk A lightweight computer disk platter that is kept in a protective envelope and can be used for file information (storage). Synonym: diskette, flexible disk.

flora (flō'rah) The bacteria living in various parts of the alimentary canal.

f., fusospirochetal The microorganisms *Fusobacterium fusiforme* and *Borrelia vincentii*. Present in most individuals as normal inhabitants of the oral cavity. Believed by some to be the primary and by others the secondary cause of acute necrotizing ulcerative gingivitis (ANUG).

f., oral The microorganisms inhabiting the oral cavity of an individual. They are usually saprophytic in nature and live together in a symbiotic relationship. Some are potentially pathogenic, assuming a pathologic role when adverse local and/or systemic factors influence the symbiotic balance of the microorganic flora.

floss tape A silk tape often incorporated with pumice and used to polish the proximal surfaces of teeth.

flow To move in a manner similar to a liquid stream.

f., dental material Continued deformation or change in shape under a static load. As with waxes and amalgam.

f., traffic The pattern of office personnel and patient movement from one area within the office to another.

flowchart A graphic representation of a sequence of operations using symbols to represent the operations. Flowcharts often symbolize the most important steps of the process without detailing the algorithm of how the work is to be performed.

flowmeter A physical device for measuring the rate of flow of a gas or liquid.

fluconazole An oral antifungal tablet used in the treatment of oral candidiasis.

fluctuation A wavelike motion produced in soft tissues in response to palpation or percussion. Due to a collection of fluids or exudates in the tissues.

fluid (floo'ĭd) A liquid or gaseous substance.

f., synovial The small amount of fluid occurring in normal joints whose principal function is to lubricate the joint surfaces and nourish the articular cartilage. Its content is approximately 95% water, with only 1% to 2% protein concentration.

f., total body All the fluids contained in the body. There are two main types: the intracellular fluid, which is contained totally within the cells, and the extracellular fluid, which is contained entirely outside the cells.

f. wax See wax, fluid.

fluorescence (flū-ō-rĕs'ĕns) Emission of radiation of a particular wavelength by certain substances as the result of absorption of radiation of a shorter wavelength.

fluorescent screen See screen, intensifying.

fluoridate (flū-or'ĭ-dāt) To add fluoride to a water supply.

fluoridation The use of a fluoride to reduce caries activity; may be by means of communal water supplies; oral hygiene preparations for home use, or topical applications for the purpose of prophylaxis.

fluoridization (flū-or"ĭ-dī-zā'shŭn) The topical application of a solution of a fluoride to teeth.

fluoroscope (flū-or'ō-skōp) A device consisting of a fluorescent screen mounted in a metal frame covered with lead glass. In the presence of a roentgen ray, the screen glows in direct proportion to the intensity of the remnant x radiation, producing visual impressions of the densities traversed.

fluorosis (flū-ō-rō'sĭs) Enamel hypoplasia due to the ingestion of water containing excess fluoride during the time of enamel formation. General term for chronic fluoride poisioning. See also fluorosis, chronic endemic dental.

f., chronic endemic dental (mottled enamel) An enamel defect caused by excessive ingestion of fluoride in the water supply (usually 2 to 8 ppm) during the period of tooth calcification. Affected teeth appear chalky white on eruption and later turn brown.

Fluothane Trade name for halothane.

flush blush (on the cheeks) due to vasodilation of small arteries and arterioles.

flutter A quick, irregular motion.

flux Any substance or mixture used to promote fusion, especially the fusion of metals or minerals. Used principally in dentistry as an inclusion in ceramic materials and in soldering and casting metals.

f., casting A flux that increases fluidity of the metal and helps to prevent oxidation.

f., ceramic A flux used in the manufacture of porcelain and silicate powders.

f., reducing A flux that contains powdered charcoal to remove oxides.

f., soldering A ceramic material such as borax, boric acid, or a combination, in paste, liquid, or granular form; used to keep metallic parts clean while they are being heated during a soldering procedure. It is a solvent for metallic oxides and will flow over the parts to be soldered at temperatures well below the fusion temperature of solder, but it becomes separated from the solid metal by the molten solder.

FMIA *See* angle, Frankfort-mandibular incisor.

focal infection *See* infection, focal.

focal spot *See* spot, focal.

focal-film distance *See* distance, target-film.

fog (fogging) *See* film fault, fogged.

f., chemical *See* film fault.

f., dyschroic *See* film fault, dyschroic fog.

f., light *See* film fault.

f., radiation Film darkening due to radiation from sources other than intentional exposure to the primary beam; for example, film may be exposed to scatter radiation, or accidental exposure may occur if stored film is not protected from radiation.

foil A very thin, flexible sheet of metal, usually gold, platinum, or tin.

f., adhesive Tinfoil that is covered on one side with powdered gum arabic or karaya gum.

f. assistant *See* foil holder.

f. cylinder A cylinder of gold foil formed by repeatedly folding a sheet of foil into a narrow ribbon, which is then rolled into cylindrical form.

f., gold (fibrous gold) Pure gold that has been rolled and beaten from ingots into a very thin sheet. Thickness usually varies from 1/40,000 inch (No. 2 foil) to 1/20,000 inch (No. 4 foil). Classified as cohesive, semicohesive, or noncohesive. One of the oldest restorative materials, the most permanent if used properly, and the yardstick by which all others are measured. It is compacted or condensed into a retentive cavity form piece by piece, using this metal's property of cold welding.

f., cohesive gold Gold foil that has been annealed or whose surface is completely pure so that it will cohere or weld at room temperature.

f., corrugated gold A gold foil made by burning gold-foil sheets between paper in the absence of air.

f., noncohesive gold Gold foil that will not cohere at room temperature due to the presence on its surface of a protecting or contaminating coating. If the coating is a volatile substance, such as ammonia, the foil may be rendered cohesive by heating or annealing it to remove the protection.

f., platinized gold A form rolled or hammered from a "sandwich" made of platinum placed between two sheets of gold; used in portions of foil restorations where greater hardness is desired.

f. holder (foil assistant) An instrument used to retain a foil pellet in place while it is being condensed or to retain a bulk of gold while additions to it are made.

f. passer (foil carrier) A pointed or forked instrument used to carry pellets of gold foil through an annealing flame or from the annealing tray to the prepared cavity for compaction.

f. pellet *See* pellet, foil.

f., platinum Pure platinum rolled into extremely thin sheets. A precious-metal foil whose high fusing point makes it suitable as a matrix for various soldering procedures; also suitable for providing the internal form of porcelain restorations during fabrication.

f., tin A base-metal foil used as a separating material, or protective covering (e.g., between the cast and denture base material during flasking and curing procedures).

fold A doubling back of a tissue surface.

f., mucobuccal (mucobuccal reflection) The line of flexure of the oral mucous membrane as it passes from the mandible or maxillae to the cheek.

f., mucolabial The line of flexure of the oral mucous membrane as it passes from the mandible or maxillae to the lip.

f., sublingual The crescent-shaped area on the floor of the mouth following the inner wall of the mandible and tapering toward the molar regions. It is formed by the sublingual gland and the submaxillary duct beneath the mucous membrane of the alveololingual sulcus.

folder Usually a heavy paper envelope in which the patient's records are kept.

folic acid A vitamin of the B complex group essential for cell growth and reproduction. It functions as a coenzyme with vitamin B_{12} and C in the breakdown and utilization of proteins and in the formation of nucleic acids.

follow-up The process of monitoring the progress of a patient after a period of active treatment.

Fones' method *See* method, Fones'.

Food and Drug Administration (FDA) An agency of the Department of Health and Human Services responsible for the enforcement of the Federal Food, Drug and Cosmetic Act and other statutes assigned.

food Ingested solids and liquids that supply the body with nutriment and energy.

f., comminution of (kom'i-noo'shun) Reduction of food into small parts.

f. impaction *See* impaction, food.

f., physical character of The consistency, as the firmness, viscosity, or density, of food substances. Soft, adhesive, and nonabrasive foods tend to cling to the teeth, whereas coarse foods leave liitle debris and create a frictional effect on the tissues, thus cleansing them. A soft diet can thus lead to calculus formation.

foot-and-mouth disease A viral disease, common to farm animals outside the United States. It occasionally affects humans exposed to infected animals or animal products. Symptoms and signs in humans, include headache, fever, and vesicles on tongue, oral mucous membranes, and hands and feet, lasting 7 to 10 days.

foramen (fō-rā′mĕn) **1:** A natural opening in a bone or other structure. **2:** A natural opening in the root, usually at or near the apical end.

f., incisive (ĭn-sī′sĭv) **(nasopalatine foramen)** **1:** The opening of the nasopalatine canal. **2:** The foramen, or opening, in the midline of the palate in the region where the premaxilla and maxillae join, which is situated palatal to the upper central incisors; contains nasopalatine vessels and nerve.

f., mandibular The opening on the medial aspect of the vertical ramus of the mandible approximately midway between the mandibular and gonial notches; may be located posterior to the middle of the ramus. It contains interior alveolar vessels and the inferior alveolar nerve.

f., mental A circular opening on the lateral aspect of the body of the mandible either below the apex of the first premolar or below the apex of the second premolar but usually between the first and second premolars inferior to their apices. The mental vessels and nerve pass through this foramen to supply the lip. In edentulous mandibles, the bone may have been resorbed, so that it is in such a position that the denture base will cover it.

f., nasopalatine See foramen, incisive.

force Any application of energy, either internal or external to a structure; that which initiates, changes, or arrests motion.

f., centrifugal Force that tends to recede from the center.

f., chewing The degree of force applied by the muscles of mastication during the mastication of food.

f., component of **1:** One of the factors from which a resultant force may be compounded or into which it may be resolved. **2:** One of the parts of a force into which it may be resolved.

f., condensing **1:** The force required to compress gold-foil pellets, facilitating their cohesion, to fabricate or build up a gold-foil restoration. **2:** The force required to compact or condense a plastic material (e. g., amalgam, wax).

f., constant Continuous force or pressure applied to the teeth.

f., denture-dislodging An influence that tends to displace a denture from its intended position on supporting structures.

f., denture-retaining An influence that tends to maintain a denture in its intended position on its supporting structures.

f., electromotive The difference in potential in a roentgen-ray tube between the cathode and anode; usually expressed in kilovolts.

f., intermittent A force or pressure applied to the teeth that is alternated with a period of passiveness or rest.

f., line of The direction of the power exerted on a body.

f., masticatory The force applied by the muscles attached to the mandible during mastication.

f., occlusal (occlusal load) **1:** The resultant of muscular forces applied on opposing teeth. **2:** The force transmitted to the teeth and their supporting structures by tooth-to-tooth contact or through a bolus of food or other interposed substance.

f. and stress Pressure forcibly exerted on the teeth and on their investing and supporting tissues that is detrimental to tissue integrity. In occlusal trauma the production of lesions of the attachment apparatas depends on an interrelationship of the strength, duration, and frequency of the application of the force.

forceps **1:** An instrument used for grasping or applying force to teeth, tissues, or other instruments. **2:** An instrument used for grasping and holding tissues or specific structures. (Objectionable term in restorative dentistry because of its association with the extraction of teeth.)

f., bone Force used for grasping or cutting bone.

f., chalazion A thumb forceps with a flattened plate at the end of one arm and a matching ring on the other. Originally used for isolation of eyelid tumors. It is useful for isolation of lip and cheek lesions (e.g., a mucocele) to facilitate removal.

f., dental extracting Forceps used for grasping teeth.

f., hemostatic An instrument for grasping blood vessels to control hemorrhage.

f., insertion See forceps, point.

f., lock See forceps, point.

f., mosquito A small hemostatic forceps.

f., point (lock forceps, insertion forceps) A device used in filling root canals that securely holds the filling cones during their placement.

f., rubber dam clamp Forceps whose beaks are designed to engage holes in the rubber dam retainer to facilitate its placement, adjustment, or removal.

f., suture See needle holder.

f., thumb Forceps used for grasping soft tissue; used especially during suturing.

f., tissue A thumb forceps; an instrument with one or more fine teeth at the tip of each blade for controlling tissues during surgery, especially during suturing.

Fordyce's spots See spots, Fordyce's.

foreign body See body, foreign.

forensic dentistry See jurisprudence, dental.

foreshortening See distortion, vertical.

forging Working or shaping heated metal; hot working a metal.

fork, face-bow The part of the face-bow assembly used to attach an occlusion rim or transfer record of maxillary teeth to the face-bow proper.

form The configuration, shape, or particular appearance of anything.

f., acquaintance A registration sheet for new patients on which data (e.g., the patient's name and address) are recorded and that contains a statement of the policies of the specific dentist's office and the responsibilities of the dentist to the patient.

f., anatomic The natural shape of a part.

f., arch The shape of the dental arch. *See also* arch, dental.

f., convenience The modifications necessary, beyond basic outline form, to facilitate proper instrumentation for the preparation of the cavity or insertion of the restorative material; also the placing of starting points or slight undercuts to retain the first portions of restorative material while succeeding portions are placed.

f., face The outline form of the face from an anterior frontal view.

f., functional The shape that permits optimal performance.

f., message A checklist form, by means of which auxiliary personnel can quickly make a record of telephone communications for the dentist to peruse later.

f., occlusal The form of the occlusal surface of a tooth, a row of teeth, or dentition.

f., outline The shape of the area of the tooth surface included within the cavosurface margins of a prepared cavity.

f., registration A form used to gather personal data about a patient other than professional information.

f., resistance The shape given to a prepared cavity to enable the restoration and remaining tooth structure to withstand masticatory stress.

f., retention The provision made in a cavity preparation to prevent displacement of the restoration.

f., root The shape of the root of the tooth; it is capable of being modified by such factors as resorption and cemental apposition.

f., tooth The characteristics of the curves, lines, angles, and contours of various teeth that permit their identification and differentiation.

f., anterior tooth The outline form and other contours of an anterior tooth.

f., posterior tooth The distinguishing contours of the occlusal surface of the various posterior teeth.

formaldehyde A toxic pungent water-soluble gas used in the aqueous form as a disinfectant, fixative, or tissue preservative.

formalin A clear aqueous solution of formaldehyde. A 37% solution is used to fix and preserve tissues for histologic and pathologic study.

format A predetermined computer arrangement of characters, fields, lines, page numbers, punctuation marks, etc.

former, angle *See* angle former.

former, crucible *See* sprue former.

former, sprue *See* sprue former.

formocresol A compound consisting of formaldehyde, cresol, glycerin, and water used in vital pulpotomy of primary teeth and as a temporary intracanal medicament during rool canal therapy. Brand name Buckley's Formo Cresol.

fortified (fŏrt-ĕ′fīd) Containing additives more potent than the principal ingredient.

forward protrusion *See* protrusion, forward.

Foshay's test *See* test, Foshay's.

fossa (fahs′ah) A pit, hollow, or depression.

f., canine The concavity, or depression, in the maxilla superior to the apex of the canine tooth.

f., depth of The distance from the top of the shorter cusp downward into the bottom of the fossa.

f., nasal *See* cavity, nasal.

foundation A structure added to a remaining tooth structure to enhance stability and retention of a cast restoration placed over it. May be pin retained of amalgam, plastic cement, or a casting.

four-handed dentistry *See* dentistry, four-handed.

Fournier's glossitis (foor-nē-āz′) *See* glossitis, interstitial sclerous.

Fox scissors *See* scissors, Fox.

Fox's knife *See* knife, Goldman-Fox.

fracture A break or rupture of a part. In the oral region it is most frequently seen in teeth and bones.

f., avulsion Loss of a section of bone.

f., blow-out A fracture involving the orbital floor, its contents, and the superior wall of the maxillary antrum, in which orbital contents are incarcerated in the fracture area, producing diplopia.

f., cementum The tearing of fragments of the cementum from the tooth root.

f., clasp Failure of a clasp arm because of stresses that have exceeded the elastic limit of the metal from which the arm was made.

f., closed reduction of Reduction and fixation of fractured bones without making a surgical opening to the fracture site.

f., comminuted A fracture in which the bone has several lines of fracture in the same region; a fracture in which the bone is crushed and splintered.

f., compound A fracture in which the bony structures are exposed to an external environment.

f., craniofacial dysjunction (transverse facial fracture) A complex fracture in which the facial bones are separated from the cranial bones; a LeFort III fracture.

f., dislocation A fracture of a bone near an articulation, with dislocation of the condyloid process.

f., fissured A fracture that extends partially through a bone, with no displacement of the bony fragments.

f., greenstick A fracture in which the bone appears to be bent; usually only one cortex of the bone is broken.

f., Guérin's A LeFort I fracture of the facial bones in which there is a bilateral horizontal fracture of the maxillae.

f., impacted A fracture in which one fragment is driven into another portion of the same or an adjacent bone.

f., indirect A fracture at a point distant from the primary area of injury due to secondary forces.

f., intra-articular A fracture of the articular surface of the condyloid process of a bone.

f., intracapsular A fracture of the condyle of the mandible occurring within the confines of the capsule of the temporomandibular joint.

f., LeFort A transverse fracture involving the orbital, malar, and nasal bones.

f., midfacial Fractures of the zygomatic, maxillary, nasal, and associated bones.

f., pyramidal A fracture of the midfacial bones, with the principal fracture lines meeting at an apex in the area of the nasion; a LeFort II fracture.

f., root A microscopic or macroscopic cleavage of the root in any direction.

f., simple A linear fracture that is not in communication with the exterior.

f., transverse facial *See* fracture, craniofacial dysjunction.

fragilitas ossium (frah-jĭl'ĭ-tās os'ē-ŭm) *See* osteogenesis imperfecta.

frambesia (frăm-bē'zē-ah) *See* yaws.

frame A structure, usually rigid, designed to give support or attachment to a part, or to immobilize a part.

f., implant *See* substructure, implant.

f., occluding A device for relating casts to each other for the purpose of arranging teeth or for use in making an index of the occlusion of dentures; an articulator. *See also* articulator.

f., rubber dam *See* holder, rubber dam.

framework The skeletal metal portion of a removable partial denture around which and to which the remaining units are attached.

franchise dentistry **1:** The practice of dentistry under a trade name, the rights of which have been purchased from another dentist or dental practice. Under a franchise license agreement the franchiser may use the trade name, marketing products, and treatment techniques for a sum of money, as long as certain rules and regulations of the franchise are adhered to. **2:**

Refers to a system for marketing a dental practice, usually under a trade name. where permitted by state laws. In return for a financial investment or other consideration, participating dentists may also receive the benefits of media advertising, a national referral system, and financial and management consultation.

Frankel appliance *See* appliance, Frankel.

Frankfort horizontal plane *See* plane, Frankfort horizontal.

Frankfort-mandibular incisor angle *See* angle, Frankfort-mandibular incisor.

fraud Intentional perversion of truth for the purpose of inducing another, in reliance on it, to part with something valuable or to surrender a legal right; deliberate deception; deceit; trickery.

fraudulent concealment The deliberate attempt to withhold information or to conceal an act in order to avoid contractual responsibility. Fraudulent concealment as applied to health care providers arises when a treating doctor conceals from an aggrieved patient the fact that a previous treating doctor may have committed malpractice.

freckle *See* ephelis.

freedom of choice A provision in a dental benefits program that permits the insured to choose any licensed dentist to provide his or her dental care and receive full benefits under the program.

free gingiva *See* gingiva, free.

free gingival margin *See* margin, gingival, free.

free mandibular movement *See* movement, mandibular, free.

free-end *See* base, extension.

free-way space *See* distance, interocclusal.

Frei's test (frīz) *See* test, Frei's.

fremitus (frĕm'ĭ-tŭs) Palpable vibrations of nonvascular origin that can be noted by placing the hand on the chest. *See also* thrill.

frenectomy (frē-nĕk'tō-mē) **1:** Excision of a frenum. **2:** Surgical detachment and/or excision of a frenum from its attachment into the mucoperiosteal covering of the alveolar processes.

frenoplasty (frēn″ō-plăs'tē) Correction of an abnormal frenum by repositioning it.

frenotomy (frē-not'ō-mē) The cutting of a frenum; especially the release of tongue-tie, or ankyloglossia.

frenulum (fren'u-lum) *See* frenum.

frenum (frē'nŭm) (frenulum) A fold of mucous membrane attaching the cheeks and lips to the mandibular and maxillary mucosa and limiting the motions of the lips and cheeks.

f., abnormal (enlarged labial frenum) A labial frenum appearing to be unusually heavy, broad, or attached too near the crest of the ridge that may be an etiologic factor in the production, perpetuation, and/or modification of lesions of the marginal gingivae.

f., buccal A fold or folds of mucous membrane connecting the residual alveolar ridge to the cheek in the premolar region. They exist in both the upper and lower jaws and separate the labial vestibule from the buccal vestibule.

f., labial The fold of mucous membrane connecting the lip of the residual alveolar ridge near the midline of both the upper and lower ridges.

f., enlarged labial *See* frenum, abnormal.

f., lingual The vertical band of mucous membrane connecting the tongue with the floor of the mouth and the alveolar or residual alveolar ridge.

frequency The number of cycles per second of a wave or other periodic phenomenon.

f. polygon A graphic representation of a frequency distribution constructed by plotti ng each frequency above the score or midpoint of a class interval laid out on a base line and connecting the points so plotted by a straight line.

Frey's syndrome (frīz) *See* syndrome, auriculotemporal.

fricative (frĭk′ah-tĭv) Any speech sound made by forcing the airstream through such a narrow orifice or opening that audible high-frequency air currents or vibrations are set up.

Friedman splint (frĕd′măn) *See* splint, cast bar.

Friedman's test (frĕd′mănz) *See* test, pregnancy.

fringe benefits Benefits, other than wages or salary, provided by an employer for employees (e.g., health insurance, vacation time, disability income).

frit (frĭt) A partly or wholly fused porcelain that is plunged into water while hot. The mass cracks and fractures, and it is from this "frit" that dental porcelain powders are made.

Frohlich's syndrome (frā′lĭks) *See* syndrome, Frohlich's.

frontal (PA) cephalometric radiograph A cephalometric radiograph made with the subject facing the film (posteroanterior or PA view); the axis between the ears is parallel to the film and perpendicular to the x-ray beam.

fulcrum line *See* line, fulcrum.

fulguration (ful-gū-rā′shŭn) Destruction of soft tissue by an electric spark that jumps the gap from an electrode to the tissue without the electrode's touching the tissue. *See also* electrocoagulation.

function The normal or special action of a part. As a noun, *function* has the following synonyms: role, capacity, task, use, purpose, service, activity, and direction. As a verb, it has the following synonyms: act, operate, work, perform, go, take effect, and serve. Use of the term to express intended purpose may be misleading.

f., auxiliary A function that is supplementary or additional to the function for which the part or organ is primarily intended.

f., dental, normal The correct action of opposing teeth in the process of mastication; sometimes referred to as normal occlusion.

f., group The simultaneous contact of opposing teeth in a segment or a group.

f., heavy (occlusal function) An increase in functional activities of the tooth, which may result in compensatory changes in the attachment apparatus (e.g., a stronger periodontal ligament) with an increase in the number of fibers; a reinforcement of the supporting bone by formation of new bone; and the formation of cemental spikes, which are calcifications of the cemental fibers. Such changes take place so that the increased stress may be withstood without damage.

f., impaired Diminished, weakened, or less-than-optimal work or action.

f., insufficiency of Hypofunction of the tooth, which may lead to regressive changes in the attachment apparatus and supporting bone. The severity of lesions varies with the degree of hypofunction. *See also* atrophy of disuse.

f., muscle The action of muscle—principally contraction.

f., occlusal *See* function, heavy.

f., physiologic The degree of activity that stimulates the physical structures but that is so limited as to stop short of irritation of those tissues.

f., skeletal The role of the skeleton in relation to the maintenance of body functions. The bony skeleton welds together and protects the softer vital visceral organs, supports and maintains the body form, and accomplishes body movement for locomotion, respiration, manual skills, and the functions associated with mandibular motion.

f., subcortical Function controlled by all the structures of the brain except the outer cortical rim of the cerebrum; most of the nonconscious activities of a sensory and motor nature.

functional 1: Pertaining to the movements and actions of a part. **2:** Of or pertaining to the functions of an organ, part, or prosthesis.

f. jaw orthopedics The objectives of activator-type appliances.

fungal infection An infection caused by a fungus or yeast organism.

fungate (fŭn′gāt) To produce funguslike growths; to grow rapidly like a fungus.

fungus (fŭn′gŭs) A class of vegetable organisms of a low order of development, including mushrooms, toadstools, and molds. Many are saprophytic and/or pathogenic for humans (e.g., *Candida albicans* and *Histoplasma, Trichophyton, Actinomyces,* and *Blastomyces* organisms. Oral and systemic moniliasis (thrush) is produced by overgrowth of *C. albicans,* which is a saprophytic resident in the oral cavity.

When physiologic processes are sufficiently impaired, the organism may gain a foothold and assume a pathogenic role.

furcation (fer-kā′shūn) Region of division of the root portion of a tooth.

f., root The interradicular bone resorption in multirooted teeth due to periodontal disease.

furnace An apparatus in which to generate heat.

f., inlay A furnace used for eliminating the wax from an inlay mold and establishing the proper condition and temperature of the investment to receive the molten casting gold.

f., porcelain A furnace used for fusing, firing, or fusion **1:** The uniting or joining together of two or more entities. The fusion temperature of an alloy lies just below the lower limit of its melting range, which is particularly important in soldering operations because temperatures near or above fusion temperature will decrease ductility. *See also* concrescence; range, melting. **2:** The process of producing fused teeth.

f. of metal *See* metal, fusion of.

f., nuclear The union of atomic nuclei to form heavier nuclei, resulting in the release of enormous quantities of energy when certain light elements unite.

Fusobacterium fusiforme (fū″zō-băk-tē′rē-ŭm) **(Vincent's bacillus)** A microorganism that, along with *Borrelia vincentii,* is implicated in the causation of necrotizing ulcerative gingivitis. Although *Fusobacterium fusiforme* and *B. vincentii* are inhabitants of the oral cavity, they may become pathogenic when tissue resistance is impaired.

Fusobacterium nucleatum A genus of schizomycetes, an anaerobic gram-negative bacterium often seen in necrotic tissue and implicated, but not conclusively, with other organisms in the causation and perpetuation of periodontal disease.

g *See* gram.

gag A surgical device for holding the mouth open.

gagging An involuntary retching reflex that may be stimulated by something touching the posterior palate or throat region.

gait (gāt) Manner of walking; a cyclic loss and regaining of balance by a shift of the line of gravity in relationship to the center of gravity. A person's gait is as characteristic and as individual as fingerprints.

  g., cerebellar An unsteady, irregular gait characterized by short steps and a lurching from one side to the other; most commonly seen in multiple sclerosis or other cerebellar diseases.

  g., festinating A gait characterized by rigidity, shuffling, and involuntary hastening. The upper part of the body advances ahead of the lower part. It is associated with paralysis agitans and postencephalitic Parkinson's syndrome.

  g., sensor ataxic An irregular, uncertain, stamping gait. The legs are kept far apart, and either the ground or the feet are watched, since there has been a loss of knowledge of the position of the lower limbs. This gait is caused by an interruption of the afferent nerve fibers and may be associated with tabes dorsalis and sometimes with multiple sclerosis and other lesions of the nervous system.

  g., spastic (creeping palsy) A slow, scuffing gait in which the patient appears to be wading in water. There is restricted movement at the knee and hip. This gait may be associated with multiple sclerosis, syphilis, combined systemic disease, or other diseases affecting the spinal pyramidal tracts.

  g., staggering A reeling, tottering, and tipping gait in which the individual appears as if he may fall backward or lose his balance. It is associated with alcoholic and barbiturate intoxication.

  g., waddling Exaggerated alteration of lateral trunk movements, with an exaggerated elevation of the hip, suggesting the gait of a duck; characteristic of progressive muscular dystrophy.

galactin (gah-lăk′tĭn) *See* hormone, lactogenic.

galvanic current *See* current, galvanic.

galvanism *See* current, galvanic.

galvanotherapy *See* ionization.

ganglion(ia) (găng′glē-on) Any collection or mass of nerve cells that serves as a center of nervous influence.

  g., basal A group of forebrain nuclei that, with the related structures of brain, play an important role in the regulation of muscle tone and motor control. The cell groups of these ganglia and their respective nerve tracts are classified as the extrapyramidal motor system to differentiate them from the pyramidal motor system, which goes directly from the cerebral cortex to the lower motor neuron. Disease associated with the basal ganglia is manifested by three principal motor abnormalities: disturbance of muscle tone, derangement of movement, and loss of associated or automatic movement.

  g., ciliary A parasympathetic nerve ganglion in the posterior part of the orbit. It receives preganglionic fibers from the region of the oculomotor nucleus and sends postganglionic fibers via short ciliary nerves to (1) the constrictor muscle of the iris (constriction of pupil) and (2) circular fibers of the ciliary muscle (accommodation for vision).

  g., otic A ganglion located medial to the mandibular nerve just below the foramen ovale in the infratemporal fossa. It supplies the sensory and secretory fibers for the parotid gland. Its sensory fibers arise from the facial and glossopharyngeal nerves.

  g., sphenopalatine One of the four ganglia of the autonomic nervous system associated with the head and neck region. It is located deep in the pterygopalatine fossa and is intimately associated with the maxillary nerve. It lies distal and medial to the maxillary tuberosity. Its fibers supply the mucous membrane of the roof of the pharynx, tonsils, soft and hard palates, and nasal cavity. The mucous and serous secretions of all the mucous membranes in the oropharynx are also mediated by this ganglion.

  g., submaxillary A ganglion located on the medial side of the mandible between the lingual nerve and the submaxillary duct. It is distributed to the sublingual and submaxillary glands. The sensory fibers arise from the lingual branch of the trigeminal nerve, i.e., the chorda tympani of the facial nerve.

ganglionitis, acute posterior (găng″glē-ō-ni,tŭs) *See* herpes zoster.

gangrene Death of tissue en masse; e.g., gangrene of the pulp is total death and necrosis of the pulp.

Gantrisin Brand name for sulfisoxazole, an antibacterial sulfonamide, effective in the treatment of acute, recurrent or chronic urinary tract infections, in the treatment of meningococcal meningitis and in the treatment of acute otitis media.

gap, interocclusal *See* distance, interocclusal.

gap arthroplasty Surgical correction of ankylosis by creation of a space between the ankylosed part and the portion in which movement is desired.

gargoylism *See* syndrome, Hurler's.

gas A fluid with no definite volume or shape whose molecules are practically unrestricted by cohesive forces.

   g., laughing *See* nitrous oxide.

   g., noble A gas that will not oxidize; the inert gases (e.g., helium, neon).

   g., olefiant *See* ethylene.

GAS *See* syndrome, general adaptation.

gasometer (găs-ahm′ĕ-ter) A calibrated instrument or vessel for measuring the volume of gases. Used in clinical and physiologic investigation for measuring respiratory volume.

gastric intrinsic factor (GIF) A substance secreted by the gastric mucosa that is essential for the intestinal absorption of vitamin ^{B12}; also known as intrinsic factor.

gate keeper system A managed-care concept used by some alternative benefit plans, in which enrollees elect a primary care dentist, usually a general practitioner or pediatric dentist, who is responsible for providing nonspecialty care and managing referrals, as appropriate, specialty and ancillary services.

Gaucher's cell, disease (gō-shāz′) *See* under appropriate nouns.

gauge An instrument used to determine the dimensions or caliber of an object.

   g., Boley A vernier type of instrument used for measuring in the metric system. It is accurate to tenths of millimeters.

   g., leaf A device for measuring the distance between two objects. It consists of a series of thin strips of plastic or metal, each calibrated and arranged in a sequential fashion in ascending or descending thicknesses, usually expressed in millimeters or fractions of millimeters. In dentistry, used to measure interocclusal space or magnitude of an interocclusal interference.

   g., undercut An attachment used in conjunction with a dental cast surveyor to measure the amount of infrabulge of a tooth in a horizontal plane.

gel (jĕl) A colloid in solid form, jellylike in character. Hydrocolloid impression materials are examples of gels.

   g. strength *See* strength, gel.

   g. time *See* time, gel.

gelation time (jĕ-lā′shŭn) *See* time, gel.

germination (jĕm″ĭ-nā′shŭn) Division of a tooth bud that results in the formation of double, or twin, crowns on a single root with a single pulp canal.

gene Fundamental unit of inheritance located in the chromosome. It determines and controls hereditarily transmissible characteristics.

   g. locus *See* locus, gene.

   g., sex-linked A gene located on a sex chromosome.

generated path (chew-in) *See* path, generated occlusal.

   g. occlusal path *See* path, occlusal, generated.

generator One who, or that which, begets, causes, or produces.

   g., electric A device that converts mechanical energy into electrical energy.

   g., x-ray A device that converts electrical energy into electromagnetic energy (photons).

genetic effects of radiation (jĕ-nĕt′ĭk) Those changes produced in the individual's genes and chromosomes of all nucleated body cells, both somatic and gonadal. The more common meaning relates to the effect produced in the reproductive cells. Radiation received by the gonads before the end of the reproductive period has the potential to add to the number of undesirable genes present in the population.

genetic counseling Advising a patient with a genetic disease, or child-bearing parents of a patient with a genetic disease, about the probabilities and risks of future genetic accidents in conception, and counseling such persons about future family planning.

genetic disease A disease that is caused by a defect or anomaly in the genetic inheritance of the patient.

genetics The science that deals with the origin of the characteristic of an individual.

genial tubercle *See* tubercle, genial.

genioplasty (jē′nē-ō-plăs″tē) A surgical procedure, performed either intraorally or extraorally, to correct deformities of the mandibular symphysis.

genome The total gene complement of a set of chromosomes found in higher life forms.

genotype (jē′nō-tīp) The aggregate of ordered genes received by offspring from both parents; e.g., a person with blood group AB is of genotype AB.

gentian violet (jĕn′shŭn) *See* violet, gentian.

geographic tongue *See* tongue, geographic.

geometric unsharpness Impairment of image definition resulting from the geometric penumbra. *See also* penumbra, geometric; x-ray beam.

geometry of x-ray beam The effect of various factors on the spatial distribution of radiation emerging from an x-ray generator or source. *See also* law, inverse-square; penumbra, geometric, and subentries; x-ray beam and subentries.

geriatrics (jĕr″ē-ăt′rĭks) The department of medicine or dentistry that treats health problems peculiar to advanced age and the aging, including the clinical problems of senescence and senility.

geriatric dentistry A branch of dentistry that deals with the special and unique dental problems of senior citizens.

germicide (jĕr′mĭ-sīd) A substance capable of killing a wide variety of microorganisms. More specifically, one capable of killing all microorganisms, except for spores, with which it is in contact for a standard period of time.

gerodontics (jĕr″ō-dahn′tĭks) **(gerodontology)** The branch of dentistry that deals with the diagnosis and treatment of the dental conditions of aging and aged persons.

gerodontology (jĕr″ō-dahn-tol′ō-jē) *See* gerodontics.

giant follicular lymphoblastoma *See* lymphoblastoma, giant follicular.

giantism (macrosomia) Excessive growth resulting in a stature larger than the range of normnal for age and race.

  g., infantile Excessive growth occurring before adolescence.

  g., primary Excessive growth not attributable to a definite cause.

  g., secondary Excessive growth secondary to a disorder of the adrenal, pineal, gonadal, or pituitary gland.

GIF *See* gastric intrinsic factor.

gift A voluntary transfer of personal property without consideration.

Gigli's wire saw (jēl′yēz) *See* saw, Gigli's wire.

Gillies' operation *See* operation, Gillies.

Gillmore needle *See* needle, Gillmore.

Gilson fixable-removable bar *See* connector, cross arch bar splint.

gingiva(e) (jĭn′jĭ-vah) The fibrous tissue covered by mucous membrane that immediately surrounds the teeth.

  g., attached The portion of the gingivae extending from the free gingival groove, which demarcates it from the free or marginal gingivae, to the mucogingival junction, which separates it from the alveolar mucosa. This tistue is firm, dense, stippled, and tightly bound down to the underlying periosteum, tooth, and bone.

    g., attached, extension *See* extension, gingiva, attached.

  g., free The unattached coronal portion of the gingiva that encircles the tooth to form the gingival sulcus.

  g. hyperplasia *See* hyperplasia, gingival, Dilantin.

  g., interdental (interproximal gingiva[e]) The soft supporting tissue, consisting of prominent horizontal collagen fibers, that normally fills the space between two contacting teeth.

  g., interproximal *See* gingiva, interdental.

  g., lymphatic drainage of Lymphatic drainage that follows the course of the gingival blood supply, i.e., from the lymphatic vessels on the gingival side of the periosteum of the alveolar process to the lymphatic vessels in the periodontal membrane to vessels leaking into the alveolar bone.

  g., marginal The free gingiva at the labial, buccal, lingual, and palatal aspects of the teeth.

  g., microscopic appearance of Stratified squamous epithelium that varies in degree of keratinization and overlies a corium of connective tissue with interspersed blood vessels and nerves. Rete pegs of epithelium project downward into the connective tissue corium, except from the base of sulcular epithelium. The gingival fiber apparatus is readily discerned.

  g., stippling A series of small depressions characterizing the surface of healthy gingivae, varying from a smooth velvet to that of an orange peel, either finely or coarsely grained.

gingival Pertaining to or in relation to the gingiva.

  g. abrasion The attrition (scraping or wearing away) of the gingival tissue by harsh irritants such as coarse foods or faulty toothbrushing.

  g. anatomy Gingiva is a dense connective tissue covered by keratinized mucosa except in the sulcus, where it is nonkeratinized. The margin is arcuate buccolingually with the peaks (papillae) interdentally. The sulcus depth normally is the apical limit to the free (unattached) gingiva, the attached gingiva extending from the free gingiva to the oral mucosa.

  g. architecture Gingival form.

  g. blanching Lightening of gingival color resulting from stretching with diminution of blood supply; usually of a temporary nature.

  g. bleeding A prominent symptom of periodontal disease produced by ulceration of the sulcular epithelium and an inflammatory process.

  g. blood supply The vascular supply to the gingivae arises from the vessels that pass on the gingival side of the outer periosteum of bone and anastomoses with blood vessels of the periodontal membrane and intra-alveolar blood vessels.

  g. color The color of the gingival tissues in health and in disease. It varies with the thickness and degree of keratinization of the epithelium, blood supply, pigmentation, and alterations produced by diseased processes affecting the gingival tissues. In health, often described as coral pink.

  g. consistency Visual and tactile characteristics of healthy gingival tissue. Visual consistency varies from a smooth velvet to an orange peel, either finely or coarsely grained. The tactile consistency of the gingival tissue should be firm and resilient.

  g. crater A concave depression in the gingival tissue. Especially seen in area of former apex of the interdental papilla as a result of the gingival destruction associated with necrotizing ulcerative gingivitis or when food impaction occurs against the tissue subjacent to the contact points of adjacent teeth.

g. discoloration A change from the normal coloration of the gingivae; associated with inflammation, diminution of blood supply, abnormal pigmentation, etc.

g. hormonal enlargement Enlargement of the gingivae associated with hormonal imbalance during pregnancy or puberty.

g. mat The gingival connective tissue composed of coarse, broad collagen fibers that serve to attach the gingivae to the teeth and to hold the free gingivae in close approximation to the teeth.

g. physiology The gingivae encircle the teeth and serve as a protective mucosal covering for the underlying tissues; the gingival fiber apparatus serves as a barrier to apical migration of the epithelial attachment and serves to bind the gingival tissues to the teeth. The normal topography permits the free flow of food away from the occlusal surfaces and from the cervical and interproximal areas of the teeth.

g. pigmentation Variations in gingival color may be correlated with the complexion of the individual or may be a reflection of pathologic influences, as in the melanin pigmentation associated with hypoadrenocorticism (Addison's disease), nevi, depositions of heavy metals, etc.

g. position The level of the gingival margin in relation to the tooth.

g. shrinkage The reduction in size of gingival tissue, principally by diminution of edema, usually as a result of therapeutic elimination of subgingival deposits and curettement of the soft tissue wall of the pocket.

g. stippling A series of small depressions characterizing the surface of healthy gingivae, varying from a smooth velvet to that of an orange peel.

g. sulcus The space between the free gingiva and the tooth.

g. surface texture The texture of the attached gingivae, which normally is stippled; in inflammatory conditions, the edema, cellular infiltration, and concomitant swelling cause loss of the surface stippling, and the gingivae take on a smooth, shiny edematous appearance.

g. third Relating to the most apical one third of a given clinical crown or of an axial surface cavity or preparation.

g. topography The form of the healthy gingival tissues. The marginal gingivae and the interdental papillae have a characteristic shape.

gingivectomy (jǐn″jǐ-věk′tō-mē) Surgical excision of un-

supported gingival tissue to the level where it is attached, creating a new gingival margin apical in position to the old.

g. in edentulous area Elimination of periodontal pockets surrounding abutment teeth; requires the removal of gingival tissue on the adjacent edentulous area.

gingivitis (jǐn″jǐ-vī′tǐs) Any inflammation of the gingival tissue.

g., bacteria in The causative organisms in gingival inflammation. The common chronic forms of gingivitis, from a bacterial standpoint, are nonspecific, with the exception of acute necrotizing ulcerative gingivitis, in which there is an apparent specificity of the bacterial flora: the fusospirochetal organisms.

g., bismuth Metallic poisoning caused by bismuth given for treatment of systemic disease; characterized by a dark, bluish line along the gingival margin.

g., chronic atrophic senile Gingival inflammation characterized by atrophy and areas of hyperkeratosis; found primarily in elderly women.

g., desquamative An inflammation of the gingivae characterized by the tendency of the surface epithelium to desquamate. The disease is a clinical entity, not a pathologic entity. It is most frequently associated with menopause but may be associated with any biologic stress.

g., eruptive (ē-rŭp′tǐv) Gingival inflammation occurring at the time of eruption of the permanent teeth.

g., fusospirochetal *See* gingivitis, necrotizing ulcerative.

g. gravidarum *See* gingivitis, pregnancy.

g., hemorrhagic Gingivitis characterized by profuse bleeding, especially that associated with ascorbic acid deficiency.

g., herpetic Inflammation of the gingivae caused by herpesvirus. *See also* gingivostomatitis, herpetic.

g., hormonal Gingivitis associated with endocrine imbalance, the endocrinopathy being modified, in most instances, by the influence of local environmental factors.

g., hyperplastic Gingivitis characterized by proliferation of the various tissue elements. May be accompanied by dense infiltration of inflammatory cells.

g., idiopathic Gingival inflammation of unknown causation.

g., inflammatory cells in Since the gingival inflammatory process is usually chronic and progressive in nature, the inflammatory cells are, for the most part, lymphocytes, plasma cells, and some histiocytes. With acute exacerbations, polymorphonuclear leukocytes are also present.

g. and malposed teeth Malposition may predispose the gingivae to inflammation by permitting food impaction or impingement, by providing irregular spaces in which calculus may be deposited, and making cleaning difficult.

g., marginal Inflammation of the gingivae localized to the marginal gingivae and interdental papillae.

g., necrotizing ulcerative (fusospirochetal gingivitis, NUG, trench mouth, ulcerative gingivitis, ulceromembranous gingivitis, Vincent's gingivitis, Vincent's infection) An inflammation of the gingivae characterized by necrosis of the interdental papillae, ulceration of the gingival margins, and the appearance of a pseudomembrane, pain, and a fetid odor.

    g., necrotizing ulcerative, inflammatory cells in Prevalent cellular infiltrate in necrotizing ulcerative gingivitis, including polymorphonuclear leukoctyes, plasma cells, and lymphocytes. In the acute phase polymorphonuclear leukocytes predominate.

g., nephritic (uremic gingivitis, uremic stomatitis) A membrane form of stomatitis and gingivitis associated with a failure of kidney function. It is accompanied by pain, ammoniacal odor, and increased salivation.

g., pregnancy (gingivitis gravidarum, hormonal gingivitis) Enlargement of hyperplasia of the gingivae resulting from hormonal imbalance during pregnancy.

g., puberty An enlargement of the gingival tissues as a result of an exaggerated response to irritation resulting from hormonal changes.

g., scorbutic Gingivitis associated with vitamin C (ascorbic acid) deficiency.

g., ulcerative *See* gingivitis, necrotizing ulcerative.

g., ulceromembranous *See* gingivitis, necrotizing ulcerative.

g., uremic *See* gingivitis, nephritic.

g., Vincent's *See* gingivitis, necrotizing ulcerative.

gingivoplasty (jĭn″jĭ-vō-plăs′tē) The surgical contouring of the gingival tissues to secure the physiologic architectural form necessary for the maintenance of tissue health and integrity.

gingivosis (jĭn″jĭ-vō′sĭs) A noninflammatory degenerative condition of the gingivae. The term is applied to desquamative gingivitis.

gingivostomatitis (jĭn″jĭ-vō-stō″mah-tī′tĭs) An inflammation that involves the gingivae and the oral mucosa.

g., herpetic An inflammation of the gingivae and oral mucosa caused by primary invasion of herpesvirus. It occurs chiefly in childhood, one attack giving immunity to generalized stomatitis but not to isolated lesions (herpetic lesions). The symptoms are red and swollen gingivae; red mucosa, which soon shows vesicles and ulcers; painful mouth; and elevated temperature. The course is about 14 days.

    g., acute herpetic *See* stomatitis, herpetic, acute.

g., membranous A disease, or group of diseases, in which false membranes form on the gingivae and oral mucosa; the membranes have a grayish white coloration and are surrounded by a narrow red margin. Detachment of the membrane leaves a raw, bleeding surface. One cause is mixed pyogenic infection in which *Streptococcus viridans* and *Staphylococcus* organisms predominate.

g., white folded *See* nevus spongiosus albus mucosa.

ginglymus (jĭng′glĭ-mŭs) (hinge joint) A joint that allows motion around an axis.

glabella (glah-bĕl′ah) The most anterior point on the frontal bone.

gland(s) An organ producing a specific product or secretion.

g., Blandin and Nuhn's Minor anterior lingual salivary glands, partly serous and partly mucous. The duct of each gland opens on the inferior surface of the tongue.

g., ectopic sebaceous *See* spots, Fordyce's.

g., endocrine Any one of the glands of internal secretion; a hormone-secreting gland (e.g., the pituitary gland, thyroid gland, parathyroid glands, adrenal glands, ovaries, and testes).

g., pituitary (hypophysis) An endocrine gland located at the base of the brain in the sella turcica. It is composed of two parts: the pars nervosa, which is an extension of the anterior part of the hypothalamus, and the pars intermedia, which is an epithelial evagination of secretory tissue from the stomodeum of the embryo. By its structural and functional relationships with the nervous system and with the endocrine glands, it acts as a mediator of both the nervous system and the endocrine system.

g., salivary Glands in the mouth that secrete saliva. Three major groups of salivary glands contribute their secretions to form the whole saliva; accessory mucous glands found within oral mucosa contribute also in small part. The prime glands are the parotid, submaxillary, and sublingual.

    g., accessory salivary Glands located at the posterior aspect of the dorsum of the tongue behind the vallate papillae and along the margins of the tongue; also located in the palate, labial mucosa, and buccal mucosa. The secretion is mucous.

    g., parotid salivary The largest of the salivary glands; situated between the ramus of the mandible in front, the mastoid process and sternocleidomastoideus behind, and the zygomatic arch above; irregularly wedge shaped, with the lateral surface flattened and the medial aspect more or less pointed toward the pharyngeal wall. Its secretion, which is serous, traverses Stensen's duct to empty into the mouth at the ductal orifice on the buccal mucosa opposite the upper molar teeth.

g., sublingual salivary The smallest of the principal salivary glands. It lies below the mucous membranes of the floor of the mouth at the sides of the lingual frenum and is in contact with the sublingual depression on the inner side of the mandible. It numerous ducts open directly into the mouth on the sides of the lingual frenum and/or join to form the duct of Bartholin (sublingual duct), which enters into the submaxillary duct (Wharton's duct). Its secretion is mucous in nature.

g., submaxillary salivary A gland that has an irregular form and is situated in the submaxillary triangle, bordered anteriorly by the anterior belly of the digastricus and posteriorly by the stylomandibular ligament. Its mucoserous section is carried by Wharton's duct, whose orifice lies at the summit of a small papilla (submaxillary caruncle) at the side of the lingual frenum.

glass, lead Lead-impregnated glass used in windows of control booths and in protective shields to protect radiologists and their assistants from primary and scattered radiation.

glaze A critical stage in the final firing of dental porcelain when complete fusion takes place, with the formation of a thin, vitreous, glossy surface (glaze).

glenoid The fossae in the temporal bone in which condyles of the mandible articulate with the skull.

glide(s) 1: The passage of one object over another as guided by their contracting surfaces. **2:** The sounds "w" and "wh" and the sound "y," which are voiced as bilabial and palatal glides, respectively. The rapid movement of the lips or tongue from a set position toward a neutral vowel ("u," as in up).

g., mandibular Side-to-side, protrusive, and intermediate movement of the mandible, occurring when the teeth or other occluding surfaces are in contact.

gliding occlusion *See* occlusion, gliding.

globulin A class of proteins.

g., antihemophilic *See* factor VIII.

g., antihemophilic A *See* factor VIII.

g., antihemophilic B *See* factor IX.

glossalgia (glah-săl′jē-ah) Painful sensations in the tongue.

glossectomy (glah-sĕk′tō-mē) Surgical removal of the tongue, a portion of the tongue, or a lesion of the tongue.

glossitis (glah-sī′tĭs) Inflammation of the tongue.

g. areata exfoliativa *See* tongue, geographic.

g., atrophic (bald tongue, smooth tongue) Atrophy of the glossal papillae, resulting in a smooth tongue. The tongue may be pallid or erythematous and may appear small or enlarged. Atrophic glossitis may be associated with anemias, pellagra, vitamin B complex deficiencies, sprue, or other systemic diseases or may be local in origin. Because atrophy may be

one phase, and circumscribed, painful, glossal excoriations may be another phase of one or more of the same systemic disease(s), much confusion in terminology has arisen (e.g., Moeller's glossitis; Hunter's glossitis; slick, glazed, varnished, glossy, or bald tongue; chronic superficial erythematous glossitis; glossodynia exfoliativa; beefy tongue; and pellagrous glossitis).

g., benign migratory *See* tongue, geographic.

g., chronic superficial erythematous *See* glossitis, Moeller's.

g., Clarke-Fournier *See* glossitis, interstitial sclerous.

g., Hunter's *See* glossitis, Moeller's.

g., interstitial sclerous (Clarke-Fournier glossitis) Nodular, lobulated, indurated tongue associated with terminal syphilis.

g., median rhomboid A developmental defect appearing as a red, slightly elevated area of the tongue just anterior to the foramen cecum. It is of no clinical significance and results from trapping of the median lobe of the tongue (tuberculum impar) at the surface during development.

g. migrans *See* tongue, geographic.

g., Moeller's (chronic superficial erythematous glossitis, glossodynia exfoliativa, Hunter's glossitis, pellagrous glossitis) Chronic, superficial, irregular atrophy of the mucosa of the tongue. It may be caused by allergy, neural disturbance, vitamin B complex deficiency, etc. A smooth, red, painful tongue associated with pernicious anemia.

g., pellagrous *See* glossitis, Moeller's.

glossodynia (glos″ō-dĭn′ē-ah) Painful sensations in the tongue; a sensation of burning in the tongue; a sore tongue.

g. exfoliativa *See* glossitis, Moeller's.

glossoplasty (glos′ō-plas″tē) A surgical procedure performed on the tongue.

glossoplegia (glos″ō-plē′jē-ah) Paralysis of the tongue; may be unilateral or bilateral.

glossoptosis A downward displacement of the tongue; a severe displacement may occlude the airway.

glossopyrosis (glos″ō-pī-rō′sĭs) Burning sensation of the tongue.

glossorraphy (glos″or′ah-fē) Suture of a wound of the tongue.

glossotomy (glah-sot′ō-mē) Excision or incision of the tongue.

glottal (glot′tăl) Pertaining to, or produced in or by, the glottis. The sound of "h" is a voiceless glottal fricative. The airstream on the exhalation phase moves unimpeded through the larynx, pharynx, and oral cavities.

glottidospasm (glot-tĭ′dō-spăzm) *See* laryngospasm.

glottis (glot′ĭs) The vocal apparatus of the larynx, consisting of the true vocal cords (vocal folds) and the opening between them (rima glottidis).

gloves or surgical gloves Latex gloves used as an essential part of barrier protection in health care delivery.

glucagon (gloo'kah-gahn) (hyperglycemic factor, hyperglycemic-glycogenolytic factor [HGF]) A hormone from the alpha cells of the pancreas that raises the blood sugar by increasing hepatic glycogenolysis.

glucocorticoids (gloo″kō-kor'tĭ-koidz) (anti-inflammatory hormone, 11-oxycorticoids) Adrenocortical steroid hormones that affect glycogenesis in the liver. They are anti-inflammatory, are active in protection against stress, and affect carbohydrate and protein metabolism. Typical of the group are cortisol and cortisone.

gluconeogenesis (gloo″kō-nē″ō-jĕn'ĕ-sĭs) The formation of glycogen or glucose from noncarbohydrate sources (e.g., the glycogenic amino acids, glycerol, lactate, and pyruvate) by pathways mainly involving the citric acid cycle and glycolysis.

glucose (gloo'kōs) A six-carbon (hexose) sugar that is the principle sugar in blood and serves as a major metabolic source of energy.

glucose tolerance test A metabolic test that measures the ability of the body to metabolize carbohydrates. A patient is administered a standard dose of glucose, and blood and urine samples are measured for glucose levels at periodic intervals following administration. The test is most often used to assist in the diagnosis of diabetes.

glucoside (gloo'kō-sīd) A glycoside in which the sugar component is glucose.

glyceride (glĭs'er-īd) An ester of glycerin with one or more aliphatic acids.

glycerite (glĭs'er-īt) A solution or suspension of a drug in glycerin.

glycogen (glī'kō-jĕn) A branched, homopolysaccharide of glucose held by alpha 1-4 and alpha 1-6 glucosidic bonds. Liver glycogen provides a ready source of blood glucose through glycogenolysis.

glycogenesis (glī″kō-jĕn'ĕ-sĭs) The synthesis of glycogen from glucose.

glycogenolysis (glī″kō-jĕ-nol'ĭ-sĭs) The formation of blood glucose by hydrolysis of stored liver glycogen.

glycolysis (glī-kōl'ĭ-sĭs) Oxidation of glucose or glycogen by cystoplasmic enzymes of the Embden-Meyerhof pathway to pyruvate and lactate.

glycoside (glī'kō-sīd) A compound that contains a sugar as part of the molecule.

glycosuria (glī'kō-sū'rē-ah) Presence of sugar in the urine. It results most commonly from diabetes mellitus but may occur from a lowered renal threshold (renal glycosuria) in pregnancy, inorganic renal disease, and in patients taking adrenocorticosteroids.

glutaraldehyde A germicidal agent for the disinfection

and sterilization of instruments or equipment that cannot be heat sterilized. An effective agent used in solution for "cold" sterilization.

Gm *See* gram.

gnathic organ (năth'ĭk) A collective organ assembled about the upper and the lower dentolingual surface and used to pronounce the consonants th, t, d, n, l, and r.

gnathion (năth'ē-ahn) The lowest point in the lower border of the mandible at the median plane. It is a point on the bony border palpated from below and naturally lies posterior to the tegumental border of the chin.

gnathodynamometer (nă″thō-dī″nah-mom'ĕ-ter) An instrument used for measuring biting pressure.

g., Bimeter A gnathodynamometer equipped with a central bearing point of adjustable height.

Gnathograph (năth'ō-grăf) An articulator designed by McCollum. Its resembles the Hanau instrument but differs chiefly by having a provision for increasing the intercondylar distance, an important determinant of groove directions in the occlusal surfaces of teeth.

Gnatholator An articulator by Granger that has since been succeeded by an improved instrument called the *Simulator* (or *Gnathosimulator*).

gnathologic instrument Term often used as a synonym for an articulator. Any dental instrument used for diagnosis and treatment, such as a probe for determining the depth of a periodontal pocket, is a gnathologic tool.

gnathology The study of the functional and occlusal relationships of the teeth; sometimes also used to identify a specific philosophy of occlusal function.

gnathoschisis (nah-thos'kĭ-sĭs) *See* jaw, cleft.

Gnathoscope Name of an articulator designed by McCollum, with tiltable remnant hinge "axles" set in stirrup mounts that can be swiveled and turned so that the setting of each condylar element provides an approximate path of travel for the condyles of the patient.

gnathostatics (năth″ō-stăt'ĭks) A technique of orthodontic diagnosis based on relationships between the teeth and certain landmarks on the skull. *See also* cast, gnathostatic.

goiter (goi'ter) Enlargement of the thyroid gland.

g., colloid (endemic goiter, iodine deficiency goiter, simple goiter) Visible enlargement of the thyroid gland without obvious signs of hypofunction or hyperfunction of the gland resulting from inadequate intake or to an increased demand for iodine.

g., endemic *See* goiter, colloid.

g., exophthalmic A disease of the thyroid gland consisting of hyperthyroidism, exophthalmos, and goiterous enlargement of the thyroid gland. A diffuse primary hyperplasia of the thyroid gland of obscure origin; may occur at any age. It produces nervousness, muscular weakness, heat intolerance, tremor, loss of weight, lid lag, and absence of winking and may lead to thyrotoxic heart disease and thyroid crisis.

g., iodine deficiency *See* goiter, colloid.

g., nodular, nontoxic Recurrent episodes of hyperplasia and involution of colloid goiter, resulting in a multinodular goiter. Symptoms are related to pressure.

g., simple *See* goiter, colloid.

goitrogens (goi′trō-jĕnz) Agents such as thiouracil and related antithyroid compounds that are capable of producing goiter.

gold A precious or noble metal; yellow, malleable, ductible, nonrusting; much used in dentistry in pure and alloyed forms.

g., crystal *See* gold, mat.

g., fibrous *See* foil, gold.

g. file *See* file, gold.

g. foil *See* foil, gold.

　g. foil cylinder *See* foil cylinder.

　g. foil pellet *See* pellet, foil.

g., inlay 1: An alloy, principally gold, used for cast restorations. Desired physical properties may be obtained by selecting those with varying ingredients and/or proportions. Acceptable alloys are classified by ADA specifications according to Brinell hardness: Type A—soft, Brinell 40 to 75; Type B—medium, Brinell 70 to 100; Type C—hard, Brinell 90 to 140. **2:** An intracoronal cast restoration of gold alloy fabricated outside the mouth and cemented into the prepared cavity.

g. knife *See* knife, gold.

g., mat (crystal gold, sponge gold) A noncohesive form of pure gold prepared by electrodeposition. Sometimes used in the base of restorations and then veneered or overlaid with cohesive foil.

g., powdered Fine granules of pure gold, formed by atomizing the molten metal or by chemical precipitation. For clinical use it is available either as clusters of the granules or as pellets of the powder contained in an envelope of gold foil.

g. saw *See* saw, gold.

g., sponge *See* gold, mat.

g., white A gold alloy with a high palladium content. It has a higher fusion range, lower ductility, and greater hardness than a yellow gold alloy.

Goldent Trade name for a direct gold restorative material. It consists basically of varying amounts of powdered gold contained in a wrapping or envelope of gold foil.

Goldman-Fox knife *See* knife, Goldman-Fox.

Golgi's corpuscles (gol′jēz) *See* corpuscle, Golgi's.

gomphosis (gahm-fō′sĭs) A form of joint in which a conical body is fastened into a socket, as a tooth is fastened into the jaw.

gonad (gō′năd, gon′ăd) An ovary or testis, the site of origin of eggs or spermatozoa.

gonadotrophin (gō-năd″ō-trŏf′ĭn) *See* gonadotropin.

gonadotropin (gō-năd″ō-trŏp′ĭn) **(gonadotropic hormone)** A gonad-stimulating hormone derived either from the pituitary gland (e.g., follicle-stimulating hormone [FSH] and a luteinizing hormone [LH], which is also an interstitial cell–stimulating hormone [ICSH]) or from the chorion (e.g., chorionic gonadotropin, which is found in the urine of pregnant women).

g., chorionic *See* hormone, pregnancy.

gonion (Go) The most posteroinferior point of the angle of the mandible near the lower border of the ramus.

good faith Honesty of intention. Generally, not a sufficient defense in a dental malpractice lawsuit.

Good Samaritan legislation Statutes enacted in some states protecting physicians, dentists, and some other health professionals from liability for aid rendered in emergency situations, unless there is a showing of willful wrong or gross negligence.

goodwill Intangible assets of a firm established by the excess of the price paid for the going concern over its book value.

gothic arch tracer *See* tracer, needle point.

gothic arch tracing *See* tracing, needle point.

gr *See* grain.

grace period A specified time, after a plan's premium payment is due, in which the protection of the plan continues subject to actual receipt of premium within that time.

graft A slip or portion of tissue used for implantation. *See also* donor site; recipient site.

g., allo A graft between genetically dissimilar members of the same species.

g., alloplast A graft of an inert metal or plastic material.

g., autogenous A graft taken from one portion of an individual's body and implanted into another portion of the individual's body.

　g., autogenous bone A bone graft taken from one part of a patient's body and transplanted to another part of the same patient's body.

g., auto- *See* graft, autogenous.

g. donor site The site from which graft material is taken.

g., filler A graft used for the filling of defects, such as bone chips used to fill a cyst.

g., free A graft of tissue completely detached from its original site and blood supply.

g., full-thickness A skin graft consisting of the full thickness of the skin with none of the subcutaneous tissues.

g., heterogenous A graft implanted from one species to another.

g., hetero *See* graft, heterogenous.

g., homogenous A graft taken from a member of a species and implanted into the body of a member of the same species.

g., homo *See* graft, homogenous.

g., iliac A bone graft whose donor site is the crest of the ilium. Various locations of the iliac crest duplicate areas of the mandible and curvatures of the midfacial skeleton.

g., iso A graft between individuals with identical or histocompatible antigens.

g., kiel Denatured calf bone used to fill defects or restore facial contour.

g., mucosal A split-thickness graft involving the mucosa.

g., onlay bone A graft in which the grafted bone is applied laterally to the cortical bone of the recipient site, frequently to improve the contours of the chin or the malar eminence of the zygomatic bone.

g., pedicle A stem or tube of tissue that remains attached near the donor site to nourish the graft during advancement of a skin graft.

g., split-thickness A graft that varies in thickness and contains only mucosal elements and no subcutaneous tissue.

g., swaging A procedure analogous to bone grafting. Also referred to as a contiguous transplant that involves a greenstick fracture of bone bordering on an infrabony defect and the displacement of bone to eliminate the osseous defect.

g., Thiersch's skin A split-thickness skin graft containing cutaneous and some subcutaneous tissues, the line of cleavage being through the rete peg layer.

grain (gr) 1: A unit of weight equal to 0.0648 g.   **2:** A crystal of an alloy.

g. boundary The junction of two grains growing from different nuclei, impinging on each other and causing discontinuity of the lattice structure. Important in corrosion and brittleness of metals.

g. growth *See* growth, grain.

gram (Gm, g) The basic unit of mass of the metric system. Equivalent of 15.432 gr.

Gram's stain *See* stain, Gram's.

granmicidin An antibacterial agent generally used in conjunction with nystatin, a specific anticandidal agent, and neomycin, a complementary antibacterial agent, in the treatment of angular cheilosis.

granules, sulfur *See* actinomycosis.

granulocytopenia (grăn″ū-lō-sī″tō-pē′nē-ah) A deficiency in the number of granulocytic cells in the bloodstream.

granuloma (grăn″ū-lō′mah) A localized mass of granulation tissue.

g., chronic (chronic apical periodontitis) Chronic inflammatory tissue surrounding the apical foramina as a result of irritation from within the root canal system.

g., dental A mass of granulation tissue surrounded by a fibrous capsule attached at the apex of a pulp-involved tooth. It produces a fairly well demarcated radiolucency.

g., eosinophilic (ē″ō-sĭn″ō-fĭl′ĭk) A granulomatous inflammatory disease of unknown etiology, usually monofocal in bone but sometimes affecting soft tissues. Sheets of histiocytes and masses of eosinophils characterize the lesion histologically.

g., giant cell reparative An abnormal reparative reaction to an injury, characterized by fibroblastic proliferation with numerous giant cells. It may be peripheral (i.e., on the gingiva, as in giant cell epulis) or central (i.e., within the bone, producing a radiolucency). Most giant cell lesions of the jaws are reparative granulomas rather than neoplasms.

g., pyrogenic A tumorlike mass of granulation tissue produced in response to minor trauma in some individuals. It is highly vascular and bleeds readily.

g., reticuloendothelial *See* disease, lipoid storage.

granulation tissue Any soft pink fleshy projections that form during the healing process in a wound that is not healing by first intent. Gradulation tissue consisting of many capillaries surrounded by fibrous collagen. Overgrowth of granulation tissue is termed *proud flesh*. Such tissue is evident at the opening to a fistulous tract.

grasp The manner in which an instrument is held.

g., finger A modification of the palm and thumb grasp; it is more useful with modern, smaller handled instruments. The handle is held by the four flexed fingers rather than allowed to rest in the palm, and the thumb is used to secure a rest. Used when working indirectly on the upper arch.

g., instrument A method of holding the instrument with the fingers in such a manner that freedom of action, control, tactile sensitivity, and maneuverability are secured. The most common grasp is the pen grasp.

g., palm-and-thumb A grasp that is similar to the hold on a knife when one is whittling wood; the handle rests in the palm and is grasped by the four fingers, while the thumb rests on an adjoining object.

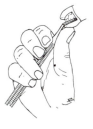

Palm-and-thumb grasp

g., pen A grasp in which the instrument is held somewhat as a pen is held, with the handle in contact with the bulbous portion of the thumb and index finger and the shank in contact with the radial side of the bulbous portion of the middle finger (not crossing the nail) while the handle rests against the phalanx of the index finger.

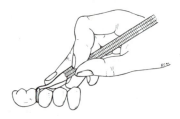

Pen grasp

gratis Free, without reward or consideration.

Graves' disease *See* goiter, exophthalmic.

gravity, specific A number indicating the ratio of the weight of a substance to that of an equal volume of water.

grid A device used to prevent as much scattered radiation as possible from reaching an x-ray film during the making of a radiograph. It consists essentially of a series of narrow lead strips closely spaced on their edges and separated by spacers of low-density material.

g., crossed An arrangment of two parallel grids rotated in position at right angles to each other. *See also* grid, parallel.

g., focused A grid in which the lead foils are placed at an angle so that they all point toward a focus at a specified distance.

g., moving A grid that is moved continuously or oscillated throughout the making of a radiograph.

g., parallel A grid in which the lead strips are oriented parallel to each other.

g., Potter-Bucky A grid using the principle of the moving grid, with an oscillating movement.

g., stationary A nonoscillating or nonmoving grid; the image of its strips will be visible on the radiograph for which it is used.

grinding, selective Modification of the occlusal forms of teeth by grinding at selected places to improve function.

grinding-in The process of correcting errors in the centric and eccentric occlusions of natural or artificial teeth.

groove A linear channel or sulcus.

g., abutment A transverse groove that may be cut in the bone across the alveolar ridge to furnish positive seating for the implant framework and to prevent tension of the tissue.

g., developmental A fine depressed line in the enamel of a tooth that marks the union of the lobes of the crown in its development.

g., gingiva, free The shallow line or depression on the surface of the gingiva at the junction of the free and attached gingivae.

g., interdental A linear, vertical depression on the surface of the interdental papillae; functions as a sluiceway for the egress of food from the interproximal areas.

g., retention A groove formed by opposing vertical constrictions in the preparation of a tooth that provides improved retention of the restoration.

ground, electrical Electrical connection with the earth (or other ground).

g. state The state of a nucleus, an atom, or a molecule when it has its lowest energy. All other states are termed *excited*.

grounded Pertaining to an arrangement whereby an electrical circuit or equipment (e.g., x-ray generator) is connected by an electrical conductor with the earth or some similarly conducting body.

group, blood *See* blood groups.

group function *See* function, group.

group practice *See* practice, group.

group purchase The purchase of dental services, either by postpayment or prepayment, by a large group of people.

growth Increase in size.

growth and development Growth is defined as an increase in size; development is defined as a progression toward maturity. Thus the terms are used together to describe the complex physical, mental, and emotional processes associated with the "growing up" of children.

growth factor One of about a hundred chemical messengers that induces cell growth by tissue type (e.g., osteoinductive factor, epidermal growth factors).

g., grain A phenomenon resulting from heat treatment of alloys. In excessive amounts this growth produces undesirable physical properties.

GTT *See* test, glucose tolerance.

guaranty A contract that some certain and designated thing shall be done exactly as it is agreed to be done.

guard, bite An acrylic resin appliance designed to cover the occlusal and incisal surfaces of the teeth of a dental arch so as to stabilize the teeth and/or provide a flat platform for the unobstructed excursive glides of the mandible. *See also* plane, bite.

guard, mouth A resilient intraoral device worn during participation in contact sports to reduce the potential for injury to the teeth and associated tissue.

guard, night *See* guard, bite.

guardian A person appointed to take care of the person or property of another; one who legally has the care and management of the person, or the property, or both, of a child until the child attains his or her majority.

Guérin's fracture (gā-rănz′) *See* fracture, Guérin's.

guidance A mechanical or other means for controlling the direction of movement of an object.

g., condylar *See* guide, condylar.

g., condylar, inclination *See* guide, condylar, inclination.

g., developmental Comprehensive dentofacial orthopedic control over the growth of the jaws and eruption of the teeth, with the objective of optimizing the achievement of the genetic potential of the individual. Requires a combination of carefully timed active appliance therapy and supervisory examinations, including radiography and other diagnostic records, at various stages of development. May be required throughout the entire period of growth and maturation of the face, beginning at the earliest detection of a developing malformation.

g., incisal The influence on mandibular movements of the contacting surfaces of the mandibular and maxillary anterior teeth.

g., incisal, angle *See* angle, incisal guidance.

guide A device for directing the motion of something.

g., anterior The part of an articulator contacted by the incisal guide pin to maintain the selected separation of the upper and lower members of the articulator. The guide influences the changing relationships of mounted casts in eccentric movements. *See also* guide, incisal.

g., adjustable anterior An anterior guide, the superior surface of which may be varied to provide desired separation of the casts in various eccentric relationships.

g., condylar (condylar guidance) The mechanical device on an articulator; intended to produce guidance in articulator movement similar to that produced by the paths of the condyles in the temporo-mandibular joints.

g., condylar, inclination (condylar guidance inclination) The angle of inclination of the condylar guide mechanism of an articulator in relation to the horizontal plane of the instrument.

g., incisal (anterior guide) The part of an articulator that maintains the incisal guide angle.

g., incisal, adjustment Occlusal adjustment that produces a minimum of overbite (vertical overlap) and a maximum of overjet (horizontal overlap), eliminates fremitus and racking effects on the anterior segment of teeth in the protrusive glide, and attains maximal incisive group function.

g., incisal, angle *See* angle, incisal guide.

g. plane A fixed or removable orthodontic appliance designed to deflect the functional path of the mandible and alter the positions of specific teeth.

gum(s) The fibrous and mucosal covering of the alveolar process or ridges. *See also* gingiva.

g. pads Edentulous segments of the maxillae and mandible that correspond to the underlying primary teeth.

gumma (gŭm′ah) A granulomatous, gummy lesion of tertiary syphilis. The palate and tongue are sites of predilection in the oral region. A similar lesion occurring with tuberculosis is designated a tuberculous gumma.

Gunning's splint *See* splint, Gunning's.

Gunn's syndrome *See* syndrome, Gunn's.

gutta-percha (gŭt″ah-per′chah) The coagulated juice of various tropical trees that has certain rubberlike properties. Used for temporary sealing of dressings in cavities; also used in the form of cones for filling root canals and in the form of sticks for sealing cavities over treatment.

g.-p., baseplate Gutta-percha combined with fillers and coloring materials and rolled into sheets that are used as temporary bases for denture construction.

g.-p. points Fine, tapered cylinders of gutta-percha used, because of their radiopacity, for radiographic ascertainment of pocket depth and topography; used also as a root canal filling material.

g.p., temporary stopping Gutta-percha mixed with zinc oxide and white wax. Used for temporary sealing of dressings in cavities.

gypsum (jĭp′sŭm) The dihydrate of calcium sulfate $(CaSO_4 \cdot 2H_2O)$. Alpha-hemihydrate and beta-hemihydrate are derived from gypsum. *See* plaster of paris.

h II *See* hemophilia B.

habit The tendency toward an act or an act that has become a repeated performance, relatively fixed, consistent, easy to perform, and almost automatic. Once learned, habits may occur without the intent of the person or may appear to be out of control and are difficult to change. In dentistry, habits such as bruxism, clenching, tongue thrusting, and lip and cheek biting may produce injury to the teeth, their attachment apparatus, oral mucosa, mandibular and temporomandibular musculature, and articulation.

habituation A state in which an individual involuntarily tends to continue the use of a drug. Generally refers to the state in which an individual continues self-administration of a drug because of psychologic dependence without physical dependence.

Hageman trait (hahg′măn) *See* factor XII.

half-life The time in which a radioactive substance will lose half of its activity through disintegration.

   h.-l., biologic The time in which a living tissue, organ, or individual eliminates, through biologic processes, half of a given amount of a substance that has been introduced into it.

   h.-l., effective Half-life of a radioactive isotope in a biologic organism, resulting from the combination of radioactive decay and biologic elimination.

$$\text{Effective half-life} = \frac{\text{Biologic half-life} \times \text{Radioactive half-life}}{\text{Biologic half-life} + \text{Radioactive half-life}}$$

   h.-l., physical The average time (t ½) required for the decay of half the atoms in a given amount of a radioactive substance.

half-value layer (HVL) The thickness of a specified material (usually aluminum, copper, or lead) required to decrease the dosage rate of a beam of x rays at a point of interest to half its initial value. A determination of the half-value layer of a given x-ray beam is used to denote the quality of the x-ray beam. The half-value layer will vary depending on kilovolt peak and the amount of filtration at the source.

halisteresis (hah-lĭs″ter-ē′sĭs) A theory of the method of bone resorption according to which bone salts can be removed by a humoral mechanism and returned to the tissue fluids, leaving behind a decalcified bone matrix; osteolysis. This is not considered to be the mechanism under which resorption occurs in periodontal disease.

halitosis (hăl″ĭ-tō′sĭs) **(bad breath, bromopnea, fetor ex ore, offensive breath)** Offensive odor of the breath resulting from local and metabolic conditions (e.g., poor oral hygiene, periodontal disease, sinusitis, tonsillitis, suppurative bronchopulmonary disease, acidosis, uremia).

Haller's plexus *See* plexus, Haller's.

halogen (hăl′ō-jĕn) An element of a closely related group of elements consisting of fluorine, chlorine, bromine, and iodine.

halothane (hăl′ō-thān) A potent nonflammable and non-explosive liquid anesthetic agent administered by inhalation. Common complications associated with other inhalation anesthetic agents are generally absent. Chemical name is 2-bromo-2-chloro-1, 1, 1-trifluoroethane.

hamartoma (hăm″ăr-tō′mah) A localized error in the composition of the tissue elements of an organ. May be automatically manifested in three ways, either singly or in combination: abnormal quantity, abnormal structure, or degree of maturation of the tissue components.

Hamberger's schema *See* schema, Hamberger's.

Hamburger's phenomenon *See* phenomenon, Hamburger's.

hamular notch *See* notch, pterygomaxillary.

hamular process *See* process, hamular.

hand air syringe *See* syringe, hand air.

hand condenser *See* condenser, hand.

hand pressure *See* pressure, hand.

handicap A disability that hinders effective function; may involve any combination of physical, emotional, or social factors.

handpiece An instrument used to hold rotary instruments in the dental engine or condensing points in mechanical condensing units. It is connected by an arm, cable, belt, or tube to the source of power (motor, air, water).

   h., air-turbine A handpiece with a turbine powered by compressed air.

h., contra-angle A binangled instrument for use with the dental engine; permits access to areas difficult or im possible to reach with a straight handpiece.

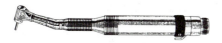

Contra-angle handpiece

h., high-speed A type of rotary or vibratory cutting tool that operates at speeds above 12,000 rpm. It is propelled by gears, a belt, or a turbine. Generally classified as an air turbine, a hydraulic turbine, or a high-speed handpiece on a conventional dental engine.

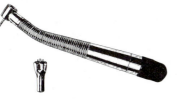

High-speed handpiece

h., high-speed, ultra A handpiece designed to permit rotational speeds of 100,000 to 300,000 rpm.

h., right-angle A monangled instrument used with mechanical condensers to reach some operating areas.

h., straight A handpiece whose axis is in line with the rotary instrument.

h., water-turbine A handpiece with a turbine powered by water under pressure.

Hand-Schüller-Christian disease (hănd-shĭl′er-krĭs′ chan) *See* disease, Hand-Schüller-Christian.

Hansen's disease *See* leprosy.

hard copy Readable output from a computer generated in a storable form such as printed on paper or on microfiche; contrast with soft copy in which the data are displayed on a videoterminal or presented in some other transitory form.

hard of hearing Term applied to persons whose hearing is impaired but who have enough hearing left for practical use.

hardener An ingredient (potassium alum) of the photographic and radiographic fixing solution that serves to harden the gelatin of the film to prevent softening and swelling of the gelatin.

hardening The process of setting or becoming firm.

h., age The precipitation of intermetallic compounds that alters certain physical properties in alloys; usually brought about through heat treatment.

h., precipitation *See* tempering.

h. solution *See* solution, hardening.

h., strain An increase in proportional limit resulting from distortion of the space lattice and fracture of grain boundaries through cold working. Ductility is markedly reduced.

h., work The hardening of a metal by cold work, such as repeated flexing.

hardness (of a substance) The ability of a material to resist an indenting type of load.

h., Mohs Relative scratch resistance of minerals based on an arbitrary scale: 10, diamond; 9, corundum; 8, topaz; 7, quartz; 6, orthoclase; 5, apatite; 4, fluorite; 3, calcite; 2, gypsum; and 1, talc.

h. (of x rays) Term used to indicate in a general way the quality of x radiation, "hardness" being a function of wavelength; the shorter the wavelength, the "harder" the x radiation.

hard palate *See* palate, hard.

hardware The mechanical, magnetic, electronic, and electric devices or components of a computer.

harelip (hăr′lĭp) (cheiloschisis, cleft lip, congenital cleft lip) Congenital nonunion or inadequacy of soft and hard tissues related to the lip. The deformity may be extensive enough to involve the nose, alveolar process, hard palate, and velum. The extent of deformity varies among individuals. Various classifications have been established to identify the extent of a cleft. A rare midline cleft may occur in the lower lip at the embryonal junction of the two mandibular processes.

harmony, occlusal The nondisruptive relationship of an occlusion to all its factors (e.g., the neuromuscular mechanism, temporomandibular joints, teeth and their supporting structures).

h., functional occlusal An occlusal relationship of opposing teeth in all functional ranges and movements that will provide the greatest masticatory efficiency without causing undue strain or trauma on the supporting tissues.

Hatch clamp *See* clamp, gingival, Hatch.

hatchet An angled cutting hand instrument in which the broad side of the blade is parallel with the angle(s) of the shank. Used to develop internal cavity form. May be bibeveled or single beveled like a chisel, in which case the instrument is paired with another.

h., enamel An angled cutting hand instrument in which the broad side of the blade is parallel with the angle(s) of the shank. May be bibeveled or single beveled like a chisel, in which case the instrument is paired with another. Used primarily with a chipping or a lateral scraping stroke to develop internal cavity form.

haversian system *See* osteon.

Hawley appliance, chart, retainer *See* under appropriate noun.

Hawley retainer *See* retainer, Hawley.

hay rake *See* appliance, hay rake.

hazard, radiation The hazard that exists in any area in which a person is subject to radiation.

HDL Abbreviation or acronym for high-density lipoproteins. HDL molecules are considered a protective factor in coronary heart disease.

head, steeple *See* oxycephalia.

headache Pain in the cranial vault resulting from intracranial, extracranial, or psychogenic causes: intracranial vascular dilation; space-occupying lesions; diseases of the eyes, ears, and sinuses; extracranial vascular dilation; sustained muscular contraction; hysteria; certain habit patterns (clenching); and reaction to stress.

h., cluster *See* neuralgia, facial, atypical.

h., lower-half *See* neuralgia, facial, atypical.

h., migraine A vascular type of headache, typically unilateral in the temporal, frontal, and retroorbital area, but may occur midface. It is described as throbbing, burning, pulsating, exploding, or as pressure and may become generalized and persist for hours or days. Onset of pain is usually preceded by prodromal symptoms that may include visual disturbances, scotomas, vomiting, and nausea. A migraine headache is usually considered to be a psychophysiologic (psychosomatic) disorder.

headcap The part of an extraoral orthodontic appliance that engages the back of the head, incorporating the skull as a source of resistance for tooth movement, and gives attachment to the intraoral element of the appliance.

h., plaster A cap, constructed of plaster-of-paris gauze, that embodies points for applying fixation and traction appliances in the treatment of mandibular and maxillofacial injuries.

headdress Protective covering for the patient's head.

headgear The apparatus encircling the head or neck and providing attachment for an intraoral appliance in use of extraoral anchorage.

h., radiologic A device used to protect the head from injury by radiation.

health A bodily state in which all parts are functioning properly. Also refers to the normal functioning of a part of the body. A state of normal functional equilibrium; homeostasis.

health maintenance organization (HMO) A legal entity that accepts responsibility and financial risk for providing specified services to a defined population during a defined period of time at a fixed price. An organized system of health care delivery that provides comprehensive care to enrollees through designated providers. Enrollees are generally assessed a monthly payment for health care services and may be required to remain in the program for a specified amount of time.

h., patient The state of bodily soundness of the patient; the patient's absolute or relative freedom from physical and/or mental disease.

h. professional A person who by education, training, certification and/or licensure is qualified to and is engaged in providing health care.

h. promotion An educational program or effort directed at a targeted population to improve, maintain, and safeguard the health of that segment of society.

hearsay 1: The testimony given by a witness who relates not what is known personally but what others have stated. **2:** Evidence that does not derive its value solely from the credit of the witness, but rests mainly on the veracity and competency of other persons and is admitted in court only in specified cases from necessity.

heart block The condition in which the muscular interconnection between the auricle and ventricle is interrupted so that the auricle and ventricle beat independently of each other.

heart defect A fault in the structural integrity of the heart.

heart disease A disorder in the normal functioning of the heart.

heart failure (hărt′ fāl-yĕr) A sudden, sometimes fatal, cessation of the heart's action.

h. f., acute A rapid and marked impairment of the cardiac output.

h f., backward Congestive heart failure in which the initiating factor is increased venous pressure resulting from ventricular failure to empty the atria.

h. f., congestive A clinical syndrome resulting from chronic cardiac decompensation associated with left-sided and/or right-sided heart failure. Left-sided failure may result from rheumatic mitral valvular disease, aortic valvular disease, systemic hypertension, or arteriosclerotic disease. Manifestations include orthopnea, paroxysmal dyspnea, pulmonary edema, cough, and cardiac asthma. Right-sided failure results most commonly from pulmonary congestion and hypertension associated with left-sided failure but may result from anemia, myocarditis, beriberi, or dysrhythmia. Manifestations include peripheral pitting edema, ascites, cyanosis, oliguria, and hydrothorax.

h. f., forward Heart failure initiated by decreased cardiac output that leads to decreased blood supply to tissues, decreased excretion of salt (Na^+) and salt retention, elevated venous pressure, and edema.

heat The state of a body or of matter that is perceived as opposed to cold and is characterized by elevation of temperature.

h., applied Therapeutic application of wet or dry heat to increase circulation and produce hyperemia, to acellerate dissolution of infection and inflammation, to increase absorption from tissue spaces, relieve pain, relieve muscle spasm and associated pain, and increase metabolism.

h., applied, and cold The most commonly employed physical agents in dental practice; they modify the physiologic processes and have both a systemic and a local effect. The principal effect on the tissues is mediated by the alteration in the circulatory mechanisms. Properly used, heat and cold have a salutary therapeutic result; improperly used, they may produce serious pathologic consequences.

h., applied, contraindications Conditions that preclude the use of heat application: peripheral neuropathy, conditions in which maximum vasodilation and inflammation are already present, acute inflammatory conditions in which more swelling will cause exquisite (acute) pain and pulpitis, septicemia, and malignancies.

h., applied, general physiologic effects The physiologic effects of generally applied wet or dry heat; increase in body temperature, generalized vasodilation, rise in metabolism, decrease in blood pressure, increase in pulse rate and circulation, and increase in depth and rate of respiration.

h., applied, local physiologic effects The physiologic effects of locally applied wet or dry heat to the intraoral and/or extraoral tissues: increase in caliber and number of capillaries, increased absorption resulting from capillary dilation, increased lymph formation and flow, relief of pain, relief of spasm, increase of phagocytes, and a rise in local metabolism.

h. loss, metabolic causes Biologic factors that influence heat loss: redistribution of blood vasodilation and vasoconstriction, variations in blood volume, tendency of fat to insulate the body, and evaporation.

h. loss, physical causes Physical factors that influence heat loss: radiation, convection, and conduction; evaporation from the lungs, skin, and mucous membranes; the raising of inspired air to body temperatures; and the production of urine and feces.

h. production, metabolic causes Chemical factors of the body that cause heat production: specific dynamic action of food, especially protein, that results in a rise of metabolism; a high environmental temperature that, by raising temperatures of the tissues, increases the velocity of reactions and thus increases heat production; and stimulation of the adrenal cortex and thyroid glands by the hormones of the pituitary glands.

h. treatment *See* treatment, heat.

heavy function *See* function, heavy.

hebephrenia (hĕb″ĕ-frē′nē-ah) A form of schizophrenia in which the individual behaves like a child (e.g., giggling, acting silly).

heel effect *See* effect, heel.

Heerfordt's syndrome *See* fever, uveoparotid.

height of contour *See* contour, height of.

helium (hē′lē-ŭm) A colorless, odorless, tasteless gas; one of the inert gaseous elements. Symbol, He; atomic number, 2; atomic weight, 4.003. Used in medicine as a diluent for other gases.

hemangioameloblastoma (hē-măn″jē-ō-ah-mēl″ō-blăstō′mah) A neoplasm in the jaw that has characteristics of ameloblastoma and hemangioma.

hemangioendothelioma (hē-măn″jē-ō-ĕn″dō-thē″lē-ō′mah) A malignant tumor formed by proliferation of endothelium of the capillary vessels.

hemangiofibroma (hē-măn″jē-ō-fī-brō′mah) A benign neoplasm characterized by proliferation of blood channels in a dense mass of fibroblasts.

hemangioma (hē-măn″jē-ō′mah) **1:** A benign neoplasm characterized by blood vascular channels. A cavernous hemangioma consists of large vascular spaces. A capillary hemangioma consists of many small blood vessels. **2:** A benign tumor composed of newly formed blood vessels.

hemangiopericytoma (hē-măn″jē-ō-pĕr″ī-sī-tō′mah) A vascular tumor composed of pericytes.

hemataerometer (hĕm″ăt-ā″er-om′ĕ-ter) A device for determining the pressure of the gases in the blood.

hematemesis (hĕm″ah-tĕm′ĕ-sĭs) Vomiting of blood.

hematocrit (hē-măt′ō-crĭt) **(packed-cell volume) 1:** The percentage of the total blood volume composed of red blood cells (erythrocytes). Normal values are 42% to 45%. **2:** The percentage of the total volume of a blood sample that is taken up by the red blood cells. Normal values: children, 32% to 65%; adult men, 42% to 53%; adult women, 38% to 46%.

hematolotgic disorders Diseases of the blood and blood-forming tissues.

hematology tests Diagnostic tests of the blood and its constituent parts.

hematoma (hē″mah-tō′mah) A mass of blood in the tissue as a result of trauma or other factors that cause the rupture of blood vessels.

hematosis (hĕm″ah-tō′sĭs) Oxygenation or aeration of the venous blood in the lungs.

hematuria (hĕm″ah-tū′rē-ah) Blood in the urine.

h., gross Visible evidence of blood in the urine. It may occur from neoplasms of the kidney and bladder, hemorrhagic diathesis, hypertension with renal epistaxis, or acute glomerular nephritis.

h., microscopic Demonstration of hematuria during the microscopic examination of centrifuged urine. It may result from the same causes as gross hematuria or to toxicity of drugs, embolic glomerulitis, vascular diseases, or chronic glomerular nephritis.

hemianesthesia (hĕm″ē-ăn″ĕs-thē′zē-ah) Anesthesia or loss of tactile sensibility on one side of the body.

hemiatrophy (hĕm″ē-ăt′rō-fē) Atrophy of one half of the body, an organ, or a part (e.g., facial hemiatrophy).

hemiglossectomy (hĕm″ē-glŏ-sĕk′tō-mē) Surgical removal of half of the tongue.

hemihypertrophy (hĕm″ē-hī-per′trō-fē) Excessive growth of half of the body, an organ, or a part (e.g., facial hemihypertrophy).

hemiplegia (hĕm″ē-plē′jē-ah) In medical jurisprudence, paralysis of one side of the body.

hemisection The complete sectioning through the crown of a tooth into the furcation region.

hemocytes A generic term referring to any cellular or formed element of the blood. Synonym: hematocyte.

hemoglobin (hē″mō-glō′bĭn) The oxygen-carrying red pigment of the red blood corpuscles. It is a reddish, crystallizable conjugated protein consisting of the protein globulin combined with the prosthetic group, heme.

h. estimation Determination of the hemoglobin content of the blood. By the Sahli method, 14 to 17 g/100 ml of blood is normal, and 15.1 Sahli units are taken as 100% for estimation of hemoglobin percentages.

hemoglobinopathy (hē″mō-glō″bĭ-nop′ah-thē) Any one of a group of genetically determined diseases involving abnormal hemoglobin (e.g., sickle cell disease, in which hemoglobin S occurs, and hemoglobin C disease).

h., paroxysmal nocturnal An acquired hemolytic anemia of unknown cause characterized by increased hemolysis during sleep, resulting in the presence of hemoglobin in the urine on awakening.

hemolysin (hē-mol′ĭ-sĭn) An antibody that causes hemolysis of red blood cells in vitro.

hemophilia (hē″mō-fĭl′ē-ah) **(bleeder's disease)** A sex-linked genetic disease manifested in males and characterized by severe hemorrhage.

h. A (classic hemophilia) A hemorrhagic diathesis resulting from a deficiency of antihemophilic globulin (AHG); inherited as a recessive sex-linked characteristic and characterized by recurrent bouts of bleeding from even trivial injury. The coagulation time is prolonged, but the bleeding time is normal.

h. B (Christmas disease, hemophilia II, hemophilioid state C) A hemorrhagic diathesis resulting from a deficiency of plasma thromboplastin component (FTC); transmitted as a sex-linked recessive characteristic and characterized clinically by the same manifestations as classic hemophilia. There is a delay in the generation of thromboplastin. The platelet count, bleeding time, tourniquet test, and thrombin and prothrombin times are normal.

h. C (plasma thromboplastin antecedent [PTA] deficiency, Rosenthal's syndrome) A hemophilia-like condition believed to result from a deficiency of plasma thromboplastin antecedent (PTA), transmitted as a simple autosomal dominant trait, and characterized by a moderate bleeding tendency after extraction of teeth or after tonsillectomy. Prothrombin consumption and thromboplastin generation are abnormal. *See also* factor XI.

h., classic *See* hemophilia A.

h., vascular A hereditary hemorrhagic disorder affecting both sexes and associated with a deficiency of antihemophilic globulin and vascular abnormalities characteristic of pseudohemophilia (von Willebrand's disease). The bleeding time is prolonged, and severity of bleeding varies considerably from one person to another.

hemophilioid state A (hē″mō-fĭl′ē-oid) *See* parahemophilia.

hemophilioid state C *See* hemophilia B.

hemoptysis (hē-mop′tĭ-sĭs) Expectoration of blood, by coughing, from the larynx or lower respiratory tract.

hemorrhage (hĕm′or-ĭj) Escape of blood from the blood vessels; bleeding.

hemorrhagic bone cyst *See* cyst, hemorrhagic.

hemosiderin (hē″mō-sĭd′er-ĭn) A dark yellow-brown pigment that contains iron.

hemostasis (hē″mō-stā′sĭs) The arrest of an escape of blood.

hemostatic (hē″mō-stăt-ĭk) An agent used to reduce bleeding from minute vessels by hastening the clotting of blood or by the formation of an artificial clot.

Henderson's test *See* test, Henderson's.

heparin Heparinic acid, an anticoagulant factor that acts with a serum protein cofactor as an antithrombin and antiprothrombin agent preventing platelet agglutination and hence clot formation.

heparinized lock system An in-dwelling intravenous system developed by which multiple daily intravenous accesses can be accomplished and multiple penetrations of the veins can be avoided. The heparin chamber prevents the formation of a clot or thrombus at the needle site.

hepatitis (hĕp″ah-tī′tĭs) Inflammation of the liver.

h., homologous serum (homologous serum jaundice, serum hepatitis, syringe jaundice, type B hepatitis) A viral hepatitis clinically difficult to distinguish from epidemic infectious hepatitis. It is transmitted by human serum (parenteral injection, transfusions, lacerations). The incubation period is 40 to 90 days or longer. Principal manifestations are jaundice, gastrointestinal symptoms, anorexia, and malaise.

h., infectious (IH, type A hepatitis) A viral hepatitis that is frequently epidemic in nature and has an incubation period of 1 to 4 or even 7 weeks. It is usually transmitted by the virus in fecal matter but may be transmitted by human serum (transfusions, lacerations, needle punctures).

h., serum *See* hepatitis, homologous serum.

Herbst appliance The only fixed, tooth-borne, functional orthodontic appliance in which jaw position is influenced by a pin and tube spring loaded appliance that is cemented or bonded to the teeth.

hereditary benign intraepithelial dyskeratosis A hereditary disease seen in triracial isolates (whites, Indians, blacks). It involves the oral mucosa and periodic seasonal keratoconjunctivitis.

hereditary opalescent dentin A developmental disturbance in the formation of dentin, better known as dentiogenesis imperfecta. The teeth range from gray to brownish violet and are translucent or opalescent. The crowns fracture easily because of an abnormal dentinoenamel junction.

heredity (hĕ-rĕd´ĭ-tē) The inheritance of resemblance, physical qualities, or disease from a familial predecessor; the passage of characteristics from one generation to its progeny by genetic linkage.

Hering-Breuer reflex (hĕr´ĭng-broi´er) *See* reflex, Hering-Breuer.

hermetic seal *See* seal, hermetic.

heroin A highly addictive alkaloid prepared from morphine, previously used for the relief of cough. Its use is prohibited by federal law because of its highly addictive properties and potential for abuse.

herpangina (her˝păn-jī´-nah) **(Coxsackie A disease)** A viral disease of children occurring usually in summer and characterized by sudden onset, fever (100° to 105° F; 38° to 40.5° C), sore throat, and oropharyngeal vesicles. It results from Coxsackie A viruses and is self-limiting.

herpes labialis (her´pēz lā˝bē-ăl´ĭs) **(cold sore)** A disease of the lips caused by herpesvirus and characterized by vesicles that rupture, leaving ulcers. The local lesions are often called *fever blisters* or *cold sores*. Herpes simplex of the lips.

herpes simplex (hĕr´pēz sĭm´plĕx) Infection caused by the herpes simplex virus. Primary infection, occurring most often in children between 2 and 5 years of age, may result in apparent clinical disease or such manifestations as acute herpetic gingivostomatitis, keratoconjunctivitis, vulvovaginitis, or encephalitis. Recurrent manifestations include herpes labialis (fever blisters or cold sores), dendritic corneal ulcers, or genital herpes simplex.

herpes zoster (hĕr´pēz zahs´tĕr) **(acute posterior ganglionitis, shingles)** An acute viral disease involving the dorsal spinal root or cranial nerve and producing vesicular eruption in areas of the skin corresponding to the involved sensory nerve. Pain is a prominent feature and may persist, although skin lesions subside in 1 to 2 weeks.

herpetic lesion *See* lesion, herpetic.

herpetic ulcer *See* ulcer, herpetic.

heteresthesia (hĕt˝er-ĕs-thē´zē-ah) Variation in the degree of cutaneous sensibility on adjoining areas of the body surface.

heterograft *See* graft, heterogenous.

heterosexual A person with a sexual orientation towards persons of the opposite gender; having erotic attraction to, predisposition to, or sexual activity, with a person of the opposite gender.

heterozygous (hĕt˝er-ō-zī´gŭs) Term indicating that genes lying at equivalent loci on chromosome pairs are different.

HGF *See* glucagon.

HIAA Health Insurance Association of America.

hiccup An involuntary spasmodic contraction of the diaphragm that causes a beginning inspiration that is suddenly checked by closure of the glottis, thus producing a characteristic sound.

hidrosis (hī-drō´sĭs) The secretion of sweat.

high labial arch *See* arch, high labial.

high lip line *See* lip line, high.

high pressuring The forcing of extensive dental treatment on a patient who is not completely convinced of its necessity.

high speed *See* speed, high.

high-pull headgear Apparatus designed to give an upward pull on the face-bow.

high-speed handpiece *See* handpiece, high-speed.

hinchazon (hĭnch˝ah-zon´) *See* beriberi.

hinge axis *See* axis, hinge.

hinge axis determination *See* axis, condylar, determination.

hinge axis–orbital plane *See* axis, hinge, orbital plane.

hinge axis point *See* point, hinge axis.

hinge movement *See* movement, hinge.

hinge position *See* position, hinge.

hinge-bow The kinematic face-bow used to determine the location of the hinge axis. It is a three-piece instrument with independently adjustable arms controlled by micrometer screws that lengthen or shorten them. Other micrometer screws raise or lower the caliper points to find the spots in or on the skin near the tragi where only rotary movements occur when the jaw is opened and closed at the rearmost point. *See also* face-bow, kinematic.

Hinton's test *See* test, Hinton's.

hippus, respiratory (hĭp´ŭs) Dilation of the pupils occurring during inspiration and contraction of the pupils occuring during expiration; often associated with pulsus paradoxus.

Hirschfeld-Dunlop file *See* file, Hirschfeld-Dunlop.

Hirschfeld's method *See* point, Hirschfeld's silver.

histidine One of the essential amino acids for infants and children; *see also* amino acid.

hirsutism (her'sūt-ĭzm) Increased body or facial hair, which is especially noted in the female.

histiocyte (hĭs'tē-ō-sīt'') A large phagocytic cell found in the interstices of the tissues; of reticuloendothelial origin.

histiocytosis, nonlipid (hĭs''tē-ō-sī-tō'sĭs) *See* disease, Letterer-Siwe.

> **h., acute disseminated, X** *See* disease, LettererSiwe)

> **h., chronic disseminated X** *See* disease, Hand-Schüller-Christian.

> **h., X** A group of diseases characterized by abnormal histiocyte activity. Includes a chronic disseminated type (Hand-Schüller-Christian disease) and a chronic localized type (eosinophilic granuloma).

histoclasia, implant (hĭs''tō-klā'zē-ah) A condition of the tissues existing in the presence of an implant in which the implant is not directly involved. It is a condition of the oral mucosal tissues in which the pathology results from some external cause (e.g., salivary calculus, attached prosthetic appliances).

histogram A bar graph; a graphic representation of a frequency distribution.

histology Microanatomy, the microscopic study of normal tissue and organs at the cellular level.

histopathology The microscopic study of abnormal tissue and organs at the cellular level

histoplasmosis (hĭs''tō-plăz-mō'sĭs) A disease caused by the fungus *Histoplasma capsulatum* and affecting the reticuloendothelial system. Ulceration of the oral mucosa may occur.

history, case A detailed and concise compilation of all physical, dental, social, and mental factors relative and necessary to diagnosis, prognosis, and treatment.

histotoxic (hĭs-tō-tahk'sĭk) Relating to poisoning of the respiratory enzyme system of the tissues.

HIV gingivitis (HIV-G) A distinct type of gingivitis found in HIV infected patients, characterized by an intensely red linear erythemic band around the free gingiva that extends 2 to 3 mm apically into the attached gingiva. The involved gingiva tends to bleed spontaneously and may be present even in AIDS patients with good plaque control.

HIV periodontitis (HIV-P) An aggressive form of periodontal disease with all of the characteristics of HIV-G combined with soft tissue ulceration and necrosis and rapid destruction of the periodontum and bone. The condition is very painful. HIV-P may resemble acute necrotizing ulcerative gingivitis (ANUG). However ANUG is limited to the soft tissue, whereas HIV-P disease extends into the crestal bone.

HIV-G *See* HIV gingivitis.

HIV-P *See* HIV periodontitis.

HIV-wasting syndrome A constitutional disease associated with AIDS also known as the slim disease. This subgroup of patients present with history of fever of more than one month, involuntary weight loss of more than 10%, nd/or diarrhea persisting for more than 1 month.

hives *See* urticaria.

Hodgkin's disease *See* disease, Hodgkin's.

hoe An angled instrument with the broad dimension of its blade perpendicular to the axis of the shank of the shaft.

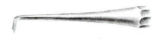

Monangle hoe

hold To possess by reason of a lawful title.

hold harmless clause A contract provision in which one party to the contract promises to be responsible for liability incurred by the other party. Hold harmless clauses frequently appear in the following contexts: 1) Contracts between dental benefits organizations and an individual dentist often contain a promise by the dentist to reimburse the dental benefits organization for any liability the organization incurs because of dental treatment provided to beneficiaries of the organization's dental benefits plan. This may include a promise to pay the dental benefits organization's attorney fees and related costs, and 2) contracts between dental benefits organizations and a group plan sponsor may include a promise by the dental benefits organization to assume responsibility for disputes between a beneficiary of the group plan and an individual dentist when the dentist's charge exceeds the amount the organization pays for the service on behalf of the beneficiary. If the dentist takes action against the patient to recover the difference between the amount billed by the dentist and the amount paid by the organization, the dental benefits organization will take over the defense of the claim and will pay any judgments and court costs.

holder An apparatus or instrument that is used to hold something.

> **h., broach** *See* broach holder.

> **h., clamp** *See* holder, rubber dam clamp.

> **h., matrix** *See* retainer, matrix.

> **h., rubber dam** An apparatus used to hold a rubber dam in place on the face and to secure the edges of the dam clear of the field of operation.

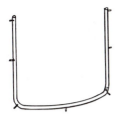

Young rubber dam holder (frame)

h., rubber dam clamp (clamp holder) *See* forceps, rubber dam clamp.

Rubber dam clamp holder

Hollenback condenser *See* condenser, pneumatic.

hollow bulb That portion of a prosthesis made hollow to minimize weight.

home care The physiotherapeutic measures employed by the patient for the maintenance of dental and periodontal health. Includes proper cleaning with a toothbrush, floss, or other device.

homeostasis (hō″mē-ō-stā′sĭs) Term used to describe the tendency toward physiologic equilibration (e.g., acid-base balance, pH level of blood, blood sugar level).

h., cell The tendency of biologic tissues and processes to maintain a constancy of environment consistent with their vitality and well being. For cells to maintain their stability or equilibrium, the cell membranes must be in continuous interaction with both the internal (intracellular) environment and the external (extracellular) environment. When the equilibrium of any component is disturbed, the interaction permits automatic readjustment by giving rise to stimuli that result in restoration of the equilibrium.

homograft *See* graft, homogenous.

homosexual A person with a sexual orientation towards persons of the same gender, having erotic attraction to, predisposition to, or sexual activity, with a person of the same gender.

homozygous (hō-mō-zī′gŭs) Term indicating that genes lying at equivalent loci on chromosome pairs are the same.

hook, skin A metallic instrument ending in a fine, sharp hook for handling soft tissues during surgery.

Hoover's sign *See* sign, Hoover's.

HOP Abbreviation for high oxygen pressure.

horizontal overlap *See* overlap, horizontal.

horizontal plane *See* plane, horizontal.

hormone(s) (hōr′mōn) Biochemical secretions of the endocrine glands that, in relatively small quantities, partially regulate the physiologic activity of the tissues, organs, organ systems, and other endocrine glands, and of the nervous system itself. The hormonal secretions are conducted and distributed throughout the body by the circulation of the bloodstream and tissue fluids.

h., adenohypophyseal Hormones secreted by the adenohypophysis. Includes seven distinct hormones: somatotropin (STH), thyrotropin (TSH), prolactin, follicle-stimulating hormone (FSH), luteinizing hormone (LH), melanocyte-stimulating hormone (MSH), and adrenocorticotropic hormone (ACTH).

h., adrenal medullary Hormones secreted by adrenal medulla, including two catecholamines: epinephrine and norepinephrine.

h., adrenocortical Steroid hormones secreted by the adrenal cortex that are biologically active in one or more of the following states: stress, inflammation, metabolism of carbohydrates, proteins, electrolytes, and water.

h., adrenocorticotropic *See* ACTH.

h., adrenotropic *See* ACTH.

h., androgenic *See* hormones, sex, male.

h., anterior pituitary-like *See* hormone, pregnancy.

h., antidiabetic *See* insulin.

h., antidiuretic (ADH, vasopressin) A hormone of the posterior pituitary gland that encourages resorption of water by acting on the epithelial cells of the distal portion of the renal tubule. The pressor-antidiuretic principle of the neurohypophysis. It raises blood pressure by its effect on the peripheral blood vessels and exerts an antidiuretic effect (antifacultative resorption of water in the renal tubules). An absence of ADH causes diabetes insipidus.

h., antiinflammatory *See* glucocorticoids.

h., corticosteroid *See* steroid, adrenocortical.

h., corticotropic Any one of the ovarian or adrenal hormones (e.g., estradiol, estrone, estriol) that is capable of stimulating changes of a cyclic nature in the genital system. One of the ovarian or adrenal hormones capable of affecting the cyclic changes of the female genital system. *See* ACTh.

h., follicle-stimulating A pituitary tropic hormone that promotes the growth and maturation of the ovarian follicle and, with other gonadotropins, induces secretion of estrogens, and possibly spermatogenesis.

h., gastrointestinal Hormones that regulate motor and secretory activity of the digestive organs, i.e., gastrin, secretin, and cholecystokinin.

h., gonadotropic *See* gonadotropin.

> **h., chorionic gonadotropic** A glycoprotein secreted by placental tissue early in normal pregnancy but also found in the urine or blood in association with chorioepitheliomas and some neoplastic diseases of the testes.

h., growth (somatotropic hormone, somatotropin) A growth, or somatotropic, hormone that is secreted by the anterior lobe of the pituitary gland and that exerts an influence on skeletal growth. As long as the growth apparatus is functional, it is responsive to the effects of the hormone.

h., ketogenic Term used to describe a factor of the anterior pituitary hormone responsible for ketogenic effect. It is probably not an entity differing from known pituitary hormones.

h., lactogenic (galactin, mammotropin, prolactin) A pituitary hormone that stimulates lactation.

h., luteal *See* hormones, progestational.

h., luteinizing A pituitary hormone that causes ovulation and development of the corpus luteum from the mature graafian follicle. It is called an *interstitial cell–stimulating hormone* because of its action on the testis in maintaining spermatogenesis and because of its role in the development of accessory sex organs.

h., melanocyte-stimulating (intermedin, MSH) A hormone of the middle lobe of the pituitary gland that increases melanin deposition by the melanocytes of the skin.

h., N *See* hormone, nitrogen; steroid, C-19 cortico-.

h., neurohypophyseal Octapeptides of the neural lobe: oxytocin and vasopressin.

h., nitrogen (N hormone) C-19 corticosteroids that have androgenic and protein anabolic effects.

h., parathyroid The secretory product of the parathyroid glands that promotes bone resorption and increases renal resorption of calcium and magnesium and diminishes that of phosphate. Excessive secretion of the parathyroid hormone produces generalized bone resorption, formation of fibrous marrow in the spongiosa, and, in young individuals, hypocalcification of the teeth.

h., pituitary Hormones of the anterior lobe of the pituitary gland, including the growth hormones (somatotropin 1; lactogenic hormone, prolactin, galactin, mammotropin) and pituitary tropins (gonadotropins, thyrotropic hormone, and ACTH). Whether or not a true diabetogenic pituitary hormone exists is a question. The melanocyte-stimulating hormone is secreted by the middle lobe of the pituitary gland, and vasopressin and oxytocin are secreted by the posterior lobe of the pituitary gland.

h., pregnancy (anterior pituitary-like hormone, antuitrin S, chorionic gonadotropin) A gonadotropic hormone found in the urine during pregnancy; it is a product of the very early placenta.

h., progestational (luteal hormone) Hormones produced during the phase of the menstrual cycle just preceding menstruation. Includes progesterone, pregnanediol, and pregneninolone.

h., proinflammatory *See* mineralocorticoids.

h., "S" (glucocorticoid factor, sugar hormone) A factor in the secretions of the adrenal cortex related to the regulation of carbohydrate metabolism.

h., sex Steroid hormones that are produced by the testes and ovaries and that control secondary sex characteristics, the reproductive cycle, development of the accessory reproductive cycle, and development of the accessory reproductive organs. Also included are the gonadotropins produced by the pituitary gland.

> **h., female sex** Hormones secreted by the ovary. They include two main types: the follicular, or estrogenic, hormones produced by the graafian follicle, and the progestational hormones from the corpus luteum.

> **h., male sex (androgenic hormone, C-19 steroids)** Hormones found in the testes, urine, or blood. Included are testosterone found in the testes, andosterone excreted into the urine, and dehydro-3-epiandrosterone found in the blood.

h., somatotropic *See* hormone, growth.

h., steroid A group of biologically active organic compounds that are secreted by the adrenal cortex, testes, ovary, and placenta, and that have in common a cyclopentanoperhydrophenanthrene nucleus.

h., sugar *See* hormone, "S"; steroid, C-21 cortico-.

h., testicular Hormones elaborated by the testes (chiefly testosterone) that promote the growth and function of the male genitalia and secondary sex characteristics and that have potent protein anabolic effects.

h., thyroid Hormonal variants, including thyroxin and triiodothyronine, derived from the thyroid gland. Thyroid hormone acts as a catalyst for oxidative processes of the body cell and thus regulates the rates of body metabolism and stimulates body growth and maturation.

h., thyroid-stimulating *See* hormone, thyrotropic.

h., thyrotropic (thyroid-stimulating hormone, TSH) A pituitary hormone that regulates the growth and activity of the thyroid gland.

horn, pulp A small projection of vital pulp tissue directly under a cusp or developmental lobe.

hospital An institution for the care of sick, wounded, infirm, or aged persons; generally incorporated as a nonprofit organization.

host site An anatomic area surgically prepared to receive an implant or graft.

Howard's method *See* method, Howard's.

Howe's silver nitrate *See* silver nitrate, ammoniacal.

Howe's silver precipitation method *See* method, Howe's silver precipitation.

h.s. Abbreviation for *hora somni,* a Latin phrase meaning "at bedtime."

humectant (hū-mĕk′tănt) A substance that prevents loss of moisture.

Hunter's glossitis *See* glossitis, Moeller's.

Hunt's syndrome *See* syndrome, Hunt's.

hurt To molest or restrain; not restricted to physical injuries; also includes mental pain, discomfort, or annoyance.

husband A man who has a wife.

Hutchinson-Gilford syndrome *See* syndrome, Hutchinson-Gilford.

Hutchinson triad *See* triad, Hutchinson.

Hutchinson's incisors *See* incisors, Hutchinson's.

HVL *See* half-value layer.

hyalinization (hī″ah-lĭn″ĭ-zā′shŭn) The appearance of an acellular, avascular, homogeneous area in the periodontal ligament in which compression of the ligament between bone and tooth occurs as a result of orthodontic forces.

    h. of periodontal ligament A degenerative process resulting from long-continued occlusal trauma in which the fibers become hyalinized into a homogeneous mass.

hyaluronic acid A mucopolysaccharide that forms the gelatinous substance in the tissue spaces. It is the intercellular cementing substance found throughout the tissues of the body.

hyaluronidase (hī″ah-lū-rŏn′ĭ-dās) An enzyme that produces hydrolysis of hyaluronic acid, the cementing substance of the tissues. Produced by certain pathogenic bacteria and also formed by sperm.

hydraulic pressure *See* pressure, hydraulic.

hydraulicity (hī″draw-lĭ′sĭ-tē) The ability of a material (cement) to set while in contact with moisture.

hydremia (hī″drē′mē-ah) Increase in blood volume caused by an increase in serum volume. This may result from cardiac failure, renal insufficiency, pregnancy, or the intravenous administration of fluids.

hydroalcoholic (hī″drō-ăl-kō-hol′ĭk) Containing both water and alcohol. *See also* solution.

Hydrocal (hī′drō-kăl) Trade name for a gypsum product, alpha-hemihydrate, known as artificial stone. It is used for making casts.

hydrocephalus (hī″drō-sĕf′ah-lŭs) Abnormal accumulation of fluid in the cranial vault, resulting in a disproportionately large cranium.

hydrocodone A semisynthetic narcotic analgesic and antitussive with multiple actions similar to those of codeine. It is an ingredient in prescription analgesics and cough medicines.

hydrocolloid (hī″drō-kol′oid) **1:** The materials listed as colloid solids with water; used in dentistry as elastic impression materials. Hydrocolloids can be reversible or irreversible. **2:** An agar-base impression material.

    h., irreversible (alginate) A hydrocolloid whose physical condition is changed by a chemical action that is not reversible. It is an impression material that is elastic when set. *See also* alginate.

    h., reversible (agar-agar type) A hydrocolloid whose physical condition is changed by temperature. The material is made fluid by heat and becomes an elastic solid on cooling.

hydrocortisone (hī″drō-kor′tĕ-sōn) **(cortisol)** A glucocorticosteroid secreted by the adrenal cortex in response to stimulation by ACTH. It is antianabolic, stimulates gluconeogenesis, and probably acts on some cellular system in response to a need for adaptation to change (stress).

hydrogen peroxide An unstable compound of hydrogen and oxygen that is easily broken down into water and oxygen. A 3% solution is used as a mild antiseptic for the skin and mucous membranes, more concentrated solutions may be used as a bleach.

hydrolysis (hī-drol′ĭ-sĭs) **1:** Reaction between the ions of salt and those of water to form an acid and a base, one or both of which is only slightly dissociated. A process whereby a large molecule is split by the addition of water. The end products divide the water, the hydroxyl group being attached to one and the hydrogen ion to the other. **2:** The splitting of a compound into two parts with the addition of the elements of water.

hydrophilic (hī″drō-fĭl′ĭk) Having an affinity for water. Opposite of lipophilic. *See also* ointment, hydrophilic.

hydroquinone (hī-drō-kwĭn′ōn) **1:** A reducing agent used as an inhibitor in resin monomers to prevent polymerization during storage. **2:** One of the two chemicals used as reducing agents in film-developing solutions. It is made from benzene (paradihydroxybenzene) and is sensitive to thermal changes. Above 70° F (21° C) its action is rapid; below 60° F (15.5° C) it becomes inactive. Its action is to control the contrast of the film.

hydrostatic pressure (hī″drō-stăt′ĭk) *See* pressure, hydrostatic.

hydrotherapy (hī″drō-thĕr′ah-pē) An empirical adjunct to oral physiotherapy where forced water irrigation is used to cleanse subgingival spaces, remove debris from interproximal spaces, and cleanse pockets.

hydroxyapatite (hī-drok″sē-ăp′ah-tīt) A mineral compound of the general formula $3Ca_3(PO_4)_2 \cdot Ca(OH)_2$, which is the principal inorganic component of bone, teeth, and dental calculus.

hygiene (hī′jēn) The science of health and its preservation.

h., oral (mouth hygiene) The practice of personal maintenance of oral cleanliness.

h., radiation The art and science of protecting human beings from injury by radiation. Since any amount of radiation is potentially harmful, the ideal objective is to prevent the exposure of any person without a definite medical purpose.

hygienist, dental A person trained in an accredited school and licensed by the state where residing to provide health services, such as scaling and polishing teeth, health education and training, radiography, etc., under the direction of a licensed dentist.

hygroma (hī-grō′mah) A sac or cyst swollen with fluid.

h. colli cysticum (cystic hygroma, cystic lymphangioma) A cavernous lymphangioma involving the neck. It may be of large size, impairing breathing and swallowing.

hygroscopic (hī″grō-skop′ĭk) Having the property of absorbing moisture. When applied to gypsum products in contact with free water during their set, the resultant expansion is implied. *See also* expansion, hygroscopic.

h. investment *See* investment, hygroscopic.

hypacusis (hī″pah-kū′sĭs) A hearing disorder associated with diminished hearing function.

hypalgesia (hī″păl jē′zē-ah) Diminished sensitivity to pain that results from a raised pain threshold.

hyper- (hī′per) A prefix signifying above, beyond, or excessive.

hyperadrenocorticism (hī″pĕr-ah-drē″nō-kŏr′tĭ-sĭzm) Adrenocortical hyperfunction resulting from neoplasia of the cortex or hyperplasia of the cortex secondary to an increase in ACTH. Manifestations include hyperglycemia, edema, hypertension, glycosuria, negative nitrogen balance, acne, and hirsutism. *See also* syndrome, adrenogenital; syndrome, Cushing's.

hyperalgesia (hī″per-ăl-jē′zē-ah) A greater-than-normal sensitivity to pain that may result from a painful stimulus or a lowered pain threshold.

hyperalgia (hī-per-ăl′jē-ah) Abnormal sensitivity to pain.

hypercalcemia (hī″per-kăl-sē′mē-ah) **(hypercalcinemia)** **1:** Elevated blood calcium level. **2:** Abnormal elevation of calcium in the blood. Causes include primary hyperparathyroidism, sarcoidosis, multiple myeloma, malignant neoplasms, prolonged androgen therapy, massive doses of vitamin D, etc. Symptoms suggestive of hypercalcemia are nausea, vomiting, constipa-

tion, polyuria, weight loss, muscular weakness, and polydipsia. The normal level of total serum calcium is 8.5 to 10.5 mg/100 ml.

hypercalcinemia *See* hypercalcemia.

hypercalcinuria *See* hypercalciuria.

hypercalciuria (hī″per-kăl″sē-ū′rē-ah) **(hypercalcinuria)** A condition in which there is an excessive increase in urinary calcium excretion. Major causes include primary hyperparathyroidism, hypervitaminosis D, excessive milk intake, metastatic malignancy, immobilization, and renal tubular acidosis. *See also* hypercalcemia for normal values.

hypercapnia (hī″per-kăp′nē-ah) Presence of more than the normal amount of carbon dioxide in the blood tissues resulting from an increase of carbon dioxide in the inspired air or a decrease in elimination.

hypercementosis (hī″per-sē″mĕn-tō′sĭs) Excessive formation of cementum on the roots of one or more teeth.

hypercenesthesia (hī″per-sĕn″ĕs-thē′zē-ah) A feeling of exaggerated well-being such as is seen in general paralysis and sometimes in mania.

hyperchloremia (hī″per-klō-rē′mē-ah) Excessive concentration of chloride in the plasma. Normal range is 98 to 100 mEq/L. It may occur in water depletion, dehydration, decreased bicarbonate concentration, or metabolic acidosis.

hyperemia (hī″per-ē′mē-ah) **(congestion)** An increased and excessive amount of blood in a tissue. The hyperemia may be active or passive.

h., active Hyperemia caused by an increased flow of blood to an area by active dilation of both the arterioles and capillaries. It is associated with neurogenic, hormonal, and metabolic function.

h., passive Hyperemia caused by a decreased outflow of blood from an area. It may be generalized, resulting from cardiac, renal, or pulmonary disorders, or it may be localized, as in the oral cavity, and caused by pressure from mechanical or physical obstruction or by pressure from a tumor, denture, filling, or salivary calculus.

hyperesthesia (hī″per-ĕs-thē′zē-ah) Excessive sensitivity of the skin or of a special sense.

hyperesthetic (hī″per-ĕs-thĕt′ĭk) Pertaining to or affected with hyperesthesia.

hyperfunction Increase in activity of a part or in the stresses applied to a part.

hypergammaglobulinemia (hī″per-găm″ah-glob″ū-līnē′mē-ah) An excess of gamma globulin in the blood. It occurs in chronic granulomatous inflammations, chronic bacterial infections, liver disease, multiple myeloma, lymphomas, and dysproteinemias.

hyperglobulinemia (hī″per-glob″ū-lĭn-ē′mē-ah) Abnormally high concentration of globulins in the blood.

hyperglycemia (hī″per-glī-se′me-ah) Increase in the concentration of sugar in the blood. It is a feature of diabetes mellitus.

hypergonadism (hī″per-gō′năd-ĭzm) Excessive secretion of hormonal agents by the testes or ovaries. Gingival changes induced by the administration of estrogens and androgens include an increase in keratinization and hyperplasia of epithelial and connective tissue.

hyperhidrosis (hī″per-hī-drō′sĭs) Excessive sweating, which may be generalized or localized.

h., gustatory Increased sweating in the preauricular region, forehead, or face associated with eating. *See also* syndrome auriculotemporal.

h., masticatory Excessive sweating associated with chewing. The cause is traumatic injury producing anastomosis of the facial nerve with a sympathetic branch.

hyperkalemia (hī″per-kah-lē′mē-ah) Abnormally elevated concentration of serum potassium. It may occur in renal failure, shock, and advanced dehydration, and in association with high intracellular potassium in Addison's disease. Normal adult range of serum potassium is 4.0 to 5.5 mEq/L.

hyperkeratosis (hī″per-ker″ah-tō′sĭs) Excessive formation of keratin (e.g., in leukoplakia).

hypermagnesemia (hī″per-măg″nĕ-sē′mē-ah) Excess of magnesium in the blood serum. Normal range is 1.5 to 2.5 mEq/L. It may result in respiratory failure and coma and may occur in untreated diabetic acidosis, renal failure, and severe dehydration.

hypernasality (hī″per-nāz-ăl′ĭ-tē) Excessive nasal resonance usually accompanied by emission of air through the nasal passageways.

hypernatremia (hī″per-nā-trē′mē-ah) Abnormally elevated concentration of serum sodium. It may occur rarely in nephrosis, congestive heart failure, and Cushing's disease and after administration of ACTH, cortisone, or deoxycorticosterone. Normal adult range of serum sodium is 135 to 145 mEq/L.

hyperocclusion (traumatic) Premature tooth contact during mouth closure.

hyperostosis (hī″per-os-tō′sĭs) **1:** Excessive growth of bone, as in infantile cortical hyperostosis. **2:** Hypertrophy of bone. *See also* exostosis.

h., infantile cortical (Caffey's disease, Smyth's syndrome) A disease of infants of unknown etiology and characterized by tender soft tissue swelling that is followed by hyperostosis of the cortex of the underlying bone. The mandible, clavicle, and ulna are most frequently affected.

hyperoxia (hī″per-ok′sē-ah) An excess of oxygen in the system.

hyperparathyroidism (hī″per-păr″ah-thī′roid-ĭzm) **(generalized osteitis fibrosa cystica, von Recklinghausen's disease of bone) 1:** Increased parathyroid function resulting from primary hyperplasia, a functioning neo-

plasm of the parathyroid glands, or secondary hyperplasia related most often to chronic renal insufficiency. Manifestations are related to abnormalities of the bones, kidneys, and blood vessels. Skeletal changes are referred to as generalized osteitis fibrosa cystica or von Recklinghausen's disease. Brown tumors, which are essentially giant cell tumors, may develop generally, as well as in the jaws. Kidney changes include renal stones and nephrocalcinosis. Calcification of muscles in arteries occurs. Renal rickets is associated with secondary hyperparathyroidism in children with chronic renal disease. Laboratory findings include high serum calcium, low phosphorus, and a normal or high alkaline phosphatase. Renal impairment, such as occurs in secondary hyperparathyroidism, tends to nullify hypercalcemia because of an increased loss of calcium in the urine. **2:** Abnormally increased activity of the parathyroid glands causing loss of calcium from the bones and resulting in tenderness in bones, spontaneous fractures, muscular weakness, and osteitis fibrosa. **3:** Excessive production of parathormone by the parathyroid gland (as in parathyroid hyperplasia and/or adenoma), resulting in increased renal excretion of phosphorus by lowering of the renal threshold for this substance. The pathologic changes produced are osteoporotic or osteodystrophic in nature as a consequence of withdrawal of calcium and phosphorus from osseous tissues.

h., brown node of *See* node, brown, of hyperparathyroidism.

hyperphosphatemia (hī″per-fos″fah-tē′mē-ah) Increased concentration of inorganic phosphates in the blood serum. May occur in childhood and also in acromegaly, renal failure, and vitamin D intoxication. Normal adult range of serum inorganic phosphorus is 2.5 to 4.2 mg/ 100 ml.

hyperphosphaturia (hī″per-fos″fah-tū′rē-ah) Excessive excretion of phosphate in the urine.

hyperpituitarism (hī″per-pĭ-tū′ĭ-tăr-ĭzm″) A condition caused by excessive production of the hormones secreted by the pituitary gland. An excess of the growth hormone results in giantism or acromegaly; an excess of ACTH produces Cushing's syndrome.

hyperplasia (hī″per-plā′zē-ah) Abnormal multiplication or increase in the number of normal cells in normal arrangement is a tissue, resulting in a thickening or enlargement of the tissue.

h., denture (denture hypertrophy) Enlargement of tissue beneath a denture that is traumatizing the soft tissue.

h., gingival 1: Enlargement of the gingival tissue resulting from proliferation of its cellular elements. Hereditary or inflammatory etiology may be involved. **2:** Proliferation of gingival epithelium to form elongated rete pegs and proliferation of fibroblasts with increased collagen formation in the underlying connective tissue; leads to nodular enlargement of the gingiva in diphenylhydantoin sodium therapy. **3:** Gingival enlargement, primarily produced by proliferation of connective tissue elements; often accompanied by gingival inflammation as a result of trauma to the hyperplastic tissues and coincidental with or following the ingestion of diphenylhydantoin sodium.

h., Dilantin gingival (dī-lăn′tĭn) (Dilantin enlargemenf) Enlargement of the gingivae caused by the use of diphenylhydantoin sodium (Dilantin sodium) in the treatment of epilepsy. **h., idiopathic gingival** *See* fibromatosis gingivae.

h., inflammatory fibrous *See* epulis fissurata.

h., papillary A growth in the midline of the hard palate, usually in the relief area of a denture; characterized by a papillary, or raspberry, appearance.

h., inflammatory papillary (inflammatory papillomatosis, multiple papillomatosis, papillary hyperplasia) A condition of unknown etiology but associated with the presence of maxillary dentures. Characterized by numerous red papillary projections on the hard palate.

hyperplastic tissue *See* tissue, hyperplastic.

hyperpnea (hī″perp-nē′ah) Abnormal increase in respiratory volume; an abnormal increase in the rate and depth of breathing.

hyperpotassemia (hī″per-pot″ah-sē′mē-ah) *See* hyperkalemia.

hyperproteinemia (hī″per-prō″tē-ĭ-nē′mē-ah) Abnormal increase in serum and plasma proteins.

hyperproteinuria (hī″per-prō″tē-ĭ-nū′rē-ah) *See* albuminuria.

hypersalivation *See* sialorrhea.

hypersensitive Abnormally sensitive.

hypersensitiveness (hī″pĕr-sĕn′sĭ-tĭv″nĕs) A state of altered reactivity in which the body reacts more strongly than normal to a foreign agent.

hypersensitivity 1: Adverse reaction to contact with specific substances in quantities that usually produce no reaction in normal individuals. **2:** Usually, an allergic tendency. In general, a tendency to react with unusual violence to stimuli. **3:** A common complaint after periodontal therapy in which dentin may be exposed, resulting in pain in the teeth or sensitivity to heat, cold, and sweet substances.

h., atopic *See* atopy.

h., bacterial Delayed inflammatory reaction resulting from previous sensitization of the host by an antigen.

hypersensitization The process of rendering abnormally sensitive or the condition of being abnormally sensitive.

hypersthenuria (hī″per-sthĕ-nū′rē-ah) Urine with an abnormally high specific gravity. It is seen in uncontrolled diabetes mellitus and in severe dehydration.

hypersusceptibility (hī″per-sŭh-sĕp″tĭ-bĭl′ĭ-tē) A condition of abnormal susceptibility to poisons, infective agents, or agents that are entirely innocuous in the normal individual.

hypersympathicotonus (hī″per-sĭm-păth″ē-kō-tō′nŭs) Increased tonicity of the sympathetic nervous system.

hypersystolic (hī″per-sĭs-tol′ĭk) Characterized by hypersystole; having heartbeats of excessive force.

hypertarachia (hī″per-ta-răk′ē-ah) Extreme irritability of the nervous system.

hypertelorism (hī″per-tē′lō-rĭzm) Excessive distance between paired organs. *See also* syndrome, Greig's for ocular hypertelorism.

hypertension (hī″per-tĕn′shŭn) Abnormal elevation of systolic and/or diastolic arterial pressure. Systolic hypertension is generally related to emotional stress, sclerosis of the aorta and large arteries, or aortic insufficiency. Diastolic hypertension may result from obscure causes (essential), renal disease, or endocrine disorders.

h., essential Elevated blood pressure of unknown etiology.

h., malignant Elevated blood pressure characterized by a progressive course uncontrollable by medication.

hypertensive agents Agents that reduce or control blood pressure.

hyperthyroidism (Parry's disease) Abnormalities of calorigenic mechanisms, body tissues, blood, and body fluids and of the circulatory, muscular, and nervous systems resulting from an excessive elaboration of thyroid hormone. Manifestations include increased sweating, increased appetite, intolerance to heat, weight loss, increased protein-bound iodine (PBI), early shedding of primary teeth and early eruption of permanent teeth, tachycardia, palpitation, tremors, nervousness, muscular weakness, diarrhea, increased excretion of calcium and phosphorus, hypocholesterolemia, creatinuria, and osteoporosis. May occur as the result of primary hyperplasia, hyperfunctioning nodular goiters, functional benign tumor, or adenoma of the thyroid gland. *See also* goiter, exophthalmic.

hypertonic (hī″per-ton′ĭk) Having an osmotic pressure greater than that of the solution with which it is compared.

hypertrichosis (hī″per-trĭ-kō′sĭs) Excessive growth of hair on the body, possibly as a result of endocrine dysfunction, as in the hirsutism accompanying excessive adrenocortical function.

hypertrophy (hī-pĕr′trō-fē) Morbid enlargement or overgrowth of an organ or part resulting from an increase in size of its constituent cells.

h., denture *See* hyperplasia, denture.

h., muscle Hypertrophy denotes an increase in the size or number of constituent fibers of a muscle. Any other condition (e.g., inflammation, tumor, fatty infiltration) that increases the size of a muscle is called *pseudohypertrophy*. True or physiologic hypertrophy results from excessive activity of muscle. Genetic and hormonal factors play a role in determining the size of muscles; e.g., muscles in a male tend to be larger than in a female in the temporal and facial regions. The histologic characteristics of hypertrophied muscle are normal. The fibrils are slightly wider in diameter than is normal, and the only change might be a slight increase in vascularity.

hyperventilation 1: Abnormally prolonged, rapid, and deep breathing; also the condition produced by overbreathing of oxygen at high pressures. It is marked by confusion, dizziness, numbness, and muscular cramps brought on by such breathing. **2:** Rapid, deep, forced breathing frequently resulting from anxiety. It results in a transient loss of carbon dioxide and respiratory alkalosis. Symptoms include anxiety, circumoral numbness, tingling sensation, faintness, and occasionally, carpopedal spasms, tetany, and syncope.

hypervitaminosis A (hī″per-vī″tah-mĭ-nō′sĭs) The effects of toxic doses of vitamin A. Manifestations include bone fragility, xeroderma, nausea, headache, and loss of hair.

hypervitaminosis D The toxic effects of ingesting large amounts of vitamin D. Manifestations include symptoms resulting from hypercalcemia, impairment of renal function, and metastatic calcification.

hypervolemia Increased blood volume.

hypnalgia (hĭp-năl′jē-ah) Pain that recurs during sleep.

hypnesthesia (hip″nes-thē′zē′ah) Sleepiness.

hypnic (hĭp′nĭk) Inducing or pertaining to sleep.

hypno (hĭp′nō) Combining form denoting a relationship to sleep.

hypnosis (hĭp-nō′sĭs) A condition of artificially induced sleep or of a trance resembling sleep induced by drugs, psychologic means, or both. Generally creating a condition of heightened suggestibility in the subject.

hypnotic (hĭp-not′ĭk) **1:** A drug that induces sleep or depresses the central nervous system at a cortical level. **2:** Causing sleep or a trance. *See also* sedative.

hypnotism (hĭp′nō-tĭzm) **1:** The method or practice of inducing sleep. **2:** In medical jurisprudence, a mental state rendering the patient susceptible to suggestion at the will and inducement of another.

hypnotize (hĭp′nō-tīz) To put into a state of hypnosis in which there is a condition of heightened suggestibility.

hypo (hī′pō) An abbreviated form of the term *hyposulfite,* which is a synonym of sodium thiosulfate ($Na_2S_2O_3$), a solution used in photography and radiography to fix and harden the manifest image. *See also* fixation.

hypo- (hī′po) A prefix signifying beneath, under, or deficient.

hypoadrenocorticalism (hī″pō-ăd-rē″nō-kor′tĭ-kăl-ĭzm) **(adrenocortical insufficiency, hypoadrenocorticism)** Acute or chronic adrenocortical hypofunction, as in Waterhouse-Friderichsen syndrome or Addison's disease.

hypoadrenocorticism (hī″pō-ah-drē-nō-kor′tĭ-sĭzm) *See* hypoadrenocorticalism.

hypoalgesia (hī″pō-ăl-jē′ze-ah) Diminished sensation of pain resulting from a raised pain threshold.

hypocalcemia (hī″pō-kăl-sē′mē-ah) Abnormally low concentration of calcium in the blood; may be associated with hypoparathyroidism, rickets, osteomalacia, renal rickets, pancreatic disease, sprue, obstructive jaundice, or tetany.

hypocalcification (hī″pō-kăl-si-fĭ-kā′shŭn) Reduced calcification, especially of enamel. It produces opaque white spots that may be discolored later. *See also* fluorosis.

h., hereditary enamel A hereditary anomaly of enamel formation affecting the primary and permanent dentition in which the enamel peels off after tooth eruption and exposes dentin, giving the teeth a yellow appearance.

hypocalciuria (hī″pō-kăl″sē-ū′rē-ah) Decrease in urinary calcium. Normal values vary considerably but are roughly related to calcium intake. Various values are given (e.g., 100 to 200 mg/day on a normal diet, or 350 to 400 mg/day for calcium intake of 10 mg/ kg of body weight in children). It may occur in hypoparathyroidism, rickets, osteomalacia, metastatic carcinoma of the prostate, and renal failure. *See also* test, Sulkowitch's.

hypocapnia (hī″pō-kăp′nē-ah) **(hypocarbia)** A deficiency of carbon dioxide in the blood.

hypocarbia *See* hypocapnia.

hypocenesthesia (hī″pō-sĕn″ĕs-thē′zē-ah) Lack of the normal sense of well-being.

hypochloremia (hī″pō-klō-rē′mē-ah) Decrease below normal of chloride concentration in the plasma. Normal range is 98 to 100 mEq/L. It may occur in adrenal insufficiency, persistent vomiting, renal failure, acute infections, and dehydration with sodium depletion.

hypochondria (hī″pō-kon′drē-ah) **(hypochondriasis)** Anxiety about disease; a type of neurosis characterized by fear of disease or by simulated disease.

hypochondriasis (hī″pō-kon-drī′ah-sĭs) *See* hypochondria.

hypochromia (hī-pō-krō′mē-ah) **(hypochromasia)** Reduced staining quality of cells, particularly palestaining red blood cells associated with hemoglobin deficiency.

hypodermoclysis (hī″pō-der-mok′lĭ-sĭs) Subcutaneous injection of fluid in large volume.

hypodontia (hīp″ō-dŏn′shē-ah) Fewer teeth than normal.

hypoesthesia (hī″pō-ĕs-thē′zē-ah) Decreased sensitivity to touch or pressure.

hypoestrogenism (hī″pō-ĕs″trō-jĕn′ĭzm) Diminished production of estrogenic substances by the ovaries, such as that which occurs during menopause. May produce desquamative lesions on the oral mucous membranes. *See also* gingivitis, desquamative.

hypofibrinogenemia (hī″pō-fī-brĭn″ō-jĕ-nē′ mē-ah) Reduction of fibrinogen in the blood. Excessive bleeding may occur following trauma. The deficiency of fibrinogen may be congenital or may result from faulty synthesis associated with liver disease and defibrinogenation resulting from disorders of pregnancy involving the placenta and amniotic fluid. The normal range is 200 to 600 mg/100 ml of plasma. Clotting deficiencies do not occur until the concentration falls below 75 mg/ 100 ml.

hypogammaglobulinemia (hī″pō-găm″ah-glahb′ū-lĭ-nē′ mē-ah) Deficiency of gamma globulin. It is usually manifested by recurrent bacterial infections.

hypogeusia (hī″pō-gū′zē-ah) Decreased sense of taste.

hypoglycemia (hī″pō-glī-sē′mē-ah) A condition existing when the concentration of blood sugar (true blood sugar) is 40 mg/ 100 ml or less. Symptoms may not occur even when the concentration is considerably less. Symptoms include nervousness, hunger, weakness, vertigo, and faintness. Hypoglycemia may occur in the fasting state and/or following the injection of insulin.

    h., fasting Hypoglycemia occurring in the postabsorptive state; occurs in renal glycosuria, lactation, hepatic disease, or central nervous system lesions.

    h., insulin Hypoglycemia resulting from improper administration of insulin. If hypoglycemia is severe, convulsions, coma, and death may occur. *See also* shock, insulin.

    h., mixed Hypoglycemia occurring during the fasting state and after the ingestion of carbohydrate; occurs in idiopathic spontaneous hypoglycemia of infancy, in anterior pituitary and adrenocortical insufficiency, and with tumors of the islet cells of the pancreas.

    h., reactive Hypoglycemia occurring after the ingestion of carbohydrate with an excessive release of insulin, as in functional hyperinsulinism.

    h., spontaneous Hypoglycemia that is functional (i.e., renal glycosuria, lactation, severe muscular exertion, etc.) or is due to organic disease (i.e., hepatic disease, adrenocortical insufficiency, etc,)

hypogonadism (hī″pō-gō′năd-ĭzm) Gonadal deficiency resulting from abnormalities of the testes and ovaries or to pituitary insufficiency. Manifestations include

eunuchism, eunuchoidism, Fröhlich's syndrome, amenorrhea, and incomplete development or maintenance of secondary sex characteristics.

hypohidrotic ectodermal dysplasia (hī″pō-hī-drŏt′ĭk ĕk-tō-dĕr′mal dĭs-plā′zē-ah) Syndrome consisting of hypodontia, hypotrichosis, hypohidrosis, and other defects related to the development of ectodermal structures.

hypokalemia (hī″pō-kă-lē′mē-ah) **(hypopotassemia)** Abnormally low serum potassium. It may occur in metabolic alkalosis, chronic diarrhea, Cushing's syndrome, primary aldosteronism, and excessive use of deoxycorticosterone, cortisone, or ACTH.

hypolarynx (hī″pō-lăr′ĭnks) The infraglottic compartment of the larynx that extends from the true vocal cords to the first tracheal ring.

hypolethal (hī″pō-lē′thal) Not quite lethal; said of dosage.

hypomagnesemia (hī″pō-măg″nĕ-sē′mē-ah) Deficiency of magnesium in the blood serum (normal values range from 1.5 to 2.5 mEq/L). It may be associated with chronic alcoholism, starvation, and prolonged diuresis in congestive heart failure. Manifestations include muscular twitching, convulsions, and coma.

hyponasality (hī″pō-nā-zăl′ĭt-ē) Lack of nasal resonance necessary to produce acceptable voice quality. The type of voice quality heard when the speaker's nose is occluded or when the speaker is suffering from a severe cold.

hyponatremia (hī″pō-nah-trē′mē-ah) Abnormally low concentration of sodium in the blood serum. It may develop in adrenocortical insufficiency and chronic renal disease or with extreme sweating.

hypoparathyroidism (hī″pō-păr″ah-thī′roid-ĭzm) Decrease in parathyroid function, usually the result of surgical removal. Symptoms include tetany, irritability, and muscle weakness. The serum calcium is low, the blood phosphorus elevated, the blood magnesium reduced, and the alkaline phosphatase normal.

hypopharyngoscope (hī″pō-fah-rĭng′gō-skōp) An apparatus devised for bringing the lower part of the pharynx or hypopharynx into view.

hypopharynx (hī″pō-făr′ĭnks) The division of the pharynx that lies below the upper edge of the epiglottis and opens into the larynx and esophagus.

hypophosphatasia (hī″pō-fos″fah-tā′zē-ah) A familial disease in which the children may have very low serum alkaline phosphatase levels, total or partial aplasia of the cementum, and an abnormal periodontal ligament in the deciduous teeth. A decreased phosphatase level that has been linked to a premature loss of deciduous teeth in children. Examination reveals absence, hypoplasia, or dysplasia of cementum.

hypophosphatemia (hī″pō-fos″fah-tē′mē-ah) Abnormally low concentration of serum phosphates. Blood phosphorus levels are low in sprue, celiac disease, and hyperparathyroidism and in association with an elevated alkaline phosphatase in vitamin D—resistant rickets and other diseases involving a renal tubular defect in resorption of phosphate.

hypophysis *See* gland, pituitary.

hypopituitarism (hī″pō-pǐ-tū′ǐ-tăr-ǐzm) Decrease in the hormonal secretions of the pituitary gland.

hypoplasia (hī″pō-plā′zē-ah) Defective or incomplete development of any tissue or structure.

  h., enamel, chronologic A prenatal or postnatal systemic hypoplasia affecting amelogenesis occurring at the time of the systemic disorder.

  h., enamel, hereditary (hereditary brown tooth) A hereditary anomaly of the enamel affecting the primary and permanent dentition in which a thin layer of hard enamel covering the yellow dentin gives the tooth a brown appearance.

  h., mandibular Abnormally small mandibular development (e.g., in micrognathia or brachygnathia).

hypopnea (hī-pop′nē-ah) Abnormally shallow and rapid respirations.

hypopotassemia (hī″pō-pot′ah-sē′mē-ah) *See* hypokalemia.

hypoproteinemia (hī″pō-prō′tē-ǐ-nē′mē-ah) A decrease in serum and plasma proteins.

hypoprothrombinemia (hī″pō-prō-throm″bǐ-nē′mē-ah) A deficiency of prothrombin in the blood. It may be congenital or associated with vitamin K deficiency, large doses of salicylates, liver disease, or excessive anticoagulant. The normal level ranges from 70% to 120% plasm a prothrombin concentration. There is little danger of hemorrhage if the prothrombin concentration is greater than 20% of normal.

hyposalivation (hī″pō-săl″ǐ-vā′shŭn) **(xerostomia)** A decreased flow of saliva. It may be associated with dehydration, radiation therapy of the salivary gland regions, anxiety, the use of drugs such as atropine and antihistamines, vitamin deficiency, various forms of parotitis, and various syndromes (Sjögren' s, Riley-Day, Plummer-Vinson, and Heerfordt's disease). *See also* asialorrhea.

hyposensitive (hī″pō-sĕn′sǐ-tǐv) Less sensitive.

hyposthenuria (hī″pōs-thē-nū′rē-ah) A condition in which the urine has an abnormally low specific gravity. It may occur in cases in which renal damage impairs concentrating power or when the kidneys are normal but lack hormonal stimulus for concentrations, as in diabetes insipidus.

hypotension (hī″pō-tĕn′shŭn) Abnormally low tension, especially low blood pressure.

hypothalamus (hī″pō-thăl′ah-mŭs) A small extension of the brain that lies in the sella turcica in the cranium. It lies just at the superior level of the body of the sphenoid bone. It is intimately related structurally and functionally with the pituitary gland, and it is important in the central regulation of the endocrine glands, including the thyroid gland, pancreas, adrenal glands, and gonads. The most important visceral functions are under control of the hypothalamus because it functions in such close coordination with the endocrine glands. The control is mediated through its structural communication with the pituitary gland.

hypothermia Body temperature significantly below normal, (i.e., 98.6° F, 37° C.)

hypothetical question Assumed or proved facts and circumstances, stated so as to constitute a specific situation or state of facts, on which the opinion of an expert is asked, in producing evidence at a trial.

hypothyroidism (hī″pō-thī′roid-ǐzm) Diminished activity of the thyroid gland with decreased secretion of thyroxin, resulting in lowered basal metabolic rate, lethargy, sleepiness, dysmenorrhea in females, and a tendency toward obesity. Occasionally there is accompanying gingival hyperplasia. The condition is called *cretinism* in children and *myxedema* in adults.

hypoxemia (hī″pŏk-sē′mē-ah) Deficient oxygenation of the blood.

hypoxia (hī-pŏk′sē-ah) Low oxygen content or tension.

  h., anemic Hypoxia brought about by a reduction of the oxygen-carrying capacity of the blood because of a decrease in the complete blood counts or an alteration of the hemoglobin constituents.

  h., anoxic Hypoxia resulting from inadequate oxygen in inspired air or interference with gaseous exchange in the lungs.

  h., histotoxic Hypoxia resulting from the inability of the tissue cells to use the oxygen that may be present in normal amount and tension.

  h., metabolic Hypoxia resulting from an increased tissue demand for oxygen.

  h., stagnant Hypoxia resulting from decreased circulation in an area.

hyrax appliance A fixed orthodontic appliance used for the bilateral expansion of the maxillary posterior teeth and/or the bilateral expansion of the palate.

hysteresis (hǐs-tĕ-rē′sǐs) A physical phenomenon whereby a material such as a reversible hydrocolloid passes from a solid to a gel state at one temperature and a gel to a solid state at another.

hysteria (hǐs-tĕr′ē-ah) **1:** A disease or disorder of the nervous system, more common in females than males, not originating in lesions and resulting from psychic rather than physical causes. **2:** A psychoneurosis characterized by lack of control over emotions or acts, exaggeration of sensory impression, and stimulation of disease or pain associated with disease. In some patients trismus, neuralgia, and temporomandibular joint disturbance may be hysterical in origin.

I and D (surgical fistulation) Incision and drainage; the procedure of incising a fluctuant mucosal lesion to allow for the release of pressure and drainage of fluid exudate.

-ia Latin suffix that indicates a condition (e.g., a disease) or a science, practice, or treatment.

iatrogenic (ī-ăt″rō-jĕn′ĭk) Originating as a result of professional care, e.g., an iatrogenic dermatitis.

ibuprofen Generic name for 2(p-isobutylphenyl) propionic acid, a nonsteroidal anti-inflammatory agent with analgesic and antipyretic properties. It is useful for the temporary relief of minor aches and pains associated with the common cold, toothache, muscular aches, minor arthritic pain, and menstrual cramps and for the reduction of fever. Brand name Advil.

I cell disease A congenital disease, also known as *mucolipidosis II* that is characterized by shortness of stature, psychomotor retardation, coarse facial features, and gingival enlargement. The progressive gingival enlargement may delay tooth eruption and may impair closure of the mouth.

-ics Indicative of a science, practice, or treatment. In dentistry the trend is from the use of *-ia* to the use of *-ics;* e.g., about 1937 the term orthodontics began to replace the term orthodontia. In ancient Greek times the adjectival ending *-ikos* was used without a following noun to indicate a practice, e.g., ethics. The ending *-ics*, unlike *-ia*, can indicate only a practice, not a condition. Preferred to *-ia*.

icterus (ĭk′ter-ŭs) See jaundice.

　i., acholuric See jaundice, hemolytic, congenital.

-id reaction See reaction, -id.

identity Sameness; the fact that a subject, person, or thing before a court is the same as it is claimed to be.

idiopathic disease See disease, idiopathic.

idiopathic enlargement (ĭd″ē-ō-păth′ĭk) See enlargement, idiopathic.

idiosyncrasy (ĭd″ē-ō-sĭng′krah-sē) Tendency to react atypically or with unusual violence to a food, drug, or cosmetic. Also, any characteristic peculiar to an individual.

ignorance of law See law, ignorance of.

illegal Not authorized by law; illicit.

illuminator (light box) A source of light with uniform intensity for viewing radiographs.

illusion A mistaken or erroneous perception of an object external to the individual. In some cases, the laws of physics explain the errors. In others, the explanation lies with the perceiver. Illusion should be distinguished from hallucinations, which are perceptions that lack external stimuli, and delusions, which are false beliefs. Illusions are seen in certain reactions to general anesthesia or intoxication.

illustration A drawing or photograph used to help clarify the patient's concept of proposed treatment and conditions present.

image, latent The invisible image produced on photographic or radiographic film by the action of light or radiation before development.

imbalance, occlusal An inharmonious relationship between the maxillary and mandibular teeth during closure or functional jaw movements.

imbedded See embedded.

imbibition (ĭm″bĭ-bĭsh′ŭn) Absorption of liquid. Gel structures are particularly susceptible to imbibition.

immediate denture See denture, immediate.

immune reaction See reaction, immune.

immunity (ĭ-mū′nĭ-tē) **1:** Exemption from service or from duties that the law ordinarily requires other citizens to perform (e.g., jury duty). **2:** Condition of an organism whereby it successfully resists or is not susceptible to injury or infection.

immunodeficiency A condition resulting from a defective immunologic mechanism. Primary immunodeficiency is due to a defect in the immune system, secondary immunodeficiency is a result of another disease process such as HIV infection.

immunoglobulins (ĭm″ū-nō-glob′ū-lĭnz) **(Ig)** Serum proteins (gamma globulins) synthesized by plasma cells that act as antibodies and are important in the body's defense mechanisms against infection. Main classes are designated as IgG, IgA, and IgM.

immunosuppressants Agents that lower or reduce immune response, useful in organ transplant surgery to prevent organ rejection.

immunosuppression The act or action of lowering or reducing the immune response.

impact strength *See* strength, impact.

impacted tooth *See* tooth, impacted.

impaction Pressed closely together so as to be immovable

   i., food Impaction of food generally interproximally because of open contact areas, uneven marginal ridge height, or "plunger" cusps.

   i., tooth Situation in which an unerupted tooth is wedged against another tooth or teeth or otherwise located so that it cannot erupt normally.

impaired function *See* function, impaired.

impeachment of witness The questioning of the veracity of a witness by means of evidence obtained for that purpose.

impetigo (ĭm″pĕ-tī′gō) An inflammatory disease of the skin characterized by pustules.

impingement The striking or application of excessive pressure to a tissue by food or a prosthesis.

implant A device, usually alloplastic, surgically inserted into or onto the jawbone. To be used as a prosthodontic abutment, it should remain quiescent and purely incidental to local tissue physiology.

   i., abutment of The portion of an implant that protrudes through the gingival tissues and is designed to support a prosthodontic appliance.

   i., arthroplastic A cast chrome-alloy glenoid fossa prosthesis available in right and left models.

   i., bone *See* graft, autogenous, bone; graft, iliac; graft, kiel; graft, onlay bone; graft, swaging.

   i., cervix of That portion of an implant that connects the infrastructure with the abutment as it passes through the mucoperiosteum.

   i., endosseous *See* implant, endosteal.

   i., endosteal An implant that is placed into the alveolar and/or basal bone and that protrudes through the mucoperiosteum.

     i., anchor endosteal An implant with a narrow buccolingual wedge-shaped infrastructure that is designed to be placed deep into the bone. The outline of the implant appears similar to a nautical anchor, and there are a variety of sizes and shapes to satisfy many anatomic and prosthodontic needs. They are cast of chromium-cobalt surgical alloy and annealed.

       i., arms of anchor endosteal The major portion of the implant infrastructure.

       i., crown of anchor endosteal The abutment part of an anchor implant.

       i., flukes of anchor endosteal The end portions of the arms that rise to the most superficial portion within the bone.

       i., seating instrument of anchor endosteal, arm type A bayonet-shaped device designed to assist in seating an anchor implant by straddling its arms over a specially designed "seating notch."

       i., seating instrument of anchor endosteal, crown type A bayonet-shaped, double-ended device designed to assist in seating an anchor implant by cupping its crown or abutment.

       i., shaft of anchor endosteal The cervix of an anchor implant.

     i., blade endosteal An implant with a narrow (buccolingually) wedge-shaped infrastructure bearing openings or vents through which tissue grows to obtain retention.

       i., complete-arch blade endosteal A blade type of implant designed to be inserted into a completely edentulous ridge as a single appliance bearing multiple abutments.

       i., shoulder of blade endosteal That unbroken surface of the wedge-shaped infrastructure that is widest and most superficial. It is this part that is tapped during the seating of the implant.

     i., ceramic endosteal An endosteal implant of a variety of designs constructed of silicate or porcelain.

     i., endodontic endosteal An implant with a threaded or nonthreaded pin that fits into a root canal and extends beyond the dental apex into the adjacent bone, thereby lengthening the clinical root.

     i., helicoid endosteal A two-piece endosteal implant consisting of a helical steel spring that is inserted into bone as a female and a male that may be placed postoperatively and serves as the abutment.

     i., needle endosteal (pin endosteal) A smooth, thin shaft (self-perforating) that serves as an implant usually in conjunction with two others, the three being placed in bone in tripodal conformity.

       i., mandrel of needle endosteal A hollow device available in full, half, and shallow depths into which needle implants fit. The mandrel, in turn, is used in the contra-angle to drive the needle implant into place.

     i., ramus endosteal A blade type of implant designed for the anterior part of the ramus. *See also* implant, endosteal, blade.

       i., frame type of ramus endosteal A prefabricated mandibular full-arch implant consisting of two posterior ramus implants: an anterior (symphyseal) endosteal component and a conjunction bar.

     i., seating instrument of endosteal A device designed to be placed on a portion of an implant so that malleting on it will seat the implant into the bone. It usually has an angled or bayoneted shaft to enable it to protrude from the mouth in a more or less vertical direction.

i., spiral endosteal A screw type of implant, either hollow or solid, usually consisting of abutment, cervix, and infrastructure.

i., C. M. (crête manche) spiral endosteal A narrow-diameter screw implant designed for thin ridges.

i., fabricated A custom-designed implant constructed for a specific operative site.

i., infrastucture of The part of an implant that is designed to give it retention.

i., intraperiosteal An artificial appliance made to conform to the shape of a bone and placed beneath the outer, or fibrous, layer of the periosteum.

i., mesostructure An intermediate superstructure. A series of splinted copings, each of which fits over an implant abutment or natural tooth and over which fits the completed prosthodontic appliance.

i., oral *See* implant.

i., polymer tooth replica An acrylic resin implant, shaped like the tooth recently extracted, that is placed into the tooth's alveolus.

i., stock An implant, usually endosteal, that is available in manufactured form in uniform sizes and shapes.

i., subperiosteal An appliance consisting of an open-mesh frame designed to fit over the surface of the bone beneath the periosteum.

i., anterior subperiosteal An implant placed in the anterior part of an edentulous mandible and designed to supply abutments in the two canine regions.

i., complete subperiosteal An implant used for an entire edentulous jaw.

i., fixation screw of subperiosteal Screws, 5 to 7 mm long, that are made of the same surgical alloy as the implant and are used to affix the implant to the underlying bone.

i., single-tooth subperiosteal An implant designed to replace a single missing tooth; usually unsupported by adjacent natural teeth.

i., strut of subperiosteal A thin, striplike component of an infrastructure.

i., superstructure of A completed prosthesis that is supported entirely or in part by an implant. It may be a removable or fixed prosthesis and may be a single crown or a complete arch splint.

i., two-piece An implant, either endosteal or subperiosteal, having its infrastructure and abutment in separate parts. Generally, the abutment, which is threaded, is screwed to the infrastructure some weeks after its incision, so that healing has taken place.

implantation, tooth *See* transplantation, tooth.

implantodontology (ĭm-plăn″tō-don-tŏl′ō-jē) The study of the placement of a foreign material into or onto the jawbones to replace or support artificial dentition.

implantology, oral (ĭm-plăn-tol′ō-jē) The art and science of dentistry concerned with the surgical insertion of materials and devices into, onto, and about the jaws and oral cavity for purposes of oral maxillofacial, or occlusal rehabilitation and/or cosmetic correction.

implied Inferred; conceded.

impression An imprint or negative likeness of an object from which a positive reproduction may be made.

i., anatomic An impression that records tissue shape without distortion.

i., area *See* area, impression.

i., boxing of an *See* boxing.

i., bridge An impression made for the purpose of constructing or assembling a fixed restoration, fixed partial denture, or bridge.

i., cleft palate An impression of the upper jaw of a patient with a cleft (incomplete closure, or union) in the palate.

i., closed mouth An impression made while the mouth is closed and with the patient's muscular activity molding the borders.

i., complete denture An impression (negative record) of an edentulous arch made for the purpose of constructing a complete denture.

i., composite An impression consisting of two or more parts.

i., correctable An impression whose surface is capable of alteration by the removal from or addition to some area of its surface or border.

i., dual *See* technique, impression, dual.

i., duplicating *See* duplication.

i., elastic An impression made in a material that will permit registration of undercut areas by springing over projecting areas and then returning to its original position.

i., final (secondary impression) An impression used for making the master cast.

i., fluid wax An impression of the functional form of subjacent structures made with selected waxes that are applied (brushed on) to the impression surface in fluid form.

i., functional An impression of the supporting structures in their functional form. *See also* structure, supporting, functional form of.

i., hydrocolloid An impression made of a hydrocolloid material.

i., lower *See* impression, mandibular.

i., mandibular (lower impression) An impression of the mandibular jaw and related tissues and dental structures.

i., material *See* material, impression.

i., maxillary (upper impression) An impression of the maxillary jaw and related tissues and dental structures.

i., mercaptan An impression made of mercaptan (polysulfide), a rubber base elastic material.

i., partial denture An impression of part or all of a partially edentulous arch made for the purpose of designing or constructing a partial denture.

i., pickup An impression made with the superstructure frame in place on the abutments in the mouth after the implant has been surgically inserted and the mouth has healed. The superstructure frame is included in the impression material, and an accurate impression of the oral mucosal tissue over the implant is obtained.

i., preliminary (primary impression) An impression made for the purpose of diagnosis or the construction of a tray for making a final impression.

i., primary See impression, preliminary.

i., secondary See impression, final.

i., sectional An impression that is made in sections.

i., silicone A rubber base, elastic, impression using a material that contains a silicone. See also silicone.

i., snap See impression, preliminary.

i., surface See denture foundation area; surface, basal.

i., surgical bone A negative likeness of the exposed bony surfaces necessary to support the implant substructure.

i., technique See technique, impression.

i. tray See tray, impression.

i., upper See impression, maxillary.

impulse A surge of electric current for a short time span; e.g., in a 60-cycle AC current, there are 120 impulses per second. See impression, maxillary.

i., muscle A wave of excitation along a muscle fiber initiated at the neuromuscular endplate; accompanied by chemical and electrical changes at the surface of the muscle fiber and by activation of the contractile elements of the muscle fiber; detectable electronically (electromyographically); and followed by a transient refractory period.

i., nerve A wave of excitation along a nerve fiber initiated by a stimulus; accompanied by chemical and electrical changes at the surface of the nerve fiber and followed by a transient refractory period during which further stimulation has no effect.

IMZ implant system An endosseous implant system provisionally accepted by the ADA.

in chief Principal; directly obtained. Evidence obtained from a witness on examination in court by the party producing the witness.

in pais (ĭn pā') A legal transaction that has been accomplished without legal proceedings.

in potestate parentis (ĭn pō-tĕst'āt pah-rĕn'tĭs) Under the authority of the parent.

inacidity Absence of acidity.

inactivate To render inactive; to destroy the activity of.

inactivator A substance added to a culture medium to prevent the activity of an inoculant. Penicillinase is added to the culture medium to prevent the activity of penicillin that might be carried over from a root canal treatment.

inadequacy, velopharyngeal (vĕl"ō-făh-rĭn'jē-ăl) A lack of functional closure of the velum to the postpharyngeal wall.

inadmissible That which cannot be admitted into evidence in a legal proceeding under the established rules of law.

incentive plan A plan whereby the insurer pays an increasing share of the claim cost provided the indiviual insured visits the dentist as stipulated during each incentive period (usually a year) and receives the prescribed treatment.

incentive program A dental benefits program that pays an increasing share of the treatment cost provided that the covered individual utilizes the benefits of the program during each incentive period (usually a year) and receives the treatment prescribed. For example a 70% to 30% copayment program in the first year of coverage may become an 80% to 20% program in the second year if the subscriber visits the dentist in the first year as stipulated in the program. Most frequently, there is a corresponding percentage reduction in the program's copayment level if the covered individual fails to visit the dentist in a given year (but never below the initial copayment level).

inchacao (ĭn-chah-kah'ō) See beriberi.

incipient (ĭn-sĭp'ē-ĕnt) Beginning, initial, commencing.

incisal (ĭn-sī'zăl) Relating to the cutting edge of the anterior teeth, incisors or canines.

i. angle See angle, incisal.

i. guidance angle See angle, incisal guidance.

i. guide See guide, incisal.

i. guide pin See pin, incisal guide.

i. rest See rest, incisal.

incision (ĭn-sĭzh'ŭn) The act of cutting or biting.

i. and drainage See I and D.

i. of food The phase of the masticatory cycle, using the incisor teeth, that cuts or separates the bolus of food.

i., preauricular The incision of the soft tissue anterior to the external ear that permits access to the temporomandibular joint.

i., relieving A cut into the soft tissues adjacent to a wound to permit a tension-free closure.

i., Risdon's The incision of the soft tissues in the area of the mandibular angle that permits access to the lateral surface of the mandibular ramus, subcondylar neck, and condylar area.

incisive foramen See foramen, incisive.

incisive papilla See papilla, incisive.

incisor(s) (ĭn-sī′zor) A cutting tooth, one of the four anterior teeth of either jaw.

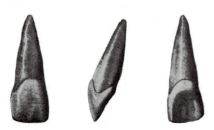

Right upper first incisor
Labial surface   Mesial surface   Lingual surface

i., central The first incisor.

i., Hutchinson's Malformed teeth caused by the presence of congenital syphilis during tooth development. The incisors usually are shorter than normal, show a single permanent notch on each incisal edge, and are screwdriver shaped.

i., lateral The second incisor.

i. point *See* point, incisor.

inclination (ĭn′klĭ-nā′shŭn) The angle of slope from a particular item of reference.

i., axial The alignment of a tooth in a vertical plane in relationship to its basal bone structure.

i., lateral condylar The direction of the lateral condyle path.

i. of tooth *See* tooth, inclination of.

inclusion cyst A epidermal cyst formed of a mass of squamous epithelium cells with concentric layers of keratin.

income The return in money from one's business, practice, or capital invested; gains, profit.

incompatibility (ĭn′kom-păt″ĭ-bĭl′ĭ-tē) Term that refers to a disharmonious relationship among the ingredients of prescriptions and other drug mixtures.

i., chemical A situation in which two or more of the ingredients of a drug interact chemically, with resulting deterioration of the mixture.

incontinentia pigmenti *See* syndrome, Bloch-Sulzberger.

incubation period The lapsed time between exposure to an infectious agent and the onset of symptoms of a disease.

incubator (ĭn′kū-bā-tor) A laboratory container with controlled temperature for the cultivation of bacteria.

incurred claims Outstanding obligations of the insurer for dental services rendered to the insured.

indemnification schedule *See* table of allowances

indemnity benefit A contract benefit which is paid to the insured to meet the cost of dental services received.

indemnity plan 1: A plan that provides payment to the insured for the cost of dental care but makes no arrangement for providing care itself. **2:** A dental plan in which a third-party-payer provides payment of an amount for specific services regardless of the actual charges made by the provider. Payment may be made to enrollees or by assignment directly to dentists. Schedule of allowances, table of allowances, or reasonable and customary plans are examples of indemnity plans.

index **1:** The ratio of a measurable value to another. **2:** A core or mold used to record or maintain the relative position of a tooth or teeth to one another and/or to a cast. *See also* splint.

i., Broders' (Broders' classification) 1: A system of grading of epidermoid carcinoma suggested by Broders. Tumors are graded from I to IV on the basis of cell differentiation. Grade I tumors are highly differentiated (there is much keratin production); Grade IV tumors are poorly differentiated (cells are highly anaplastic, with almost no keratin formation). **2:** Classification and grading of malignant neoplasms according to the proportion of malignant cells to normal cells in the lesion.

i., cardiac The minute volume of blood per square meter of body surface.

i., carpal The degree of ossification of the carpal bones noted in radiographs of the wrist; a method of determining the state of skeletal maturation.

i., cephalic Head shape and size.

i., DEF A dental caries index applied to the primary dentition in somewhat the same manner as the DMF index is used for classifying permanent teeth. The letter D stands for decayed; E for extraction indicated because of caries; and F for filled. Missing primary teeth are ignored in this index because of the uncertainty in determining whether they were extracted because of advanced caries or exfoliated normally.

i., DMF A technique for managing statistically the number of decayed, missing, or filled teeth in the mouth. Analysis may be based on the average number of DMF teeth (sometimes called DMFT) per person or the average number of DMF tooth surfaces (DMFS).

i., gingiva–bone count (Dunning-Leach index) An index that permits differential recording of both gingival and bone conditions to determine gingivitis and bone loss.

i., gnathic Relationship of jaw size to head size.

i., icterus *See* test, Meulengracht's.

i., malocclusion A measure of the severity of a malocclusion, obtained by assigning values to a series of defined observations.

i., measuring An expression of relationship of one measurable value to another, or a formula based on measurable values.

i., oral hygiene, simplified (Greene-Vermillion index) An index made up of two components, the debris index and the calculus index, which are based on numerical determination representing the amount of debris or calculus found on six preselected tooth surfaces.

i., periodontal disease (Russell index) An index that measures the condition of both the gingiva and the bone individually for each tooth and arrives at the average status for periodontal disease in a given mouth.

i., periodontal (Ramfjord index) A thorough clinical examination of the periodontal status of six teeth:

$$\frac{6}{41} \quad \frac{14}{6}$$

with an evaluation of the gingival condition, pocket depth, calculus and plaque deposits, attrition, mobility, and lack of contact.

i., PMA (Schour-Massler index) An index used for recording the prevalence and severity of gingivitis in schoolchildren by noting and scoring three areas: the gingival papillae (P), the buccal or labial gingival margin (M), and the attached gingiva (A).

i., Pont's The relation of the width of the four incisors to the width between the first premolars and the width between the first molars.

i., Russell *See* index, periodontal disease.

i., salivary lactobacillus A count of the lactobacilli per milliliter of saliva; used as an indicator of present dental caries activity. The test is of questionable value in individual patients, although its use in large groups led to valuable information on caries activity.

i., saturation A number indicating the hemoglobin content of a person's red blood cells as compared with the normal content.

i., therapeutic The ratio of toxic dose to effective dose.

i., ventilation The index obtained by dividing the ventilation test by the vital capacity.

indication That which serves as a guide or warning.

indicator diseases Opportunistic infectious diseases or neoplastic diseases that are associated with a primary immunodeficiency disease such as caused by the retrovirus HIV-I.

indirect method *See* method, indirect.

indirect pulp capping *See* capping, pulp, indirect.

indirect retention *See* retention, indirect.

individual practice association (IPA) 1. Organization for the maintenance of the solo private practitioner as a lobbying force and vocal springboard. **2.** A legal entity organized and operated on behalf of individual participating dentists for the primary purpose of collectively entering into contracts to provide dental services to enrolled populations. Dentists may practice in their own offices and may provide care to patients not covered by the contract as well as to IPA patients.

inositol An essential growth factor in tissue culture with no known human requirement. It has been used therapeutically in the management of diseases associated with the metabolism of fat.

individual retirement account (IRA) A savings certificate exempt from income tax until the time of withdrawal. There are limits to the amount that can be saved annually under this plan, and there are conditions of withdrawal for maximal interest and tax advantage.

induced Produced artificially.

induction The act or process of inducing or causing to occur.

indurated Hardened.

i. tissue Soft tissue that is abnormally firm because of an influx of exudate or fibrous tissue elements.

industrial dentistry 1: Dentistry that is concerned with the dental health of the worker as it affects the working environment. **2:** Dental service provided in the plant, usually restricted to emergency care.

inertia (ĭn-er'shuh) According to Newton's law of inertia, the tendency of a body that is at rest to remain at rest and a body that is in motion to continue in motion with constant speed in the same straight line unless acted on by an outside force.

infantilism (ĭn-făn'tĭ-lĭsm) A disturbance marked by mental retardation and retention of childhood characteristics into adult life. Teeth may be delayed in eruption or absent.

infarct (ĭn'farkt) Death of a tissue due to partial occlusion of a vessel or vessels supplying the area.

infection (ĭn-fĕk'shŭn) Invasion of the tissues of the body by disease-producing microorganisms and the reaction of these tissues to the microorganisms and/ or their toxins. The mere presence of microorganisms without reaction is not evidence of infection.

i., focal The process in which microorganisms located at a certain site (focus) in the body are disseminated throughout the body to set up secondary sites (foci) of infection in other tissues.

i., hemolytic streptococcal 1: Infection usually caused by Group A hemolytic streptococci. Such infections include scarlet fever, streptococcal sore throat, cellulitis, and osteomyelitis. **2:** An infection caused by streptococci that produce a toxic substance (hemolysin) that will lyse the erythrocytes and liberate hemoglobin from red blood cells.

i. resistance The ability of an individual to fight off the detrimental effects of microorganisms and their toxic products. A complexity involving individual and interacting factors, e.g., antibody formation, adequate nutrition, tissue tone, circulation, and emotional stability.

i. susceptibility The degree of capability of being influenced by or involved in the pathologic processes produced by microorganisms and/or their toxins.

i., Vincent's *See* gingivitis, necrotizing ulcerative.

infection control Procedures and protocols designed to prevent of limit cross contamination in the health care delivery environment.

infectious mononucleosis A benign lymphadenosis caused by the Epstein-Barr virus and characterized by fever, sore throat, enlargement of lymph nodes and spleen, and prolonged weakness with a characteristic shift in the white blood cells during the course of the disease.

infiltrate (ĭn-fĭl'trāt) Material deposited by infiltration.

infiltration (ĭn"fĭl-trā'shŭn) Accumulation in a tissue of a substance not normal to it.

i., inflammatory Influx or accumulation of inflammatory elements (cellular and exudative) in the interstices of the tissues as a result of tissue injury by physical, chemical, microbiologic, and other irritants. Cellular elements include lymphocytes, plasma cells, polymorphonuclear leukocytes, and/or the macrophages of reticuloendothelial origin.

i., local The prevention of excitation of the free nerve endings by literally flooding the immediate area with a local anesthetic solution.

inflammation (ĭn"flah-mā'shŭn) The cellular and vascular response or reaction to injury. It is characterized by pain, redness, swelling, heat, and disturbance of function. It may be acute or chronic. The term is not synonymous with infection, which implies an inflammatory reaction initiated by invasion of living organisms.

i., gingival *See* gingivitis.

i., granulomatous Chronic inflammation in which there is formation of granulation tissue.

i., periodontal *See* periodontitis. inflation (infla'shun) The act of distending with air or with a gas.

influences, local environmental Factors or agents within the oral cavity that are responsible for the initiation, perpetuation, or modification of a pathologic state within the stomatognathic system.

influences, systemic environmental Systemic factors that may initiate, perpetuate, or modify disease processes within the stomatognathic system. Generally, the oral manifestations of systemic disease are modified by the influence of local environmental factors.

information A meaningful collection of data as perceived by its user.

i. retrieval The methods and procedures for recovering specific information from stored data.

i. system A computerized system with the capability of manipulating and processing data in different ways to facilitate their interpretation and use.

informed consent Agreement by a patient, verbal or written, to have a procedure performed after being told in sufficient detail of possible risks.

infrabony pocket (ĭn'frah-bō-nē) *See* pocket, infrabony.

infrabulge (ĭn'frăh-bulj) The surface of the crown of a tooth cervical to the clasp guide line, survey line, or surveyed height of contour.

infraclusion (ĭn"frah-kloo'zhŭn) **(infraversion)** The position occupied by a tooth when it has failed to erupt sufficiently to reach the occlusal plane.

infracrestal pocket (ĭn"frah-krĕs'tal) *See* pocket, infrabony.

infradentale (ĭn"frah-dĕn-tă'lē) The most anterior point of the alveolar process of the mandible.

infraversion (ĭn"frah-ver'zhŭn) *See* infraclusion.

infusion **1:** Therapeutic introduction of a fluid, e.g., saline solution, into a vein. In contrast to injection, infusion suggests the introduction of a larger volume of a less concentrated solution over a more protracted period. **2:** A term used in pharmacy for a liquid extract prepared by steeping a plant substance in water.

ingate *See* sprue.

inhalant (ĭn-hā'lănt) A medicine to be inhaled.

inhalation (ĭn-hah-lā'shŭn) The drawing of air or other vapor into the lungs.

i., endotracheal Inhalation of an anesthetic mixture into the lungs through an endotracheal catheter at low or atmospheric pressure.

inhaler, nasal A device that is placed over the nose to permit inhalation of anesthetic agents.

inhibition (ĭn"hĭ-bĭsh'ŭn) A neurologic phenomenon associated with the transmission of an impulse across a synapse. An impulse can be blocked from passing a synapse in a reflex situation by the firing of another, more dominant nerve. Inhibition can be achieved directly by preventing the passage of an impulse along an axon, or it can be achieved by liberation of a chemical substance at the nerve ending. This chemical inhibition is demonstrated by the sympathetic-parasympathetic control over smooth muscle activity in a blood vessel. Inhibition is the restraining of a function of a tissue or organ by some nervous or hormonic control. It is the opposite of excitation.

inhibitor of cholinesterase (ĭn-hĭb'ĭ-tor, kō"lĭn-ĕs'terās) A chemical that interferes with the activity of the enzyme cholinesterase.

inhouse A computer located onsite, in the building where used, instead of being located remotely.

inion (ĭn'ē-on) The most elevated point on the external occipital protuberance in the midsagittal plane.

initialize To set counters, switches, and addresses to 0 or other starting values at the beginning of, or at prescribed points in, a computer routine.

initiator (ĭ-nĭsh'ē-ā"tor) A chemical agent added to a resin to initiate polymerization.

injection (ĭn-jĕk´shŭn) The act of introducing a liquid into a part such as the bloodstream or tissue.

i. molding *See* molding, injection.

injury The insult, harm, or hurt applied to tissues; may evoke dystrophic and/or inflammatory response from the affected part.

i., root Damage to the root, especially to the cementum, when an excessive force is placed on the tooth.

i., toothbrush Insult or damage to the teeth and their investing structures produced by faulty toothbrushing,

inlay restoration of metal, fired porcelain, or plastic made to fit a tapered cavity preparation and fastened to or luted into it with a cementing medium.

i. furnace *See* furnace, inlay.

i., setting The procedure of fitting a casting to a preparation; adjusting the occlusal function and contact areas; securing the proper, clean dry field; cementing the cleaned, polished casting in an aseptic, dry prepared cavity; and completing the final finishing and polishing of the restoration.

i. wax *See* wax, inlay.

innervation (ĭn″er-vā´shŭn) Distribution or supply of nerves to a part.

i., reciprocal The simultaneous excitation of one muscle with the inhibition of its antagonist. Rhythmic chewing is achieved efficiently when the masticatory muscles are reciprocally innervated, permitting alternate elevation and depression of the mandible in a smooth, coordinated sequence of actions.

input, computer The data to be processed.

input/output control (I/O control) The portion of the central processor of some computer systems that contains electronics for supervising data flow between memory and the input/output devices connected to the CPU.

inquiry A request for information from storage in a computer.

insert, intramucosal (ĭn″trah-mū-kō´săl) **(mucosal insert, implant button)** A nonreactive metal appliance that is affixed to the tissue-bone surface of a denture and offers added retentive qualities to the denture. An intramucosal insert consists of a base, cervix, and head.

insert, mucosal *See* insert, intramucosal.

insertion (ĭn-ser´shŭn) The act of implanting, placing, or introducing the needle into the tissues.

i., path of The direction in which a prosthesis is inserted and removed.

insidious (ĭn-sĭd´ē-ŭs) Coming on in a stealthy manner.

insoluble Not susceptible to being dissolved.

inspection Visual examination of the body or portions thereof, which is an integral phase of the physical or dental examination procedure.

inspiration The act of drawing air into the lungs.

inspirator (ĭn´spĭ-rā″tor) A form of inhaler or respirator.

inspirometer (ĭn-spĭ-rom´ĕ-ter) An instrument for measuring the force, frequency, or volume of the inspirations.

instruction A set of characters, together with one or more addresses, that defines a computer operation and, as a unit, causes the computer to operate accordingly on the indicated quantities; a term associated with software operation.

i. of partial denture patient *See* denture, partial, instruction of patient.

instrument(s) A tool or implement, especially one used for delicate or scientific work.

i., carving *See* carver.

i., classification of, names Classification of instruments by name to denote purpose (e.g., excavator), to denote position or manner of use (e.g., hand condenser), to describe the form of the point (e.g., hatchet), or to describe the angle of the blade in relation to the handle.

i., cutting An instrument used to cut, cleave, or plane the walls of a cavity preparation; the blade ends in a sharp, beveled edge. Unless otherwise specified, it refers to a hand instrument rather than to a rotary type.

i., bibeveled cutting (bi´bĕv-ĕld) An instrument in which both sides of the end of the blade are beveled to form the cutting edge, as in a hatchet.

i., rotary cutting A power-activated instrument used in a dental handpiece, e.g., a bur, mounted diamond point, mounted carborundum point, wheel stone, or disk.

i., single-beveled cutting An instrument in which one side of the end of the blade is beveled to form the cutting edge, as in a wood chisel.

i., diamond A rotary abrasive instrument, wheel, or mounted point. Made of fine diamond chips bonded into a desired form; used to reduce tooth structure.

i., double-plane An instrument with the curve of the blade in a plane perpendicular to that of the angles of the shank.

i., formula name of Method of naming and describing dental hand instruments. Measurements are in the metric system. The working point is described first, and then the formula is given in three (or sometimes four) units. The first figure denotes the width of the blade in tenths of millimeters, the second shows the length of the blade in millimeters, and the third indicates the angle of the blade in relation to the shaft in centrigrades or hundredths of a circle. Whenever it is necessary to describe the angle of the cutting edge of a blade with its shaft, the number is entered in brackets as the second number of the formula. Paired instruments are also designated as right or left. In lateral cutting instruments the one used to cut from right to left is termed right; in direct cutting instruments with right and left bevels, the one having the bevel on the right side of the blade as it is held with the cutting edge down and pointing away from the observer is termed right.

i. grasp *See* grasp, instrument.

i., hand An instrument used principally with hand force.

i., holding An instrument used to support gold foil while a foil restoration is inserted.

i., McCall's Periodontal instruments designed by John Oppie McCall; used for gingival curettage and for removing accretions from the tooth surfaces.

i., parts Handle or shaft, blade or nib, and shank.

i. blade The part bearing a cutting edge; it begins at the terminal angle of the shank and ends at the cutting edge.

i. nib The counterpart of the blade in the condensing instrument; the end of the nib is the face.

i. shaft or handle The part that is grasped by the operator's hand while using the instrument.

i. shank The part that connects the shaft and the blade or nib.

i., plastic An instrument used to manipulate a plastic restorative material.

i., screwdriver An instrument made of surgical alloy; it may have a screw holder at its tip designed to drive screws into the bone.

i. sharpening *See* sharpening, instrument.

i., single-plane An instrument with all its angles and curves in one plane; when the instrument lies on a flat surface, the cutting edge and the blade will parallel the surface.

i. stop A device, usually metal, that can be placed on a reamer or file to mark the measurement of the root.

instrumentation (ĭn″stroo-mĕn-ta′shŭn) The use of, or work done by, instruments in the treatment of a patient.

insufficiency, adrenocortical (ah-drē″nō-kor′tĭ-kăl) *See* hypoadrenocorticalism.

insufficiency, functional Inadequacy of usage of, stimulation to, a part of the body, often resulting in atrophic tissue changes.

insufflation (ĭn″sŭ-flā′shŭn) The act of blowing a powder, vapor, gas, or air into a cavity, e.g., into the lungs.

i., endotracheal The forcing of an anesthetic mixture into the lungs through an endotracheal catheter under pressure.

i., mouth-to-mouth The oldest recorded procedure for artificially ventilating the lungs. The lungs are inflated by blowing into the mouth, and expiration either is passive or is assisted by compressing the thorax. Adequate ventilation is produced, and the procedure should be used when other techniques are not applicable, e.g., in thoracic injury. Auxiliary airway tubes are available for use when mouth-to-mouth insufflation is required. Such tubes maintain the airway and prevent the tongue from obstructing the glottis.

insufflator (ĭn′suh-flā″tor) An instrument used in insufflation.

insulator, thermal A material having a low thermal conductivity.

insulin (antidiabetic hormone) A hormone produced by the beta cells of the islets of Langerhans in the pancreas. It promotes a decrease in blood sugar. Its action may be influenced by the pituitary growth hormone, ACTH, "S" hormones of the adrenal cortex, epinephrine, glucagon, and thyroid hormone.

i. shock *See* shock, insulin.

insurance A contract (policy) whereby, for a stipulated consideration (premium), one party (insurer or underwriter) promises to compensate the other (insured or assured) for loss on a specified subject (insurable interest) by specified perils (risks).

i., group Insurance covering a group of persons, usually employees of a single employer or members of a union local, under one contract for the benefit of the members of the group.

i., guaranteed renewable A policy that is renewable at the option of the insured until a stated time, such as the 70th birthday of the insured. *See* noncancellable insurance.

i., health Insurance that provides financial return when the dentist is unable to practice due to prolonged illness.

i., liability Insurance protecting the dentist from financial loss due to liability suits.

i., life A protective contract providing for compensation to the beneficiaries of the insured.

i., malpractice In dentistry, insurance covering accidents or catastrophes that may occur during the performance of professional duties.

i., retirement Life insurance that carries, as an additional benefit, payments to the insured when he or she reaches a specific age.

insurer An organization that bears the financial risk for the cost of defined categories or services for a defined group of beneficiaries; *see* third party.)

insured person covered by the program. (*See* Beneficiary)

intake The substance or quantities thereof taken in and used by the body.

intelligence Mental potential or capacity; an individual's total repertoire of those problem-solving and cognitive discrimination responses that are usual and expected at a given age level and in the large population unit; that which is measured by an intelligence test.

i. quotient (IQ) An estimate of intelligence level; an index determined by dividing the mental age in months by the chronological age in months and multiplying the result by 100. Thus, the IQ of a child of 100 months with a mental age of 110 months would be 110.

  i., dental, quotient An estimated appraisal of a patient's knowledge and appreciation of dental services.

intensifying screen *See* screen, intensifying.

intensity of an x-ray beam The amount of energy in an x-ray beam per unit volume or area.

  i., radiation Energy flowing through a unit area perpendicular to the beam per unit of time. It is expressed in ergs per square centimeter or in watts per square centimeter.

interaction According to Newton's law of interaction, the phenomenon in which every force is accompanied by an equal and opposite force. For every force there are two bodies—one to exert the force and one to receive it. Furthermore, whenever there is one force, another force must also be involved. If there is force to the right on one body, there is force to the left on another. Since the one force acts as long as the other, the impulses are equal. The total momentum of the two interacting bodies cannot change. Continuous interaction is demonstrated between the food that is masticated and the force applied to the food.

interalveolar space (ĭn″ter-ăl-vē′ō-lar) *See* distance, interarch.

interarch distance *See* distance, interarch.

interceptive occlusal contact *See* contact, interceptive occlusal.

interceptive orthodontics An extension of preventive orthodontics that may include minor local tooth movement in an otherwise normally developing dentition.

intercondylar distance (ĭn″ter-kon′dĭ-lar) The distance between the vertical axes of a pair of condyles.

intercuspation (ĭn″ter-kŭs-pā′shŭn) The cusp-to-fossa relationship of the upper and lower posterior teeth to each other.

interdental (ĭn″ter-dĕn′tal) Situated between the proximal surfaces of adjacent teeth.

  i. canal *See* canal, interdental.

  i. embrasure *See* embrasure, interdental.

  i. septum *See* septum, interdental.

  i. splint *See* splint, interdental.

interdigitation (ĭn″ter-dĭj″ĭ-tā′shŭn) *See* intercuspation.

interface (ĭn′ter-fās) The surface, such as a plane surface, formed between the walls of a prepared cavity or extracoronal preparation and a restoration. It forms a common boundary between the tooth structure and the restorative material.

  i., computer A common boundary (connection) between automatic data processing systems or parts of a system.

interfacial surface tension *See* tension, interfacial surface.

interference, cuspal *See* contact, deflective occlusal.

interference, occlusal Any tooth-to-tooth contact that interferes with jaw movement.

interincisal angle The A-P angle made by the intersection of the long axis of the maxillary central incisor with the mandibular central incisor. Statistically a normal angle is about 130 degrees. A more acute angle may indicate proclined incisor, a more obtuse angle may indicate a retracted incisor.

interferon A small class of glycoproteins capable of exerting antiviral activity in homologous cells through metabolic processes involving synthesis of RNA.

  i. alpha Formed by leukocytes in response to viral infection and/or by stimulation with double-stranded RNA. These protein products are used as antineoplastic agents. Specifically used as an antineoplastic agent for the treatment of Kaposi sarcoma in AIDS patients.

  i. beta Formed by fibroblasts by similar stimulation as the alpha form.

  i. gamma Formed by lymphocytes in response to mitogenic stimulation.

interleukin-2 A hormone produced by T helper and suppressor lymphocytes that function to control the expansion and reactivity of T lymphocytes. Used to boost the immune system in HIV-positive patients.

Integral endosseous implant system An endosseous implant system provisionally accepted by the ADA.

International classification of diseases (ICD) Diagnostic codes designed for the classification of morbidity and mortality information for statistical purposes, and for the indexing of hospital records by disease and operations, for data storage and retrieval.

interocclusal contacts Tooth contact between maxillary and mandibular teeth in closure.

interocclusal distance The distance between the maxillary and mandibular teeth when the mandible is in the rest position or other defined position of the mandible to maxillary.

interradicular osseous defect Radiographic evidence of a discontinuity in the bony image in the area between the roots of a multirooted tooth.

interim denture *See* denture, interim.

intermaxillary Between the maxillae and mandible.

  i. anchorage *See* anchorage, intermaxillary.

  i. elastic *See* elastic, maxillomandibular.

  i. fixation *See* fixation, maxillomandibular.

  i. relation *See* relation, maxillomandibular.

  i. traction *See* traction, maxillomandibular.

intermedin (ĭn-ter-mē′dĭn) *See* hormone, melanocytes-timulating.

intern A dental or medical college graduate serving and residing for 12 months in a hospital, usually during the first year after receiving a D.D.S., D.M.D., or M. D. degree.

interocclusal (ĭn″ter-ŏ-kloo′sal) Between the occlusal surfaces of the maxillary and mandibular teeth.

i. clearance *See* clearance, interocclusal.

i. distance *See* distance, interocclusal.

i. gap *See* distance, interocclusal.

i. record *See* record, interocclusal.

i. rest space *See* distance, interocclusal.

interoceptors (ĭn″ter-ŏ-sĕp′torz) Those sensory nerve end receptors lining the mucous membrane of the respiratory and digestive tracts. They are similar to exteroceptors but differ from them essentially in their location, which is in the viscera.

interpolate (ĭn-ter′pō-lāt) To insert intermediate terms in a series according to the trend of the series; to calculate intermediate values according to observed values.

interposition arthroplasty (ăr′thrō-plăs″tē) The surgical correction of ankylosis by the separating of the immobile fragment from the mobilized fragment and the interpositioning of a substance—such as fascia, cartilage, metal, or plastic—between them. *See also* ankylosis.

interpretation Translation of radiographic changes seen by the dentist into real variations in the object radiographed for diagnostic purposes.

i., radiographic (radiologic interpretation, roentgenographic interpretation) An opinion formed from the study of a radiograph.

i., radiologic *See* interpretation, radiographic.

interproximal Between the proximal surfaces of adjoining teeth.

interradicular alveoloplasty (ĭn″ter-rah-dĭk′ū-lar ălvē′ōlō-plăs″tē) **(intraseptal alveoloplasty)** Removal of the interradicular bone and the collapsing of the cortical plates to a more normal alveolar contour. *See also* alveolectomy.

interridge distance *See* distance, interarch.

interview A question-and-answer conference, at which time the parties concerned state the principles and facts regarding their relationship. In dental practice, this usually refers to the relationship between dentist and employee, and between dentist and patient.

intolerance Inability to endure or withstand.

intra-arterial Situated within an artery or arteries.

intracellular (ĭn″trah-sĕl′ū-lar) Situated or occurring within a cell or cells.

intracoronal (ĭn″trah-kō-rō′nal) Pertaining to the inside of the coronal portion of a natural tooth.

i. attachment *See* attachment, intracoronal

i. retainer *See* retainer, intracoronal.

intramaxillary anchorage *See* anchorage, intramaxillary.

intramaxillary elastic *See* elastic, intramaxillary.

intramucosal insert *See* insert, intramucosal.

intramuscular (ĭn″trah-mŭs′kū-lar) Situated in the substance of a muscle.

intraoral (ĭn″trah-or′al) Within the mouth.

i. tracing *See* tracing, intraoral.

intraosseous fixation (ĭn″trah-os′ē-ŭs) *See* fixation, intraosseous.

intrapulmonary (ĭn″trah-pul′mō-ner″ē) Situated in the substance of a lung.

intrapulmonic (ĭn″trah-pul-mon′ĭk) Occurring in the substance of the lungs.

intravenation (ĭn″trah-vē-nā′shŭn) The act of injecting anything into a vein.

intravenous (ĭn″trah-vē′nŭs) In, into, or from within a vein or veins.

intraversion Indicating teeth or other maxillary structures that are too near the medial plane.

intrinsic coloring Coloring from within; the incorporation of pigment within the material of a prosthesis.

intrude To move a tooth apically.

intrusion A depression; an inward projection.

intubate (ĭn′tū-bāt) To treat by intubation.

intubation (ĭn″tū-bā′shŭn) Insertion of a tube; especially the introduction of a tube into the larynx through the glottis for the introduction of air, etc.

intubator (ĭn′tū-bāt-or) An instrument used in intubation.

inunction (ĭn-ŭngk′shŭn) Local application of a drug in an oily or semisolid vehicle, such as an ointment, or the preparation that is thus applied.

invagination of enamel *See* dens in dente.

i., epithelial Downgrowth of epithelium along the cervical tract of an implant.

inventory An itemized compilation of materials on hand.

i., equipment A detailed listing of all the nonexpendable items owned by the dentist and used in the practice of the profession.

i., materials A detailed listing of expendable supplies that are on hand in the practice. This is a constantly fluctuating list, depending on the quantity of the various materials presently on hand.

inverse-square law *See* law, inverse-square.

inversion The state of being upside down.

invest (ĭn-vĕst′) To surround, envelop, or embed in an investment material. e.g., a gypsum product.

investing (ĭn-vĕst′ĭng) The process of covering or enveloping wholly or in part an object.

i., vacuum The investing of a pattern within a vacuum to form a mold.

investment (ĭn-vĕst′mĕnt) The material used to enclose or surround a pattern of a dental restoration for casting or molding or to maintain the relations of metal parts during soldering.

i., casting Material from which the casting mold is made in fabrication of gold or cobalt-chromium castings.

i., gypsum-bonded casting Casting investment that can be bonded by alpha-hemihydrate, a derivative of gypsum, because the fusion temperatures of the metal alloys to be cast in it are relatively low. All gold alloy investments and some low-fusing cobalt-chromium alloy investments are gypsum bonded.

i., phosphate-bonded casting Casting investment that is bonded by a phosphate and a metallic oxide that react to form a hard mass; generally used for high-fusing alloys.

i., silica-bonded casting Casting investment that is bonded by a silica gel that reverts to cristobalite in heating and is generally used for highfusing alloys.

i., hygroscopic An investment specially designed for use with the hygroscopic investing techniques.

i., refractory An investment material that can withstand the high temperatures used in soldering or casting.

i., sectional A mold made in sections.

i., soldering A quartz investment, preferably one with a very low thermal expansion, used for the investment of appliances during the soldering procedure.

involucrum (ĭn″vō-lū′krŭm) A covering; usually a covering of new bone around a sequestrum.

involuntary Performed independently of the will.

involute (ĭn′vō-loot) To decrease normally, in size and functional activity, an organ whose role in the body economy is temporary or confined to certain periods of life. Involute should be distinguished from atrophy, which means to waste away from abnormal causes.

involvement The state of becoming involved.

i., bifurcation (bī″fŭr-kā′shŭn) The extension of pocket formation into the interradicular area of multirooted teeth in periodontitis.

i., pulp A condition wherein consideration of the vitality or health of the dental pulp is a factor.

i., trifurcation *See* involvement, bifurcation.

iodine A halogen element that is nonmetallic in nature; atomic weight, 126.91. Essential as a nutritional element because it is vital to the production of thyroxin by the thyroid gland. In radioactive form, it is used as a diagnostic substance to determine the ability of the thyroid gland to take up iodine. In tincture form it is used as a locally applied antiseptic, germicide, and disclosing solution.

i., protein-bound (PBI) Iodine bound to protein, mainly thyroxin in the plasma. The thyroid hormone is precipitated by protein-denaturing agents, and, in general, the amount of iodine in a protein precipitate indicates the amount of thyroid hormone present and is thus an index of thyroid activity. Various values are given for thyroid function: hypothyroidism, 0 to 3.5 μg/ml of protein-bound iodine; euthyroidism, 3.5 to 8 μg/ml; hyperthyroidism, values higher than 8 μg/ml.

iodism (iodine poisoning, iodine stomatitis) Acute or chronic intoxication due to the ingestion or absorption of iodides. Manifestations of acute poisoning include abdominal pain, nausea, vomiting, hypersalivation, conjunctivitis, and collapse. Chronic manifestations include hypersalivation, fever, coryza, swelling and tenderness of the salivary glands, and dermatitis and stomatitis in hypersensitive individuals. It is a toxic condition that sometimes follows the use of preparations containing iodine.

iodophor (ī-ō′dō-for) A loose chemical compound of iodine with certain organic compounds, e.g., polyvinylpyrrolidone.

ion (ī′on) An atomic particle, atom, or chemical radical bearing an electric charge, either negative or positive.

i. pair Two particles of opposite charge, usually the electron and the positive atomic residue resulting after the interaction of ionizing radiation with the orbital electrons of atoms. The average energy required to produce an ion pair is approximately 33 (or 34) electron volts.

ionization (ī″on-ĭ-zā′shŭn) The process or the result of a process by which a neutral atom or molecule acquires either a positive or a negative charge.

i. chamber *See* chamber, ionization.

i., air-equivalent, chamber *See* chamber, ionization, air-equivalent.

i. density The number of ion pairs per unit volume.

i. path (ionization track) The trail of ion pairs produced by ionizing radiation in its passage through matter.

i. potential The potential necessary to separate one electron from an atom, resulting in the formation of an ion pair.

ionizer *See* electrolyzer.

iontophoresis (ī-on″tō-fō-rē′sĭs) Application, by means of an appropriate electrode, of a galvanic current to an ionizable agent in contact with a surface to hasten the movement into the tissue of the ion of opposite charge to that of the electrode. *See also* ionization.

IQ *See* intelligence quotient.

irradiation (ĭ-rā″dē-ā′shŭn) **1:** The exposure of material to roentgen or other radiation. (One speaks of radiation therapy but of irradiation of the patient.) **2:** Exposure to radiation.

irresuscitable (ĭr″rē-sŭs′ĭ-tah-bl) Beyond the possibility of being revived.

irreversibility (ĭr″rē-ver″sĭ-bĭl′ĭ-tē) The quality of being incapable of being revived.

irreversible (ĭr″rē-ver′sĭ-bl) Incapable of being reversed or returned to the original state.

i. hydrocolloid *See* hydrocolloid, irreversible.

irrigation (ĭr″ĭ-gā′shŭn) The technique of using a solution to wash or flush debris from the root canal or from a wound.

irritability The quality of being irritable or of responding to a stimulus.

irritant 1: An agent that causes an irritation or stimulation. **2:** An agent (toxic, bacterial, physical, chemical, etc.) that is capable of inducing functional derangements or organic lesions of the tissues.

    i., chemical A chemical agent that causes irritation. The primary agents that have an etiologic relationship to periodontal disease are plaque and calculus. Other agents that serve as a medium for the growth of microorganisms include food debris, sloughed cells, and necrotic material.

irritation The act of stimulating. Any condition of functional derangement and nervous irritability.

    i. of gingival tissues *See* impingement.

    i., mechanical Tissue damage, injury, or insult by physical forces directed against the tissue, e.g., the tissue irritation produced by faulty toothbrushing.

    i. from overstimulation *See* impingement.

ischemia (ĭs-kē′mē-ah) A focal deficiency of blood to a part of the body or simply a local anemia. It results from encroachment of the lumen of an artery or the capillaries supplying the affected area. The reduction in the lumen may be caused by allergic hypersensitivity, degeneration of the tunica intima (atherosclerosis), inflammation, physical pressure, pharmacologic and toxic agents, and/or neurogenic disorders.

isobar (ī′sō-bahr) In radiochemistry, one of two or more different nuclides having the same mass number.

isolation of tooth A technique to protect the tooth against contamination from oral fluids during a surgical or restorative procedure, usually through the application of a rubber dam or the use of cotton roles.

isoleucine One of the essential amino acids. *See* amino acid.

isomers (ī′sō-merz) **1:** Organic compounds having the same empirical formula, i.e., the same number of the same atoms, but different structural formulas and therefore different physical and chemical properties.

2: One of several nuclides having the same number of neutrons and protons but capable of existing, for a measurable time, in different quantum states with different energies and radioactive properties. The isomer of higher energy commonly decays to one with lower energy by a process known as isomeric transition.

    i., optical Two isomers whose structures, dextro- and levo-, differ only in a spatial arrangement that makes them mirror images. This occurs only when there is an asymmetric carbon atom, i.e., one attached to four different substituents. The pharmacologic activity often resides very largely in one of the two forms.

    i., stereo- Molecules that differ only in the spatial arrangement of the atoms. This term includes optical isomers.

isometric muscle contraction (ī″sō-mĕt′rĭk) *See* contraction, muscle, isometric.

isosthenuria (ī″sos-thĕ-nū′rē-ah) Excretion of urine with fixed specific gravity. It may occur in terminal renal disease when the specific gravity reaches that of the glomerular filtrate, 1.010.

isotone (ī′sō-tōn) One of several different nuclides having the same number of neutrons in their nuclei, but different mass numbers.

isotonic (ī″sō-ton′ĭk) Equivalent in osmotic pressure. Specifically used in reference to a solution whose osmotic pressure is equal to that of a body fluid, such as blood plasma or tears, to which it is compared.

    i. muscle contraction *See* contraction, muscle, isotonic.

isotope (ī′sō-tōp) One of several nuclides having the same number of protons in their nuclei, and hence having the same atomic number but differing in the number of neutrons, and therefore in the mass number. The isotopes of a particular element have virtually identical chemical properties.

    i., stable A nonradioactive isotope of an element.

Ivalon sponge Polyvinyl alcohol sponge.

Ivy loop wiring *See* wiring, Ivy loop.

Ivy's test *See* test, Ivy's.

jacket *See* crown, complete, veneer, acrylic resin; crown, complete, veneer, porcelain.

jackscrew A threaded device used in appliances for separation or approximation of teeth or jaw segments.

Jackson's sign *See* sign, Jackson's.

Janet's test *See* test, Janet's.

jaundice (jawn'dĭs) A condition characterized by an abnormal accumulation of bilirubin (red bile pigment) in the blood and manifested by a yellowish discoloration of the skin, mucous membranes, and cornea. Seen in hemolytic anemias, biliary obstruction, hepatitis, cholangiolitis, cirrhosis of the liver, etc. Oral mucous membranes may be pigmented.

j., acholuric Jaundice without bile in the urine.

j., epidemic *See* disease, Weil's.

j., hemolytic (prehepatic jaundice) Excess bile pigments in the blood resulting from increased destruction of erythrocytes.

j., congenital hemolytic (acholuric icterus, spherocytic anemia, hereditary spherocytosis) A familial hemolytic anemia transmitted as a mendelian dominant. The intrinsic defects of the red blood cells include a spheroidal shape (which allows them to be trapped by the spleen) and increased mechanical fragility.

j., hepatic *See* jaundice, hepatocellular.

j., hepatocellular (hepatic jaundice, infective jaundice, medical jaundice, toxic jaundice) Jaundice resulting from disease of liver cells by infectious agents or toxins, decreasing the ability of the liver to handle the bile pigments that are continually produced by the destruction of red blood cells.

j., homologous serum *See* hepatitis, homologus serum.

j., infective *See* jaundice, hepatocellular.

j., latent Increased bilirubin in the blood without clinical signs of jaundice.

j., medical *See* jaundice, hepatocellular.

j., obstructive (posthepatic jaundice) Extrahepatic and intrahepatic obstruction of the biliary tract, resulting in retrograde retention of bile pigments and jaundice.

j., posthepatic *See* jaundice, obstructive.

j., prehepatic *See* jaundice, hemolytic.

j., regurgitating Jaundice resulting from reentry of conjugated bilirubin into the blood as a result of obstruction of the biliary tract or hepatocellular damage and failure to excrete conjugated bilirubin from liver cells.

j., retention An increase in bilirubin in the blood from hemolysis; failure of the liver cells to conjugate bilirubin or remove free bilirubin.

j., surgical Extrahepatic obstruction of the biliary tract.

j., syringe *See* hepatitis, homologous serum.

j., toxic *See* jaundice, hepatocellular.

jaw A common name for either the maxillae or the mandible; the meaning is usually extended to include their soft tissue covering.

j., cleftz (gnathoschisis) *See* palate, cleft.

j.-to-jaw relationship *See* relation, jaw.

j., lumpy *See* actinomycosis.

j. movement *See* movement, jaw.

j., phossy *See* poisoning, phosphorus.

j. reflex *See* reflex, jaw.

j. relation *See* relation, jaw.

JCAHO An acronym for the Joint Commission on Accreditation of Healthcare Organizations.

jelly, petroleum *See* petrolatum.

Johnston's method *See* method, chloropercha.

joint(s) The junction of union between two or more bones or cartilages of the skeleton.

j., Charcots (shar-cōz') A manifestation of late syphilis in which there is degeneration, hypertrophy, hypermobility, and loss of contour of a joint, usually a weight-bearing joint. It is most common in tabes dorsalis.

j., diarthrosis (dīärth'rō-sĭs) A joint that moves freely in contact. The adjacent bone surfaces are typically covered by a film of cartilage and are bound by stout connective tissues, frequently enclosing a liquid-filled joint cavity.

j., hinge *See* ginglymus.

j. mice Cartilaginous material present in the synovial spaces of a joint.

j., synarthrosis (sĭn"ăr-thrō'sĭs) **(junctura fibrosa, fibrous joint)** A joint in which the bony elements are connected by thin intervening layers of cartilage, connective tissue, or direct contact of bone to bone such as the rigid unions in the adult skull.

j., temporomandibular *See* articulation, temporomandibular.

Joint Commission on Accreditation of Health Care Organizations (JCAHO). Formerly the Joint Commission on Accreditation of Hospitals/ Formerly, Joint Commission on Accreditation of Hospitals. The JCAHO conducts accreditation programs for most of the health care facilities in the United States. The American Dental Association is a corporate member of the JCAHO. Hospitals and clinics are surveyed on a regular basis for compliance with the standards and criteria for accreditiation.

Joint Commission on Accreditation of Hospitals. *See* Joint Commission on Accreditation of Healthcare Organizations.

Jones protein *See* protein, Bence Jones.

Jorgensen's drug administration principles Principles employed in the selection and administration of intravenous sedative agents that have a wide margin of safety and predictable effects and which in combination can elevate the pain threshold, produce euphoria, have an antisialogogue effect, and promote an amnesic response. The principles include the sequence and rate of administration while monitoring patient response signs.

junction (jŭngk'shŭn) A place of coming together or union.

j., cementoenamel (cervical line) The junction of the enamel of the crown and the cementum of the root of a tooth. The area above the junction corresponds to the anatomic crown of the tooth; the area apical to the junction constitutes the anatomic root of the tooth.

j., dentinocemental The line of union or apposition of the cementum and dentin of a tooth.

j., dentinoenamel (dentoenamel junction) The interface of enamel and dentin of the tooth crown, conforming in a general way to the shape of the crown.

j., dentoenamel *See* junction, dentinoenamel.

j., dentogingival The junction between the gingival attachment, a nonkeratinized epithelium, and the tooth surface.

j., mucogingival The scalloped linear area denoting the approximation or separation of the gingivae and alveolar mucosa.

jurisprudence The philosophy of law.

j., dental (forensic dentistry) 1: The science that teaches the application of every branch of dental knowledge to the purposes of the law, including the elucidation of doubtful legal questions. **2:** The state laws and codes covering the legal limitations of the practice of the profession of dentistry.

j., medical The science that applies the principles and practice of the different branches of medicine in the elucidation of doubtful questions in a court of justice. Synonym: forensic medicine.

jury A certain number of citizens selected according to law and sworn to inquire of certain matters of fact and to declare the truth on evidence submitted to them.

just Right; according to law and justice.

justice The constant and perpetual disposition to render every man his due. Also, the conformity of one's actions and will to the law.

juvenile periodontitis A distinct form of periodontal disease that may present with either localized or generalized inflammatory changes in the periodontium of prepubertal children. The disease is characterized by severe pocketing and rapid destruction of alveolar bone. Several subtypes of the disease are recognized (formerly called *periodontosis*).

juxtaposition Adjacent situation; apposition or contact.

K

Kahn's test *See* test, Kahn's.

kakke (kahk'kā) *See* beriberi.

Kanamycin An aminoglycoside antibiotic which acts by inhibiting the synthesis of protein in susceptible organisms. Kanamycin requires close clinical supervision because of its potential toxicity and adverse side effects to the auditory and vestibular branches of the eighth cranial nerve and to the renal tubules.

kaolin (kā'ō-lĭn) A fine, pure-white clay (hydrated aluminum silicate) used in porcelain teeth.

Kaposi's sarcoma *See* sarcoma, Kaposi's.

Kazanjian's operation (kah-zăn'jē-ŭnz) *See* operation, Kazanjian's.

Kazanjian's procedure *See* operation, Kazanjian's.

keloid (kē'loid) A dense, proliferative growth on the skin (hypertrophy of scar tissue) that appears to be an abnormal reaction to trauma, especially burns. Keloids tend to recur after excision and occur more frequently in blacks than in whites.

keloplasty (kē'lō-plăs'tē) Excision of scar tissue in the skin.

Kendall's compound B *See* corticosterone.

Kendall's compound E *See* cortisone.

Kennedy bar *See* connector, minor, secondary lingual bar.

Kennedy classification A method of classifying partially edentulous conditions and partial dentures; based on the location of the edentulous spaces in relation to the remaining teeth.

keratin (kĕr'ăh-tĭn) An insoluble sulfur-containing protein with a high content of the amino acids tyrosine and leucine; the main component of epidermis, hair, nails, keratinized epithelium, etc.

keratinization (kĕr"ăh-tĭn"ĭ-zā-shŭn) The process of becoming keratinized.

keratoacanthoma (ker"ah-tō-ăk"ăn-thō'mah) A rapidly growing papular lesion with a superficial crater filled with keratin.

keratoconjunctivitis sicca (kĕr"ah-tō-kon-jŭnk"tĭ-vī-tĭs sĭ-k'ah) *See* syndrome, Sjögren's.

keratocyst (ker-ah'tō-sĭst) A hornified cyst.

keratohyalin granules (ker"ah-tō-hi'ah-lin) Basophilic granules (0.2 to 4.5 μ) found in cells of the stratum granulosum that are presumed to play a role in keratinization.

keratosis (ker"ah-tō'sĭs) **1:** A horny or cornified growth (e.g., wart, callosity). **2:** A condition characterized by cornification, or hyperkeratinization, of the tissues.

k. blennorrhagia A skin condition found in Reiter's syndrome characterized by pustules and crusting; once incorrectly associated with gonorrhea; more recently considered a genetic disorder occuring mostly in men between the ages of 20 and 25.

k., focal Localized areas of increased cornification (hyperkeratinization). Such lesions are seen particularly on the lips.

k. follicularis *See* disease, Darier's.

k., seborrheic (basal cell papilloma, verruca senilis) Benign, pigmented, superficial epithelial tumors that clinically appear to be pasted on the skin of the trunk, arms, or face. Characterized histologically by marked hyperkeratosis, with keratin cyst formation, acanthosis of basal cells, and melanin pigmentation, all above the level of the adjacent epidermis.

k., senile Small firm lesions occurring principally on the face and back of the hands in elderly people or those exposed to the sun. There is hyperkeratosis with irregular and atypical proliferation of the cells of the rete Malpighi. The condition is one of premalignancy with tendency toward epidermoid carcinoma. *See also* leukoplakia.

k., chronic senile Keratosis of the lips in elderly individuals. These lesions should be considered precancerous.

keratolytic agents Agents the loosen or remove the horny outer layer of the skin.

keratoplasty Corneal transplantation.

ketaconazole A broad-spectrum synthetic antifungal agent applied to the skin to inhibit the growth of dermatophytes and yeasts, effective in *Candida* infections and in the treatment of seborrheic dermatitis.

ketoacidosis (kē"tō-ăs"ĭ-dō'sĭs) A form of acidosis characterized by an increased accumulation of ketone bodies (acetoacetic acid, beta-hydroxybutyric acid, acetone) in the blood (e.g., the acidosis of uncontrolled diabetes mellitus).

ketone body *See* body, ketone.

ketosis *See* ketoacidosis.

kev Abbreviation for 1000 electron volts.

keyway The slot into which the male portion of precision attachments fits.

kg *See* kilogram.

KHN Abbreviation for Knoop hardness number. *See also* test, Knoop hardness.

kilo- (kĭl′ō) Prefix meaning 1000.

kilocalorie One thousand calories, a unit of measure of the energy value in foodstuffs.

kilogram (kĭl′ō-grăm) **(kg)** 1000 Gm; or equivalent to about 2.2 pounds avoirdupois.

kilovolt (kĭl′ō-vōlt) **(kv)** Unit of electrical potential equal to 1000 volts.

   k. peak (kvp) The crest value of the potential wave in kilovolts in an alternating current cycle. When only half of the wave is used, the value refers to that of the useful half of the wave.

kilovoltage (kĭl′ō-vōl″tĭj) The electrical potential difference between the anode and cathode of an x-ray tube.

   k., constant potential The potential of a constant voltage generator, in constant potential kilovolts (kvcp).

   k., equivalent (effective kilovoltage) The kilovoltage of monoenergetic radiation having the same half-value layer (HVL) as the heterogeneous beam produced by a peak kilovoltage in question.

   k., peak The crest value of the potential wave, in peak kilovolts (kvp).

kinanesthesia (kĭn″ăn-ĕs-thē′zē-ah) Loss of the power to perceive the sensation of movement resulting from derangement of deep sensibility.

kinematic face-bow (kĭn-ē-măt′ĭk) *See* face-bow, kinematic.

kinesiology (kĭ-nē″sē-ŏl′ō-jē) The study of human motion that attempts to explain the manner in which movements of the body occur. The principles of kinesiology may be used to describe the laws of articulation and the several theories of mandibular movement.

kink A bend or twist.

Kirkland cement dressing, knife *See* under appropriate noun.

Kirschner wire *See* wire, Kirschner.

Kirstein's method *See* method, Kirstein's.

kissing disease A vernacular term for infectious mononucleosis, a viral infection frequently occuring in teenages and young adults. *See* infectious mononucleosis.

Kline's test *See* test, Kline's.

Kloehn headgear An extra-oral orthodontic appliance consisting of a facebow and a cervical strap used to retract maxillary teeth or to reinforce the anchorage during tooth retraction.

knife An instrument used for cutting that consists of a sharp-edged blade provided with a handle.

   k., buck A periodontal knife possessing spearshaped cutting points; used for interdental incision during gingivectomy.

   k., electronic An electrosurgical scalpel used to incise or shave tissue.

   k., gold An instrument sometimes contra-angled, with a blade or cutting edge; used to trim excess metal and develop contour in foil restorations.

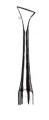

Gold knife

   k., Goldman-Fox Any of a group of surgical instruments designed for the incision and contouring of gingival tissue.

   k., Kirkland A heart-shaped knife, sharp on all edges, used for the primary gingivectomy incision.

   k., Merrifield's A knife that has a long, narrow, triangular blade in a shank; used for gingivectomy incisions.

Knoop hardness test *See* test, Knoop hardness.

Kobayashi ties Orthodontic ligature ties used to fix an orthodontic arch wire to the brackets attached to the teeth, that also provides attachment for the use of inter and intra maxillary elastic traction.

Koeber's saw *See* saw, Koeber's.

koilcytosis A histologic feature of the mucosal changes associated with the intraoral use of smokeless tobacco. The spinous cells of the squamous epithelium present with pyknotic, irregularly shaped nuclei surrounded by a perinuclear clear zone.

Koplik's spots *See* spots, Koplik's.

Kramer-Rhodes periodontal collection system A plaque-scoring and record-keeping system used to monitor plaque accumulation and to motivate patients to improve oral hygiene. It is based upon a surface-by-surface, tooth-by-tooth assessment using a 0-3 scale. *0* means no plaque is present, *3* means there is full surface heavy plaque accumulation.

Krause's corpuscles *See* corpuscle, Krause's.

KS *See* Kaposi's sarcoma

K ties *See* Kobayashi ties.

Kurer anchor system An endodontic post system with parallel sides, threaded and made of stainless material.

Kryptex *See* cement, silicophosphate.

Küstner's test (kĭst′nerz) *See* test, skin, indirect.

kv *See* kilovolt.

kvcp *See* kilovoltage, constant potential.

kvp *See* kilovolt peak.

kyphosis (kĭ-fō′sĭs) **(humpback)** An abnormal curvature of the spine with the convexity backward.

label (lā′bĕl) **1:** The portion of the prescription in which the directions for use are stated. **2:** One or more characters used to identify an item of data. Synonym: key. *See also* signa.

labial (lā′bē-ăl) Of or pertaining to a lip.

l. notch *See* notch, labial.

labile (lā′bīl) Unstable, as labile fever.

labioversion (lā′bē-ō-ver′zhŭn) Any deviation of a tooth toward the lips from the line of occlusion.

labium superius oris (lā′bē-ŭm sū-pē′rē-ŭs ō′rĭs) Point of the upper lip lying in the midsagittal plane and a line drawn across the boundary of the mucous surface tangent to the curves.

laboratory The room in which the dentist or auxiliaries perform technical procedures related to dental treatment but not done directly in the patient's mouth.

laceration A wound produced by tearing; the process of tearing.

laches (lătch′ĭz) Negligence; inexcusable delay; a failure to claim or enforce a claim or right at a proper time.

lacrimation, gustatory *See* syndrome, auriculotemporal.

Lactobacillus acidophilus A species of the genus *Lactobacillus* of the family Lactobacillaceae characterized by Grampositive rods found in cultured buttermilk and in the gastrointestinal track of persons on a high milk, lactose-, or dextrin-containing diet. *Lactobacillus acidophilus* preparations may be effective in the treatment of some recurrent aphthous ulcers and for the prevention of candidiasis secondary to tetracycline and/or steroid therapy.

lactoflavin (lăk′tō-flā-vĭn) *See* vitamin B_2.

lacuna (lah-kū′nah) A term used in anatomic nomenclature to designate a small hollow cavity or pit.

l., absorption (Howship's lacuna) An area (pit) of bone resorption, usually irregular in outline, and often containing osteoclasts.

l., osteocyte Hollow cavity within bone, containing osteocytes, from which canaliculi, containing protoplasmic processes of the osteocytes, radiate.

lambda (lăm′dah) The point in the skull at which the sagittal and lambdoid sutures meet. The strap of a rubber dam holder placed at this level will hold its position without slipping up or down.

lameila, cemental (lah-mĕl′ah) The arrangement and deposition of cementum in incremental layers more or less parallel to the root configuration.

lamina (lăm′ĭ-nah) A flat, thin plate.

l. dura Radiographic term denoting the plate of compact bone (alveolar bone) that lies adjacent to the periodontal membrane.

l. propria The zone of connective tissue subjacent to the epithelium of a mucous membrane.

laminagraphy (lăm′ĭ-năg′rah-fē) Body section radiography.

laminate veneer restorations A conservative esthetic restoration of anterior teeth to mask discoloration, restore malformed teeth, close diastemas, and correct minor tooth alignment. The materials of choice are acrylic veneers, processed composite resin veneersn and/or porcelain veneers that are bonded directly to a properly prepared tooth.

lamp, mouth A device to produce light or illumination directly in the oral cavity and to transilluminate the dental tissues.

lance To cut open with a lancet; to incise.

lancinating Pertaining to a stabbing pain (e.g., the pain occurring in tic douloureux).

landmark An anatomic structure used as a guide for anatomic relationships.

l., cephalometric (sĕf′ah-lō-mĕt′rĭk) One of the points located on oriented head radiographs from which lines, planes, and angles may be constructed to analyze the configuration and relationship of elements of the craniofacial skeleton.

language A defined set of characters that is used to form symbols and words and the rules and connections for combining these into meaningful communications.

l., machine A language designed for interpretation and use by a computer system without translation. Synonym: machine code.

laryngismus (lar″ĭn-jĭz′mŭs) Spasm of the larynx.

laryngopharyngeal (lah-rĭng″gō-fah-rĭn′jē-al) Related jointly to the larynx and the pharynx.

laryngopharynx (lah-rĭng″gō-făr′ĭngks) The lower portion of the pharynx, which extends from the corner of the hyoid bone or the vestibule of the larynx to the lower border of the cricoid cartilage.

laryngoscope (lah-rĭng′gō-skōp) An instrument for examining the larynx.

laryngospasm (lah-rĭng′gō-spăzm) Spasmodic closure of the larynx, sometimes noted during the induction phase of general anesthesia or during the recovery period.

laser High energy coordinated light source used in surgery, including for the experimental removal of the hard tissues of the teeth.

last will and testament The legal document describing the desires of a person for the distribution of worldly goods after death.

latent image *See* image, latent.

latent period *See* period, latent.

lateral (lăt′ĕr-ăl) A position either to the right or the left of the midsagittal plane.

> **l. checkbite** *See* record, interocclusal.
> **l. condylar inclination** *See* inclination, lateral condylar.
> **l. condyle path** *See* path, lateral condyle.
> **l. excursion** *See* excursion, lateral.
> **l. movement** *See* movement, lateral.
> **l. protrusion** *See* protrusion, lateral.

laterodetrusion (lăt″ĕr-ō-dē-trū′zhŭn) Noun that describes precisely the directions in which the muscles thrust a condyle outward and downward in the side shift preparatory to handling a large bolus of food.

lateroprotrusive (lăt′er-ō-prō-trū′sĭv) Pertaining to a movement direction of the jaw that has both sideward and forward components of movement.

lateroretrusive (lăt′er-ō-rē-trū′sĭv) Pertaining to a movement direction in cusp or condyle thrusts that has both lateral and backward components of movement.

laterotrusion (lăt″ĕr-ō-trū′zhŭn) The outward thrust given by the muscles to the rotating condyle or the condyle on the bolus side.

> **l., precurrent** Laterotrusion in which the working side condyle is rotated as it is thrust laterally.

latex (lā′tĕks) Natural rubber.

latitude (lăt′ĭ-tūd″) The range between the minimum and maximum film exposures to radiation that yield images of structures whose photographic density differences are discernible under normal viewing conditions. Latitude chiefly varies directly with kilovoltage and inversely with contrast. *See also* contrast.

lattice, space (lăt′ĭs) An arrangement of atoms in a definite relationship to each other, forming a lattice.

lavage (lah-vahzh′) Irrigation, or washing out, as in oral lavage.

law(s) 1: That which is laid down or established. An enforceable rule of conduct. **2:** That which must be obeyed and followed by citizens, subject to sanctions or legal consequences. The term is also used in opposition to *fact*; e.g., in a lawsuit questions of law are to be decided by the court, whereas the jury decides questions in fact.

> **l., Charles′** The principle that states that all gases on heating expand equally and on cooling contract equally.
> **l., Dalton′s** The principle that states that the pressure of a mixture of gases equals the sum of the partial pressures of the constituent gases.
> **l., ignorance of** Want of knowledge or acquaintance with the laws of the land insofar as they apply to the act, relation, duty, or matter under consideration.
> **l., inverse-square** The principle that states that the strength of x radiation from a point source varies inversely as the square of the distance.
> **l., moral** The aggregate of those rules and principles of ethics that relate to right and wrong conduct and prescribe the standards to which the actions of persons should conform in their dealings with each other.
> **l., neurologic** *See* law of specific energy.
> **l., Pascal′s** The principle that states that pressure applied to a liquid at any point is transmitted equally in all directions.
> **l. of specific energy (neurologic law)** The principle that states, in essence, that sensory quality is perceived according to the nerve that is excited, not according to the object that excites. If pressure placed on the eyeballs stimulates the retina, light is perceived, not pressure; similarly, electrical stimulation will produce sensations of smell, taste, touch, or pain in accordance with the nerve stimulated but not a sensation of electricity as such. The special, as well as the general, senses maintain this principle.
> **l., Wolff′s** The principle that states that all changes in the function of bone are attended by definite alterations in its internal structure.
> **l., written** Law or laws created by express legislation or enactment, as distinguished from unwritten or common law, which includes all law or laws from any other legal source.

lay Nonprofessional.

layer, Beilby′s (bīl′bēz) An amorphous layer formed on the surface of metals by a disorientation of the crystalline structure during polishing.

LD$_{50}$ *See* dose, lethal, median.

LD$_{50}$ time *See* time, median lethal.

lead apron *See* apron, lead.

lead glass *See* glass, lead.

lead poisoning *See* plumbism.

leaf gauge *See* gauge, leaf

learning disability The inability to learn at a rate comparable to a peer group. Some learning disorders have been traced to nutritional and behavioral causes, others stem from trauma or disease, whereas others have a genetic origin.

lease 1: A conveyance of lands or tenements to a person

for life, for a stated number of years, or at will, in consideration of rent or some other recompense. **2:** Any agreement that gives rise to a landlord and tenant relationship.

least expensive alternative treatment (LEAT) A limitation in a dental benefits plan that will only allow benefits for the least expensive treatment. Also referred to as least expensive professionally acceptable alternative treatment (LEPAAT).

lecithin (lĕs′ĭ-thĭn) **(phosphatidylcholine)** A class of phosphatides containing glycerol, phosphate, choline, and fatty acids. Lecithins are widely distributed in cells and possess both metabolic and structural functions in membranes. Dipalmityl lecithin is an important surface-active agent in the lungs.

ledger sheet An accounting form for keeping track of debits, expenditures, credits, and charges.

Leede's test *See* test, capillary resistance.

leeway space The arch circumference difference between the primary canine, first primary and second primary molars and the permanent canine and the first and second premolars. According to Black's means, the maxillary arch leeway space is 1.9 mm and the mandibular arch leeway space is 3.4 mm.

LeFort fracture *See* fracture, LeFort.

left justified Data are left justified when the leftmost digit or character occupies the leftmost position of the space allotted for those data.

legal 1: In compliance with the law. **2:** Not forbidden by law.

leiomyoma (lī″ō-mī-o′mah) A benign tumor derived from smooth muscle.

length The longest measure of an object, or the measurement between the two ends.

   l., muscle The variable end-to-end measurement of a muscle. The physical changes in muscle observed in the isotonic and isometric states of contraction are related to the alteration in the striated bands of muscle.

   l.-of-stay The expected length of time—usually a median—for which institutionalized patients in a hospital or other health care facility of similar age and diagnosis or condition would be expected to remain.

   l., tooth The distance along the long axis of the tooth from the apex of the root to the tip, or incisal edge, of the tooth.

lentula (lĕn-too′lah) A flexible spiral-wire instrument used in a handpiece to apply paste filling materials in root canals.

leontiasis ossea (lē″ŏn-tī′ah-sĭs ŏs′ē-ah) An enlargement of the bones of the face leading to a lionlike appearance. Osseous encroachment may cause obliteration of sinuses, blindness, and malocclusion.

leproma Nodular lesion of leprosy Seen on the skin, mu-

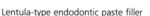

Lentula-type endodontic paste filler

cous membranes (including those of the eyes), upper respiratory tract, tongue, and palate.

leprosy (lĕp′rō-sē) **(Hansen's disease)** A chronic granulomatous infection caused by *Mycobacterium leprae*. It may exist in lepromatous (contagious), tuberculoid (noncontagious), and intermediate forms.

leptocytosis, hereditary (lĕp″tō-sī-tō′sĭs) *See* thalassemia.

Leptothrix (lĕp′tō-thrĭks) A filamentous microorganism, apparently not directly capable of pathogenicity, that may act as a nidus for the formation of dental calculus and its attachment to the tooth structure. Some investigators have associated this organism with the presence of periodontitis in human beings.

lesion (lē′zhŭn) Any pathologic disturbance of a tissue, with loss of continuity, enlargement, function, etc.

   l., extravasation *See* cyst, traumatic.

   l., herpetic A vesicle and/or ulceration of the mucosa caused by the herpes virus.

   l., herpetiform A painful ulceration of the oral mucosa with a red center and yellow border; occurs as a solitary lesion or in groups and appears similar to those lesions caused by herpesvirus. The term *herpetiform* is used as a clinical designation unless the viral cause has actually been demonstrated.

   l., indefinite bone *See* cyst, extravasation.

   l., traumatic bone *See* cyst, traumatic.

Lesser's triangle *See* triangle, Lesser's.

LET *See* transfer, linear energy.

Letterer-Siwe disease *See* disease, Letterer-Siwe.

leucine One of the essential amino acids; *see* amino acid.

leucovorin, calcium The calcium salt of folinic acid used in the treatment of megaloblastic anemias.

leukemia (lū-kē′mē-ah) A usually fatal disease of the blood-forming tissues characterized by the abnormal proliferation of leukocytes and their precursors and attended by fatigue, weakness, fever, lymphadenopathy, splenomegaly, and a tendency toward profuse tissue hemorrhage. Oral lesions include gingival enlargement, severe gingivitis, and necrosis. Lymphatic, monocytic, and myelogenous leukemias are the chief types.

l., aleukemia A phase of the leukemic state marked by proliferation of leukocytes within the bloodforming tissues, but without an increase in the white blood cell count: relatively few precursor cells are found in the blood smear until the phase passes and the blood becomes flooded with white cells. Oral lesions, when present, are ulceronecrotic and hypertrophic.

l., lymphatic (lymphoid leukemia) A hyperplasia, of undetermined origin, affecting lymphoid tissue. Predominating cells are lymphocytes and lymphoblasts. Generally assumes a more chronic course than other forms of leukemia but may be acute. Oral lesions include swollen and hyperplastic gingivae, ulceronecrotic lesions, marked tendency to gingival hemorrhage, etc.

l., monocytic A form of leukemia characterized by an abnormal increase in the number of monocytes. Manifestations include progressive weakness, anorexia, lymphadenopathy, hepatomegaly, splenomegaly, secondary anemia, etc. Oral lesions may be ulceronecrotic and hemorrhagic.

l., myelogenous Leukemia in which the leukocytes are of bone marrow origin (e.g., polymorphonuclear leukocytes, myelocytes, myeloblasts). Oral manifestations may include gingival enlargement and necrosis.

leukocyte (loo'kō-sīt) **1:** A white blood cell. **2:** White blood cell; a nucleated ameboid mass of protoplasm circulating in the blood. *See also* lymphocyte; monocyte.

l., basophilic A basophil; a leukocyte that has coarse granules stainable with basic dyes and a bent lobed nucleus.

l., eosinophilic An eosinophil; a leukocyte that has coarse granules stainable with eosin and a bilobed nucleus.

l., immature One of several forms of leukocyte usually found in disease (e.g., myelocytes, myeloblasts, lymphoblasts).

l., polymorphonuclear 1: A neutrophil; a white blood cell with finely granular cytoplasm, an irregularly lobulated nucleus, and the appearance of a microphage. It is found in the tissues during acute inflammatory processes and in the superficial surface aspects of a lesion during subacute or chronic inflammation. It is the predominating leukocyte of the blood. Blood levels may be increased during acute inflammatory states, myelogenous leukemia, etc., and decreased in agranulocytosis (malignant neutropenia). **2:** A neutrophil; a polymorph; a leukocyte that has fine granules stainable with neutral dyes and an irregularly lobed nucleus.

leukocytosis (loo″kō-sī-tō'sīs) An increase in the normal number of white blood cells; may be a defensive reaction, as in inflammation, or may result from a disturbance in white blood cell formation, as in leukemia. Various limits are given; e.g., leukocytosis in the adult is indicated when there are more than 10,000 white blood cells per cubic millimeter. *See also* eosinophilia; lymphocytosis; neutrophilia.

leukoedema (loo″kō-ĕ-dē'mah) An innocuous oral condition characterized by a filmy, opalescent, white covering of the buccal mucosa consisting of a thickened layer of parakeratotic cells. It is most commonly associated with mechanical and chemical irritation.

leukopenia (loo″kō-pē'nē-ah) A decrease in the normal number of white blood cells in the circulating blood. Various lower limits are given; e.g., leukopenia signifies less than 4000 white blood cells per cubic millimeter. *See also* lymphocytopenia; neutropenia.

leukoplakia (loo″kō-plā'kē-ah) **1:** A white plaque formed on the oral mucous membrane from surface epithelial cells. It is leathery, opaque, and somewhat thickened. Excluded from this are the white lesions of lichen planus, white sponge nevus, burns, thrush, and other clinically recognizable entities. Histologically, hyperkeratosis, acanthosis, subepithelial and perivascular infiltrate of round cells, etc., may be seen. Dyskeratosis may be present. Leukoplakia lesions may progress to malignancy, with cellular atypicism, dyskeratosis, epithelial pearl formation, infiltration of malignant cells into connective tissue corium, etc. **2:** A premalignant surface lesion of the mucous membrane characterized by hyperkertosis and dyskeratosis of the stratified squamous epithelium. See also dyskeratosis; hyperkeratosis.

leukotaxine (loo″kō-tăk'sīn) A substance that appears when tissue is injured and can be removed from inflammatory exudates. Increases capillary permeability and the diapedesis of leukocytes.

lev- *See* levo-.

levarterenol The official (USP) drug name for norepinephrine. The British (BP) name is noradrenaline. In contrast to epinephrine, levarterenol produces its pressor effect primarily through vasoconstriction in certain areas rather than by cardiac excitatory action. See also norepinephrine.

level (lĕv'ĕl) To reduce the curve of Spee by intrusion and/or extrusion of the teeth in an arch.

leveling arch wire Arch wire used to align teeth in the same plane.

lever (lĕv'er) A bar or rigid body that is capable of turning about one joint or axis and in which are two or more other points where forces are applied. There are three classes of levers, and each has its own most effective use.

l., second-class A lever in which the force arm is longer than the work-producing arm; thus the work produced is always greater than the energy used, with a resultant high efficiency.

l., third-class A lever in which the axis is at one end, the load at the other end, and the effort is exerted in between, as in a treadle.

leverage (lĕv′er-ĭj) The mechanical advantage gained by the use of a lever. A factor in the magnification of stresses generated by an extension-base partial denture, etc.

levo- (lev) Prefix applied to the name of optical isomers that rotate the plane of polarized light to the left.

liabilities All the claims against a corporation. Liabilities include accounts and wages and salaries payable, dividends declared payable, accrued taxes payable, and fixed or long-term liabilities such as mortgage bonds, debentures, and bank loans.

l., current Short-term debts and obligations that must be paid within a period of 1 year.

liability (lī″ah-bĭl′ĭ-tē) The state of being bound by law or justice to do something or to make something good; legal responsibility.

libel (lī′bĕl) **1:** That which is written and published, calculated to injure the character of another by ridicule or contempt. **2:** Defamation expressed by print, writing, pictures, or signs.

license Permission, accorded by a competent authority, granting the right to perform some act or acts that without such authorization would be contrary to law.

lichen planus (lī′kĕn plā′nŭs) **1:** A disease of unknown etiology affecting the skin and oral mucous membranes, either alone of concomitantly. The oral lesions are most common on the buccal mucous membrane, where they appear as a lacy pattern or bilateral network of raised white or bluish white, porcelain-like fine lines or a series of small, similarly appearing dots. The lesions are painless. On the tongue the lesions may appear as flat white plaques resembling leukoplakia. **2:** A dermatologic disease affecting the skin and mucous membranes; of unknown etiology but often associated with nervousness, fatigue, emotional depression, and allergy and considered to be a manifestation of quinacrine (Atabrine) therapy. Oral lesions often appear as white or blue-white striae forming an interweaving lacelike network of lines of epithelial thickening. Associated with the striated network; bullous or erosive lesions may be found. Histologically, varying degrees of hyperkeratosis and epithelial aconthosis may be found, with formation of sawtooth-shaped rete pegs of epithelium projecting into connective tissue corium. Subjacent to the epithelium is a bandlike infiltrate of round cells with perivascular accumulation of leukocytes. Treatment is symptomatic.

lidocaine A local anesthetic that is effective topically, by infiltration through subcutaneous injection and regionally using a nerve block technique. Brand name Xylocaine.

lien (lēn) A qualified right of property that a creditor has in specific property of the debtor as security for the debt or for performance of some act.

life, radioactive *See* half-life.

l., effective half- *See* half-life, effective.

ligament (lĭg′ah-mĕnt) Any tough, fibrous connective tissue band that connects bones or supports viscera. Some of the ligaments are distinct fibrous structures; others are folds of fascia or of indurated peritoneum; still others are the relics of unused fetal organs.

l., periodontal (PDL) The mode of attachment of the tooth to the alveolus. The ligament consists of numerous bundles of collagenous tissue (principle fibers) arranged in groups, between which is loose connective tissue, together with blood vessels, lymph vessels, and nerves. It functions as the investing and supportive mechanism for the tooth.

l., biologic width of periodontal The width of the periodontal ligament in normal, functioning teeth. It varies with the age of the individual and the functional demands made on the tooth, and in normalcy it is about 0.25 and 0.1 mm in width, narrowest at the center of the alveolus and widest at the margin and apex.

l., sphenomandibular The ligament extending from the spine of the sphenoid bone to the mandibular lingula.

l., stylohyoid A fibroelastic cord attached superior to the styloid process of the sphenoid bone.

l., stylomandibular A ligament extending from the styloid process of the temporal bone and attached to the mandibular gonial angle.

l., temporomandibular A triangular-shaped fibrous band extending from the lateral aspects of the root of the zygomatic process of the temporal bone to the mandibular subcondylar neck.

ligate (lī′gāt) To tie or bind with a ligature or suture.

ligation (lī-gā′shŭn) The binding together of tissue or teeth with wire, string, thread, etc., for stabilization and immobilization.

l., surgical Exposure of an unerupted tooth with placement of a metal ligature around its cervix. The free ends of the ligature are fixed to a fine, preciousmetal chain, which in turn is fixed to an orthodontic appliance for the purpose of placing traction on the unerupted tooth to cause its eruption.

ligature (lĭg′ah-tūr) **1:** A cord, thread, or fine wire tied around teeth for the purpose of holding a rubber dam in place on retained teeth with fractured roots or split crowns or on teeth that have been replanted. **2:** A wire or threadlike substance used to tie a tooth to an orthodontic appliance or to another tooth.

l., grass-line A ligature composed of the fibers of a grass-cloth plant (ramie); used for minor tooth movement. It depends for its activation in movement on the property of shrinkage of the ligature when it is wetted by the saliva of the patient.

l., steel A form of ligature, available as steel filaments in several useful diameters.

light box *See* illuminator.

light, operating A light with a strong beam that may be directed for concentrated illumination of a part being operated on.

light pen A pointerlike device available with some computer terminals. It is used to select data displayed on the screen by being pointed at any desired item.

light touch *See* touch, light.

limit Restriction.

l., elastic (proportional limit) The greatest stress to which a material may be subjected and still be capable of returning to its original dimensions when the forces are released.

l., proportional *See* limit, elastic.

limited treatment Treatment directed at a limited objective not involving the entire dentition. It may be directed at the only existing problem, or at only on aspect of a larger problem in which a decision is made to defer more comprehensive therapy.

limitations Restrictive conditions stated in a dental benefits contract, such as age, length of time covered, and waiting periods, which affect an individual's or group's coverage. The contract may also exclude certain benefits or services, or it may limit the extent or condition under which certain services are provided. *See* Exclusions.

lincomycin An antibiotic effective against susceptible strains of streptococci, pneumococci, and staphylococci. It should be reserved for pencillin-allergic patients. Close clinical supervision is required because severe colitis has been associated with Lincomycin therapy. Brand name Lincocin.

linea alba buccalis A normal variation in the buccal mucosa that appears as a white line beginning at the corners of the mouth and extending posteriorly at the level of the occlusal plane.

line Boundary; demarcation.

l. angle *See* angle, line.

l., basophilic A group of microscopic sections of bone that stains darkly with hematoxylin. Represents periods of bone inactivity.

l., Camper's The line running from the inferior border of the ala of the nose to the superior border of the tragus of the ear.

l., cement The line of cement exposed at the margin of an inlay or crown.

l., cemental (cementing line) Basophilic line distinguishing adjacent lamellae of bone; represents periods of inactivity of bone formation and resorption.

l., cementing *See* line, cemental.

l., cervical *See* junction, cementoenamel.

l. of credit An arrangement whereby a financial institution (bank or insurance company) commits itself to lend up to a specified maximum amount of funds during a specified period. Sometimes the interest rate on the loan is specified; at other times it is not. Sometimes a commitment fee is imposed for obtaining the line of credit.

l., cross arch fulcrum *See* line, fulcrum, cross arch.

l. of draw The direction or plane of withdrawal or seating of a removable or cemented restoration.

l., external oblique A ridge of osseous structure on the body of the mandible extending from the anterolateral border to the mandibular ramus, passing downward and forward, after covering the buccocervical portion of the third molar, and ending by blending into the molar teeth.

l., finish In cavity preparations, a minimal line of demarcation of the wall of the preparation at the cavosurface angle; usually results from a slice made by an abrasive disk.

l. focus A principle employed in the design of x-ray tubes, by which the effective focal spot is sharply reduced relative to the actual (larger) focal spot desirable to deal with the heat generated. It involves focusing the cathode stream, in the pattern of a thin rectangle, onto an anode truncated at about 20 degrees to the transverse axis of the tube. *See also* spot, focal, effective.

l. of force *See* force, line of.

l., fulcrum Any imaginary line around which a removable partial denture tends to rotate.

l., fulcrum, anteroposterior An imaginary line of rotation extending through the rest and other support areas along the same side of a removable partial denture.

l., cross arch fulcrum An imaginary line through the tooth-supported rest areas that are nearest to soft tissue—supported areas and around which the partial denture will tend to rotate when forces are applied to the soft tissue—supported areas.

l., lead A bluish black patch on the gingival tissues, usually about 1 mm from the gingival crest. Caused by the deposition of fine granules of lead sulfide in the tissues. A sign of lead absorption in lead poisoning (plumbism).

l., median The intersection of the midsagittal plane with the maxillary and mandibular dental arches. The center line divides the central body surface into right and left.

l., mercurial A linear area of abnormal pigmentation of the gingival tissues associated with mercury poisoning. Seen along the gingival margin, it has been variously described as bluish, brownish, dirty reddish, or purplish in coloration.

l. of occlusion The alignment of the occluding surfaces of the teeth in the horizontal plane. *See also* plane, occlusal. line

l. printer A fast printing device. It prints on paper each line of characters in one operation, rather than character by character.

l., protrusive One of the three tracings made on each of the six projection planes of a jaw motion data recorder.

l., survey A line produced on the various portions of a dental cast by a surveyor scriber or marker. It designates the greatest height of contour in relation to the orientation of the cast to the vertical scriber.

l., vibrating The imaginary line across the posterior part of the palate marking the division between the movable and relatively immovable tissues of the palate.

linear energy transfer (LET) The linear rate of loss of energy by an ionizing particle traversing a material medium.

linen strip *See* strip, abrasive.

liner, cavity *See* varnish, cavity.

lines Elongated marks traced by a stylus on a gnathic projection plane, indicating direction of movement related variously to condyle movements.

lingua alba *See* tongue, white hairy.

lingua nigra *See* tongue, black hairy.

lingua villosa alba *See* tongue, white hairy.

lingual (lĭng′gwahl) Pertaining to the tongue.

l. bar, major connector *See* connector, major, lingual bar.

l. button Attachment welded to the lingual side of the canine, premolar, or molar bands.

l. peak, gingival A lingual peak that characterizes the normal interproximal tissue, which is composed of a lingual papilla and a buccal papilla connected interdentally in a triangular ridge depression termed a *col*.

l. plate *See* connector, major, linguoplate.

lingula (lĭng′gū-lah) A small, tonguelike projection of bone forming the anterior border of the mandibular foramen.

lingual appliances Orthodontic appliances that apply force from the lingual aspect of the anterior teeth. This mode of treatment is used to reduce the visibility of the appliance and thus improve the appearance of the smile during treatment.

lingual arch A space-holding arch or the basic arch for an active lingual orthodontic appliance. The arch usually spans around the inside of the dental arch from one first permanent molar to its antimere.

linguoclusion (lĭng-gwō-klū′zhŭn) An occlusion in which the dental arch or group of teeth is lingual to normal.

linguoplate *See* connector, major, linguoplate.

linguoversion The state of being displaced toward the tongue.

linkage (lĭngk′ĭj) The connection between two or more objects. In computer programming, coding that connects two separately coded routines.

l., cross polymerization, cross.

l., sex Inheritance of certain characteristics that are determined by genes located in the sex chromosomes.

linoleic acid An unsaturated fatty acid essential to nutrition. Linoleic acid occurs in many plant glycerides.

lip biting An oral habit in which either lip is placed between the teeth with more or less forcible application of the teeth to the lips.

lip, cleft *See* harelip.

l., congenital cleft *See* harelip.

lip, double A redundant fold of tissue on the mucosal side of the upper lip that gives the appearance of a second lip and that may become accentuated by habitually being sucked between the teeth.

lip line, high The greatest height to which the lip is raised in normal function or during the act of smiling broadly.

lip line, low The lowest position of the lower lip during the act of smiling or voluntary retraction. The lowest position of the upper lip at rest.

lip pits (congenital lip fistulas) Congenital depressions, usually bilateral and symmetrically placed, on the vermilion portion of the lower lip. These pits may be circular or may be present as a transverse slit. The depression represents a blind fistula that penetrates downward into the lower lip to a depth of 0.5 to 2.5 cm. They often exude viscid saliva on pressure.

lip retractors Apparatus to retract the lips when taking intraoral photographs.

lipid (lĭp′ĭd) A heterogeneous group of substances related actually or potentially to the fatty acids that are soluble in nonpolar solvents such as benzene, chloroform, and ether and are relatively insoluble in water. Included are the fatty acids, acylglycerols, phospholipids, cerebrosides, and steroids.

l., plasma The various plasma lipid classes include triacylglycerols, phospholipids, cholesterol, cholesterol esters, and unesterified fatty acids. Due to their hydrophobic nature, plasma lipids are carried in association with specific plasma proteins, the lipoproteins.

lipidosis (lĭp″ĭ-dō′sĭs) *See* disease, lipid storage.

Lipiodol (lĭp-ē′ō-dahl) Trade name for an iodized oil used as an opaque contrast medium in radiography. When it is laced within periodontal pockets and radiographs are made, the depth and topography of periodontal pockets may be ascertained.

lipoids (lĭp'oidz) A fatlike substance that may not actually be related to the fatty acids, although *lipid* and *lipoid* are occasionally used synonymously.

lipoma (lĭ-pō'mah) A benign tumor characterized by fat cells.

lipophilic (lĭp-ō-fĭl'ĭk) **1:** Showing a marked attraction to, or solubility in, lipids. **2:** Having an affinity for oil or fat.

Lipschütz body (lĭp'shĭtz) *See* body, Lipschütz.

lipoproteins Biochemical compounds that contain both lipid and protein. Most lipids in plasma are present in the form of lipoproteins.

litigation The act or process of engaging in a lawsuit.

LJP *See* localized juvenile periodontitis

load An external force applied to an object.

    l., occlusal The stresses generated by functional or habitual contacting of the occlusal surfaces of the upper and lower teeth. There are two components of such stress loads—the vertically directed components and those components that tend to move a tooth or denture laterally. *See also* force, occlusal.

loading The amount included in the premiums to meet liabilities beyond anticipated claims payment to provide administrative costs and contributions to reserve funds and to cover contingencies such as unexpected loss or adverse fluctuation.

lobectomy (lō-bĕk'tō-mē) Excision of a lobe of an organ such as the submandibular gland or the lung.

Lobstein's disease (lōb'stīnz) *See* osteogenesis imperfecta.

local analgesia Loss of pain sensation over a specific area, caused by local administration of a drug that blocks nerve conduction.

localization A direct, exact site or restriction to a limited area, such as localization of abscess.

    l., radiographic Determination, by means of radiographs, of the location of an object or structure in the body or head. Usually accomplished by obtaining radiographs made from different angulations to the part in question.

    l., tactile The property of localization associated with the sense of touch. Perception of the location of a stimulus is more precise in the regions of the lips and the fingertips than elsewhere. This more precise perception results from a greater density of special touch receptors in a given area.

localized juvenile periodontitis (LJP) A localized periodontal tissue breakdown in young children in the primary or mixed dentition stage, apparently resulting from gingival pocket infection with *H. actinomycetemcomitans*. *See also* juvenile periodontitis

location The geographic spot in which the equipment is set up to practice dentistry.

locking gate A portion of the peripheral frame of a maxillary subperiosteal implant; attached by a hinge. This device permits the implant to be placed into an area of undercut. After the implant is seated, the gate is closed and locked, and wire is wrapped about two locking buttons.

lockpin A soft metal pin used to attach an archwire to an orthodontic bracket.

locomotor ataxia *See* tabes dorsalis.

locus, gene The position of a gene on the chromosome.

locus minoris resistentiae (lō'kŭs mī-nor'ĭs rĕ-sĭs-tĕn'chē-ē″) An area offering little resistance to invasion by microorganisms and/or their toxins. The junction between reduced enamel epithelium and oral epithelium within the epithelial wall of the gingival sulcus has been described as a weak link, providing a portal of entry for microorganisms and their toxins with initiation of pocket formation.

loempe (lĕm'pē) *See* beriberi.

logopedics (log″ō-pe'dĭks) The study and treatment of speech defects in children, involving habilitation or rehabilitation of speech.

long face syndrome A malocclusion characterized by a long, narrow face; steep mandibular plane angle; and Class II Division 1 dental/skeletal relationship with anterior crowding; and associated mouth breathing. A contemporary name for *adenoid facies*.

loop, programming A programming technique whereby a group of instructions is repeated with modification of some of the instructions in the group and/or with modification of the data being operated on.

loop, vertical A U-shaped bend in the archwire that aids in the opening or closing of spaces in the arch.

loose premaxilla *See* premaxilla, loose.

lordosis (lor-dō'sĭs) An anteroposterior curvature of the spine with the convexity facing forward.

loss of bone *See* resorption of bone.

loss ratio The relationship between the money paid out in benefits and the amount collected in premiums.

loupe, binocular (loop) A magnifier that consists of lenses in an optical frame; it is worn like spectacles and is used with both eyes.

low lip line *See* lip line, low.

lower ridge slope *See* slope, lower ridge.

lozenge (lahz'ĕnj) (troche) A medicated, disk-shaped tablet designed to dissolve slowly in the mouth.

Ludwig's angina (lood'vĭgz) *See* angina, Ludwig's.

luetic (loo-ĕt'ĭk) Pertaining to or affected by syphilis.

lumen (loo'mĕn) The space within a tube structure, such as a blood vessel, tube, or duct.

lupus (loo'pŭs) A disease of the skin and mucous membrane.

    l. erythematosus (systemic lupus erythematosus, disseminated lupus erythematosus) A chronic inflammatory disease of unknown etiology affecting skin, joints, kidneys, nervous system, serous membranes, and often other organs of the body. The classical facial "butterfly rash" facilitates diagnosis, although the rash need not be present. Other skin areas, particularly those exposed to the sun, may be involved by a scaly lesion that is referred to as *discoid lupus erythematosus*.

l. vulgaris Cutaneous tuberculosis with characteristic nodular lesions on the face, particularly about the nose and ears.

luting agents Agents that bond, seal, or cement particles or objects together.

luxate Be forced out of place or joint; to be displaced; to dislocate.

luxation 1: The act of luxating or state of being luxated, as in the dislocation or displacement of a tooth or of the temporomandibular joint.   **2:** Dislocation or displacement of a tooth or of the temporomandibular articulation.

lymphadenitis 1: Inflammation of a lymph node or nodes.   **2:** Inflammation of the lymph glands, characterized chiefly by swelling, pain, and redness.

lymphadenopathy Any disease process that involves a lymph node or nodes.

l., generalized Involvement of all or several regionally separated groups of lymph nodes by a systemic disorder.

l., regional Involvement of nodes draining a specific region (e.g., submental nodes draining the middle of the lower lip, floor of the mouth, skin of the chin).

lymphangioma (lĭm-făn-jē-ō′mah) A benign neoplasm characterized by lymph vessel proliferation. A benign tumor of the lymph vessels.

l., cystic *See* hygroma, cystic.

lymphoblastoma, giant follicular (Brill-Symmers disease) A malignant disease characterized by enlargement of the spleen and lymph nodes throughout the body. Lymphoblasts and reticular cells proliferate within lymphoid follicles, producing an increase in both the number and size of germinal follicles.

lymphocyte (lĭm′fō-sīt) A form of white blood cell originating in lymphoid tissues; possesses a single spherical nucleus and a nongranular cytoplasm. The lymphocytes comprise 25% of the white blood cells. Some lymphocytes, along with plasma cells and histiocytes, are found in clinically normal gingivae. Their numbers within the gingival connective tissue are increased in gingivitis and periodontitis. With progress of gingival inflammation to the underlying bone, lymphocytes are found within the marrow spaces of the supporting bone.

lymphocytopenia (lĭm″fō-sī″tō-pē′nē-ah) A decrease in the normal number of lymphocytes in the circulating blood. Various limits are given (e.g., a total number less than 600/mm³). It may be associated with agranulocytosis, hyperadrenocorticism, leukemia, advanced Hodgkin's disease, irradiation, and acute infections with neutrophilia.

lymphocytosis (lĭm″fō-sī-tō′sĭs) An absolute or relative increase in the normal number of lymphocytes in the circulating blood. Various limits are given; e.g., *absolute* lymphocytosis is said to be present if the total number of cells exceeds 4500/mm³, whereas *relative* lymphocytosis is said to be present if the percentage of lymphocytes is greater than 45% and the total number of cells is less than 4500/mm³. Lymphocytosis may be associated with infancy, exophthalmic goiter, mumps, rubella, infectious mononucleosis, sunburn, lymphatic leukemia, pertussis, and pyogenic infections in childhood.

lymphoepithelial lesion, benign (lĭm″fō-ĕp′ ĭ-thē′lē-al) *See* disease, Mikulicz′.

lymphoepithelioma (lĭm″fō-ĕp′ĭ-thē″lē-ō′mah) A malignant neoplasm arising from the epithelium and lymphoid tissue of the nasopharynx and characterized by cells of both tissues; may occur in the palate.

lymphoma (lĭm-fō′mah) Any neoplasm made up of lymphoid tissue.

lymphoreticulosis, benign inoculation (lĭm″fō-rĕ tĭk″ū-lō′sĭs) *See* fever, cat-scratch.

lymphosarcoma (lĭm″fō-sar-kō′mah) A malignant disease of the lymphoid tissues characterized by proliferation of atypical lymphocytes and their localization in various arts of the body. The jaws may be the sites of lymphosarcomas.

lysin (lī′sĭn) *See* plasmin.

lysine One of the essential amino acids found in many proteins. *See* amino acids.

lysing effect *See* effect, lysing.

lysis (lī′sĭs) Gradual abatement of the symptoms of a disease. Disintegration or dissolution of cells by a lysin.

lysokinase (lī″sō-kī′nās) *See* fibrinokinase.

lysozyme (lī′sō-zīm) An enzyme in major salivary secretions that may rupture bacterial cell walls and may regulate the oral flora.

ma Abbreviation for milliampere.

macro- A prefix meaning excessively large or big.

macrocheilia (măk″rō-kī′lē-ah) Abnormally large lip.

macrodontia (măk-rō-don′shē-ah) **(megadontismus)** Abnormally large teeth. One, several, or all teeth in a given individual may be involved.

macrofill resins *See* resins, composite

macrogingivae (măk″rō-jĭn′jĭ-vē) Abnormally large gingivae resulting from inflammation, heredity, scurvy, leukemia, neoplasia, diphenylhydantoin (Dilantin) therapy (in epilepsy), or hormonal stimulation of puberty or pregnancy.

macroglossia (măk″rō-glahs′ē-ah) An enlarged tongue resulting from muscle hypertrophy, vascular or neurogenic tumor, or endocrine disturbance.

   m., amyloid *See* tongue, amyloid.

macroglossic Descriptive of macroglossia.

macrognathia (măk″rō-năth′ē-ah) A definite overgrowth of the maxillae and mandible.

macrognathic (măk-rō-năth′ĭk) Descriptive of macrognathia.

macromolecule Any substance with molecules of colloidal size, notably proteins, nucleic acids, and polysaccharides.

macrophage (măk′rō-fāj) *See* histiocyte.

macroscopic Relating to macroscopy or the examination of areas such as surfaces of teeth without magnification.

macrosomia *See* giantism.

macrostomia An abnormally large oral opening.

macule A lesion of the mucous membrane or cutaneous tissue that is not elevated above the surface.

magnesium An elemental metal; atomic weight, 24.32. An essential nutritional substance. Deficiency produces irritability of the nervous system, trophic disturbances, etc.

magnetic disk A storage device, consisting of magnetically coated disks, on the surface of which information is stored in the form of magnetic spots arranged in a manner to represent binary data.

magnetic resonance imaging Also known as nuclear magnetic resonance imaging. A diagnostic technique in which the phosphorus in cellular tissues is excited by magnetic force. The distribution and alignment of these cellular elements can be captured on phosphorus nuclear magnetic resonance instruments forming a-high resolution tissue image. A higher degree of resolution of soft tissues is possible using this technique than from radiographic techniques. The word nuclear has been dropped from the term because it result in the incorrect inference that radioactivity is involved in the imaging process.

magnetic tape A continuous, flexible, recording medium whose basic material is impregnated or coated with a magnetic-sensitive material ready to accept data in the form of magnetically polarized spots.

maintenance, space *See* space maintainer.

major connector *See* connector, major.

making the turn The step in the procedure of inserting and condensing foil in a Class 3 cavity preparation at which the line of force is changed from an incisogingival direction to a gingivoincisal direction.

mal- Prefix denoting a bad or unfavorable condition.

malaise (mă′lāz) A general feeling of discomfort or uneasiness, often the first indication of an infection or other disease.

malar (mā′lar) Pertaining to the cheek or the zygomatic bone.

   m. bone *See* bone, malar.

malare Midpoint of the intersection between the projection of the coronoid process and the lower contour of the malar bone.

Malassez, debris of *See* debris of Malassez.

Malassez, rests of *See* debris of Malassez.

maldevelopment Abnormal, imperfect, or deficient formation or development.

malfeasance (măl-fē′zĕns) An act that one should not do at all or the unjust performance of some act that the party had no right to do.

malfunction A disorder in function or performance, which may or may not be related to a malformation of tissues, organs or organ systems. *See* dysfunction.

malice A state of mind that disregards the law and legal rights of others but that does not necessarily involve personal hate or ill will.

   m. in the law of libel and slander An evil intent arising from spite or ill will; willful and wanton disregard of the rights of the person defamed.

malignant (mah-lĭg′ nănt) **1:** Resistant to treatment. **2:** Able to metastasize and kill the host.

malingering Feigning of illness.

malleability (măl″ē-ah-bĭl′ĭ-tē) Ability of a material to withstand permanent deformation under compressive forces without rupture.

mallet A hammer instrument.

    m., hard A small hammer with a leather-, rubber-, fiber-, or metal-faced head; used to supply force or to supplement hand force for the compaction of foil or amalgam and to seat cast restorations.

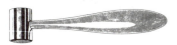

Mallet

malnutrition Any disorder concerning nutrition. It may result from a poor diet or from impaired utilizations of foods ingested.

malocclusion (relationship of teeth in occlusion) A deviation in intramaxill ary and/or intermaxillary relations of teeth that presents a hazard to the individual's well-being. Often associated with other dentofacial deformities. *See* Angle's, classification.

    m., deflective A type of malocclusion occurring in persons who cannot close all their teeth while holding their condyles in the rearmost position. Instead, in closure they first contact one or two pairs of poorly coupled teeth. To gain occlusal contacts of the other teeth, they must move the jaw anteriorly, laterally, or anterolaterally, as the deflectors demand in their guidance.

malposed (măl-pōzd′) In an abnormal position.

malposition A faulty or abnormal position of a part of the body.

    m. of jaw Any abnormal position of the mandible.

    m. of teeth Improper position of teeth in relationship to the basal bone of the alveolar process, to adjacent teeth, and/or to opposing teeth.

malpractice In medicine and dentistry, a professional person's act or failure to act that was the proximate cause of an injury to a patient and that was below the standard of care required.

malrelation (of tooth, teeth, jaws, or facial structures) Malalignment, malocclusion, and malposition are interrelated, so that one term frequently implies concurrent malrelationships of related teeth or structures.

mammotropin (măm″ō-trō′pĭn) *See* hormone, lactogenic.

manage To control and direct; to administer.

managed care Refers to a cost containment system that directs the utilization of health benefits by (1) restricting the type, level, and frequency of treatment; (2) limiting the access to care; and (3) controlling the level of reimbursement for services.

management The planning, organizing, directing, and controlling of the enterprises' operation so that objectives can be achieved economically and efficiently through others.

    m. information system (MIS) The specific type of data processing system that is designed to furnish management with information that may be of assistance in making decisions.

mandible Lower jawbone.

    m., inferior border of Lower edge of the mandible. Begins anterior to the insertion of the masseter muscle at the inferior surface of the angles of the mandible and is continuous anteriorly with the incisor region.

    m., movements of *See* movement, mandibular.

    m., posture of The physiologic rest position or the rest vertical relation of the mandible.

mandibular Pertaining to the lower jaw.

    m. angle *See* angle of the mandible.

    m. axis *See* axis, mandibular.

    m. border *See* border, mandibular.

    m. canal *See* canal, mandibular.

    m. centric relation The closing relation of the mandible with the fixed craniofacial complex as determined clinically by jaw motion recording instruments.

    m. condyle *See* condyle, mandibular.

    m. foramen *See* foramen, mandibular.

    m. glide *See* glide, mandibular.

    m. guide prosthesis A prosthesis with an extension designed to direct a resected mandible into a functional relation with the maxillae.

    m. hinge position *See* position, hinge, mandibular.

    m. movement *See* movement, mandibular.

    m. notch *See* notch, mandibular.

    m. pain-dysfunction syndrome *See* temporomandibular joint pain-dysfunction syndrome

    m. rest position *See* position, rest, mandibular.

    m. retraction *See* retraction, mandibular.

mandibulofacial dysostosis (măn-dĭb″u-lō-fā′shŭl) *See* syndrome, Treacher-Collins.

mandrel (măn′drĕl) A shaft that supports or holds any object to be rotated. An instrument, held in a handpiece, that holds a disk, stone, or cup used for grinding, smoothing, or polishing.

Mann-Whitney U-test *See* test, Mann-Whitney U-.

manual Performed by the hand; used in the hand.

margin 1: The extreme edge of something. **2:** Boundary of a surface. **3:** In a cavity preparation for a restoration it is the outside limit of the surgical preparation. Synonym: cavosurface angle.

    m., bone The peripheral edge of a bone.

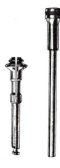

Mandrels

m., thickened bone *See* bone, thickened margin of.

m., enamel The part of the margin of a preparation that is laid in enamel.

m., free gum *See* margin, free gingival.

m., gingival 1: The cavosurface angle of the wall of a cavity preparation closest to the apex of the root. **2:** The crest or tip of the gingival tissues.

m., free gingival (free gum margin) The edge or summit of the gingival tissue immediately adjacent to the cervical portion of the crown of a natural tooth. The tissue is normally unattached to a depth of 2 to 2.5 mm.

m. of safety The margin between lethal and toxic doses.

marginal ridge *See* ridge, marginal.

marginal spinning The burnishing of the margins of a casting during the initial setting of the cement to close the space between the margin and the preparation, resulting from the slight lifting of the marginal gold from its seat by the interposition of the cement. The rounded edge of the spinning tool must always be drawn along the margin and not across it.

margination Adhesion of the leukocytes to the luminal surface of blood vessel walls in the early stages of inflammation.

Marie's disease *See* acromegaly.

marketing Set of human activities directed at facilitating and consummating exchanges. The following three elements must be present to define a marketing situation: two or more parties who are potentially interested in exchange; each party possessing things of value to others; and each party capable of communication and delivery.

marking medium *See* medium, marking.

marsupialization (măr-su″pē-ah-lĭ-zā′shŭn) The opening of a cyst to establish communication with the external environment. *See also* operation, Partsch's.

MAS (MaS, mas, milliampere-second) The product of the milliamperes and the exposure time in seconds (e.g., 10 ma × ½ sec = 5 MAS).

mask 1: *n.,* Something that conceals from view, **2:** *v.,* To cover up. **3:** *n.,* A protective covering, especially for the face.

m., rubber dam *See* pad, rubber dam.

m., Wanscher's A mask for ether anesthesia.

m., Yankauer's An open type of mask for administering ether.

masking An opaque covering used to camouflage the metal or other parts of a prosthesis.

Maslow's hierarchy of human needs A term from sociology or social anthropology based upon the hierarchical hypothesis of Abraham Maslow of the basic needs of man. The first need is for air, food, and water, the second for safety, including protection and freedom from fear and anxiety, followed in order by the need to love, and to be loved, the need for self-esteem, and ultimately, the need for self-actualization. The Maslow hypothesis states that the high needs cannot be fully satisfied until the lower needs are met.

mass number (A) The number of nucleons (protons and neutrons) in the nucleus of an atom.

mass storage A storage medium in which data may be organized and maintained both sequentially and nonsequentially. Usually used for storage of files.

massage Manipulation of tissues for remedial or hygiene purposes (as by rubbing, stroking, kneading, or tapping) with the hand or other instrument.

m., cardiac A systematic, rhythmic application of pressure to the heart to cause a significant blood flow in the treatment of a cardiac arrest; may be an open or closed chest procedure.

m., gingival Massage of the gingival tissues for cleansing purposes, increasing tissue tone, increasing the circulation of blood through the tissues, and increasing the keratinization of the surface epithelium.

Masseter muscle One of the four muscles of mastication. The thick rectangular muscle in the cheek that functions to close the jaw. It arises from the zygomatic arch and inserts into the mandible at the corner of the jaw.

master One having authority; one who directs, instructs, or superintends; an employer.

m. file A file of semipermanent information that is usually updated periodically.

masticate 1: To grind or crush food with the teeth to prepare it for swallowing and digestion. **2:** Chew.

masticating apparatus *See* apparatus, masticating.

masticating cycle *See* cycle, masticating.

mastication 1: The process of chewing food in preparation for swallowing and digestion. **2:** The act of chewing accomplished by the coordinated activity of the tongue, mandible, mandibular musculature, structural components of the temporomandibular joints, etc., and controlled by the neuromuscular mechanism.

m., components of The various jaw movements made during the act of mastication as determined by the neuromuscular system, temporomandibular articulations, teeth, and food being chewed. For purposes of analysis or description, the components of mastication may be categorized as opening, closing, left lateral, right lateral, or anteroposterior jaw movements.

m., forces of See force, masticatory.

m., insufficiency of Inefficiency or inadequacy of the chewing act.

m., organ of See system, stomatognathic.

m., physiology of The movements of the mandible during the chewing cycle, which are controlled by neuromuscular action and correlated to the structural attributes of the temporomandibular joints and the proprioceptive sense of the periodontal membranes. There are three phases in the physiology of mastication: the incision of food, mastication of the bolus, and the act of swallowing. Accessory activity by the tongue and facial musculature facilitates the masticatory actions.

m., saliva in Increase in salivation, which serves to wet and lubricate the food to facilitate deglutition.

m., tongue in The muscular organ in the floor of the mouth whose function in the masticatory process consists in crushing some food by pressing it against the hard palate, forming it into a compact bolus, and assisting in placing it on the occlusal platform for tooth action.

masticatory force See force, masticatory.

masticatory movements (măs′tĭ-kah-tor″ē) See movements, mandibular, masticatory.

mastoidale Lowest point on the contour of the mastoid process.

materia alba A soft white deposit around the necks of the teeth usually associated with poor oral hygiene; composed of food debris, dead tissue elements, and purulent matter; serves as a medium for bacterial growth.

materia medica The study of drugs and their use.

material(s) Substance(s).

m., dental All the substances used to assist in rendering dental service.

m., duplicating Materials used to copy casts, models, etc.; usually hydrocolloids.

m., filling Gutta-percha, silver cones, paste mixtures, or other substances used to fill root canals.

m., impression Any substance or combination of substances used for making a negative reproduction or impression.

m., silicone rubber impression A dimethyl polysiloxane material whose polymerization is affected by an organ-metal compound and some type of alkyl silicate.

matrix (mā′trĭks) **1:** An intergranular substance that acts somewhat as a cementing material for other particles; e.g., zinc phosphate cement is made of undissolved zinc oxide particles, surrounded and held or cemented together by phosphate compounds. The phosphate compounds make up the matrix. See also bone; splint. **2:** A mechanical or artificial wall to complete the mold into which plastic material may be inserted. **3:** Also a mold into which something is formed.

m., amalgam A metal form, usually of stainless steel, about 0.0015 to 0.002 in. thick, adapted to a prepared cavity to supply the missing wall so that the plastic amalgam will be confined when it is condensed into the cavity.

m., Celluloid A strip of Celluloid used to mold cement into the desired shape. See also strip, plastic.

m., custom A matrix made especially for a given location, tooth, or preparation.

m. holder See retainer, matrix.

m., mechanical (proprietary matrix) A patented or manufactured type of matrix.

m., plastic A matrix of resin or plastic for use with cold-curing resin or cement.

m., platinum A matrix of wrought platinum foil, usually 0.001 in. or thinner, adapted to a die of a preparation for a fired porcelain restoration; serves as a vehicle to carry and maintain the applications of porcelain when they are placed in a furnace for firing.

m., proprietary See matrix, mechanical.

m. retainer See retainer, matrix.

m., T-band Matrix material cut with a T-shaped projection at one end; the lugs are bent over to engage the band as it encircles the tooth.

maxilla (măk-sĭl′ah) The irregularly shaped bone forming half of the upper jaw. The upper jaw is made up of the two maxillae.

maxillary (măk″sĭ-lĕr′ē) Pertaining to the superior jaw.

m. arch The upper dental arch and its supporting bone.

m. retrusion See retrusion, maxillary.

m. sinus See sinus, maxillary.

m. tuberosity See tuberosity, maxillary.

maxillofacial (măk-sĭl″ō-fā′shŭl) Pertaining to the jaws and the face.

m. pain Any pain in the region or the jaws or face. Usually coupled with oral pain, i.e., oral and/or maxillofacial pain. Maxillofacial pain frequently is associated with functional disorders of the temoromandibular joint and/or the muscles of mastication, which in turn may arise from structural problems in the occlusion of the teeth. Determining the cause of maxillofacial pain may require comprehensive study of many possible factors or agents.

m. prosthetics See prosthetics, maxillofacial.

maxillomandibular relation (măk-sĭl″ō-măn-dĭb′ū-lar) See relation, maxillomandibular.

maxillotomy (măk″sĭ-lot′ō-mē) Surgical sectioning of the maxilla to allow movement of all or a part of the maxilla into the desired portion.

maximum allowance As specified in a fee schedule or table of allowances, the maximum dollar amount a dental plan will pay toward the cost of a dental service.

maximum benefit The maximum dollar amount a dental plan will pay toward the cost of dental care incurred by an individual or family in a specified policy year.

maximum fee schedule A compensation arrangement in which a participating dentist agrees to accept a prescribed sum as the total fee for one or more covered services.

Mazzini's test (mah-zē′nēz) *See* test, Mazzini's.

MCHC *See* mean corpuscular hemoglobin concentration.

MCH *See* mean corpuscular hemoglobin.

MCV *See* mean corpuscular volume

MDS *See* temporomandibular joint pain-dysfunction syndrome.

MDR Minimum daily requirement, especially the Minimum Daily Requirements for Specific Nutrients compiled by the United States Food and Drug Administration.

mean (x̄) A measure of central tendency that is the calculated arithmetic average of a series of scores.

mean corpuscular hemoglobin A measure of the weight of hemoglobin in a single red blood cell. The value is obtained by multiplying the hemoglobin by 10 and dividing by the number of red blood cells. The normal range is between 27 and 31.

mean corpuscular hemoglobin concentration A measure of red blood cells useful in identifying the type of anemia. MCHC is obtained by multiplying the value of hemoglobin by 100 and dividing by the value of the hematocrit. The normal range is between 31.5 and 35.5.

mean corpuscular volume Indicates the size of the red blood cells. MCV is obtained by multiplying the hematocrit by 10 and dividing by the number of red blood cells. The normal range is between 82 and 98.

mean foundation plane *See* plane, mean foundation.

mean life *See* average life.

measles (mē′zĕlz) An infectious disease caused by a virus. There are two types: rubeola and rebella (German measles). Both have oral manifestations.

m., German *See* rubella.

m., three-day *See* rubella.

mechanically balanced occlusion *See* occlusion, balanced, mechanically.

mechanism A structure of working parts functioning together to produce an effect.

m., cough A short inspiration, closure of the glottis, forcible expiratory effort, and then release of the glottis, with a rush of air at a flow rate of 3000 to 4000 cc/sec. A cough is essentially used or regarded as a process for removing foreign material from the lungs. It involves two phases. In the first, the combined action of the cilia and bronchiolar peristalsis moves the material up to the main bronchi and the bifurcation of the trachea. Further movement out of the respiratory system depends on the cough mechanism. In all medical conditions in which this mechanism is abolished or reduced, secretions and foreign material accumulate in the alveoli, with a resultant reduction in the aerating surface and a predisposition to infection. Since ventilation of the lungs depends on a patent airway, the cough mechanism should always be used by patients whose inadequate ventilation of lungs may be related to obstruction of the airway.

m., inhibitory-excitatory A mechanism that provides coordinated and continuous stimuli to the lower motor neuron for smooth, facile, and rapidly adjustable muscle contraction. This mechanism operates on every level of the central nervous system, from the final common pathway back up the spinal cord to the cerebrum. The excitatory phase of stimulation is transmitted directly to the nerve. Inhibition, however, is effected not by stimulating the motor output directly, as is done in the parasympathetic nerves, but rather by the interaction of inhibitory mechanisms on the excitatory impulses.

m., respiratory control The mechanism by which the respiratory functions are controlled. There are three major factors in the control of respiration that concern the dentist: neurogenic control of respiration, chemical regulation of respiration, and mechanical events leading to pulmonary ventilation. These three factors are significant in practice procedures because the dentist influences each of these factors in routine dental care; e.g., the patency of the airways is always subject to alteration by instrumentation, dental prostheses, and the use of pharmacologic agents, and the physically induced responses modify the rate and magnitude of the respiratory mechanism.

m., suspensory The hammocklike arrangement of the structures comprising the attachment apparatus.

media (mē′dē-ah) The plural form of medium.

median (mē′dē-ăn) **(md)** **1:** Pertaining to the middle. **2:** A measure of central tendency attained by a calculation or count that separates all cases in a ranked distribution into halves. The median may be used as an average score.

m. lethal dose *See* dose, lethal, median.

m. line *See* line, median.

m. mandibular point *See* point, median mandibular.

m. palatine suture *See* suture, intermaxillary.

m. retruded relation *See* relation, centric.

m. rhomboid glossitis A patch of papillae free mucosa located in the center of the tongue immediately behind the circumvallate papillae. The area appears as a red, smooth, depressed area that is rhomboidal in shape. Generally the lesion is asymptomatic and is thought to result from a fault in embryonic development of the tongue. The tissue may be susceptible to candidal infections. Some writers refer to this condition as central papillary atrophy of the tongue.

m. sagittal plane *See* plane, median sagittal.

mediation Intervention; the act of a third person who interferes between two contending parties to reconcile them or to persuade them to adjust or settle their differences.

Medicaid A federal assistance program established as Title XIX under the Social Security Amendments of 1965 which provides payment for medical care for certain low income individuals and families. The program is funded jointly by the state and federal governments and administered by states. ADA

medical alert warning A coding of the patient's medical or dental record to indicate the presence of a serious medical condition that requires treatment planning consideration before initiating treatment of any kind; usually a pressure-sensitive red warning label containing a notation as to the exact nature of the compromising condition is placed on the record jacket.

medically necessary care The reasonable and appropriate diagnosis, treatment, and follow-up care (including supplies, appliances and devices) as determined and prescribed by qualified appropriate health care providers in treating any condition, illness, disease, injury, or birth developmental malformations. Care is medically necessary for the purpose of: controlling or eliminating infection, pain, and disease; and restoring facial configuration or function necessary for speech, swallowing, or chewing.

Medicare A federal insurance program enacted in 1965 as Title XVIII of the Social Security Amendments that provides certain in-patient hospital services and physician services for all persons age 65 and older and eligible disabled individuals. The program is administered by the Health Care Financing Administration.

medication (mĕd″ĭ-kā′shŭn) **1:** Impregnation with a medicine; a remedy. **2:** A drug; the administration of drugs.

m., complete Combination of synergistic drugs used in dental procedures for difficult children; the patient is in a state of sleep or light anesthesia.

m., intracanal A drug used in the root canal system during the course of therapy.

m., official *See* drug, official.

m., officinal *See* drug, officinal.

m., repository Slowly soluble drug mixtures intended for parenteral injection and gradual absorption into the blood and hence into other tissues of the body.

m., sustained release Oral dosage forms designed to be absorbed at various levels in the gastrointestinal tract, thus prolonging action.

medicine (mĕd′ĭ-sĭn) A remedy. Also, the art of healing.

m., oral The discipline of dentistry that deals with the significance and relationship of oral and systemic disease.

m., practice of A pursuit that includes the application and use of medicines and drugs for the purpose of curing or alleviating bodily diseases; surgery is usually limited to manual operations generally performed by means of surgical instruments or appliances.

mediotrusion A thrusting of the mandibular condyle inward (toward the median plane). When the right condyle is thrust outward (in laterotrusion) before it is rotated, the left condyle is thrust inward before it is orbited and is thus said to be in precurrent mediotrusion. If the left condyle is thrust outward before it is rotated, the right condyle is in precurrent mediotrusion.

mediostrusive Nonfunctional side tooth contacts during lateral jaw movements.

Mediterranean anemia *See* thalassemia major.

Mediterranean disease *See* thalassemia major.

medium (ia) (mē′dē-ŭm) An interposed agent or material; a carrier; a material serving as an environment for the growth of microorganisms.

m., computer The material on which data are recorded (e.g., punched cards, magnetic tape, disks, diskettes).

m., marking 1: Any of several agents, such as carbon paper or inked ribbon, used to indicate an occlusal interference. **2:** Any of several agents, such as stencil correction fluid, rouge and alcohol, or pressure indicator paste, used to determine areas of interference or pressure related to a removable prosthesis.

m., radiopaque A substance that may be injected into a cavity or region to increase its density in xray examination and thereby aid in diagnosis. Lipiodol, Iodochloral, Parabodril, and Ioduron are examples of such materials.

m., Sabouraud's A nutrient agar used to grow fungi. It is especially useful for the growth and identification of *Candida albicans*, the causative agent of thrush.

m., separating Any coating that is used on a surface and serves to prevent another surface or material from adhering to the first (e.g., tinfoil, cellophane, or alginate, all of which are used to protect an acrylic resin from the moisture in the gypsum mold).

MEDLARS A computerized literature retrieval service offered by the National Library of Medicine in Bethesda, Maryland. Medlars contains more than 4.5 million references to medical and dental articles in professional journals and books published since 1966. The references are made available on-line to more than 1000 hospitals, universities, medical centers and governmental agencies.

MEDLINE A National Library of Medicine computer data base of current references published during the past 2 years. The files duplicate the contents of the Unabridged Index Medicus, which contains medical and dental reports from 3,000 professional journals from more than 70 countries.

medulla oblongata (mĕ′dūl′ah ŏb-lŏng-gah′tah) The direct upward extension of the spinal cord that lies at the junction between the cerebrum and spinal cord and is considered to be in a group with the pons and midbrain because the nuclei of all the cranial nerves except one are situated within this structural group. The medulla functions are associated with the nuclei of the glossopharyngeal, vagal, spinal accessory, and hypoglossal nerves. The medulla controls the reflex actions of the pharynx, larynx, and tongue, which are related to deglutition, mastication, and speech, as well as the visceral reflexes of coughing, sneezing, sucking, vomiting, and salivation, and other secretory functions.

megadontismus (mĕg-ah-don-tĭz′mŭs) *See* macrodontia.

Meissner's corpuscles (mīs′nerz) *See* corpuscle, Meissner's.

melanin (mĕl′ah-nĭn) The dark amorphous pigment of melanotic tumors, skin, hair, choroid coat of the eye, and substantia nigra of the brain.

melanocytes (mĕl′ah-nō-sīts″) Dendritic cells of the gingival epithelium that, when functional, cause pigmentation regardless of race.

melanoma (mĕl″ah-nō′mah) A malignant neoplasm characterized by pigment-producing cells. It usually is dark in color but may be amelanotic, i.e., free of pigment.

melanosis (mĕl″ah-nō′sĭs) The condition in which melanin pigments appear in the tissues. Melanosis is normal in the gingivae of most dark-skinned individuals and occasionally in those with light skin.

melena (mĕ-lē′nah) The passage of dark or black stools; the color is produced by altered blood and blood pigments.

melituria (mĕl″ĭ-tū′rē-ah) Presence of any sugar in the urine (e.g., glucose, lactose, pentose, fructose, maltose, galactose, sucrose).

melting range *See* range, melting.

Member An individual enrolled in a dental benefits program; *See* beneficiary.).

membrane A thin layer of tissue that covers a surface or divides a space or organ.

  m., basement The delicate, PAS-positive, noncellular membrane on which the epithelium is seated.

  m. bone *See* bone, membrane.

  m., mucous *See* mucosa.

  m., Nasmyth's *See* cuticle, primary.

  m., periodontal *See* ligament, periodontal.

  m., subimplant The fibrous connective tissue that regenerates from the periosteum and that forms between the inner surface of the implant framework and the bone surface.

memory A general term for a device that stores data in binary code on electronic or magnetic media in computers.

  m. cycle The time it takes to access a character in memory.

  m. location A place in the memory where a unit of data may be stored or retrieved.

  m. register A register in storage of a computer, in contrast with a register in one of the other units of the computer.

menarche The beginning of the menstrual function.

Mendelian inheritance Better known as Mendel's laws or Mendelian laws. The basic principles of genetics based on the experiments of Gregor Mendel in the nineteenth century. Two basic genetic principles were established: the law of segregation and the law of independent assortment. According to the law of segregation, the genetic characteristics of a species are represented in the somatic cells by a pair of units called *genes* that separate during meiosis so that each gamete receives only one gene for each trait. According to the law of independent assortment, the members of a gene pair on different chromosomes segregate independently from other pairs during meiosis, so that the gametes offer all possible combinations of factors.

meniscectomy (mĕn″ĭ-sĕk′tō-mē) The surgical removal of the meniscus or condylar disc, also referred to as discetomy. A popular treatment of dysfunctional maxillofacial pain in the 1950s, somewhat discredited today.

Meniscus The cartilaginous intracapsular disc interposed between the mandibular condyle and the glenoid fossa of the temporal bone.

menopause Cessation of menstruation in the human female occurring variably from approximately 45 to 50 years of age. It is accompanied by diminution of estrogen formation, often with atrophic changes occurring in the oral mucous membranes and gingivae.

  m., oral symptoms of Burning sensation and dryness of the mouth; salty taste; edematous, reddened, atrophic-appearing, tender mucosa; glossitis; and often desquamative gingivitis.

menstruation The shedding of the necrotic mucosa of the endometrium and associated bleeding that occurs in the final phase of the menstrual cycle. The average duration of menstruation is 5 days in which approximately 30 cc of blood is lost. The average duration of the entire menstrual cycle is 28 days.

mental foramen *See* foramen, mental.

mental retardation A disorder of general intellectual function impairing the ability to learn and to adapt socially.

mental retardate An individual who is intellectually inadequate in society.

menton The most inferior point on the chin in the lateral view; a cephalometric landmark.

meperidine hydrochloride (mĕ-per′ĭ-dēn) Ethyl 1methyl-4-phenyl 4-piperidine carboxylate hydrochloride; a narcotic employed for its analgesic, sedative, and spasmolytic effect. The usual dose for adults is 500 to 100 mg. The brand name is Demerol.

mephenesin (mĕ-fĕn′ĭ-sĭn) An antispasmodic drug, 3ortho-toloxy1,2-propanediol. Used for the preparation of apprehensive patients for dental and periodontal procedures because of its ability to produce muscular relaxation and euphoria. Usual dosage for an adult is 1 Gm in either tablet or elixir form 20 minutes prior to the dental appointment.

meprobamate An anxiolytic agent used in the short-term treatment of acute anxiety and/or tension associated with anxiety. It is not recommended for the treatment of stress associated with everyday living. The brand name is Miltown.

merbromin (mer-brō′mĭn) A mercury-bromine compound used as a germicide for disinfection of the skin, mucous membrane, and wounds. Used in 10% alcoholic solution (Scott-Wilson reagent) in the treatment of moniliasis.

mercaptan (mer-kăp′tăn) The basic ingredient of the polysulfide polymer employed in rubber base impression materials. *See also* Thiokol.

mercurial (mer-kū′rē-ăl) A compound that owes its activity to the mercury it contains.

    m. line *See* line, mercurial.

mercurialism (mercury poisoning) 1: Poisoning resulting from the ingestion of pure mercury, its salts, or its vapor. Manifestations of acute intoxication include nausea, vomiting, abdominal cramps, oral and pharyngeal pain, uremia, dehydration, diarrhea, and shock. Manifestations of chronic poisoning include hypersalivation, diarrhea, vertigo, depression, intention tremor, and stomatitis. *See also* acrodynia; stomatitis, mercurial. **2:** Poisoning by ingestion or absorption of mercury compounds. *See also* line, mercurial.

Mercurochrome Trade name for merbromin.

merge To produce a single sequence of items, ordered according to some rule, from two or more sequences previously ordered according to the same rule. Merging does not change the items in size, structure, or total number.

Merkel's corpuscles *See* corpuscle, Merkel's.

Merkel's disks *See* corpuscle, Merkel's.

Merrifield's knife *See* knife, Merrifield's.

mes- (meso-) In the middle; intermediate as in position, size, type, and time degree.

mesial (mē′zē-ăl) Situated in the middle; median, toward the middle line of the body or toward the center line of the dental arch.

    m. migration The drifting teeth toward the midline or forward in the dental arch.

mesioclusion An occlusal relationship in which the lower teeth are positioned mesially, similar to the relationship in an Angle Class III malocclusion. Antonym: distoclusion.

    m., unilateral Mesioclusion on one side.

mesiodens (mē′zē-ō-dĕnz) A supernumerary tooth appearing in an erupted or unerupted state between the two maxillary central incisors.

mesioversion (mē-zē-o-ver′zhŭn) When applied to a tooth, a term indicating that the tooth is closer than normal to the median plane or midline. When applied to the maxillae or mandible, it means that the jaw is anterior to its normal position.

meso- *See* mes-.

mesocephalic (mēz″ō-sĕ-făl′ĭk) Descriptive term applied to a head size between dolichocephalic and brachycephalic (cephalic index 76 to 81).

mesodontia (mēz-ō-don′shē-ah) Medium-sized teeth.

mesognathic (mē-sō-năth′ĭk) Having an average relationship of jaws to head.

mesostomia (mēz-ō-stō′mē-ah) An oral fissure of medium size.

mesostructure conjunction bar A connecting bar joining implant abutment copings together. Bar and copings together make up the mesostructure.

metabolic disease Any disorder that causes dysfunction of the metabolic action of the body, resulting in loss of control of homeostasis.

metabolism (mĕ-tăb′ō-lĭzm) The sum of chemical changes involved in the function of nutrition. There are two phases: anabolism (constructive or assimilative changes) and catabolism (destructive or retrograde changes).

    m., basal *See* basal metabolic rate.

    m., bone The continual complex of anabolism and catabolism taking place in bone when it is in physiologic equilibrium. Bone is a highly labile substance the reflects the adequacy of general body metabolism. *See also* bone, alveolar, metabolism.

    m., cell The complexity of anabolic and catabolic processes occurring within cellular structures.

    m., energy The transformation of energy in living tissues, consisting of anabolism (storage of energy) and catabolism (the dissipation of energy).

    m., substance The sum of all the physical and chemical processes by which living organized tissues are produced and maintained.

metachysis (mĕ-tăk′ĭ-sĭs) Blood transfusion; the introduction of any substance directly into the bloodstream by mechanical means.

metal An element possessing luster, malleability, ductility, and conductivity of electricity and heat.

m., base Archaic term referring to nonprecious metals or alloys (e.g., iron, lead, copper, nickel, chromium, zinc). In dentistry, a term usually referring to the stainless steel and chrome-cobaltnickel alloys.

m., fusion of Blending of metals by melting together.

m. insert teeth *See* tooth, metal insert.

m., noble A precious metal, usually one that does not readily oxidize (e.g., gold, platinum).

m., solidification of The change of metal from the molten to the solid state.

m., wrought A cast metal that has been cold worked in any manner.

metalloid (mĕt′ăh-loid) A nonmetallic element that behaves as a metal under certain conditions. Carbon, silicon, and boron are three examples. These elements may be alloyed with metals.

metaphen, tincture of (mĕt′ah-fĕn) Trade name for tincture of nitromersol.

metaphysis (mĕ-tăf′ĭ-sĭs) The line of junction of the epiphysis with the diaphysis of a long bone.

metaplasia (mĕt″ah-plā′zē-ah) Change in the type of adult cells in a tissue to a form that is not normal for that tissue.

metastasis (mĕ-tăs′tah-sĭs) The transfer of a disease by blood vessels, lymph vessels, or the respiratory tract (aspiration) from one organ or region to another not directly contiguous with it. Usually used in reference to malignant tumor cells, but bacteria can also metastasize (e.g., in focal infection).

meter, dose rate Any instrument that measures radiation dose rate.

m., d. r., integrating Ionization chamber and measuring system designed for determining the total accumulated radiation administered during an exposure.

meter, radiation An instrument for the measurement of exposure to radiation.

m., dosimeter, radiation An instrument used to detect and measure an accumulated exposure to radiation—commonly a pencil-sized ionization chamber with built-in self-reading electrometer used in personnel radiation monitoring.

methemoglobinemia (mĕt-hē″mō-glō″bĭ-nē′mē-ah) An abnormality of hemoglobin in which the iron is in the ferric state as a result of exposure to industrial substances or the ingestion of toxic agents such as phenacetin, sulfonamides, aniline nitrates, and nitrates. A rare congenital form is seen most commonly in Greeks. Symptoms include generalized cyanosis,

headache, drowsiness, and confusion. Methemoglobin does not carry oxygen.

methionine One of the essential amino acids; *see* amino acid.

method A manner of performing an act or operation; a technique.

m., Callahan's *See* method, chloropercha.

m., Charters' A method of toothbrushing in which the brush is held horizontally, with the bristles lying against the teeth and gingivae and pointed in a coronal direction at 45 degrees so that the bristles lie half on the teeth and half on the gingivae. A vibratory cycle of a very constricted diameter is negotiated so that the brush head moves in a circular movement but the brush bristles remain fairly stationary while being agitated. The circular vibration loosens debris and pumps the bristles into interproximal areas to massage the tissues.

m., chloropercha (Callahan's method, Johnston's method) The method of filling root canals in which gutta-percha cones are dissolved in a chloroform-rosin solution in the root canal. The canal is flooded with the chloroform solution. A preselected gutta-percha cone is then pumped carefully into and out of the canal. As the cone dissolves, the material is forced into the apex as a plastic mass. Other cones and occasionally additional chloroform solution are added until the canal is sealed.

m., Fones' (Fones' technique) A toothbrushing technique in which, with the teeth occluded and with the brush at more or less right angles to the teeth, large sweeping, scrubbing circles are described. With the jaws parted, the palatal and lingual surfaces of the teeth are scrubbed using smaller circles. Occlusal surfaces are brushed in an anteroposterior direction.

m., Hirschfeld's A toothbrushing method in which the bristles are placed against the axial surfaces of the teeth, with slight incisal or occlusal inclination from a right-angled application, in simultaneous contact with teeth and gingivae, and then rotated in a circle of exceedingly small diameter. Occlusal surfaces are brushed energetically.

m., Howard's A method of artificial respiration. The patient is placed on the back, with the hands placed under the head, and a cushion is placed so that the head is lower than the abdomen. The physician applies rhythmical pressure upward and inward with the hands against the lower lateral parts of the patient's chest.

m., Howe's silver precipitation A method of depositing silver in enamel and dentin by the application of ammoniacal silver nitrate solution and its reduction with formalin or eugenol.

m., indirect restorative The technique of fabrication of a restoration on a cast or model of the original (e.g., the indirect method of inlay construction, in which a die of amalgam or other material is made from an impression of the prepared tooth, a wax pattern formed, and the cast inlay fitted and finished on the die, then cemented to the tooth).

m., Johnston's *See* method, chloropercha.

m., lateral condensation The method in which a preselected gutta-percha cone is sealed into the apex of the root. The balance of space is filled with other gutta-percha cones forced laterally with a spreader.

m., segmentation The method in which a preselected gutta-percha cone is cut into segments. The tip section is sealed into the apex of the root. The other segments are usually warmed and condensed against the first piece with a plugger. Additional pieces are then used until the space is obliterated.

m., silver cone The method in which a prefitted silver cone is sealed into the apex of the root canal. The space not sealed with the cone is obliterated with gutta-percha or sealer.

m., split cast 1: A procedure for checking the ability of an articulator to receive or be adjusted to a maxillomandibular relation record. **2:** A procedure for indexing casts on an articulator to facilitate their removal and replacement on the instrument.

methyl methacrylate (mĕth′ ĭl mĕth-ak′rĭ-lāt) An acrylic resin, $CH_2 = C(CH_3)COOCH_3$, derived from methyl acrylic acid. Monomer is the single molecule and polymer is the polymerization product.

Meticorten Trade name for prednisone.

metric system *See* system, metric.

metronidazole A generic synthetic antibacterial compound available for both oral and intravenous use. Metraonidazole is indicated in the treatment of serious infections caused by susceptable anaerobic bacteria. In dentistry used in the treatment of HIV gingivitis and HIV periodontitis.

mev One million electron volts.

micelle (mī-sĕl′) Any one of the spaces formed by the brush structure of fibrils in colloidal gels. The spaces are occupied by water in hydrocolloid impressions.

microcephalus (mī″krō-sĕf′ah-lŭs) An abnormally small head.

Micrococcus gazogenes (mī″krō-kahk′ŭs gah′zō-jēnz) *See Veillonella alcalescens.*

microcomputer A very small computer, usually with only one user for personal, home, or office use.

microcurie One millionth of a curie.

microcytosis, hereditary (mī″krō-sīō′sĭs) *See* thalassemia; thalassemia major.

microdontia (mī″krō-don′shē-ah) Abnormally small teeth. Term may apply to one, several, or all the teeth of a given individual.

microgenia (mī″krō-jē′nē-ah) Abnormal smallness of the chin.

microglossia (mī″krō-glahs′ē-ah) An abnormally small tongue.

microglossic Descriptive of microglossia.

micrognathia (mī″krō-năth′ē-ah) An abnormally small jaw (e.g., in brachygnathia). *See also* brachygnathia; retrognathism.

micrognathic Descriptive of micrognathia.

microleakage The seepage of fluids, debris, and microorganisms along the interface between a restoration and the walls of a cavity preparation.

micrometer (mī′krō-mē″ter) A millionth of a meter (10^{-6} meter).

micron *See* micrometer.

microbiology A division or branch of biology that deals with the study of microorganisms including: algae, bacteria, fungi, protozoa, rickettsiae, and viruses.

microorganism (mī″krō-ŏr′găn-ĭzm) A minute living organism, such as a bacterium, virus, rickettsia, yeast, or fungus. These organisms may exist as part of the normal flora of the oral cavity without producing disease. With disturbance of the more or less balanced interrelationship between the organisms or between the organisms and host resistance, individual forms of microorganisms may overgrow and induce disease in the host's tissues. Of course, organisms foreign to the individual may invade and produce pathologic processes.

microradiography A process by which a radiograph of a small object is produced on fine-grained photographic film under conditions that permit subsequent microscopic examination.

microscope An instrument containing a powerful lens system for magnifying and viewing near objects.

m., phase A microscope through which living microbes can be viewed. An excellent aid in the education and motivation of patients in the understanding and control of dental plaque.

microstomia (mī″krō-stō′mē-ah) A small oral fissure.

microtia (mī-krō′shē-ah) Aplasia or hypoplasia of the pinna of the ear, with a closed or missing external auditory meatus.

midbrain (mĭd′brān) The portion of the brain located superior to the pons and medulla and containing the motor nuclei of the ocular motor and trochlear nerves. It also contains the major pathways and decussations of fibers from the cerebrum and cerebellum.

midface That portion of the face comprised of the nasal, maxillary, and zygomatic bones and the soft tissues covering these bones.

midline The line equidistant from bilateral features of the head.

migraine *See* headache, migraine.

migration, tooth *See* tooth, drifting.

migratory glossitis Also known as geographic tongue *See* tongue, geographic.

Mikulicz' aphtha, disease, syndrome (mĭk'ū-lĭch) *See* disease.

Mikulicz' ulcer *See* periadenitis mucosa necrotica recurrens.

milled-in curve *See* path, milled-in.

milled-in path *See* path, milled-in.

Miller's organism *See* organism, Miller's.

milliampere (mĭl"ē-ăm'pēr) In radiography, milliamperage signifies the amount of current flowing in the tube circuit. With time (seconds) it is an indication of roentgen-ray quantity.

millicurie One thousandth of a curie.

milliliter (ml) (mĭl'ĭ-lē'ter) The preferred unit of volume used in prescription writing. It is based on the fundamental unit, the liter. One liter equals 1000 milliliters. In prescriptions the terms *ml* and *cc* are often used interchangeably because they are so nearly equal.

milling-in The procedure of refining or perfecting the occlusion of removable partial or complete dentures by placing abrasives between their occluding surfaces while the dentures make contact in various excursions on the articulator.

milliroentgen (mĭl'ĭ-rĕnt'gĕn) A submultiple of the roentgen, equal to one thousandth of a roentgen.

mineral oil *See* oil, mineral.

mineralization Bioprecipitation of inorganic substance.

mineralocorticoids (mĭn"er-ăl-ō-kor'tĭ-koidz) **(proinflammatory hormones)** Adrenal corticosteroids that are active in the retention of salt and in the maintenance of life of adrenalectomized animals. Typical are deoxycorticosterone and aldosterone. Aldosterone is a natural hormone for salt retention but also has some regulatory effect on carbohydrate metabolism.

minim (mĭn'ĭm) A unit of volume in the traditional apothecary system. It equals 0.0016 ml. A drop is sometimes used as a crude approximation of the minim.

minor A person of either sex under the age of majority; i.e., one who has not attained the age at which full civil rights are granted; an infant.

    m. connector *See* connector, minor.

Miltown *See* meprobamate

minocycline A semisynthetic derivative of tetracycline used in the treatment of Rickettsiae, such as tick fevers, psittacosis, and in the treatment of some periodontal infections generally in conjunction with mechanical therapy.

miotic (mī-ah'tĭk) A drug that constricts the pupil.

misconduct A deviation from duty by one employed in a professional capacity; a transgression of an established rule.

misfeasance (mĭs-fē'zĕns) The improper performance of some act that one may lawfully do.

misrepresentation An intentionally false statement regarding a matter of fact.

MIST An acronym for Medical Information Service via Telephone. A consultation service offered by some state-operated university medical centers.

mistake Some unintentional act, omission, or error resulting from ignorance, surprise, or misplaced confidence.

mithridatism (mĭth'rĭ-dā"tĭzm) *See* tolerance, acquired.

mitigation (mĭt"ĭ-gā'shŭn) Alleviation; abatement of diminution of a penalty imposed by law.

    m. of damages A reduction of damages based on facts that show the plaintiff's course of action does not entitle the plaintiff to as large an amount as the evidence would otherwise justify the jury in allowing.

mix To form by combining ingredients.

mixed dentition *See* dentition, mixed.

mixing, vacuum A method of mixing materials, such as gypsum products and water, in a vacuum.

MLD *See* dose, lethal, minimum.

MLT *See* time, median lethal.

Mo cavity A cavity on the mesial and occlusal surfaces of a tooth. *See* cavity, Class 2.

mobility Loosening of a tooth or teeth. An important diagnostic sign that may result not only from a decrease in root attachment or changes in the periodontal ligament but also from destruction of the gingival fiber apparatus and transseptal fibers.

    m. of tooth *See* tooth mobility.

MOD cavity A cavity on the mesial, occlusal, and distal surfaces of a tooth. *See* cavity, Class 2.

mode (mo) A measure of central tendency that is the most frequently occurring score or value in a group of scores. The mode may be used as an average score.

model 1: A replica, usually in miniature. *See* cast, *n.* **2:** A positive replica of the dentition and surrounding or adjoining structures used as a diagnostic aid and/or base for construction of orthodontic and prosthetic appliances.

    m., casting *See* cast, refractory.

    m., implant *See* cast, implant.

    m., of prepared cavity *See* die.

    m., study *See* cast, diagnostic.

modeling compound *See* compound.

modem (modulator/demodulator) A device that converts data from a form compatible with computer manipulation to a form compatible with transmission equipment and vice versa.

moderator A chairman; one who presides over an assembly, group, or panel.

modiolus (mō-dī'ō-lŭs) A point distal to the corner of the mouth where several muscles of facial expression converge.

modulus A constant that numerically indicates the amount in which a certain property is possessed by any object.

    m. of elasticity *See* elasticity, modulus of.

m. of resilience *See* resilience, modulus of.

m. of rigidity *See* rigidity.

m., Young's *See* elasticity, modulus of.

Moeller's disease (mě′lerz) *See* scurvy, infantile.

Moeller's glossitis (mě′lerz) *See* glossitis, Moeller's.

Mohs scale *See* hardness, Mohs.

molar 1: A reference solution in which the concentration is stated with regard to the number of gram molecular weights per liter of solution. **2:** A tooth adapted for grinding by having a broad, somewhat ridged surface. In the human it is one of the twelve teeth located in the posterior aspect of the upper and lower jaws.

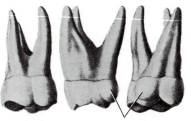

Carabelli's tubercle

Right upper first molar
Buccal surface   Mesial surface   Lingual surface

m., mulberry A malformed first molar with a crown, suggesting the appearance of a mulberry. It may be a manifestation of congenital syphilis, although other diseases affecting the enamel organ during morphodifferentiation may produce a similar lesion.

m. sheath A rectangular metallic tube soldered or welded to the molar bands.

mold (mould) A form in which an object is cast or shaped. The process of shaping a material into an object. The term used to specify the shape of an artificial tooth or teeth.

molding Shaping.

m., border border molding. **m., compression** The act of pressing or squeezing together to form a shape in a mold.

m., injection Adaptation of a plastic material to the negative form of a closed mold by forcing the material into the mold through appropriate gateways. *See also* molding, compression.

m., tissue *See* border molding.

mole A pigmented nevus.

molecular weight *See* weight, molecular.

molecule A unit of matter that is the smallest particle of an element or chemical combination of atoms (as a compound) capable of retaining chemical identity with the substance in mass.

molimina, menstrual (mō-lĭm′ĭ-nah) Circulatory symp-

toms, psychic tension, irritable behavior, belligerence, and other personality alterations prior to or during menstruation. The cause is unknown.

moliuscum fibrosum *See* neurofibromatosis.

momentum Quantity of motion, expressed as the product of mass and velocity.

money General term for the representation of value; currency; cash.

money market fund A mutual fund that invests only in high-yielding short-term money market instruments (U.S. Treasury bills, bank certificates of deposit, commercial paper, etc.)

mongolism (mon′gō-lĭzm) **(Down's syndrome) 1:** Extreme mental deficiency of a congenital type associated with features of the Mongolian race, such as slanted eyes. **2:** Clinical syndrome (Down's) associated with the autosomal abnormalities trisomy-21 or translocations 13-15/21-22, or 21/22. Affected children have almond-shaped eyes, a rather roundish head, and increased susceptibility to infection. They are mentally retarded, commonly suffer from acute leukemia, and often have congenital heart disease, a heavily fissured and protruding tongue, delayed dentition, an underdeveloped nose, short fingers, and broad simian-like hands.

Monilia albicans (mō-nĭl′ē-ah ăl′bĭ-kănz) *See Candida albicans.*

moniliasis (mō″nĭ-lī′ah-sĭs) Infection by a fungus of the genus *Candida,* usually *Candida albicans.* May involve the mouth (thrush), female genitalia, skin, hands, nails, and/or lungs. Oral moniliasis refers to thrush or to mycotic stomatitis. The latter term is sometimes applied to erythematous patches that are not typical of the usual white patches of thrush. *See also* thrush.

monitoring Periodic or continuous determination of the dose rate in an occupied area by a person.

m., area Routine monitoring of the level of radiation of any particular area, building, room, equipment, or outdoor space.

m., personal Monitoring of any part of an individual (e.g., breath or excretions or any part of the clothing).

m., personnel A systematic, periodic check of the radiation dose each person receives during working hours.

monkey An animal often used for experimental purposes in medicine and stomatology. Its dental and oral structures are morphologically and functionally similar to those of human beings, permitting an associated correlation of experimental findings.

monobloc *See* activator.

monocyte (mon′ō-sīt) A large nongranular leukocyte containing a single oval or indented nucleus and more protoplasm than a lymphocyte.

monocytosis (mon″ō-sī-tō′sĭs) Increase in the number of monocytes in the peripheral bloodstream. Various limits are given (e.g., a total number in excess of 800/mm³, regardless of the percentage, or a total greater than 8% with the total number less than 800). In both cases the presence of monocytosis is indicated. It may be associated with chronic pyogenic infections, subacute bacterial endocarditis, infectious hepatitis, monocytic leukemia, rickettsial disease, and protozoan infections.

monomer (mon′ō-mer) A single molecule. In commercial resin products, the term applies to the liquid, which is usually a mixture of monomers.

　m., residual The unpolymerized monomer remaining in the appliance or restoration after processing.

mononucleosis, infectious (mŏn″ō-nū′klē-ō′sĭs) **(acute benign lymphadenosis, "kissing disease," "student's disease")** An acute infectious viral disease most commonly affecting young adults and older children. Manifestations include fever, sore throat, cervical lymphadenopathy, petechial hemorrhages of the soft palate, and, at times, purpura with thrombocytopenia. Early leukopenia and relative lymphocytosis occur, with later increases in the number of large leukocytoid lymphocytes. The heterophil (usually sheep cell) antibody titer is significantly increased in most instances.

monostotic Affecting a single bone.

Monson curve *See* curve, Monson.

moot 1: Subject to argument; undecided. **2:** In law, in a moot case one seeks to determine an abstract question does not arise on existing facts or rights.

moral Relating to the conscience or moral sense or to the general principles of correct conduct.

morbidity State of being diseased; can be used as an outcome measure such as number of decayed, missing, and filled teeth.

morphology The branch of biology that deals with the form and structure of an organism or part, without regard to function.

　m., determinants of occlusal Variable factors that determine the forms given to the crowns of teeth restored in metals, such as mandibular centricity; the intercondylar distance; the distance of teeth from the sagittal plane; the character of lateral and protrusive paths of the condylar axes; and the overlaps of the anterior teeth and wear.

mortality Death rate.

mortgage A right given to the creditor over the property of the debtor for the security of the debt; invests the creditor with the power of having the property seized and sold in default of payment.

　m., chattel A mortgage of goods or personal property.

mortgagee The person who takes or receives a mortgage.

motion, envelope of The three-dimensional space circumscribed by border movements and by occlusal contacts of a given point of the mandible. Synonym: movement space. *See also* movement, border, posterior.

motivation The stimulus, incentive, or inducement to act or react in a certain way. Purposeful human behavior is motivated behavior, which means that either physiologic or social stimuli activate or motivate a person to do something.

motor Pertaining to a muscle, nerve, or center that produces or effects movement.

　m. output The activity that results from the integrative phenomena associated with brain activity. It is expressed in function as muscle contraction of the smooth and striated muscle and as secretion of the exocrine and endocrine glands, and, in effect, represents the total behavioral activity of human life. Whereas sensory phenomena have many avenues that feed into the brain, motor activity is expressed in terms of the simple, direct state of muscle contraction and glandular secretion. Thus muscle activity is expressed in terms of locomotion, hand-learned skills, speaking, mastication, and all forms of human activity that involve motion.

　m. pathway All reflex actions of muscle are achieved by the passage of nerve impulses through the final common pathway—the muscle fibers. The lower motor neuron (the motor route of the cranial nerve) is the final pathway for the structures that are innervated by the cranial nerves. Impulses traverse these nerves to their respective muscles from every level of the spinal cord, hindbrain, midbrain, and cerebral cortex. The cranial motor neurons collate these multiple stimuli and transmit sequences of stimuli to the motor end-plate, which in the normal muscle effects a smooth, continuous, controlled contraction.

　m. unit The entity consisting of the lower motor neuron, motor end-plate, and muscle fibers supplied by the end-plate. The final motor activity resulting from a sequence of stimulations to the lower motor neuron is considered a function of the motor unit. The proportion of nerve fibers to the muscle fibers in motor units is designated as the innervation ratio. Motor units may have ratios ranging from 1:4 to 1:150. The closer the ratio approximates unity, the greater the finesse of specificity of the muscular action. The eye muscles have the highest ratio of striated muscles, and the tongue, facial, masticatory, and pharyngeal muscles succeed in that order.

mottled enamel *See* fluorosis, chronic endemic dental.

moulage A model of a part or a lesion (e.g., a model of the face). It may be of wax or plaster and usually is colored by painting.

mould *See* mold.

mount, x-ray A windowed, stiff material on which radiographs are arranged in a specific order to correspond with the charts of the teeth.

mounting The laboratory procedure of attaching the maxillary and/or mandibular cast to an articulator or similar instrument.

m. board A jig used in mounting the maxillary cast on the top articulator frame. The mounting board enables the dentist to determine the patient's axis so that the maxillary cast can be positioned accurately.

m., split cast A cast with the margins of its base or capital beveled or grooved to permit accurate remounting on an articulator. Split remounting metal plates may be used instead of beveling or grooving in the casts.

mouth breathing *See* breathing, mouth.

mouth, denture-sore Traumatization and inflammation of the oral mucous membranes produced by ill-fitting dentures, hypersensitivity to the chemical components of the denture, and/or proliferation of *Candida albicans* with subsequent monilial infection.

mouth guard *See* guard, mouth.

mouth hygiene *See* hygiene, oral.

mouth lamp *See* lamp, mouth.

mouth preparation *See* preparation, mouth.

mouth rehabilitation *See* rehabilitation, mouth.

mouth, trench *See* gingivitis, necrotizing ulcerative.

mouth-to-mouth insufflation *See* insufflation, mouth-to-mouth.

mouthwash A mouth rinse possessing cleansing, germicidal, and/or palliative properties.

movement(s) Any change of place or of position of a body.

m., Bennett The bodily lateral movement or lateral shift of the mandible resulting from the movements of the condyles along the lateral inclines of the mandibular fossae during lateral jaw movement.

m., bodily Movement of a tooth so that the crown and root apex move the same amount in the same direction, thus maintaining the same axial inclination; opposed to tipping movement.

m., border Any extreme muscular movement limited by bone, ligaments, or other soft tissues.

m., posterior border Any movement of the mandible occurring while the mandible is in its most posterior relation to the maxillae. This movement occurs in the vertical plane from the level of occlusal contact to the level of maximal opening of the jaws.

m., hinge An opening or closing movement of the mandible on the hinge axis. A movement around a single axis.

m., intermediary (intermediate movement) All mandibular movements between the extremes of mandibular excursions.

m., jaw All changes in position of which the mandible

is capable.

m., lateral A movement of a body to one side of its established position.

m., mandibular Any movement of the lower jaw.

m., mandibular gliding Side-to-side, protrusive, and intermediate movement of the mandible, occurring when the teeth or other occluding surfaces are in contact.

m., free mandibular Mandibular movement made without tooth interference. An uninhibited movement of the mandible.

m., functional mandibular All natural, proper, or characteristic movements of the mandible made during speaking, chewing, yawning, swallowing, and other associated movements.

m., masticatory mandibular The translatory and rotary movements of the mandible that are used in the course of chewing food.

m., nonfunction mandibular Movement of the mandible for other than the accepted range of functional movements, i.e., movements dictated by tension, emotion, or aggression. Also mandibular movements may be misused to hold objects in either indulgent or work habits. These nonfunctional movements may result in a variety of pathologic manifestations.

m., opening mandibular The movement of the mandible executed during jaw separation.

m., tipping The movement of a tooth in any direction while its apex remains in almost the original position.

m., tooth Temporary or permanent deviation of a tooth from its normally fixed position in the dental arch. Also, mobility of teeth. When teeth exhibit mobility patterns, movement may be buccolingual, mesiodistal, occlusoapical, rotational, etc. Movement of teeth into different positions in the dental arch may be produced by repositioning them mesially, distally, buccally, lingually, occlusally, etc.

m., translatory Motion of a body at any instant when all points within the body are moving at the same velocity and in the same direction.

MPD *See* dose, maximum permissible.

MSH *See* hormone, melanocyte-stimulating.

mucobuccal fold *See* fold, mucobuccal.

mucobuccal reflection *See* fold, mucobuccal.

mucocele (mu′kō-sēl) *See* cyst, mucous.

mucolabial fold *See* fold, mucolabial.

mucopolysaccharides A generic term for a group of compounds comprised of protein and complex sugars (polysaccharides), many of which are found in blood group substances.

mucopolysaccharidosis (MPS) Genetic disorder involving mucopolysaccharide metabolism and leading to excess storage of the material in the tissues. Forms include

MPS I, II, III, IV, V, and VI. Eponymic designations are Hurler, Hunter, Sanfilippo, Morquio, Scheie, and Maroteaux-Lamy syndromes.

mucosa (mucous membrane) (mū-kō′sah) A membrane, composed of epithelium and lamina propria, that lines the oral cavity and other canals and cavities of the body that communicate with external air.

　　m., alveolar The covering on the alveolar process loosely attached to bone; extends from the mucogingival junction to the vestibular fomix and from the lower jaw to the sublingual sulcus.

　　m., oral Lining of the oral cavity; composed of the stratified squamous epithelium and the underlying lamina propria.

　　m., palatine The mucous membrane covering the palate.

mucositis (mū″kō-sī′tĭs) Inflammation of the mucous membrane.

　　m., chronic atrophic senile Mucosal inflammation characterized by atrophy and found primarily in elderly women.

　　m., fusospirochetal Mucosal inflammation associated with fusiform and spirochetal microorganisms.

mucostatic 1: Pertaining to the normal, relaxed condition of mucosal tissues covering the jaws. **2:** An agent that arrests the secretion of mucus.

mucous membrane *See* mucosa.

mucous patch *See* patch, mucous.

mucoviscidosis (mū″kō-vĭs″ĭ-dō′sĭs) *See* disease, fibrocystic.

mulberry molars First permanent molars in which the occlusal surface is composed of an aggregate of enamel nodules. All four molars are involved, usually as the result of congenital syphilis.

mulling (mŭh′lĭng) The final step of mixing dental amalgam; a kneading of the triturated mass to complete the amalgamation.

multiprocessing The use of two or more processors in a system configuration. One processor controls the system, and the others are subordinate to it.

multiprogramming A technique for permitting more than one program to time-share machine components. This technique permits the concurrent handling of numerous programs by one computer.

mumps (parotitis) A contagious parotitis caused by the mumps virus (paramyxovirus) and characterized by swelling of the parotid gland and sometimes swelling of the pancreas, ovaries, and testicles. The incubation period is 12 to 20 days; transmission is by droplet spread and direct contact; communicability begins about 2 days prior to the appearance of symptoms and lasts until swelling of the glands has abated. *See also* parotitis.

　　m., iodide (iodine mumps) Enlargement of the thyroid gland resulting from iodides.

　　m., iodine *See* mumps, iodide.

murmur A humming or blowing sound heard on auscultation.

　　m., aortic A murmur resulting from insufficiency of the aortic valve secondary to involvement by rheumatic fever or tertiary syphilis.

　　m., apical diastolic A murmur heard over the apex of the heart and caused by mitral stenosis, relative mitral stenosis, or aortic insufficiency.

　　m., apical systolic A murmur heard at the apex of the heart in systole and caused by mitral insufficiency, which may result from rheumatic heart disease, or by relative mitral insufficiency, which may result from congestive heart failure associated with arteriosclerosis or hypertension. The murmur may also have a functional basis.

　　m., basal diastolic A murmur heard over the base of the heart and caused by aortic insufficiency resulting from rheumatic heart disease or syphilis, relative aortic insufficiency associated with diastolic hypertension, or a patent ductus arteriosus.

　　m., basal systolic A murmur heard over the base of the heart and caused by aortic stenosis resulting from rheumatic heart disease or by relative stenosis of the aortic valve resulting from aortic dilation secondary to arteriosclerosis or hypertension. The murmur may also be functional or may result from congenital heart or vascular defects.

　　m., cardiac (heart murmur) An abnormal sound heard in the region of the heart at any time during the heart's cycle. Murmurs may be named according to the area of generation (mitral, aortic, pulmonary, or tricuspid) and according to the period of the cycle (diastolic or systolic).

　　m., functional (innocent murmur, inorganic murmur) A murmur resulting from the position of the body, severe anemia, or polycythemia. Not related to structural changes in the heart.

　　m., heart *See* murmur, cardiac.

　　m., innocent *See* murmur, functional.

　　m., inorganic *See* murmur, functional.

　　m., mitral Heart murmur produced by a defect in the mitral valve. The most common form of murmur in rheumatic heart disease.

　　m., organic A murmur resulting from structural changes in the heart or in the great vessels of the heart.

muscle(s) An organ that, by cellular contraction, produces the movements of life. There are two varieties of muscle structure: striated, including all the muscles in which contraction is voluntary and the heart muscle (in which contraction is involuntary), and unstriated, smooth, or organic, including all the involuntary muscles (except the heart), such as the muscular layer of the intestines, bladder, and blood vessels.

m., ciliary Tiny smooth muscle at the junction of the cornea and sclera, consisting of two groups of fibers: circular fibers (which exert parasympathetic control through the oculomotor nerve and the ciliary ganglion) and radial fibers (which exert sympathetic control). Responsible for accommodation for far vision through flattening of lens.

m. contraction *See* contraction, muscle.

m., concentric, contraction *See* contraction, muscle, concentric.

m., eccentric, contraction *See* contraction, muscle, eccentric.

m., isometric, contraction *See* contraction, muscle, isometric.

m., isotonic, contraction *See* contraction, muscle, isotonic.

m., elasticity of, physical The physical quality of being elastic, of yielding to passive physical stretch.

m., elasticity of, physiologic The biologic quality, unique for muscle, of being able to change and resume size under neuromuscular control.

m., facial The muscles of expression, frequently called the *mimetic muscles*. They are quite variable in contour, are widely distributed over the scalp and face, and tend to be especially concentrated about the orbits, outer ear, and lips. It is the mobility of the lips that has extended the usefulness of the facial muscles in expressing emotion, speech, and intelligence. The facial muscles, as a group, have only one bony origin in the facial skeleton. The muscles form a circular rim around the perimeter of the facial bones and extend anteriorly as a tube of tissue in which the lumen narrows and terminates in the orbicularis oris. The structure of the facial muscles may be regarded as a truncated cone in which the base rests on the skeleton (origin) in a fixed position, whereas the truncated top of the cone (insertion in the orbicularis oris) is variable in diameter and height. The lips are thus extensible and retractable and can constrict like a purse string.

m., functional changes of Asymmetric modifications in length, diameter, and bulk of muscle fibers as a result of variations in function. Muscle responds to normal function by maintenance of bulk. An increase in bulk is caused by an increase in the number of capillaries and in the mean diameter of individual muscle fibers. It is the response to function that accounts for the asymmetry of musculature, which is frequently found when the growth patterns have been influenced by a traumatogenic agent such as disease, injury, or surgery, and also by the functional processes of the body itself, such as posture and habit. Asymmetry is not necessarily pathologic; e.g., it may be the result of differences in habits of chewing, incision, speech sounds, and facial gestures.

m., hypertenseness Increased muscular tension that is not easily released but that does not prevent normal lengthening of the muscle. Hypertenseness is found in patients with general nervousness.

m., innervation of, reciprocal A phenomenon of antagonistic muscles demonstrated during a concentric contraction such as that of the temporal muscle. Innervation of the antagonist, the external pterygoid muscle, is partially inhibited, so that freedom of action in flexing the temporomandibular joint is possible. This phenomenon demonstrates inhibition of antagonistic skeletal muscles in a reflex arc brought about automatically by a reduction of the motor discharges from the central nervous system. One of the two muscles in the reflex arc is activated, and the activity of the other is depressed.

m., masticatory (măs′tĭ-kah-tō″rē) The powerful muscles that elevated and rotate the mandible so that the opposing teeth may occlude for mastication.

m. memory A kinesthetic phenomenon by which a muscle or set of muscles may involuntarily produce movement that follows a pattern that has become established by frequent repetition over a long period of time.

m., mimetic (mĭ-mĕt′ĭk) The facial muscles by which emotion and intelligence are expressed. The facial nerve provides neurologic control over the muscles of the face.

m., ocular, function The action of the eye muscles in moving the eyeballs. The eyes are in a position of rest (their primary position) when their direction is maintained simply by the tone of the ocular muscles. This condition prevails when the gaze is straight ahead into distance and not directed to any particular point in space. The visual axes are then parallel. When the eyes view some distant definite object, they are turned by contraction of the ocular muscles and converge so that the visual axes meet at the observed object, and an almost identical image of the object falls on a corresponding point on each fovea, the centralis of the retina. The adjustment of the eye movements for acute observation is called *fixation,* and the point where the visual axes meet is the fixation point. Thus the interplay of the ocular muscles permits rapid, reciprocally controlled movement of the eyeballs for fixation.

m., physical characteristics of Primarily, elasticity. A muscle is an elastic body. Its individual fibers follow Hooke's law of elastic bodies; i.e., the amount of elongation is proportional to the streching force. The muscle organs contain tissue other than muscle fibers and thus deviate slightly from this law. The human muscle fiber can contract to about half its total length.

m., regeneration of Reproduction or repair of muscle fiber, which is a sequela to many types of muscle damage. Reparation is always associated with the proliferation of sarcolemmic nuclei. Connective tissue elements do not participate in this process except to bridge the gap and to offer support for the regenerative fibers. The regenerative process takes place in two forms: regeneration by budding from the surviving parts of the muscle fibers, which occurs when segments of the muscle fiber and its sheath are destroyed, and regeneration by proliferation of cellular bands, which occurs when the sarcolemmic nuclei are spared and can form a sarcoplasmic band by linkage of the cytoplasmic processes.

m., sequence of, development The pattern of embryologic muscular development. The muscles of the neck and trunk are the first to develop; they are followed by the lingual and facial musculature and then by the distal and proximal appendicular musculature.

m., smooth The simplest of the three types of muscle (smooth, striated, and cardiac). It is the muscle of the lining of the digestive tract, ducts of glands, and viscera associated with the gut. It also supplies the muscles for the genitourinary tract, structures of the blood vessels, connective tissues of the mucous membranes, and skin with its appendages. A typical smooth muscle fiber is a slender spindle-shaped body averaging a few tenths of a millimeter in length. There is a single centrally striated nucleus. The cytoplasm appears homogeneous. The cells are arranged in bands, or bundles, with interspersed connective tissue fibers uniting them into an effective common mass. Smooth muscle fibers are innervated in part by nerve fibers and in part by the contraction of adjacent muscle tissues. The digestive tract, particularly, demonstrates waves of contraction that pass along a band of smooth muscle.

m., spasticity of Increased muscular tension of antagonists that prevents normal movement; caused by an inability to relax (a loss of reciprocal inhibition) resulting from a lesion of the upper motor neuron.

m., striated Skeletal muscles forming the bulk of the body; the voluntary muscles derived from the myotomes of the embryo. Generally, they are organized as formed muscles that attach to and move the skeletal structures. The cells are large, elongated, and cylindrical, with lengths ranging from 1 mm to several centimeters. The cells have multiple nuclei that are peripherally situated and scattered along the length of the fiber. The fiber contains a large number of elongated fibers which, under the microscope, appear as the alternating light and dark bands

that give the characteristic striated appearance of the striated muscle. The dimensional relationships between these light and dark bands are altered during contraction of the muscle fiber. The potential interaction between these bands permits the wide range of selective purposeful, and rapid activity of the skeletal muscles.

m., suprahyoid and infrahyoid The muscles grouped about the hyoid bone. They aid in depressing and fixing the mandible, hyoid bone, and larynx in the performance of their several respective functions.

m., tongue, extrinsic Muscles of the tongue that provide a scaffolding by which the intrinsic muscles can be moved about in the oral cavity while the latter are continuously modifying their dimension and contour. The extrinsic muscles are paired and originate from both sides of the cranial skeleton, mandible, and hyoid bone to radiate medially and insert into the body of the tongue, which consists principally of the intrinsic muscles.

m., tongue, intrinsic Muscles of the tongue that have no attachments in bone, terminating either within each other or in the extrinsic muscle group. The fibers of the intrinsic muscles also lie in all three planes of space and are called *longitudinal, vertical, and transverse fibers* to describe their distribution. They are capable of assuming an infinite variety of shapes. They depend, however, on the activity of the extrinsic muscles to be moved bodily through space.

m. trimming *See* border molding; impression, correctable.

muscular dystrophy (mŭs′kū-lar dĭs′trō-fē) *See* dystrophy, muscular.

musculature (mŭs′kū-lah-tūr) Any part of the muscular apparatus of the body; the source of power for the movement of the body or its parts.

m., cheek The muscles giving support, form, and function to the cheeks. Should disequilibrium exist between the functional forces exerted on the dentition by the tongue and cheek musculature, deviations in tooth alignment may occur.

m., lip The muscles that perform the physiologic or functional activities of the lips. The primary muscles include the orbicularis oris, quadratus labii superiorus, risorius, buccinators, etc. If the tongue and the musculature of the lips do not exert equivalent forces against the teeth, movement of the teeth may occur.

musculoskeletal system (mŭs″kū-lō-skĕl′ĕ-tal) *See* system, musculoskeletal.

mushbite An obsolete type of maxillomandibular record made by introducing a mass of soft wax into the patient's mouth and instructing the patient to bite into it to the desired degree. Not a generally accepted procedure. *See* record, maxillomandibular.

mutant An individual showing a mutation.

mutation (mū-tā′shŭn) A departure from the parent type, as when an organism differs from its parents in one or more heritable characteristics; caused by genetic change.

    m., gene A sudden and permanent change in a gene. The term mutation is sometimes used in a broader sense to include chromosome aberrations.

    m., lethal A mutation leading to death of the offspring at any stage.

mutual Interchangeable; reciprocal; joint.

myalgia Pain in the muscles.

mycelium (mī-sē′lē-ŭm) The filamentous network of hyphae of a fungus.

Mycobacterium tuberculous The microorganism responsible for tuberculosis, generally a respiratory infection in man; nonrespiratory tuberculosis is considered an indicator disease for AIDS.

mycology That branch of microbiology that deals with yeasts and fungi.

mycoses Any disease caused by a yeast or fungus.

mydriatic (mĭd″rē-ăt′ĭk) A drug that dilates the pupil.

myelin (mī′ĕ-lĭn) A fatlike substance forming a sheath around certain nerve fibers. It is associated with volitional nervous system fibers and is believed to be related to the capacity of nerve structures for rapid transmission of nerve impulses.

myeloma (mī″ĕ-lō′mah) A neoplasm characterized by cells normally found in the bone marrow.

    m., multiple A primary malignant neoplasm of bone marrow characterized by proliferation of cells resembling plasma cells. Circumscribed radiolucencies are seen within the bones, and Bence Jones protein is usually found in the urine.

    m., plasma cell A malignant neoplasm characterized by plasma cells. Solitary lesions may appear as radiolucencies in the bone and are sometimes considered benign, although most authorities believe that even these lesions become multiple and terminate fatally.

        m., solitary plasma cell An incompletely understood monostotic neoplasm of bone that is histologically identical with multiple myeloma. Laboratory findings, positive in multiple myeloma, are usually negative in solitary plasma cell myeloma. Behavior of the myeloma, although usually benign, may be malignant.

myelophthisis (mī″ĕ-lō-thī′sĭs) A displacement of bone marrow by fibrous tissue, carcinoma, leukemia, etc.

mylohyoid region *See* region, mylohyoid.

mylohyoid ridge, cantilevered A condition in which a major undercut occurs inferior to a broad mylohyoid ridge; creating a vertical groove into such an area often causes perforation of the medial cortical plate.

myoblastoma (mī″ō-blăs-to′mah) A benign neoplasm characterized by large polyhedral cells resembling young muscle cells. Occurs most frequently in the tongue.

    m., granular cell A benign soft tissue tumor of disputed origin. The tumor cells are large and have a granular eosinophilic cytoplasm and a small nucleus.

myocardial infarction An occlusion or blockage of arteries supplying the muscles of the heart resulting in injury or necrosis of the heart muscle.

myodysfunction (mī″ō-dĭs-fŭngk′shŭn) Imbalance or disturbance of muscle function.

myofascial pain Pain associated with inflammation or irritation of muscle or of the fascia surrounding the muscle.

myofascial pain dysfunction syndrome MPD A subset of the TMJ pain dysfunction syndrome that present with the triad of symptoms of unilateral pain in the muscles of mastication, clicking of the joint, and limitation of movement but without clinical or radiographic evidence of organic changes in the joint and the lack of tenderness in the joint when palpated from the external auditory meatus.

myofunction Normal muscle function.

myolipoma (mī″ō-lĭ-pō′mah) A myxoma containing fatty tissue.

myoma (mī-ō′mah) A neoplasm characterized by muscle cells.

myopia (mī-ō′pē-ah) A form of defective vision resulting from excessive refractive power of the eye. In this condition, commonly called *nearsightedness* or *shortsightedness*, light rays coming from an object beyond a certain distance are focused in front of the retina.

myotomy (mī-ŏt′ō-mē) Cutting or resection of a muscle.

myxedema (mĭk-sĕ-dē′mah) A condition associated with hypothyroidism (primary myxedema) or hypopituitarism (secondary or pituitary myxedema). Characteristics include dry hair and skin; thickened skin of the lips; puffy eyelids; thinning of the eyebrows, especially the lateral half; slow, low-pitched, and hoarse speech; and slowness of thinking.

myxofibroma (mĭk″sō-fī-brō′mah) A benign neoplasm characterized by mucous and fibroblastic tissues.

myxoma (mĭk-sō′mah) A benign tumor composed of fibroblastic cells that have reverted to embryonic growth and produce a mucoid matrix containing widely dispersed stellate cells that have multipolar processes.

myxosarcoma (mĭk′sō-sar-kō′mah) A sarcoma containing myxomatous tissue.

N (n) In statistics, the number of cases or observations.

N2 A single-visit endodontic technique better known as the *Sargenti technique* in which the paraformaldehyde is the principal ingredient in the endodontic paste. The technique is not approved by the Council on Dental Therapeutics, and it is not taught at any accredited dental school in the United States.

nafcillin A semisynthetic pencillin designed as an antistaphylococcal penicillin also effective in the treatment of infections caused by pneumococci and Group A beta-hemolytic streptococci.

name A word or combination of words by which a person, object, or idea or a group of persons, objects, or ideas is regularly known or designated.

    n., generic A name that is usually descriptive of the substance. Strictly speaking, it is a name used to designate a class relationship. Often used synonymously with *nonproprietary name*.

    n., nonproprietary A drug name that is not restricted by a trademark. Nonproprietary names are now selected in the United States by the USAN Council.

    n., official The title under which a drug is listed in *The United States Pharmacopeia (USP)* or *The National Formulary (NF)*.

    n., proprietary A name assigned by the manufacturer that is restricted by trademark. A drug made by several companies may have more than one proprietary name.

    n., United States Adopted (USAN) A name selected by the USAN Council (jointly sponsored by the American Medical Association, American Pharmaceutical Association, and United States Pharmacopeial Convention, Inc) when a new drug is placed on the market. A nonproprietary or generic name.

Nance analysis of arch length A method of determining whether there is sufficient arch length to accommodate the permanent dentition.

nanometer (nm) A billionth of a meter (10^9 meter). This term is now preferred over *millimicron*.

Naproxen A nonsteroid antiinflammatory drug with analgesic and antipyretic properties used in the treatment of rheumatoid arthritis and osteoarthritis.

narcoma Coma or stupor from narcotics.

narcosis (nar-kō′sĭs) Drug-induced unconsciousness.

narcotic (nar-kŏt′ĭk) A drug, usually with strong analgesic action and an addiction potential, which may be synthesized or derived from natural sources. Especially one of the opium alkaloids.

narcotism (nar′kō-tĭzm) State of stupor induced by a narcotic.

narcotize (nar′kō-tīz) To render unconscious by use of narcotics.

nasal cavity *See* cavity, nasal.

nasal septum *See* septum, nasal.

nasality The quality of speech sounds when the nasal cavity is used as a resonator, especially when there is too much nasal resonance.

nascent (nās′ĕnt) Literal meaning: recently born. Also, just released from chemical combination.

nasion (nā′zē-on) The point at the root of the nose that is intersected by the median sagittal plane. The root of the nose corresponds to the nasofrontal suture, which is not necessarily the lowest point on its dorsum and which can usually be located with the finger.

Nasmyth's membrane (nās′mĭths) *See* cuticle, primary.

nasoalveolar cyst (nā″zō-ăl-vē′ō-lar) An intraosseous cyst. A form of globulomaxillary cyst in which the epithelial inclusion is in the soft tissue fusion line.

nasolabial angle The angle formed by the labial surface of the upper lip at the midline and the inferior border of the nose. It is a measure of the relative protrusion of the upper lip.

nasomandibular fixation *See* fixation, nasomandibular.

natal teeth The presence of teeth in the mouth at birth, usually caused by the premature eruption of primary teeth but may be an extra or supernumerary tooth. The presence of natal teeth may cause discomfort in nursing.

national health plan Modification of the present method of delivering health care on a national scale, involving the professions, consumers, and government.

Nealon's technique *See* technique, Nealon's.

necessaries Things indispensable or useful for the sustenance of human life (e.g., food, shelter, clothing).

    n. contracts of infants (minors) Things suitable to each child according to the child's circumstances.

necessary treatment A dental procedure or service determined by a dentist to be necessary to establish or maintain a patient's oral health. Such determinations are based on the professional diagnostic judgment of the dentist and the standards of care that prevail in the professional community.

neck of condyle *See* process, condyloid, neck of.

necrosis (nē-krō′sĭs)   **1:** Death of a cell or group of cells in contact with living tissue.   **2:** Local death of cells resulting from, for example, loss of blood supply, bacterial toxins, physical and chemical agents.

    n., caseous (kā′sē-ŭs) A change commonly associated with tuberculosis and characterized by dry, soft, and cheesy tissue.

    n. of epitheliai attachment Death of cells composing the epithelial attachment. In a specific periodontitis produced by *Actinomyces*-like organisms, there may be necrosis of the epithelial attachment, permitting a rapid apical shift of the base of the pocket.

    n., exanthematous An acute necrotizing process involving the gingivae, jawbones, and contiguous soft tissues. It is of unknown cause, affects primarily children, and resembles noma. It differs from noma, however, in that it has a slight odor, tendency for self-limitation, low mortality rate, and normal leukocyte count. *See also* noma.

    n., gingival Death and degeneration of the cells and other structural elements of the gingivae (e.g., necrotizing ulcerative gingivitis).

    n., ischemic Death and disintegration of a tissue resulting from interference with its blood supply, thus depriving the tissues of access to substances necessary for metabolic sustenance. It may occur in the periodontal membrane resulting from occlusal trauma.

    n., periodontal membrane Necrosis of a portion of the periodontal membrane, usually resulting from traumatic injury (e.g., in occlusal traumatism). Much of this necrotic change is the result of ischemia.

    n., radiation Death of tissue caused by radiation.

needle A sharp, metal shaft in a variety of forms for penetrating tissue (e.g., in carrying sutures or injecting solutions).

    n., Gillmore An instrument used in a penetration type of test for measuring the setting time of materials such as plaster or stone. A ¼-pound needle is used for determining the initial set, and a 1-pound needle is used for defining the final set.

    n. holder A forceps used to hold and pass the needle through the tissue while suturing with a suture forceps.

    n. point tracer *See* tracer, needle point.

    n., Vicat An instrument used for measuring setting time by means of a penetration test.

neglect Failure to do something that one is bound to do; lack of due care.

negligence Failure to observe, for the protection of another person, thE degree of care and vigilance that the circumstances demand, whereby such other person suffers injury.

    n., contributory Negligence by an injured party that combines as a proximate cause with the negligence of the injurer in producing the injury. May bar recovery or mitigate damages.

    n., imputed That which is not directly attributable to a person but which is the negligence of a person employed by or in association with him or her and with whose fault he or she is chargeable (e.g., a dental assistant or other dental employee).

neighborhood An adjoining or surrounding district; an immediate vicinity.

Nembutal Trade name for pentobarbital sodium.

neomycin (nē″ō-mī′sĭn) An antibiotic secured from cultures of *Streptomyces fradiae,* used for preoperative sterilization. It is a constituent of topically applied ointments, solutions, troches, etc., for its antibacterial action against Gram-negative organisms.

neonatal teeth The presence of teeth within 1 month of birth. *See* natal teeth.

neoplasia (nē″ō-plā′zē-ah) The disease process responsible for neoplasm formation.

neoplasm (tumor) An abnormal mass of tissue, the growth of which exceeds and is uncoordinated with that of the normal tissues. It persists in the same excessive manner after cessation of the stimuli that evoked the change. Benign and malignant forms are recognized. *See also* tumor.

NeoSynephrine Brand name for phenylephrine, a vasoconstrictor and pressor drug chemically related to epinephrine and ephedrine. Commonly used as a decongestant. Contraindicated for prolonged use or in patients with severe hypertension.

nerve(s) A cordlike structure that conveys impulses between a part of the central nervous system and some part of the body and consists of an outer connective tissue sheath and bundles of nerve fibers.

    n., abducent (VI) The sixth cranial nerve; a small, completely motor nerve arising in the pons, supplying the lateral rectus muscle of the eye.

    n., accessory *See* nerve, spinal accessory.

    n., acoustic (VIII) The eighth cranial nerve; the vestibulocochlear nerve; a sensory nerve consisting of a vestibular position and an auditory (or cochlear) portion.

    n., branchial One of five cranial nerves that supply the derivatives of the branchial arches: trigeminal (V), facial (VII), glossopharyngeal (IX), vagus (X), and spinal accessory (XI). Each branchial nerve may have a variety of functions, including visceral motor and visceral and somatic sensory.

    n., chiasma, optic The decussation, or crossing, of optic nerve fibers from the medial side of the retina on one side to the opposite side of the brain.

n., chorda tympani A parasympathetic and special sensory branch of the facial nerve supplying the submandibular and sublingual glands and the anterior two thirds of the tongue (taste).

n., cochlear One of the two major branches of the eighth cranial nerve; a special sensory nerve for the sense of hearing that transmits impulses from the organ of Corti to the brain.

n., cranial Any one of twelve paired nerves, classified in three sets, arising directly in the brain and supplying various tissues of the head and neck. The cranial nerves are the *special somatic sensory nerves:* olfactory (I), optic (II), and acoustic (VIII); the *somatic motor nerves:* oculomotor (III), trochlear (IV), abducent (VI), and hypoglossal (XI); and the *brancial nerves:* trigeminal (V), facial (VII), glossopharyngeal (IX), vagus (X), and spinal accessory (XI).

n., facial (VII) The seventh cranial nerve; a mixed nerve supplying motor fibers to the facial muscles, the stapedius, and posterior body of the digastricus; sensory fibers from the taste buds in the anterior two thirds of the tongue (via the chorda tympani); and general visceral autonomic fibers for submaxillary and sublingual salivary glands.

n., glossopharyngeal (IX) The ninth cranial nerve; a mixed motor and sensory nerve arising in the medulla and supplying motor efferents to stylopharyngeal muscles and other pharyngeal muscles; visceral motor efferents via the otic ganglion for the parotid gland; special visceral afferents from the taste buds in the posterior third of tongue; and general sensory afferents from the pharynx and posterior aspects of the oral cavity.

n., hypoglossal (XII) The twelfth cranial nerve; a motor nerve that arises in the medulla and supplies extrinsic and intrinsic muscles of the tongue.

n., inferior alveolar A motor and general sensory branch of the mandibular nerve, with mylohyoid, inferior dental, mental, and inferior gingival branches.

n., intermediate The parasympathetic and special sensory division of the facial nerve with chorda tympani and greater petrosal branches.

n., lingual A general sensory branch of the mandibular nerve having sublingual and lingual branches and connections with the hypoglossal nerve and chorda tympani.

n., mandibular The mandibular division of the trigeminal nerve, arising in the trigeminal ganglion and supplying general sensory and motor fibers via mesenteric, pterygoid, buccal, auriculotemporal, deep temporal, lingual, inferior alveolar, and meningeal branches.

n., maxillary The maxillary division of the trigeminal nerve arising in the trigeminal ganglion and supplying general sensory fibers via zygomatic, posterosuperior alveolar, infraorbital, pterygopalatine, and nasopalatine branches.

n., oculomotor (III) The third crancial nerve; primarily a motor nerve arising from the midbrain and supplying motor efferents to the superior rectus, medial rectus, inferior rectus, and inferior oblique eye muscles, as well as autonomic fibers via the ciliary ganglion to the ciliary body and the iris.

n., olfactory (I) The first cranial nerve; a special sensory nerve for the sense of smell.

n., ophthalmic The ophthalmic division of the trigeminal nerve, arising in the trigeminal ganglion and supplying general sensory fibers via the frontal, lacriminal, and nasociliary branches.

n., optic (II) The second cranial nerve; a special sensory nerve for vision passing from the retina of the eye to the optic chiasma.

n., somatic motor (cranial) The somatic motor nerves—oculomotor (III), trochlear (IV), abducent (VI), and hypoglossal (XII)—largely comparable to the ventral motor roots of the spinal nerves. They are composed almost entirely of somatic motor fibers that emerge ventrally from the brainstem. Their arrangement is closely correlated to the distribution of the myotomes in the head. The oculomotor, trochlear, and abducent nerves, which supply the eye musculature, have the same myotomic origin and arrangement as the somatic muscles of the trunk and extremities.

n., special somatic sensory The structural arrangements from typical sensory nerves by which the three main sense organs—nose, eyes, and ears—are innervated. The sensory nerves are the olfactory (I), optic (II), and acoustic nerves (VIII).

n., spinal Any one of 31 pairs of mixed peripheral nerves (8 cervical, 12 thoracic, 5 lumbar, 5 sacral, and 1 coccygeal), being connected segmentally with the spinal cord, dorsal sensory trunk, and ventral motor root.

n., spinal accessory (XI) The eleventh cranial nerve; a motor nerve that derives its origin in part from the medulla and in part from the cervical spinal cord. Its internal ramus joins with the vagus nerve to supply some of the muscles of the larynx. Its external ramus joins with the spinal nerves to supply the sternocleidomastoid and trapezius muscles. The dentist's principle interest in the spinal accessory nerve is its relationship to head posture, which is important in maintaining stable occlusal relationships of vertical dimension and centric relation.

n., tensor tympani A small motor branch of the mandibular nerve.

n., trigeminal (V) The fifth cranial nerve; a mixed motor and sensory nerve connected with the pons through three roots (motor, proprioceptive, and large sensory), the latter root expanding into the trigeminal ganglion, from which arise the ophthalmic, masseteric, and mandibular divisions.

n., trochlear (IV) The fourth cranial nerve; a small motor nerve arising ventrally in the midbrain and supplying the inferior oblique muscle of the eye.

n., vagus (X) The tenth cranial nerve; a mixed parasympathetic, visceral, afferent, motor, and general sensory nerve with laryngeal, pharyngeal, bronchial, esophageal, gastric, and many other branches.

n., vestibular (VIII) One of the two major branches of the eighth cranial nerve; a special sensory nerve for the sense of balance and the transmission of space-orientation impulses from the semicircular canals to the brain.

n., vestibulocochlear (VII) The seventh cranial nerve; acoustic nerve; a sensory nerve consisting of a vestibular portion and an auditory, or cochlear, portion.

net Devoid of anything extraneous; free from all deductions, such as charges, expenses, taxes; remaining after expenses.

neuralgia (nū-răl′jē-ah) Pain associated with a nerve or nerves (e.g., trigeminal and glossopharyngeal neuralgia).

n., auriculotemporal (auriculotemporal causalgia neuralgia) Sharp pain in the distribution of the auriculotemporal nerve.

n., buccal A throbbing, burning, and boring type of pain involving the cheeks, lips, gingivae, nose, and jaws. It may last a few minutes or several days. No trigger zones are present, although the pain may be initiated by chewing or thermal changes.

n., causalgia Neuralgia characterized by an intense, diffuse burning sensation in a limited area.

n., facial *See* neuralgia, trigeminal.

n., atypical facial (cluster headache, lower-half headache, sphenopalatine neuralgia) Severe unilateral pain behind the eye that spreads to the temple and behind the ear. It lasts 30 minutes to 3 hours and occurs once to several times a day and in cycles or clusters lasting several weeks. The clusters may be separated by several months or years. No trigger zones exist.

n., glossopharyngeal Pain in the nerves of the tongue, pharynx, ear, and neck precipitated by swallowing, sneezing, coughing, talking, or blowing the nose.

n., Sluder's Irritation of the sphenopalatine ganglion. Diffuse pain may affect the eye, root of the nose, teeth, and ear. Also, slight anesthesia and paralysis of the soft palate and palatine arch on the affected side may be present.

n., sphenopalatine *See* neuralgia, facial, atypical.

n., trifacial *See* neuralgia, trigeminal.

n., trigeminal (facial neuralgia, tic douloureux, trifacial neuralgia) An excruciating paroxysmal, stabbing, searing, or lancinating pain usually occurring on the right side of the face and involving the distribution of the three divisions of the trigeminal nerve. It may last for a few seconds followed by additional episodes spontaneously or from stimulation of trigger zones. Intervals between attacks vary from a few hours to months or years.

neurasthenia (nū-răs-thē′nē-ah) A neurotic reaction characterized by chronic physical fatigue, listlessness, mental sluggishness, and often phobias.

neurectomy (nū-rĕk′tō-mē) The surgical excision of a nerve or the more traumatic tearing away of nervous tissue from its anatomic position.

neurilemma (nū-rĭ-lĕm′ah) **(nucleated sheath, primitive sheath, sheath of Schwann)** The thin membranous outer covering surrounding the myelin sheath of a medullated nerve fiber or the axis cylinder of a nonmedullated nerve fiber. It is associated with the booster mechanisms for the rapid transmission of impulses.

neurilemoma (nū″rĭ-lĕ-mō′mah) **(neurinoma, perineural fibroblastoma, schwannoma)** A benign tumor of the neurilemma of disputed origin (Schwarin cell vs. fibroblasts). May occur in soft tissue arid bone. Composed of characteristic Antoni type A and Antoni type B tissue and contains Verocay bodies. A malignant form occurs. *See also* body, Verocay; tissue.

neurinoma (nū-rĭ-nō′mah) *See* neurilemoma.

neuritis (nū-rī′tĭs) The inflammation of a nerve attended by pain and tenderness over the nerves, anesthesia, disturbance of sensation, paralysis, wasting, and disappearance of reflexes.

n., endemic multiple *See* beriberi.

neuroblastoma (nū″rō-blăs-tō′mah) A malignant neoplasm characterized by proliferating nerve cells.

neurofibroma (nū″rō-fī-brō′mah) **(neurogenic fibroma, perineural fibroblastoma) 1:** A benign neoplasm characterized by the various cells of a peripheral nerve (axon cylinders, Schwann cells, fibroblasts). *See also* neurilemoma. **2:** A connective tissue tumor of the nerve fiber fasciculi. Formed by the proliferation of the perineurium and endoneurium.

neurofibromatosis (nū″rō-fī″brō-mah-tō′sĭs) **(molluscum fibrosum, multiple neuroma, von Recklinghausen's disease of skin)** A disease characterized by multiple neurofibromas most frequently seen on the skin but possibly involving the oral mucosa.

neuroma (nū-rō′mah) Technically, a benign neoplasm of nerve cells. As used in oral disease, the term usually refers to a traumatic neuroma, which is not a true tumor but an overgrowth of nerves associated with injury. The mental foramina and extraction scars are possible oral sites of this painful lesion.

n., amputation *See* neuroma, traumatic.

n., multiple *See* neurofibromatosis.

n., traumatic (amputation neuroma) Hyperplasia of

nerve fibers and their supporting tissues in an exuberant attempt at repair after damage to, or the severing of, a nerve.

neuron (nū′rŏn) Nerve cell; the basic structural unit of the nervous system. There is a wide variation in the shape of nerve cells, but they all have the same basic structures: cell body, protoplasmic processes, axons, and dendrites. The neuron is the only body cell whose principle function is the conduction of impulses. It cannot regenerate when the cell body is destroyed; however, cell processes such as axons and dendrites often can regenerate.

neuropathy An abnormal condition characterized by inflammation and degeneration of peripheral nerves.

neurosis A diffusely defined term referring to a mental disorder for which professional help may be needed but that is milder than a psychosis; generally a functional disorder in which there is no gross personality disorganization but in which there is an inability to cope effectively with some routine frustrations, anxieties, and daily problems. Somatic conditions may be factors in the cause and may be symptoms in a neurosis; however, the use of the term to describe a dysfunction of the nervous system is obsolete. Synonym: psychoneurosis.

neurostomatosis (nū″rō-stō″mah-tō′sĭs) An oral condition associated with psychosomatic or other psychologic factors; For example, lichen planus and benign migratory glossitis may be considered types of neurostomatoses.

neurosyphilis, paretic (nū″rō-sĭ′fĭ-lĭs) *See* paresis.

neurotomy (nū-rot′ō-mē) The severance of a nerve process.

neutral A solution that has a pH level of 7. Equal numbers of hydrogen and hydroxyl ions are formed on dissociation.

n. zone *See* zone, neutral.

neutralization The reaction of an acid with a base.

neutroclusion Normal mesiodistal occlusal relationships of the buccal teeth, similar to Angle class I.

neutron (nū′tron) An elementary particle with approximately the mass of a hydrogen atom but without any electrical charge; one of the constituents of the atomic nucleus.

n. ray *See* rays, neutron.

neutropenia (nū″trō-pē′nē-ah) A relative or absolute decrease in the normal number of neutrophils in the circulating blood. Various limits are given; for example, absolute neutropenia may exist when the total is less than 1700 cells/mm^3 regardless of the percentage, whereas relative neutropenia may exist when the total percentage of neutrophils is less than 38% and the total number is not less than 1500/mm^3. May be associated with viral infections, pernicious anemia, sprue, aplastic anemia, bone marrow, neoplasms, chronic intoxication with drugs and heavy metals, malnutrition,

and nonpyogenic and overwhelming infections.

n., cyclic A condition in which there is a depression in the number of circulating white cells, especially the neutrophils, at an interval of about 21 days. The neutropenia lasts for approximately 10 days; during this time, gingival inflammation and aphthous ulcer occur.

neutrophil A polymorphonuclear granular leukocyte. The circulating white blood cell essential for phagacytosis and protelysis.

neutrophilia (nū″trō-fĭl′ē-ah) An absolute or relative increase in the normal number of neutrophils in the circulating blood. Various limits are given; for example, an absolute neutrophilia may exist, regardless of percentage, if the total number of neutrophils exceeds 7000/mm^3, whereas a relative neutrophilia may exist if the percentage of neutrophils is greater than 70% and the total number of neutrophils is less than 7000/mm^3. May be associated with acute infections, chronic granulocytic leukemia, erythemia, therapy with ACTH or cortisone, uremia, ketosis, hemolysis, drug or heavy metal intoxication, or malignancy, or may follow severe hemorrhage.

nevus (nē′vŭs) A circumscribed new growth of congenital origin that may be vascular (resulting from hypertrophy of blood or lymph vessels) or nonvascular (with epidermal and connective tissue predominating).

n., blue A benign neoplasm characterized by heavily pigmented spindle cells deep in the corium; appears clinically as a dark mole.

n., cellular pigmented A nevus composed of melanin-producing ″nevus″ cells.

n., compound A nevus in which the melanin-producing ″nevus″ cells are found in the epidermis and dermis; the intradermal nevus plus the junctional nevus.

n., intradermal A nevus in which the melanin-producing ″nevus″ cells are found only in the dermis.

n., junctional A nevus in which the melanin-producing ″nevus″ cells are found within the epidermis at the junction with the dermis.

n., pigmented A dark-colored, benign neoplasm characterized by nevus cells. Junctional, intradermal, and compound types are recognized. Melanomas (malignant neoplasms) may develop from junctional or compound nevi.

n. spongiosus albus mucosa (white folded gingivostomatitis, white sponge nevus) An inherited disease of the oral mucosa characterized by generalized white mucosal surfaces with a spongelike appearance.

Ney surveyor *See* surveyor, Ney.

NF *The National Formulary.*

niacin (nī′ah-sĭn) *See* acid, nicotinic.

nib The part of a condensing instrument corresponding to the blade of a cutting instrument. The end is called the *face of the condenser*.

nickel-chromium alloy *See* alloy, nickel-chromium.

nicotine A poisonous alkaloid found in tobacco and responsible for many of the effects of tobacco. It is first a stimulant (in small doses) and then a depressant (larger doses).

nicotinic stomatitis An inflammation caused by the intraoral use of smokeless tobacco.

Niemann-Pick disease (nē'măn pĭk) *See* disease, Niemann-Pick.

night guard *See* guard, night.

night-grinding *See* bruxism.

Nikolsky's sign (nĭ-kol'skēz) *See* sign, Nikolsky's.

nitrogen, nonprotein *See* nonprotein nitrogen.

nitrogen monoxide *See* nitrous oxide.

nitrogen monoxidum *See* nitrous oxide.

nitromersol, tincture (nī-trō-mer'sol) A solution used in 1:200 strength as a topically applied antiseptic to temporarily minimize the bacterial count on an area of tissue.

nitrous oxide (N_2O, laughing gas, nitrogen monoxide, nitrogen monoxidum) A gas with a sweet odor and taste used with oxygen as an analgesic and sedative agent for the performance of minor operations. It is sometimes called *laughing gas* because it may excite a hilarious delirium preceding insensibility.

NMR (nuclear magnetic resonance) *See* magnetic resonance imaging.

noble An archaic term referring to inert gases and precious metals.

   n. metal *See* metal, noble.

nocardiosis (nō-kar-dē-ō'sĭs) Any of the pathologic entities that may follow infection with the bacterium *Nocardia*.

node(s) (nōd) A swelling or protuberance.

   n., brown, of hyperparathyroidism A central giant cell lesion of the bone seen in hyperparathyroidism. Its microscopic appearance is similar to giant cell reparative granuloma and giant cell tumor.

   n. of Ranvier Gaps distributed at regularly spaced intervals along a myelinated nerve fiber. The intervals are 1 mm or more in length and function essentially as relay stations to facilitate the passage of an impulse.

nodule, pulp (nod'ŭl) *See* denticle.

nodules, Bohn's (Epstein's pearls) Multiple white, ricelike lesions of the mucous membrane seen in newborn infants. Microscopically each lesion shows a keratin-filled cyst that lies close to the mucosal surface. It disappears spontaneously in 2 to 3 months.

noma (nō'mah) A progressive necrotizing process originating in the cheek with secondary involvement of the gingiva and jawbone. Occurs primarily in debilitated children, and the mortality rate is high. There is a strong, foul odor; marked surrounding edema; absence of a specific erythematous halo; marked changes in the white blood cell count; and a high temperature. *See also* necrosis, exanthematous; stomatitis, gangrenous.

nomenclature (nō"měn-klā'tūr) The formally adopted terminology of a science, art, or discipline; the system of names or terms used in a particular branch of science.

non rep. (non repetatur) Abbreviation of Latin term; placed on prescriptions that are not to be refilled.

noncohesive Lacking the property of sticking together, or cohesion.

noncontributory plan A method of payment for group insurance coverage in which the entire premium is paid by the employer or the union. Also referred to as *noncontributory program*.

nonduplication of benefits This may apply if a subscriber is eligible for benefits under more than one plan. A dental benefits contract provision relieving the third-party payer of liability for cost of services if the services are covered under another program. Distinct from a coordination of benefits provision because reimbursement would be limited to the greater level allowed by the two plans rather than a total of 100% of the charges Also referred to as *benefit less-benefit* or *carve-out*.

nonfeasance (non-fē'zěnz) The failure of a person to do some act that should be done.

non-Hodgkin's lymphoma A form of lymphoma associated with AIDS. One of the indicator diseases of AIDS. *See* lymphoma.

nonocclusion A situation in which the tooth or teeth in one arch fail to make contact with tooth or teeth of the other arch.

nonparticipating dentist 1: Any dentist with whom the underwriter (insurer) does not have an agreement to render dental care to members of the plan. **2:** Any dentist who does not have a contractual agreement with a dental benefits organization to render dental care to members of a dental benefits program.

nonprofit insurers Service corporations organized under nonprofit laws for the purpose of providing dental care insurance.

nonprotein nitrogen (NPN) The nitrogen of whole blood or serum exclusive of that of the proteins. The concentration of nonprotein nitrogen is a gross measure of renal function. The upper limit of normal is 35 mg/100 ml.

nonsuit A failure on the part of a plaintiff to continue the prosecution of the suit; abandonment of a suit.

nor- A prefix that indicates lack of a methyl group.

norepinephrine (nor'ěp-ĭ-něf'rĭn) The neurohormonal transmitter for neuroeffector junctions of adrenergic nerve fibers. Its official drug name in the United States is levarterenol. *See also* levarterenol.

norm(s) 1: A statistical unit representative of the human species as a whole. **2:** Numerical or statistical measures of usual observed performance when related to health care provided to a given number of patients over time; often used in the building of profiles; can be the average or the median or some other cutoff point in a series.

normal distribution A curve representing the frequency with which the values of a variable are obtained or observed when the number is infinite and variation is subject to only chance factors. The curve is a symmetrical, bell-shaped curve with the highest frequency occurring in the middle and gradually tapering toward the extremes. In a normal distribution, 68.2% of all scores cluster around the mean within ±1 standard deviation, 95.4% within ±2 standard deviations, and 99.7% within ±3 standard deviations. Synonyms: normal curve, Gauss' curve.

normality A reference solution in which the concentration is stated with regard to the number of gram equivalent weights present per liter of solution.

normoblast (nŏr′mō blăst) A nucleated red blood cell found in the peripheral bloodstream in severe pernicious anemia and in some leukemias.

nosebleed *See* epistaxis.

notch An indentation.

    n., buccal The notch in the flange of a denture that accommodates the buccal frenum.

    n., hamular *See* notch, pterygomaxillary.

    n., labial The notch in the labial flange of an upper or lower denture that accommodates the labial frenum.

    n., mandibular A depression of the inferior border of the mandible anterior to the attachments of the masseter muscle where the external facial vessels cross the lower border of the mandible. This landmark may be accentuated by arrested condylar growth and developmental disturbances of the mandible.

    n., pterygomaxillary (hamular notch) The notch or fissure formed at the junction of the maxilla and the hamular, or pterygoid, process of the sphenoid bone.

    n., sigmoid The concavity on the superior surface of the ramus of the mandible lying between the coronoid and condyloid processes.

note, promissory A written promise to pay to another, at a specified time, a stated amount of money or other articles of value.

not-for-profit third-parties Service corporations or dental benefits organizations established under not-for-profit state statutes for the purpose of providing health care coverage (e.g., Delta Dental, Blue Cross, Blue Shield Plans).

notice 1: Knowledge; information; awareness of facts. **2:** Knowledge of facts that would naturally lead an honest and prudent person to make inquiry constitutes "notice" of everything which such inquiry pursued in good faith would disclose.

Novocain Trade name for procaine hydrochloride.

noxious (nok′shŭs) Hurtful; not wholesome.

NPN *See* nonprotein nitrogen.

NSAIDs Acronym for nonsteroidal antiinflamatory drugs. *See* Naproxen.

nucleoprotein (nū″klē-ō-prō′tē-ĭn) Any one of a special group of protein substances in combination with nucleic acid. The essential component is the phosphoric acid radical. The nucleoproteins are generally confined to the nucleus of the cell and are intimately associated with chromosome and gene function.

nucleus (nū′klē-ŭs) **1:** The small, central part of an atom in which the positive electric charge and most of the mass (protons and neutrons) are concentrated. **2:** An easily recognized structural component of most cells, surrounded by a membrane and containing chromosomes and nucleoli.

Nuhn's gland (noonz) The anterior lingual gland embedded in the substance of the tongue near the apex and the midline on the inferior surface of the tongue. *See also* gland, Blandin and Nuhn's.

nuisance That which endangers life or health, offends the senses, vilolates the laws of decency, or obstructs reasonable and comfortable use of property.

number, Brinell hardness (BHN) A numerical expression of the hardness of a material, determined by measuring the diameter of a dent made by forcing a hard steel or tungsten carbide ball of standard dimension into the material under specified load in a Brinell machine (devised by J.A. Brinell, a Swedish engineer). The larger the indention, the smaller the Brinell hardness number. *See also* test, Brinell hardness.

number, Vickers hardness Hardness as measured by the Vickers hardness test. *See also* test, Vickers hardness.

nursing bottle caries Dental caries of the maxillary primary teeth caused by the oral retention of milk or formula in the mouth.

nutrient canal (nū′trē-ĕnt) *See* canal, interdental.

nutrition The process of assimilation and use of essential food elements from the diet (e.g., carbohydrates, fats, proteins, vitamins, mineral elements).

nutriture (nū′trĭ-tūr) The nutritional status of a patient.

Nuva-Lite Brand name for an ultraviolet light used as a catalyst in the polymerization of Nuva-seal, a bonding agent used as a pit and fissure sealant.

Nuva-seal Brand name of a bonding agent used as a pit and fissure sealant.

nystagmus (nĭs-tăg′mŭs) The state of oscillatory movements of an organ or part, especially the eyeballs; irregular jerking movement of the eyes. Each movement of the cycle consists of a slow component in one direction and a rapid component in the opposite direction.

nystatin An antifungal antibiotic obtained from *Streptomyces noursei;* useful as an oral rinse in the treatment of candidiasis.

oath An affirmation of truth of a statement that renders one who is willfully asserting untrue statements punishable for perjury.

obesity (ō-bēs′ĭ-tē) A bodily condition marked by excessive generalized deposition and storage of fat.

    o., adrenocortical (buffalo obesity) One of the symptoms characteristic of Cushing's syndrome; an obesity that is confined chiefly to the trunk, face, and neck.

    o., buffalo *See* obesity, adrenocortical.

object-film distance *See* distance, object-film.

obligation The binding power of a promise, oath, or contract or of law. Independent of a promise; a legal or moral duty that renders a person liable to punishment for neglecting it.

obtain Exists; is found.

obtund (ob-tŭnd′) To diminish the ability to perceive pain and/or touch.

obtundent (ob-tŭn′dĕnt) An agent that obtunds.

obturation (ob″tū-rā′shŭn) The act of closing or occluding.

    o., retrograde *See* filling, retrograde.

    o., root canal filling technique The procedure used for filling and sealing the root canal.

obturator (ob″tū-rā′tor) A prosthesis used to close a congenital or acquired opening in the palate. *See also* aid, prosthetic speech.

    o., hollow That portion of an obturator made hollow to minimize its weight.

occipital anchorage (ok-sĭp′ĭ-tăl) *See* anchorage, occipital.

occlude To close together. To bring together; to shut. To bring the mandibular teeth into contact with the maxillary teeth.

occluder A name given to some articulators. *See also* articulator.

occluding frame *See* articulator; frame, occluding.

occluding relation *See* relation, occluding.

occlusal Pertaining to the contacting surfaces of opposing occlusal units (teeth or occlusion rims). Pertaining to the masticating surfaces of the posterior teeth.

    o. adjustment *See* adjustment, occlusal.

    o. analysis *See* analysis, occlusal.

    o. balance *See* balanced, occlusion.

    o. contacts *See* contacts teeth.

    o. contouring *See* contouring, occlusal.

    o. correction *See* correction, occlusal.

    o. curvature *See* curve of occlusion.

    o. disharmony *See* disharmony, occlusal.

    o. disturbances *See* disturbances, occlusal.

    o. embrasure *See* embrasure, occlusal.

    o. equilibration *See* equilibration, occlusal.

    o. force *See* force, occlusal.

    o. form *See* form, occlusal.

    o. function *See* function, heavy.

    o. glide *See* glide, occlusion.

    o. guard *See* occlusal splint

    o. harmony *See* harmony, occlusal.

    o. load *See* load, occlusal.

    o. path *See* path, occlusal.

    o. path registration *See* path, occlusal.

    o. pattern *See* pattern, occlusal.

    o. perception *See* perception, occlusal.

    o. pivot *See* pivot, occlusal.

    o. plane *See* plane, occlusal.

    o. position *See* position, occlusal.

    o. pressure *See* pressure, occlusal.

    o. recontouring *See* contouring, occlusal.

    o. rest *See* position, rest.

    o. splint A bite plane designed and fabricated for patients with some types of functional temporomandibular joint disorders. Provides a stable occlusal platform from which to reconstruct a functional occlusion. *See also* Splint.

    o. stop *See* rest, occlusal.

    o. surface *See* surface, occlusal.

    o. system *See* system, occlusal.

    o. table *See* table, occlusal.

    o. template *See* template, occlusal.

    o. therapy A treatment to establish and maintain a comfortable, stable, and functional occlusion for patients with one of several types of occlusal problems. Treatment may be limited to the teeth, the neuomuscular mechanisms of chewing, or a combination of both.

    o. trauma *See* trauma, occlusal.

    o. unit One of two kinds of cusps: (1) a stamp cusp coupled with a fossa and (2) a shear cusp. The occlusal edges of the shear cusp are coupled with the edges of a stamp cusp, by which it passes closely without sliding contacts.

o. wear *See* wear, occlusal.

occlusion 1: The act of closure or state of being closed. **2:** Any contact between the incising or masticating surfaces of the upper and lower teeth.

o., acentric *See* occlusion, eccentric.

o., adjustment *See* adjustment occlusion.

o., anatomic The ideal relation of the mandibular and maxillary teeth when closed.

o., anterior determinants of cusp The characteristics of the anterior teeth—occlusion, alignment, overlaps, and capacity to disclude conjointly with the trajectories given the condyles—that determine the cusp elevations and the fossa depressions of the postcanine teeth.

o., attritional An occlusion in which each tooth of the dentition wears occlusally and proximally as it erupts.

o., balanced 1: An occlusion of the teeth that presents a harmonious relation of the occluding surfaces in centric and eccentric positions within the functional range of mandibular positions and tooth size.   **2:** The simultaneous contacting of the upper and lower teeth on both sides and in the anterior and posterior occlusal areas of the jaws. This occlusion is developed to prevent a tipping or rotating of the denture base in relation to the supporting structures. This term is used primarily in connection with the mouth, but it may be used in relation to teeth on an articulator.

o., bilateral balanced The closure suitable for worn dentitions that are cuspless or have flat-sided cusps; it permits an increase of the amount of surface contact in centric closure and provides as much closure contact as possible for horizontal chewing. This kind of occlusion is a therapeutic form designed to keep dentures seated when fine-textured foods are chewed horizontally. It is not found in young, unworn natural dentitions.

o., centrically balanced A centrically related centric occlusion in which the teeth close with even pressures on both sides of the mouth but have no occlusion of the postcanine teeth in attempted eccentric closures.

o., mechanically balanced An occlusion balanced without reference to physiologic considerations (e.g., on an articulator).

o., physiologically balanced A balanced occlusion in harmony with the temporomandibular joints and the neuromuscular system. *See also* occlusion, balanced.

o., central *See* occlusion, centric.

o., centric (central occlusion) The relation of opposing occlusal surfaces that provides the maximum planned contact and/or intercuspation. Should exist when the mandible is in centric relation to the maxilla.

o., faulty centric A condition in which centric occlusion does not correspond to a patient's centric jaw relationship, resulting in premature or interceptive or deflective tooth contacts in the centric path of closure.

o., components of The various factors involved in occlusion (e.g., temporomandibular joint, associated neuromusculature, and teeth). In denture prosthetics, also the denture-supporting structures.

o., convenience (convenience jaw relation, convenience relationship of teeth) The assumed position of maximum intercuspation when there is occlusal interference in the centric path of closure. The convenience occlusion may be anterior, lateral, anterolateral, etc. to the true centric occlusion.

o., coronary A coronary thrombosis resulting in closure of the coronary artery.

o., cross-bite An occlusion in which the lower teeth overlap the upper teeth.

o., determinants of The classifiable factors in the gnathic organ that influence occlusion. These factors are divided into two groups: those that are fixed and those that can be modified by reshaping or repositioning the teeth. The fixed factors most mentioned are the intercondylar distance; anatomy, which influences the paths of the mandibular axes; mandibular centricity; and the mating of the jaws. The changeable factors most mentioned are tooth shape, tooth position, vertical dimension, height of cusps, and depth of fossae.

o., eccentric Any occlusion other than centric occlusion.

o., edge-to-edge An occlusion in which the anterior teeth of both jaws meet along their incisal edges when the teeth are in centric occlusion.

o., end-to-end *See* occlusion, edge-to-edge.

o., functional 1: Occlusion in which attention is directed specifically to performance and is differentiated from structure and appearance.   **2:** Any tooth contacts made within the functional range (according to the size) of the opposing tooth surfaces. An occlusion that occurs during function.

o., gliding Used in the sense of designating contacts of teeth in motion. A substitute for the term *articulation*.

o., ideal 1: The relationship existing when all the teeth are perfectly placed in the arches of jaws and have a normal anatomic relationship to each other. When the teeth are brought into contact, the cusp-fossa relationship is considered the most perfect anatomic relationship that can be attained.   **2:** The normal relationships of the inclines of the cusps of opposing teeth to each other in occlusion, when the alignment, proximal contacts, and axial positions of the teeth in both arches have resulted from normal growth and development in relation to all associated tissues and parts of the head. occlusion

o., locked An occlusal relationship of such nature that lateral and protrusive mandibular movements are limited.

o., malfunctional A disturbance in the normal or proper action of the masticatory apparatus produced by such factors as missing teeth or tilting and drifting of teeth.

o., normal *See* occlusion, ideal.

o., pathogenic An occlusal relationship capable of producing pathologic changes in the teeth, supporting tissues, and/or other components of the stomatognathic system.

o., physiologic 1: An occlusion in harmony with functions of the masticatory system. **2:** An occlusion that operates in harmony and presents no pathologic manifestation in the supporting structures of the teeth; the stresses placed on the teeth are dissipated normally, with a balance existing between the stresses and adaptive capacity of the supporting tissues. **3:** An acceptable occlusion found in a healthy gnathic system.

o., plane of *See* plane, occlusal.

o., protrusive An occlusion of the teeth existing when the mandible is protruded forward from a centric position. *See also* position, rest, physiologic.

o., rim *See* rim, occlusion.

o., spherical form of An arrangement of teeth that places their occlusal surfaces on the surface of an imaginary sphere (usually 9 inches [22.5 cm] in diameter) with its center above the level of the teeth, as suggested by Monson.

o. table *See* table, occlusal.

o., terminal The relation of opposing occlusal surfaces that provides the maximum natural or planned contact and/or intercuspation.

o., traumatic An occlusion that results in overstrain and injury to teeth, periodontal tissues, or the residual ridge or other oral structures.

o., traumatogenic *See* occlusion, traumatic.

o., working The occlusal contacts of teeth on the side toward which the mandible is moved. From the mesial or distal view, the buccal and lingual cusps of the upper teeth appear to be end to end with the buccal and lingual cusps of the lower teeth, respectively. Viewed from the side, each upper cusp is distal to the corresponding lower cusp. The mesial incline of each upper cusp makes contact with the distal incline of the opposing cusp in front of it, and the distal incline of each upper cusp makes contact

with the mesial incline of the opposing cusp distal to it.

occupational risk A hazard found or likely to occur in the workplace. The number and types of hazards a health care worker may encounter in the routine conduct of health care delivery.

Occupational Safety and Health Administration (OSHA) A federal agency charged with establishing guidelines and regulations regarding worker safety. These guidelines include storage and disposal of toxic chemicals and hazardous materials and the safety and proper usage of clinical and office equipment.

odontalgia (ō″don-tăl′jē-ah) Pain in a tooth; toothache.

o., phantom (ghost pain) Pain in the area from which a tooth has been removed.

odontectomy (ō″don-těk′tō-mē) The removal of a tooth.

odontoblasts (ō-don′tō-blasts) The cells that form the dentin of the tooth.

odontodysplasia (ghost teeth) A developmental anomaly characterized by deficient tooth development. Deficiencies are noted in enamel and dentin formation. *See also* tooth, shell.

odontogenesis (ō-don′tō-jĕn′ĕ-sĭs) The process of tooth formation.

o. imperfecta A generic term that includes simultaneous defects in epithelial and mesenchymal tissue involved in tooth development.

odontoma (ō″don-tō′mah) **(gestant anomaly)** An anomaly of the teeth resembling a tumor of hard tissue (e.g., dens in dente, enamel pearl, complex or composite odontoma). It is composed of enamel, dentin, cementum, and pulp tissue that may be arranged in the form of teeth.

o., ameloblastic (ă-mel′ō-blas″tĭk) An dontogenic tumor characterized by the occurrence of an ameloblastoma within an odontoma. *See also* ameloblastoma; odontoma.

o., composite (kom-pos′ĭt) Complex odontoma; an odontogenic tumor characterized by the formation of calcified enamel and dentin in an abnormal arrangement because of lack of morphodifferentiation. Compound odontoma: a tumor of enamel and dentin arranged in the form of anomalous miniature teeth. Several small abnormal teeth surrounded by a fibrous sac.

o., cystic An odontoma associated with a follicular cyst.

o., gestant *See* dens in dente.

odontotomy, prophylactic (ō″don-tot′ō-mē, prō″fi-lak-′tik) The removal of precarious pits and fissures in posterior primary and permanent molars and their restoration with amalgam restorations.

office hours *See* business hours.

office planning The physical arrangement of the rooms

available within the limitations of space designed to enable the dentist to practice.

office routine *See* routine, office.

off-line Pertaining to the operation of input/output devices or auxiliary equipment not under direct control of the central processor.

offset A deduction; a counterclaim; a contrary claim or demand by which a given claim may be lessened or cancelled.

oil An unctuous, combustible substance that is liquid, or easily liquefiable on warming, and soluble in either but insoluble in water.

  o., essential (volatile oil) A volatile, nonfatty liquid of vegetable origin having a distinct aroma and flavor, often pleasant.

  o., fixed A nonvolatile oil consisting chiefly of glycerides.

  o., mineral Any one of the various grades of liquid petrolatum.

  o., volatile *See* oil, essential.

ointment (oynt′ment) A soft, bland, smooth, semisolid mixture that is used as a lubricant and as a vehicle for external medication.

  o., hydrophilic An ointment that is miscible with water.

oligodontia (ol′ĭ-gō-don′shē-ah) The condition of having only a few teeth.

oligodynamic (ol′ĭ-gō-dī-năm′ĭk) Effective in extremely small quantities.

oliguria (ol′ĭ-gū′rē-ah) Decreased output of urine (usually less than 500 ml/day) possibly associated with dehydration from diarrhea or excessive sweating, low fluid intake, lower nephron nephrosis resulting from burns, heavy metal poisoning, terminal renal disease, or an increase in extracellular fluid volume in untreated renal, cardiac, or hepatic disease.

Ominipen *See* amipicillin.

omission A phoneme left out at a place where it should occur.

on account In partial payment; in partial satisfaction of an amount owed.

on or about Phrase used in stating the date of an occurrence or conveyance to avoid being bound by the statement of an exact or certain date.

oncocytoma (ong″kō-sī-tō′mah) **(acidophilic adenoma, oxyphilic adenoma)** A rare, benign tumor usually occurring in the parotid glands in older patients. The lesion is encapsulated and composed of sheets and cords of large eosinophilic cells with small nuclei.

One Stage Oratronics Weis Standard Blade Implant System, an ADA acceptable endosseous dental implant system.

onlay 1: A cast type of restoration that is retained by frictional and mechanical factors in the preparation of the tooth and restores one or more cusps and adjoining occlusal surfaces of the tooth. **2:** An occlusal rest portion of a removable partial denture that is extended to cover the entire occlusal surface of the tooth.

  o. bone *See* graft, onlay bone.

on-line A system of data processing under control of the central processing unit. Data reflecting current activity are introduced into the processing system as soon as they occur.

ontogeny (ŏn tŏj′ĕ-nē) The natural life cycle of an individual as contrasted with the natural life cycle of the race (phylogeny).

opacification (ō-pas″ĭ-fĭ-kā′shŭn) **1:** The process of making opaque. **2:** The formation of opacities.

opacity, optical The reciprocal of transmission, which is in turn the ratio of transmitted incident light intensity. (Do not confuse with radiopacity.) *See also* density, radiopacity.

opalescent (ō″pal-es′ent) Resembling an opal in the display of various colors, as in opalescent dentin.

  o. teeth A translucent or opal-like appearance of teeth, usually associated with a genetic defect in odontogenesis.

opaque Relatively impenetrable to light. *See also* opacity, optical.

open bite *See* bite, open.

open enrollment The annual period in which employees can select from a choice of benefits programs.

open panel A dental benefits plan characterized by three features: (1) Any licensed dentist may elect to participate. (2) The beneficiary may receive dental treatment from among all licensed dentists with the corresponding benefits being payable to the beneficiary or the dentist. (3) The dentist may accept or refuse any beneficiary. *See also* panel, open.

open-end contract *See* contract, open-end.

opening movement *See* movement, mandibular, opening.

opening, vertical *See* dimension, vertical.

operate To work on the body with the hands or by means of cutting or other instruments to correct a deformity, remove an anatomic part, or remove pathologic processes and/or tissues.

operating field *See* field, operating.

operating light *See* light, operating.

operating procedure *See* procedure, operating.

  o., Abbé-Estlander The transfer of a full-thickness section of one lip of the oral cavity to the other lip, using an arterial pedicle to ensure survival of the graft.

  o., blind A procedure in which the surgeon operates by using the sense of touch and knowledge of surgical anatomy without making a significant mucous membrane or cutaneous incision.

  o. system (OS) An integrated set of software modules that provide the framework for orderly assignment of a computer's resources to perform a variety of tasks. It is usually written in the assembler language of the computer.

operation 1: Any surgical procedure.   **2:** The action of a drug or other remedy.   **3:** An act or series of acts performed on the body of a patient for relief or cure.

  o., computer The program step undertaken or executed by a computer (e.g., addition, multiplication, comparison, data movement). The operation is usually specified by the operator part of an instruction.

  o., exploratory A surgical procedure used to establish a diagnosis.

  o., Gillies' A technique for reducing fractures of the zygoma and the zygomatic arch through an incision in the temporal hairline.

  o., Kazanjian's (Kazanjian's procedure) A technique of surgical extension of the vestibular sulcus for improved prosthetic foundation of edentulous ridges. *See also* extension, ridge.

  o., modified flap A variation of the flap procedure in oral and periodontal surgery. In this variation the vertical incisions of the flap procedure are not made, but the labial and/or lingual gingival walls are distended as far as possible to ensure sufficient access and an unobstructed view for instrumentation.

  o., open A procedure in which the surgeon operates with full view of the structures through mucous membrane or cutaneous incisions.

  o., Partsch's The name applied to a technique of marsupialization.

  o., pedicle flap A procedure in mucogingival surgery designed to relocate or slide gingival tissue from a donor site in close proximity to an isolated defect, usually a tooth surface denuded of attached gingiva.

  o., Sorrin's A type of flap approach in the treatment of a periodontal abscess; especially suitable when the marginal gingiva appears well adapted and gives no access to the abscess area. A semilunar incision is made below the involved area in the attached gingiva, leaving the gingival margin undisturbed; a flap is raised, allowing access to the abscessed area for curettage. Suturing follows.

operative dentistry The branch of dentistry that deals with the esthetic and functional restoration of the hard tissues of individual teeth.

operatory (op'er-ah-tor"ē) The room or rooms in which the dentist performs professional services.

operculectomy (ō-per-kū-lĕk'tō-mē) The surgical removal of the mucosal flap partially or completely covering an unerupted tooth.

operculitis (ō-per"kū-lī'tĭs) *See* pericoronitis.

operculum (ō-per'kū-lŭm) A cover or lid.

opiate (ō'pē-at) A remedy containing or derived from opium; also any drug that induces sleep.

opinion In the law of evidence, an inference or conclusion drawn by a witness from information known to him or her or assumed.

opisthion (ō-pĭs'thē-on) The hindmost point on the posterior margin of the foramen magnum.

opisthocheilia (ō-pĭs"thō-kē'ĭl-ĭ-ah) A condition of receding lips.

opisthocranion (ō-pĭs"thō-krā'nē-on) The point in the midline of the cranium that projects farthest backward.

opium Concrete juice of the poppy, *Papaver somniferum*. It contains morphine, codeine, nicotine, narceine, and many other alkaloids.

opportunistic infection An infection by a microbial organism to which the patient is usually resistant; however because of reduced vitality or through suppression of the immune system, the patient has become infected.

optimal (ŏp'tĭ-mal) The best or most favorable.

Orabase Brand name of a topical dental paste containing an adrenocorticoid. The base consists of gelatin, pectin, mineral oil, and sodium carboxymethylcellulose in a hydrocarbon gel. The adrenocorticoid is hydrocortisone acetate. It is used for temporary relief of symptoms associated with oral inflammation and ulcerative lesions.

oral Pertaining to the mouth.

  o. environment *See* environment, oral.

  o. evacuator (vacuum) A suction apparatus used to remove fluids and debris from an operating field.

  o. hairy leukoplakia A filamentous, white plaque found on the lateral borders of the tongue that can spread across the entire dorsum of the tongue and onto the buccal mucosa. The Epstein-Barr virus has been identified in biopsy specimens of these lesions. An indicator disease for AIDS. *See* leukoplakia.

  o. health diet score A motivational aid to good nutrition. Merit points are earned by an adequate intake of foods from the recommended food groups. Demerits are awarded for frequent intake of foods high in sugars. The difference is the oral health diet score. The technique is applicable to children with a high incidence of dental caries.

  o. health index A statistical measure that quantifies one or more aspects of a person's or group's oral health status.

  o. hygiene *See* hygiene, oral.

  o. medicine *See* medicine, oral.

  o. mucosa *See* mucosa, oral.

  o. physiology *See* physiology, oral.

  o. surgery *See* surgery, oral.

  o. warts Warts caused by human papillomavirus that may be scattered throughout the mouth or localized in one area. They frequently recur. Oral warts are associated with AIDS infection.

orbital (or'bĭ-tăl) Pertaining to the orbit.

o. exenteration Surgical removal of the entire contents of the orbit.

o. marker A projecting part of a face-bow that marks the location of the orbitale. Used in the orientation of casts on an articulator in relation to cranial planes.

o. plane *See* plane, orbital.

orbitale (or″bĭ-tā′lē) The lowest point in the margin of the orbit (directly below the pupil when the eye is open and the patient is looking straight ahead) that may readily be felt under the skin. The eye-ear plane passes throug the orbitale and tragion.

orbiting condyle The condyle that arcs around the vertical axis of the rotating condyle (i.e., the opposite condyle from the center of rotation). Aids the opposite canine to disclude all other teeth.

orders Written or verbal directions of a physician or dentist to a nurse or other assistant detailing the care to be given to a patient.

organism(s) (or′gah-nĭzm) Any organized body of living economy.

o., Miller's The fusospirochetal organisms in the flora or oral microorganisms, found by Willoughby D. Miller and Hugo Karl Plaut to be the causative agents in nondiphtheritic membranous angina (necrotizing ulcerative gingivitis, necrotizing ulcerative gingivostomatitis, Vincent's infection, ″trench mouth,″ etc.).

o., Vincent's The fusospirochetal organisms associated with the initiation of necrotizing ulcerative gingivitis, necrotizing ulcerative stomatitis, and/or Vincent's angina.

orifice (ōr′ĭ-fĭs) The entrance or outlet of any body cavity; any foramen, meatus, or opening.

orodigitofacial dysostosis (OFD syndrome) Syndrome characterized by abnormal development of the jaws and tongue, cleft lip and palate, hypoplasia of bones of the skull with ocular hypertelorism, nasal alar deformity, malformation of digits (frequently manifested as brachydactyly and syndactyly), mental retardation, granular skin, and alopecia of the scalp.

orofacial abnormality A structural and functional disorder of the mouth and face, usually arising from genetic or congential defects.

orofacial muscles The muscles of facial expression.

orofacial pain Pain within the structures of the mouth and face, usually of a diffuse pattern.

oronasal Pertaining to the mouth and nose.

oropharynx (o″rō-far′inks) The portion of the pharynx associated with the mouth; usually described as bounded above by the uvula, below by the epiglottis, in front by the tongue, and behind by the posterior pharyngeal wall.

ortho A prefix denoting straight or correct.

orthodontic Related to the orthopedic correction of abnormal dental relationships, including related abnormalities in facial structures.

orthodontics (dentofacial orthopedic) The area of dentistry concerned with the supervision, guidance, and correction of the growing and mature dentofacial structures, including conditions that require movement of the teeth or correction of malrelationships and malformations of related structures by the adjustment of relationships between and among teeth and facial bones by the application of forces and/or the stimulation and redirection of functional forces within the craniofacial complex. Major responsibilities of orthodontic practice include the diagnosis, prevention, interception, and treatment of all forms of malocclusion of the teeth and associated alterations in their surrounding structures; design, application, and control of functional and corrective appliances; and guidance of the dentition and its supporting structures to attain and maintain optimum occlusal relations in physiologic and esthetic harmony among facial and cranial structures.

orthodontist A dental specialist who has completed an approved, advanced course of at least 2 years in the special area of orthodontics.

orthognathic (or″thog-na′thik) Pertaining to the normal relationships of the jaws.

o. surgery Surgery to alter relationships of dental arches and/or supporting bones, usually accomplished with orthodontic therapy.

orthognathus (or-thō-năth′ŭs) Straight jaws; no projection of the lower part of the face. The facial angle is 85 to 90 degrees.

orthopantograph (or″thō-păn′tō-grăf) A panoramic radiographic device (Panorex) that permits visualization of the entire dentition, alveolar bone, and other contiguous structures on a single extraoral film.

orthopantomograph (or′thō-pănt′ō-mō-grăf) A radiographic system (manufactured by Siemens) that uses three axes of rotation to obtain a panoramic radiograph of the dental arches and their associated structures.

orthopedic (or″thō-pē′dik) A correction of abnormal form or relationship of bone structures. May be accomplished surgically (orthopedic surgery) or by the application of appliances to stimulate changes in the bone structure by natural physiologic response (orthopedic therapy). Orthodontic therapy is orthopedic therapy applied through the teeth.

orthopnea (or″thop-nē′ah) An inability to breathe except in an upright position.

Osler's disease *See* erythremia.

Osler-Weber disease *See* telangiectasia, hereditary hemorrhagic.

osmosis The passage of pure solvent from the lesser to the greater concentration when two solutions are separated by a membrane that selectively prevents the passage of solute molecules but is permeable to the solvent. The principles of osmosis, with the selective permeability of the cell membrane, help regulate the transfer of fluids and metabolites to and from the cells. Thus they also maintain the stability of the salt/ion concentration in the extracellular and intracellular fluids.

osmotic Pertaining to osmosis.

o. pressure *See* pressure, osmotic.

ostectomy (os-tĕk'tō-mē) **(osteoectomy)** The excision of a bone or a portion of a bone.

o., periodontal The removal of alveolar bone from around the tooth root to eliminate an adjacent pocket and to secure physiologic osseous and gingival form.

osteitis (ŏs″tē-ī'tĭs) An inflammation of the bone; an inflammation of the haversian spaces, canals, and their branches but generally not of the medullary cavity. The disease is characterized by tenderness and a dull, aching pain. Enlargement of the bone may occur. Osteitis of the alveolar process after tooth extraction is commonly referred to as a *dry socket*.

o., alveolar localized *See* socket, dry.

o., condensing A chronic inflammation associated with some nonvital teeth or located in the site of extraction of such teeth, resulting in abnormally dense bone.

o. deformans (Paget's disease) 1: A disease of the bone of unknown cause characterized by enlargement of the cranial bones and often of the maxillae or the mandible. The x-ray appearance is characterized by a cotton-wool appearance. **2:** A localized or generalized disease of bone of unknown origin characterized by the replacement of normal bone with soft, poorly mineralized osteoid tissue. In later stages, affected bone is replaced by densely sclerotic bone. Bony enlargement, deformities, and sometimes fractures occur. **3:** A generalized disease of bone characterized by the concurrent destruction and formation of bone. The etiology is unknown. **4:** A bone disease characterized by thickening and bowing of the long bones and enlargement of the skull and maxillae. represented radiographically by a cotton-wool appearance of the bone and microscopically by a mosaic bone pattern. Hypercementosis and loosening of the teeth may be significant manifestations.

o. fibrosa cystica, generalized (von Recklinghausen's disease of bone) 1: A disease caused by parathyroid adenomas and characterized by cystlike radiolucencies in the bones (including the jaws), loosening of teeth, localized swellings, giant cell lesions, increased blood calcium and phosphatase levels, and lowered blood phosphorus levels. The term *von Recklinghausen's disease (of skin)* is also used as a synonym for neurofibromatosis. **2:** Increased resorption and destruction of bone caused by primary and secondary hyperparathyroidism. *See also* hyperparathyroidism.

osteoarthritis (ŏs tē-ō-ăr-thrī'tĭs) Chronic degeneration and destruction of the articular cartilage leading to bony spurs, pain, stiffness, limitation of motion, and change in the size of joints. Considered to result from chronic traumatic injury and wear and tear. Heberden's nodes occur in a special form of the disease. Symptoms may be associated with hormonal, vascular, and/or nutritional disorders. The structural changes of advanced osteoarthritis may involve erosion of the articular cartilages or the subchondral bone. Osteoarthritis rarely affects the temporomandibular joint beyond the "creaking" state.

osteoarthropathy, hypertrophic pulmonary (ŏs″tē-ōarthrop'ah-thē) A clubbing of the fingers and toes resulting from deposition of calcium in the subperiosteal tissues around the joint. Related to chronic pulmonary disease and occasionally to circulatory and digestive disease.

osteoblast (os'tē-ō-blăst″) The cell associated with the growth and development of bone; Cuboidal in shape and about 15 to 20 μm in width. In active growth, osteoblasts form a continuous layer on old bone like a sheet of epithelial cells; when the bone growth is arrested, the cells assume an elongated appearance like fibroblasts.

osteocementum (os″tē-ō-sē-měn'tŭm) Secondary cementum; the hard, bonelike cementum deposited after root formation is completed. *See also* atrophy of disuse.

osteoclasia, traumatic (os″tē-ō-klā'zē-ah) *See* cementoma; dysplasia, osseous, focal; fibroma, periapical.

osteoclast (ŏs'tē-ō-klăst″) **1:** A large multinucleated giant cell associated with the resorption of bone; the nuclei resemble the nuclei of the osteoblasts and osteocytes; the cytoplasm is often foamy, and the cell frequently has branching processes. Osteoclasts may arise from stromal cells of the bone marrow, they may represent fused osteoblasts, or they may include fused osteocytes liberated from resorbing bone. They are usually found in close relationship to the resorption of bone and frequentiy lie in grooves (Howship's lacunae). **2:** A large multinucleated cell associated with the resorption of bone. Seen in irregular concavities within marginal areas of bone undergoing resorption.

osteoclastoma *See* granuloma, giant cell reparative, peripheral.

osteocyte (os'tē-ō-sīt″) An osteoblast that has been surrounded by a calcified interstitial substance; the cells are enclosed within lacunae, and the cytoplasmic processes extend through apertures of the lacunae into canaliculi in the bone. Like the osteoblast, the osteocyte may undergo transformations and assume the form of an osteoclast or reticular cell.

osteodystrophy (os″tē-ō-dĭs′trō-fē) A condition marked by defective or deficient bone formation.

 o., renal A form of dwarfism associated with osteoporosis produced by renal insufficiency during childhood. Periodontal changes include widening of the periodontal membrane space and marked osteoporosis of the mandibular and maxillary bones. Similar to renal rickets. *See also* rickets, renal.

oteoectomy (os″tē-ō-ĕk′tō-mē) *See* ostectomy.

osteofibroma (os″tē-ō-fī-brō′mah) **(calcifying fibroma, fibroosteoma, ossifying fibroma)** A benign neoplasm characterized by bone developing in a connective tissue mass. A benign neoplasm that develops in the spongiosa of the bone through proliferation of fibroblasts. A benign neoplasm of the bone characterized by unilateral swelling and fibroblastic and osteoclastic activity in marrow spaces. *See also* dysplasia, fibrous; dysplasia, osseous.

osteogenesis imperfecta (os″tē-ō-jĕn′ĕ-sĭs) **(brittle bone disease, fragilitas ossium, Lobstein's disease, osteopsathyrosis idiopathica)** A congenital disease of unknown cause characterized by fragile, brittle, and easily fractured bones; presumed to stem from a failure in the formation of bone matrix. Variants are often hereditary or familial and include manifestations such as blue sclerae, dentinogenesis imperfecta, and otosclerosis.

osteoid (os′tē-oid) The mucopolysaccharide-protein complex laid down by the osteoblasts. It is later calcified, with inclusion of osteoblasts as osteocytes within lacunae, into bone.

osseointegration (os″ē-ō-in″tē-grā′shun) A specific endosseous dental implant technique involving extraslow and precise bone drilling to minimize heat production; use of biocompatible metal and a defined healing environment. Synonym: Branemark technique.

osteolysis (os′tē-ol′ĭ-sĭs) A process of bone resorption whereby the bone salts can be withdrawn by a humoral mechanism and returned to the tissue fluids, leaving behind a decalcified bone matrix. Synonym: halisteresis

osteoma (os″tē-o ′mah) A benign neoplasm of bone or bone tissue.

osteomalacia (os″tē-ō-mah-lā′shē-ah) **(adult rickets)** A systemic disorder of bone characterized by decreased mineralization of bone matrix possible resulting from vitamin D deficiency, inadequate calcium in the diet, renal disease, and/or steatorrhea. Manifestations include incomplete fractures and gradual resorption of cortical and cancellous bone.

osteomyelitis (os′tē-ō-mī″ĕ-lī′tĭs) An inflammation of the bone marrow or of the bone, marrow, and endosteum. *See also* osteitis.

osteon (os′tē-on) The three-dimensional reconstruction of concentric lamellae arranged circumferentially about the course of a central blood vessel.

osteopetrosis (ostē-ō-pĕ-trō′sĭs) **(Albers-Schönberg disease, marble bone)** Osteosclerosis of unknown origin that obliterates the bone marrow regions with resultant anemia. Delayed tooth eruption and severe osteomyelitis or necrosis after dental infection may be associated with the disease.

osteoplasty (ŏs′tē-ō-plăs″tē) A surgical procedure to modify or change the configuration of a bone.

osteoporosis (os″tē-ō-po-rō′sĭs) **(Schüller's disease)** Enlargement of the soft marrow and haversian spaces resulting from a decreased rate of formation of the hard bone matrix. With the exception of immobilized parts, it is a systemic disorder that occurs in advanced age (senile osteoporosis), during ACTH and cortisone therapy, during and after menopause, in limited physical activity, in Cushing's syndrome, during malnutrition, and in other disorders of matrix formation such as hyperadrenalism, hyperthyroidism, vitamin C deficiencies, and deficiency of androgenic steroids. *See also* atrophy, bone; bone rarefaction.

osteopsathyrosis idiopathica (os″tē-op-săth″ĭ- rō′sĭs) *See* osteogenesis imperfecta.

osteoradionecrosis (os″tē-ō-rā″dē-ō-nĕ-krō′sĭs) Bone necrosis secondary to irradiation and superimposed infection.

osteosarcoma (os′tē-ō-sar-kō′mah) A malignant neoplasm of the bone-forming tissues.

osteosclerosis (os″tē-ō-sklē-rō′sĭs) An increased bone formation resulting in reduced marrow spaces and increased radiopacity.

osteotomy (os″tē-ot′ō-mē) The surgical cutting or transection of a bone.

otalgia dentalis (ō-tăl′jē-ah) A reflex pain in the ear resulting from dental disease; usually propagated along the auriculotemporal nerve.

otic ganglion *See* ganglion, otic.

otitis media (ō-tī′tĭs mē′dē-ah) An inflammation of the middle ear that may be marked by pain, fever, abnormalities of hearing, deafness, tinnitus, and vertigo that may originate in the pharynx and be transmitted by the eustachian tubes.

otolaryngology The branch or specialty of medicine that deals with diseases of the ear, nose, and throat.

otosclerosis (ō″tō-sklē-rō′sĭs) A disorder of the middle ear that generally results in hardening and fusion of the ossicles of the ear, with resultant immobilization so that sound waves cannot be conducted along their paths.

outline form *See* form, outline.

output The transfer or exit of processed or in-process information from a computer to printers, video terminals, and other peripheral devices.

ovalocytosis (ō-văl″ō-sī-tō′sĭs) *See* elliptocytosis.

overbilling A nondisclosure of waiver of patient copayment.

overbite A vertical overlapping of upper teeth over lower teeth, usually measured perpendicular to the occlusal plane. *See* overjet; overlap, vertical.

overclosure Raising of the mandible too far before the teeth make contact; loss of occlusal vertical dimension is the cause. *See also* distance, large interarch.

overcoding Reporting a more complex and/or higher cost procedure than was actually performed.

overdenture A compete or partial removable denture supported by retained roots to provide improved support, stability, and tactile and proprioceptive sensation and to reduce ridge resorption. *See* root retention; root submersion.

overextended 1: When any prosthetic appliance is inadvertently constructed in such a way that part of the oral mucosa is injured by the appliance. **2:** Pertaining to any extrusion beyond the apical opening into the periapical area. May be with instrumentation, medication, or root canal filling.

overfilled *See* overextended.

overhang An excess filling material projecting beyond cavity margins.

overhead Production costs required to be expended by the dentist to practice the profession (e.g., rent, utilities, salaries, laundry). Costs involved in management, supplies, equipment, salaries (taxes), and maintenance. Amounts deducted from the gross receipts of a dental practice before the dentist's net income (take-home pay) is received.

overjet Horizontal projection of upper teeth beyond the lower teeth, usually measured parallel to the occlusal plane. When not otherwise specified, the term is generally assumed to refer to central incisors and is measured from the labial surface of the lower central incisors to the labial surface of the upper central incisors at the level of the upper incisor edge. Unique conditions may sometimes require other measuring techniques. *See* overlap, horizontal.

overjut *See* overlap, horizontal.

overlap, horizontal (overjet, overjut) Projection of the anterior and/or posterior teeth of one arch beyond their antagonists in a horizontal direction.

overlap, vertical (overbite) Extension of the upper teeth over the lower teeth in a vertical direction when the opposing posterior teeth are in contact in centric occlusion. This term is used especially to designate the distance that the upper incisal edges drop below the level of the lower ones, but it may also be used to describe the vertical relations of opposing cusps of posterior teeth.

    o., deep vertical (closed bite, deep bite, deep overbite) Excessive vertical overlap of the anterior teeth.

overlay *See* onlay.

    o., computer A technique for bringing routines into memory from magnetic storage during processing so that several routines will occupy the same storage locations at different times. Overlay techniques are used when the total storage requirements for instructions exceed the available storage in memory.

overshooting accident The result of seating an endosteal implant beyond its normal host site (through the inferior mandibular border, into the mandibular canal or nasal or antral floor).

ovoid arch *See* arch, ovoid.

owner The person holding ownership, dominion, or title of property.

Owren's disease *See* parahemophilia.

oxacillin (oks″ah-si′lin) An orally administered antistaphylocccal penicillin recommended for use in treatment of resistant strains of *Staphylococcus aureus* infections.

oxidation The combination of oxygen with other elements to form oxides. The process in which an element gains electrons.

    o. of metal The formation of a surface oxide during the casting or soldering of a metal or during subsequent use by the patient.

oxide divinyl *See* ether, divinyl.

oxycephaly (ŏk″sē-sĕ-fălē) **(steeple head)** A high conical crown resulting from early closure of sutures and disturbed cranial development.

oxycodone (ŏk″sē-kō-dōn) A potent semisynthetic derivative of codeine found in Percodan, Percocet, and Tylox.

oxygenate (ŏk′sē-jĕ-nāt) To saturate with oxygen.

oxyhemoglobin (ŏk″sē-hē″mō-glō′bĭn) A compound of hemoglobin with two atoms of oxygen.

oxytocin (ŏk″sē-tō′sĭn) A hormone of the posterior pituitary gland that is the principal uterus-contracting hormone. Used in obstetrics to induce uterine contractions.

PA skull *See* examination, radiographic, extraoral, posteroanterior.

PAB, PABA Abbreviation for paraaminobenzoic acid.

PAC *See* aspirin, phenacetin, caffeine.

pacemaker An electrical device used to maintain a normal sinus rhythm in heart muscle contraction. Pacemakers can be permanent in-dwelling appliances. It is not advisable to use electronic devices on patients with pacemakers. Synonym: cardiac pacemaker.

pachyderma oralis (păk″ĭ-der′mah ō-rā′lĭs) An appearance of the buccal mucosa suggestive of elephant hide.

pachyderma oris (păk′ĭ-der′mah or′ĭs) **(focal keratosis, hyperkeratosis)** A benign white lesion of the mucous membrane characterized by a thick layer of keratin overlying stratified squamous epithelium, the cells of which are normal.

pachymucosa alba (păk″ĭ-mū-kō′sah ăl′bah) An appearance of the buccal mucosa resembling elephant hide with a white surface.

Pacini's corpuscle (pah-chē′nēz) *See* corpuscle, Pacini's.

pack A material used to protect tissue, fill space, or prevent hemorrhage.

  p., periodontal A surgical dressing applied to the necks of teeth and the adjacent tissue to cover and protect the surgical wound.

packing The act of filling a mold.

  p., denture The laboratory procedure of filling and compressing a denture base material into a mold in a flask.

pad, Passavant's (pas′ah-vants) **(Passavant's bar, Passavant's ridge)** The bulging "cross roll" of the posterior pharyngeal wall produced by the upper portion of the superior pharyngeal constrictor muscle during the act of swallowing or during vocal effort. (An objectionable term.) *See* pharynx, activities of posterior and lateral pharyngeal wall.

pad, retromolar (pear-shaped area) A mass of soft tissue, frequently pear shaped, that is located at the distal termination of the mandibular residual ridge. It is made up of fibers of the buccinator muscle, pterygomandibular raphe, superior constrictor muscle, temporal tendon, and mucous glands.

pad, rubber dam (rubber dam mask) An absorbent piece of flannelette, bird's-eye cloth, or gauze of suitable shape to interpose between a rubber dam and the face to protect the face from contact with the rubber and with the clips of the dam holder.

Paget's disease (păj′ĕtz) *See* osteitis deformans.

pain (pān) An unpleasant sensation created by a noxious stimulus mediated along specific nerve pathways to the central nervous system, where it is interpreted as such. The sensation of pain is a protective mechanism that warns of danger without giving too much information about the specific nature of the danger. It gives rise to nociceptive reflexes.

  p., chest Pain that occurs in the chest region because of disorders of the heart (e.g., angina pectoris, myocardial infarction, pericarditis), pulmonary artery (pulmonary embolism or hypertension), lungs (pleuritis), esophagus ("heartburn"), abdominal organs (aerophagia, biliary tract disease, splenic infarction, and gaseous distention in splenic flexure), or the chest wall (neoplasia, costochondral strains, and trauma, hyperventilation, and muscular tension).

  p., deep Dull, aching, or boring pain originating in muscles, tendons, and joints. It is poorly localized and tends to radiate.

  p. dysfunction syndrome A phrase used in dentistry to describe a condition in patients who appear to have a psychophysiologic basis for stress overload on the temporomandibular joint. The preferred term is *mandibular stress syndrome*.

  p., ghost *See* odontalgia, phantom.

  p. nerve ending A receptor nerve ending that is relatively primitive and ends in an undifferentiated arborization. The nerve ending for the sensation of pain is essentially a protective mechanism that warns of danger without giving too much information about the specific nature of the danger. The danger stimuli give rise to nociceptive reflexes, which are characterized by defensive, protective, or withdrawal movements. The nociceptive reflexes supercede other, less urgent, reflexes that are thus inhibited.

  p., projected pathologic Pain erroneously perceived to arise in a peripheral region because of a stimulus from end-organs supplying the region (e.g., sciatic pain). Actually, the stimulus has occurred somewhere along the pain pathway from the nerve to the cortex.

p. reaction The individual's manifestation of the unpleasant sensation.

p., referred Pain caused by an agent in one area but manifested in another; e.g., pain caused by caries in the maxillary third molar may be referred to the mandible so that the source of pain appears to be in the mandible.

p. and suffering An element in a claim for damages in a liability suit that allows an individual to recover for mental and physical pain and discomfort as a result of an injury.

p. threshold The point at which a stimulus causes pain. The threshold level varies widely among individuals.

pair, ion See ion.

palatal (pa′ah-tal) Relating to the palate.

p. bar See bar, palatal.

p. perforation See perforation, palatal.

p. plate See connector, major.

p. seal See seal, posterior palatal.

palate (pal′at) The bone and soft tissue closing the space encompassed by the upper alveolar arch, with a posterior extension to the pharynx. Forms the "roof" of the mouth and is connected to the nasal septum and floor of the nose in the midline.

p., cleft 1: A deformity of the palate from improper union or lack of union during the second month of intrauterine development of the maxillary process with the median nasal process. **2:** A cleft in the palate between the two palatal processes. If both hard and soft palates are involved, it is a uranostaphyloschisis; if only the soft palate is divided, it is a uranoschisis. The term *cleft palate* is often erroneously applied to clefts between the median nasal and maxillary processes through the alveolus. This type of cleft is properly termed *cleft jaw,* or *gnathoschisis.*

p., acquired cleft Noncongenital defect of soft and/or hard tissues of the hard and soft palate.

p., congenital cleft Congenital nonunion or inadequacy of soft and hard tissues related to the lip, nose, alveolar process, hard palate, and velum. The extent of these deformities varies among individuals. Varieties of classifications are available to identify the extent of the cleft.

p., hard The anterior part of the palate that is supported by and includes the palatal extensions of the maxillary and palatine bones.

p., soft The part of the palate lying posterior to the hard palate, composed only of soft tissues without underlying bony support.

p., soft, redivision Surgical incision or removal of a

V-shaped area of tissue from the soft palate to facilitate the proper placement of the pharyngeal section of the prosthetic speech aid.

p.-splitting appliance An orthodontic appliance cemented to buccal teeth on either side, incorporating a jackscrew that is progressively extended to accomplish forceful separation of the two lateral halves of the bony palate. Similar corrections are also accomplished with removable split-palate appliances.

palatine arch (păl′ah-tīn) See arch, palatine.

palatine mucosa See mucosa, palatine.

palatine suture, median See suture, intermaxillary.

palato- (păl′ah-tō) Prefix meaning pertaining to the palate.

palatoplasty (păl′ah-tō-plăs″tē) Surgical repair of palatal defects.

palatorrhaphy (păl″ah-tor′ah-fē) Surgical closure of a cleft palate with suturing.

palatoschisis (păl″ah-tos′kĭ-sĭs) See palate, cleft.

palliate (păl′ē-āt) To reduce the severity of.

palliative (păl′ē-ā″tĭv) An alleviating measure.

pallor (păl′or) Paleness; absence of skin coloration.

p., perioral Paleness of soft tissues surrounding the mouth; an indication of impending syncope.

Palmer's tooth notation A system for designating teeth by number and quadrant. The mouth is divided into quadrants and each tooth is numbered from 1 to 8 starting with the central incisor in each quadrant and continuing back to the third. The quadrant is indicated by a right angle symbol oriented right or left and up or down. The system was popular in the 1950s but is no longer in general use.

palpate (păl′pāt) To examine the soft tissues digitally.

palpation (pal-pā-shŭn) **1:** The act of feeling with the hand or fingers. **2:** A phase of the examination procedure in which the sense of touch is used to gather data essential for diagnosis.

palpitation (păl″pĭ-tā′shŭn) Unduly rapid action of the heart that is perceptible to the patient.

palsy (pawl′zē) Synonym for *paralysis* but preferred by some to refer to certain types of paralysis.

p., Bell's Facial paralysis believed to result from inflammation in or around the facial nerve. One side of the face sags, the corner of the mouth droops, the eyelid will not close, and saliva dribbles from the corner of the mouth on the affected side. See also paralysis, facial.

p., cerebral 1: Collective term for neurologic defects with associated disturbances of motor function. The disturbances vary in cause and anatomic type (e.g., acquired, hereditary, natal, postnatal, congenital palsy). **2:** Nonspecific term standing for a group of pathologies having the following common related characteristics: agenesis or a lesion of nervous tissue within the cranium; interference with voluntary muscular movements; disabling disorders of a chronic nature, neither acute nor progressive; and occurrence of the original lesion at the date of birth of the patient or before the development of learned human muscular function. **3:** A condition caused by damage to the motor centers of the brain, resulting in varying disturbances of motor function and often accompanied by mental subnormality.

p., creeping *See* gait, spastic.

p., facial Paralysis of the muscles supplied by the seventh cranial nerve. It may be associated with peripheral lesions, neoplasms invading the temporal bone, herpes zoster involving the geniculate ganglion, acoustic neuromas, and pontine disease. Bilateral paralysis may occur in uveoparotid fever and polyneuritis.

p., lead Weakness and paralysis of the hand, wrist, and fingers associated with lead poisoning.

panel, open A group dental plan characterized by three features: any licensed dentist may elect to participate, the beneficiary may choose from among all licensed dentists, and the dentist may accept or refuse any beneficiary.

pamplegia (păm-plē′jē-ah) Total paralysis.

panesthesia (păn″ĕs-thē′zē-ah) The sum of the sensations experienced.

pangamic acid There is no evidence that this substance is a vitamin. It is a derivative of apricot pits and contains some potentially toxic substances. Synonym: vitamin B$_{15}$.

panhypopituitarism (păn-hī″pō-pĭ-tū′ĭ-tăr-ĭzm°) A deficiency involving all the hormonal functions of the pituitary gland. *See also* disease, Simmonds′.

panneuritis endemica (păn″nū-rī′tĭs ĕn-dĕm′ē-kah) *See* beriberi.

panoral Literally, all of the oral region. A term used in diagnostic oral radiography to describe a technique that includes all of the oral structures on one film.

panoramic radiograph A radiographic tomograph of the jaws, taken with a specialized machine designed to present a panoramic view of the full circumferential length of the jaws on a single film. Also known by several trade names of machines, most of which incorporate "pan" into the name.

Panoramix A radiographic system in which the source of radiation is placed inside the mouth to expose a large film placed extraorally around the face.

Panorex A radiographic system (manufactured by the S.S. White Co.) that uses two axes of rotation to obtain a panoramic radiograph of the dental arches and associated structures. *See also* pantomography.

pansinusitis (păn″sī-nŭ-sī′tĭs) Inflammation of all the sinuses, as of the facial bones.

pantograph (păn′tō-grăf) Figurative term given to a pair of face-bows fixed to both jaws and designed to in-

scribe centrically related points and arcs leading to them on segments of planes relatable to the three craniofacial planes of space. The maxillary planes are attached to the maxillary bow, and the inscribing styluses are attached to the mandibular bow.

pantomography (păn-tō-mŏg′rah-fē) Panoramic radiography by which radiographs of the maxillary and mandibular dental arches and their associated structures may be obtained.

pantothenic acid (pan-tō-then′ik) Fatty acids. *See also* acid, pantothenic.

paper, articulating Paper strips coated with ink or dye-containing wax used for marking or locating occlusal interferences or deflecting occlusal contacts prior to making occlusal contacts. *See also* articulating paper.

paper point A cone of absorbent paper so formed that it can be inserted into the length of the root canal and used to absorb fluid, carry medication into the canal, or inoculate cultures.

papilla(e) (pah-pĭl′ah) Any small, nipple-shaped elevation.

p., incisive The elevation of soft tissue covering the foramen of the incisive or nasopalatine canal.

p., interdental The part of the gingivae filling the interproximal spaces between adjacent teeth, consisting partly of free and partly of attached gingivae.

p., interproximal The cone-shaped projection of the gingiva filling the interdental spaces up to the contact areas when viewed from the labial, buccal, and lingual aspects. When viewed buccolingually or labiolingually, the crest of the interproximal papilla appears as a rounded concavity at an area below the contact point of the teeth. If recession has occurred, this concavity may become an area of pathology, and the entire papilla may require reshaping to restore health. *See also* papilla, interdental.

p., palatine A convexly rounded and elliptically shaped pad of soft tissue lying palatal to the upper central incisors.

papillary-marginal-attached (păp′ĭ-lăr″ē) *See* PMA.

papilloma (păp′ĭ-lō′mah) A benign neoplasm of epithelium often having a warty appearance. A benign, exophytic, pedunculated, cauliflower-like neoplasm of epithelium.

p., basal call *See* keratosis, seborrheic.

papillomatosis, inflammatory (păp″ĭ-lō″mah-tō′sĭs) *See* hyperplasia, papillary, inflammatory.

papillomatosis, multiple *See* hyperplasia, papillary, inflammatory.

Papillon-Lefévre syndrome (pap″ĭ-yon′ lĕ-fa′) *See* syndrome, Papillon-Lefèvre.

papule (păp′ūl) A small, circumscribed, solid elevation of the skin.

p., split A secondary lesion of syphilis seen at the angle of the lips, resulting from the formation of a papule that becomes fissured because of its position.

paradontosis (par″ah-don-tō′sis) *See* periodontosis.

parafunction Movements (such as bruxism, clenching, and rocking of teeth) that are considered outside or beyond function and that result in worn facets.

parahemophilia (par″ah-hē″mō-fīl′ē-ah) **(ac-globulin deficiency, hemophilioid state A, Owren's disease)** A hemorrhagic disorder resulting from a deficiency of proaccelerin. Manifestations include mild to severe bleeding after extraction of teeth or other surgical procedures, epistaxis, easy bruisability, monorrhagia, and hematomas. The one-stage prothrombin time is prolonged, but the bleeding time is ordinarily normal.

parakeratosis (par″ah-kĕr″ah-tō′sīs) Persistence of nuclei in the stratum corneum of stratified squamous epithelium.

paralgesia (păr″al-jē′zē-ah) **(paraigia)** Any condition marked by abnormal and painful sensations; a painful paresthesia.

paralgia (păr-ăl′jē-ah) *See* paralgesia.

parallax (par″ah-laks) The apparent change in position of an object when viewed from two different positions. The phenomenon is useful in determining the relative position of an object in a radiograph. Two or more radiographs are made from slightly different positions and the direction and amount of shift of the object is observed and measured.

parallel attachment *See* attachment, parallel.

parallelism The condition of two or more surfaces that, if extended to infinity, could never meet. In removable partial prosthodontics, such a condition is created on vertical tooth surfaces to act as guiding planes.

parallelometer (par″ah-lĕl-om′ĕ-ter) An apparatus used to determine parallelism or a lack of parallelism or to make a part or an object parallel with some other part or object. *See also* surveyor.

paralysis (pah-răl′ĭ-sīs) **1:** Cessation of cell function. **2:** Loss or impairment of the motor control or function of a part or region.

> **p., facial** Paralysis of the muscles of facial expression resulting from supranuclear, nuclear, or peripheral nerve disease. With a mild case, when the face is at rest, the disorder is not readily observed. However, during muscular contraction (e.g., wrinkling the forehead, blinking the eyes, pursing the lips, speaking), the disorder is very noticeable. Only one lid may close, and the asymmetry of the mouth is pronounced because the normal buccinator muscle contracts and is unopposed by the weakness on the paralyzed side. This imbalance produces a significant asymmetry. The affected side remains smooth, and the normal side shows contraction. *See also* palsy, Bell's.

> **p., infantile** *See* poliomyelitis.

> **p., motor** A loss of the power of skeletal muscle con-

traction resulting from interruption of some part of the pathway from the cerebrum to the muscle.

parameter (pah-ram′-ĕ-ter) Values that refer to a population; characteristics of a population. Because a parameter is a value of a hypothetical, infinite, unknown population, it is always an estimate.

paramolar A supernumerary tooth located buccal, lingual, or distal to a normal molar.

paranesthesia (par″ăn-ĕs-thē′zē-ah) Anesthesia of the lower part of the body and limbs.

paranoia (par″ah-noi′ah) **1:** Psychosis characterized by delusions and hallucinations that are well systematized. **2:** The irrational belief that one is the object of special persecution by others or by fate.

parasympatholytic (par″ah-sīm″pah-thō-līt′ĭk) *See* anticholinergic.

parasympathomimetic (par″ah-sīm″pah-thō-mī-mĕt-ĭk) *See* cholinergic.

Para-thor-mone (păr″ah-thor′mōn) Trade name for parathyroid hormone.

Parathyrin (păr″ah-thī′rĭn) Trade name for parathyroid hormone.

parenteral (pah-rĕn′ter-ăl) Not through the alimentary canal (literally, aside from the gastrointestinal tract) (i.e., by subcutaneous, intramuscular, intravenous, or other nongastrointestinal route of administration).

paresis (pah-rē′sīs) **(dementia paralytica, paretic neurosyphilis)** A progressive psychosis associated with neurosyphilis.

paresthesia (păr″ĕs-thē′zē-ah) An altered sensation reported by the patient in an area where the sensory nerve has been afflicted by a disease or an injury; the patient may report burning, prickling, formication, or other sensations.

parol (pah-rōl′) Oral or verbal; expressed by speech only; not expressed in writing.

parotid gland (pah-rot′id) One of the largest pairs of salivary glands that lie at the side of the face just below and in front of the external ear along the posterior border of the ramus of the mandible.

parotitis (par″ō-tī′tīs) Inflammation of the parotid land. *See also* mumps.

> **p., endemic (epidemic parotitis, infectious parotitis, mumps)** An acute viral infection characterized by unilateral or bilateral swelling of the salivary glands, especially the parotid.

> **p., epidemic** *See* parotitis, endemic.

> **p., infectious** *See* parotitis, endemic.

paroxysmal (păr′ok-sĭz′mal) Recurring in paroxysms.

Parry's disease *See* goiter, exophthalmic; hyperthyroidism.

partial anodontia *See* oligodontia.

partial denture retention *See* retention, denture, partial.

partial thromboplastin time (PTT) A test for detecting

coagulation defects of the intrinsic system by adding activated partial thromboplastin to a sample of test plasma and to a control sample of normal plasma. The time required for the formation of a clot is compared with the normal plasma. It is also used to monitor the activity of heparin in patients who are being treated for a variety of cardiovascular disorders.

participating dentist Any dentist who has a contractual agrement with a dental benefits organization to render care to eligible persons.

particle A small amount of material.

p., alpha (alpha ray, alpha radiation) Positively charged particulate ionizing radiation consisting of helium nuclei (two protons and two neutrons) traveling at high speeds. Such rays are emitted from the nucleus of an unstable element.

p., beta (beta ray, beta radiation) Particulate ionizing radiation consisting of either negative electrons (negatrons) or positive electrons (positrons) emitted from the nucleus of an unstable element. Such a phenomenon is called *beta decay.*

particulate bone grafts Better known as particulate bone and cancellous marrow grafts (PBCM). A type of autogenous bone graft that consists of small particles of cortical and cancellous bone, as well as hematopoietic and mesenchymal marrow.

parties The persons who take part in the performance of any act, who have a direct interest in any contract or conveyance, or who are actively involved in the prosecution and defense of any legal proceeding.

partnership 1: The association of two or more persons for the purpose of carrying on business (or practice) together and dividing its profits. **2:** A legal, binding agreement for sharing all aspects of a professional dental practice.

p., notice of dissolution of Intelligence, by whatever means communicated, to creditors and the public that a partnership has been dissolved.

partnership A contract defining the association of two or more persons in a business or professional relationship.

Partsch's operation *See* operation, Partsch's.

parulis (pah-roo′lĭs) **(gumboil)** An elevated nodule at the site of a fistula draining a chronic periapical abscess. These nodules occur most frequently in relation to pulpally involved deciduous teeth.

Pascal's law *See* law, Pascal's.

Passavant's bar *See* pad, Passavant's.

Passavant's pad *See* pad, Passavant's.

Passavant's ridge *See* pad, Passavant's.

passer, foil *See* foil passer.

passive Referring to an orthodontic appliance that has been adjusted to apply no effective tooth-moving force to the teeth.

passive-aggressive behavior Behavior that reflects hostility or resentment through indirect nonviolent means such as procrastination, inefficiency, forgetfulness, and stubbornness.

passive reciprocation *See* reciprocation, passive.

passivity The quality or condition of inactivity or rest assumed by the teeth, tissues, and denture when a removable denture is in place but is not under masticatory pressure.

paste A soft, smooth, semifluid mixture, often medicated.

p. filler A semisoft mixture of materials used to fill the root canal system, as opposed to solid filling material such as silver or guttapercha cones.

p., pressure-indicating A soft mixture used to disclose areas of contact or pressure in restorations.

patch, mucous Multiple gray-white patch overlying an area of ulceration and occurring on the oral mucosa as an expression of secondary syphilis. Highly infectious. *See also* syphilis.

path A certain course that is ordinarily followed.

p. of appliance insertion and removal *See* insertion, path of.

p. of closure *See* closure, centric path of.

p., condyle *See* condyle path.

p., lateral *See* condyle path, lateral.

p., idling The path that a stamp cusp travels when the bolus is being treated on the other side of the mouth.

p. of insertion *See* insertion, path of.

p., milled-in Any one of the contours carved by various mandibular movements into the occluding surface of an occlusion rim by teeth or studs placed in the opposing occlusion rim. The curves or contours may be carved into wax, acrylic resin, modeling compound, or plaster of paris.

p., occlusal A gliding occlusal contact. The path of movement of an occlusal surface.

p., generated occlusal A registration in the mouth of the paths of movement of the occlusal surfaces of teeth on a wax, plastic, or abrasive surface attached to the opposing dental arch.

p. of placement The direction in which a removable dental restoration is positioned in relation to the planned location on its supporting structures. The restoration is removed in the opposite direction. *See also* placement, choice of path of.

p., working The path that the stamp cusps make when working on the bolus. At first the bolus deflects the direction of these cusps, but after the fibers of the food have been reduced enough to be almost ready for swallowing, the travel coincides directionally with the working groove.

pathfinder *See* broach, smooth.

pathogenic occlusion (păth-ō-jĕn′ĭk) *See* occlusion, pathogenic.

pathognomonic (păth″ŏg-nō-mŏn′ĭk) A sign or symptom significantly unique to a disease; one that distinguishes it from other diseases.

pathology (pah-thol′ō-jē) **1:** The branch of science that deals with disease in all its relations, especially with its nature and the functional and material changes it causes. **2:** In medical jurisprudence, the science of diseases; the part of medicine that deals with the nature of disease, their causes, and their symptoms.

p., experimental The study of disease processes induced usually in animals; undertaken to ascertain the effect of local environmental changes and/or systemic disorders on particular tissues, parts, and organs of the body. This branch of medical science also attempts to correlate the interplay of local and systemic factors in the production, modification, and continuance of a disease.

p., speech The study and treatment of all aspects of functional and organic speech defects and disorders.

pathosis (pah-thō′sĭs) A disease entity. A pathologic condition. A patient is said to have a pathosis rather than pathology, which is the study of disease.

pathway of inflammation The route of extension of chronic gingival inflammation into the subjacent structures, extending into the interdental septum from the gingivae, along the interdental vessels, and/ or following the course of these blood vessels onto the periosteal side of the bone as well as into the bone marrow spaces.

patient A person under medical or dental care.

patient compliance The degree or extent to which a patient follows or completes a prescribed diagnostic, treatment, or preventive procedure.

patient education The process of informing a patient about a health matter in order to secure informed consent, patient cooperation, and a high level of patient compliance.

p. load The number of patients treated by a dentist or a group of dentists within a specified period of time.

p. satisfaction As an outcome measure of quality, refers to the perception of the patients(s) of one or more aspects of a dental care system.

pattern A form used to make a mold, as for a denture, an inlay, or a partial denture framework. **p., occlusal** The form or design of the occluding surfaces of a tooth or teeth. These forms may be based on natural or modified anatomic or nonanatomic concepts of teeth.

p., trabecular The trabecular arrangement of alveolar bone in relation to marrow spaces; may be radiographically interpreted.

p., wax 1: A wax model for making the mold in which the metal will be formed in casting. **2:** A wax form of a denture that, when it is invested in a flask and the wax is eliminated, will form the mold in which the resin denture is formed.

p., wear The topographic attributes and distribution of areas of tooth wear (facets) resulting from attritional effects of food, tooth contacts during swallowing, terminal aspects of the masticatory cycle, and habits of occlusal neuroses. Wear patterns may be used to determine many of the functional and afunctional movements the mandible has been passing through in preceding years. Occlusal wear occurs with aging. The type of wear is termed the *wear pattern.*

Paul-Bunnell test *See* test, Paul-Bunnell.

pauperissimus (paw-per-ĭs′sē-mŭs) **(Pp)** Latin term meaning "poorest." Sometimes written on prescriptions to indicate to the pharmacist that the patient is being charged less than the usual fee by the dentist or physician.

payable Pertaining to an obligation to pay at a future time; when used without restriction or modification, the term means that the debt is payable at once.

payback period The length of time required for the net revenues of an investment to return the cost of the investment.

payer In health care, generally refers to entities; other than the patient, that finance or reimburse the cost of health services. In most cases, refers to insurance carriers, other third-party payers and/or health plan sponsors (employers or unions).

payment The performance of a duty or promise, or the discharge of a debt or liability by the delivery of money or something else of value.

p., progress Interim payments by the purchaser of a dental plan contract to the carrier for use as an operating fund. There is always a final accounting when actual costs are paid.

payroll record A printed form on which detailed records are kept of the amounts of money paid to auxiliaries. The record has columns for all the necessary tax deductions so that a detailed record is available for tax reporting and cost accounting.

PBI *See* iodine, protein-bound.

p.c. (post cibum) Latin term meaning "after meals." The abbreviation may be used in writing prescriptions.

PCP An abbreviation for *Pneumocystis carinii* pneumonia, an opportunistic infection in AIDS and an indicator of AIDS.

PDL *See* ligament, periodontal.

PDS *See* temporomandibular pain-dysfunction syndrome

peak, buccal Outer high point of the normal interproximal tissue that rises to a peak; connected interdentally to a lingual peak by a triangular ridge, with a depression termed a *col.*

pearl, enamel (enameloma) A small focal mass of enamel formed apical to the cementoenamel junction and resembling pearls. The bifurcation of molar roots is a favorite site for this aberration in tooth development.

pearls, Epstein's *See* nodules, Bohn's.

pedicle flap *See* flap, pedicle.

pedodontics (pē″dō-don′tĭks) **(dentistry for children)** The branch of dentistry that includes training the child to accept dentistry; restoring and maintaining the primary, mixed, and permanent dentitions; applying preventive measures for dental caries and periodontal disease; and preventing, intercepting, and correcting various problems of occlusion.

peer review 1: A retrospective consideration or an examination by one or more individuals of equal standing or rank. **2:** A process established to provide for review by licensed dentists of the care by a dentist for a single patient; disputes regarding fees; cases submitted by carriers and initiated by patients or dentists; and quality of care and appropriateness of treatment.

peer review organization (PRO) An organization established by an amendment of the Tax Equity and Fiscal Responsibility Act of 1982 (TEFRA) to provide for the review of medical services furnished primarily in a hospital setting and/or in conjunction with care provided under the Medicare and Medicaid programs. In addition to their review and monitoring functions these entities can invoke sanctions, penalties, or other corrective actions for noncompliance in organization standards.

p. r. system A professionally sponsored and operated system for the rendering of professional judgment on disagreements between or among dentists, patients, or fiscal intermediaries, respecting quality of care and related matters.

pegs, epithelial (rete pegs) Papillary projections of epithelium into the underlying stroma of connecting tissue that normally occur in mucous membrane and dermal tissues subject to functional stimulation. They occur to exc ss where epithelium-lined tissues are irritated and inflamed.

pegs, rete *See* pegs, epithelial.

pellagra (pĕl-lăg′rah) A nutritional deficiency resulting from faulty intake or metabolism of nicotinic acid, a vitamin B complex factor. It is characterized by glossitis, dermatitis of sun-exposed surfaces, stomatitis, diarrhea, and dementia. Thiamine, riboflavin, and tryptophan deficiencies may be associated.

pellet A small, rounded mass of material.

p., cotton A rolled ball of cotton varying in diameter from approximately ⅜ to ⅛ inch (larger size is cotton ball; smaller size is pledget).

p., foil A loosely rolled piece of gold foil of various thicknesses; prepared from a portion—$1/128$, $1/96$, $1/64$, $1/48$, $1/32$, $1/16$—cut from a 4-inch (10 cm) square of foil.

pellicle (pel′ĭ-k′l) A film or membrane.

p., brown A specific name for a brownish gray to black film formed over a period of time on the surfaces of the teeth of 20% to 25% of the population as a result of not using an abrasive-containing dentifrice.

pemphigoid, benign mucous membrane (pem′fĭ-goid) A bullous disease that resembles pemphigus but is more chronic in nature. The oral mucosa, especially the gingiva where it resembles desquamative gingivitis, and conjunctiva are the sites of predilection. Skin is involved in about 20% of the cases.

pemphigus (pĕm′fĭ-gŭs) A rare, grave skin disease of unknown etiology characterized by the development of bullae on the skin and mucous membrane. *See also* bulla; sign, Nikolsky's.

p., acute disseminated A dread disease of unknown etiology, temporarily controlled by the administration of corticosteroids. Manifested by bullous formation on the skin and mucous membranes. Desquamation of the epithelium exposes a raw, burning, oozing submucosa. Adequate nutritional status is difficult to maintain; secondary infection is common; with progressive debility, pneumonia is common and is usually the cause of death.

pen grasp *See* grasp, pen.

penetrability (pĕn′ĕ-trah-bĭl′ĭ-tē) The ability of a beam of x radiation to pass through matter. The degree of penetrability is determined by kilovoltage and filtration.

penetrating (pĕn′ĕ-trā-tĭng) Piercing; entering deeply.

penetration (pĕn″ĕ-trā′shŭn) The ability of radiation to extend down into and go through substances. The degree of penetration is determined by the kilovoltage.

penetrometer (pĕn″ĕ-trom′ĕ-ter) An aluminum step wedge or ladder exposed over a film to determine the quality or penetrating ability of a specific beam of x radiation.

penicillin (pĕn′ĭ-sĭl′lin) An antibiotic secured from cultures of *Penicillium notatum*, being bacteriocidal for gram-positive cocci, some gram-negative cocci (gonococcus and meningococcus), and clostridia and spirochetal organisms. Its topical application to the oral mucous membranes is discouraged because of the high risk of sensitization from local application of antibiotic substances.

p. G. An acid-sensitive form of penicillin prepared as penicillin G benzathine and penicillin G procaine used for deep intramuscular administration. The pencillin is slowly released, resulting in prolonged effective blood levels of penicillin G. In dentistry, used prophylactically for patients predisposed to bacterial endocarditis prior to any invasive dental procedure.

p. V A form of penicillin that is resistant to inactivation by gastric acid and widely used in oral solution for infants and young children and in tablet form for adults.

pension plans Saving and investment programs designed to provide income at the time of retirement, that may be employer or individual based, in which portions of the funds may be protected from taxation at the time of earning but subject to taxation at the time of withdrawal.

pentamidine (pen-tam′ĭ-dēn) An antiprotozoal agent effective against *Pneumocystis carinii* pneumonia (PCP), an opportunistic infection in HIV positive patients.

pentobarbital sodium (pĕn″tō-bar′bĭ-tal) Monosodium ethyl (1-methylbutyl) barbiturate, used for its sedative and hypnotic effects; usual dosage, ¾ to 1½ gr. Useful as a preoperative sedative in dentistry. Pentobarbital is a controlled substance.

penumbra, geometric (pĕ-nŭm′brah) Partial or imperfect shadow about the umbra, or true shadow, of an object. In radiography, it is influenced by the size of the focal spot, focal-film distance, and object-film distance. *See also* geometric unsharpness.

peptic ulcer (pep′tik) A sharply circumscribed lesion of the mucous membrane of the stomach or small intestine or any part of the gastrointestinal system exposed to gastric acid and pepsin.

percentile (per-cen′tīl, per-sen′til) The number in a frequency distribution below which a certain percentage of fees will fall. For example, the 90th percentile is the number that divides the distribution of fees into the lower 90% and the upper 10%, or that fee level at which 90% of dentists charge that amount or less and 10% charge more.

perception, occlusal The patient's cognizance of occlusal patterns and disharmonies, mediated by the proprioceptive sense of the nerve fibers of the periodontal membrane.

Percodan Brand name for oxycodone, a semisynthetic narcotic analgesic oxycodone. Percodan is a controlled substance.

percolation Extraction of the soluble parts of a drug by causing a liquid solvent to flow slowly through it.

percussion (per-kŭsh′ŭn) The act of striking an area, a structure, or an organ as an aid in diagnosing a diseased condition by the sensations reported by the patient and by the sounds heard by the examiner.

perforation, palatal (per″fō-rā′shŭn) A perforation that exists in the palatal area after the surgical repair of a cleft.

perforation, radicular An artificial opening or hole made by boring or cutting through the lateral aspect of the root. Also occurs as the result of internal or external resorption.

perforation, sublabial A perforation existing in the upper labial sulcus after surgical repair of the area. The per-foration communicates between the oral and nasal cavities.

performance Fulfillment of a promise, contract, or other obligation.

periadenitis mucosa necrotica recurrens (per″ē-ăd-ĕni-′tĭs) **(Mikulicz' aphthae, Mikulicz' ulcer, recurrent scarring aphthae, Sutton's disease)** Involvement of the oral mucosa with deep-seated aphthous-like ulcers that tend to heal with scars. It may be impossible to differentiate the disease from Behçet's syndrome in the absence of a diagnosis of cyclic neutropenia.

perialveolar wiring *See* wiring, perialveolar.

periapex (per″ē-ā′pĕks) That area of tissue that immediately surrounds the root apex.

periapical (per″ē-ā′pĭ-kal) Enclosing or surrounding the apical area of a tooth root.

p. abscess An acute or chronic inflammation of the periapical tissues characterized by a localized accumulation of pus at the apex of a tooth. It is generally a sequela of pulp death of the tooth.

p. granuloma An accumulation of mononuclear inflammatory cells with an encircling aggregation of fibroblasts and collagen at the apex of the root of a tooth caused by chronic inflammation. Synonym: chronic apical periodontitis.

p., radiograph A radiograph demonstrating tooth apices and surrounding structures in a particular intraoral area.

p., radiographic survey A series of intraoral radiographs depicting periapical areas of interest. A complete mouth radiographic survey may consist of 17 or more intraoral radiographs that demonstrate all areas of the oral cavity.

periauricular (per″ē-aw-rĭk′ū-lar) Surrounding the external ear.

pericementitis (per″ē-sē″mĕn-tī′tĭs) *See* periodontitis.

pericervical saucerization *See* saucerization, pericervical.

pericoronitis (per″ē-kor″ō-nī′tĭs) **(operculitis)** Inflammation of the operculum or tissue flap over a partially erupted tooth, particularly a third molar. Inflammation around a crown, particularly the inflammation of a partially erupted tooth.

peri-implant space The space between an implant and its investing tissues.

perinatal The period of time surrounding the birth process.

perineural fibroblastoma (per″ĭ-nū′ral) *See* neurilemoma; neurofibroma.

period, latent The area of delay between the time of exposure of an organism to radiation and the manifestation of the changes produced by that radiation. This delay is dependent on many factors, but particularly on the magnitude of the dose. The larger the dose, the earlier the appearance of the injury. In some instances the latent period for some effects may be as long as 25 years or more.

periodontal (per″ē-ō-don′tal) Relating to the periodontium.

p. abscess A localized area of acute or chronic inflammation found in the gingival corium, infrabony pockets, or periodontal membrane. If it is located at the apex of the tooth, it is known as a periapical abscess. If located between the apex and the alveolar crest, it is known as a lateral abscess.

p. atrophy *See* atrophy, periodontal.

p. pack *See* pack, periodontal.

p. pocket *See* pocket, periodontal.

p. probe *See* probe, periodontal.

p. prosthesis *See* prosthesis, periodontal.

p. therapy *See* therapy, periodontal.

p. treatment planning The sequential arrangement of therapeutic procedures required to obtain a healthy gingival attachment and an intact, functioning attachment apparatus. Periodontal therapy cannot be performed on an empiric basis but rests on an integrated knowledge of the theory and practice of periodontology.

periodontia (per″ē-ō-don′shē-ah) *See* periodontics.

periodontics (per″ē-ō-don′tĭks) The art and science of examination, diagnosis, and treatment of diseases affecting the periodontium; a study of the supporting structures of the teeth, including not only the normal anatomy and physiology of these structures, but also the deviations from normal.

p., concept of cure in The idea that a successful result in periodontal therapy consists of restoring any tooth or collection of teeth to functional capability, regardless of whether they are able to function alone or require stabilization to survive.

periodontitis (per″ē-ō-don-tī′tĭs) **(periodontal inflammation)** The alterations occurring in the periodontium with inflammation. Gingival changes are those of gingivitis, with the clinical signs described under gingivitis. Periodontitis has histologic characteristics such as ulceration of the sulcular epithelium, epithelial hyperplasia, proliferation of epithelial rete pegs into the gingival corium, apical migration of the epithelial attachment after lysis of the gingival fiber apparatus, cellular and exudative infiltrate into tissues, and increased capillarity. With resorption of bone in an apical direction, attachment of the periodontal fibers to the bone is progressively lost. A transseptal band of reconstituted periodontal fibers walls off the gingival inflammation from the underlying bone. A chronic, progressive disease of the periodontium.

p., acute A sharply localized acute inflammatory process involving the interproximal and marginal areas of two or more adjacent teeth, characterized by severe pain, purulent exudate from edematous inflamed gingivae, general malaise, fever, and sequestration of the crestal aspects of the alveolar process.

p. in children *See* periodontitis, juvenile.

p., chronic periapical Periapical inflammation characterized by dental granuloma formation.

p., juvenile Marginal periodontitis present in children or adolescents, with radiographic and clinical findings similar to those observed in the adult, including gingivitis, periodontal pocket formation, bone resorption, etc.

p., marginal The sequela to gingivitis in which the inflammatory process has spread apically to involve the alveolar process. An inflammation of the marginal periodontium with resorption of the crest of alveolar bone; there is apical migration of the epithelial attachment with suprabony and/or infrabony pocket formation and cuplike resorptions and marginal translucence of the alveolar crest. In children the process may be more rapid and destructive than in adults.

periodontium (per″ē-ō-don′shē-ŭm) The tissues that invest (or help to invest) and support the teeth, i.e., the gingivae, cementum of the tooth, periodontal ligament, and alveolar and supporting bone.

periodontosis (per″ē-ō-don-tō′sĭs) **(diffuse alveolar atrophy)** A rare disease of young people (occurring primarily in women) that represents an idiopathic destruction of the periodontium.

perioral structures The anatomic elements around the mouth, generally the lips and muscles of facial expression within the lips.

periorbital Surrounding the eyes. The periorbital soft tissues are easily contused and will produce marked inflammatory responses to trauma.

periosteal elevator (per″ē-os′tē-al) *See* elevator, periosteal.

periosteum (per″ē-os′tē-ŭm) The layer of connective tissue that varies considerably in thickness in the different areas of bone. It is thick over the surfaces that do not serve as areas of muscle attachment, especially on surfaces that are covered only by skin and subcutaneous tissue. In these areas it is loosely connected with the bone itself and is easily lifted from it. Muscles are attached to bones directly, or they end on the periosteum. When muscles or tendons are attached to the bone itself, connective tissue extends into the bone as Sharpey's fibers. In such areas a periosteum may be lacking. When muscles are attached to the periosteum and thus are indirectly attached to the bone, the periosteum is relatively thin but is strongly fixed to the bone. The periosteum consists of two layers: an outer layer, which is rich in blood vessels and nerves and shows a dense arrangement of collagenous fibers, and an inner layer, the cambium, in which the fibers are loosely arranged, the cells numerous, and the blood vessels relatively sparse. During active growth, this layer of osteoblasts covers the periosteal surface of the bone. In the quiescent state in the adult the periosteum primarily provides support. However, the inner layer retains its osteogenetic potencies and in fractures is activated to form osteoblasts and new bone.

periostitis (per″ē-os-tī′tĭs) An inflammation of the periosteum in which the membrane may become detached from the underlying bone resulting from exudates produced by inflammation or infection.

peripheral circulation (pĕ-rĭf′er-al) *See* circulation, peripheral.

periphery (pĕ-rĭf′er-ē) *See* border, denture.

peritonsillar Surrounding the tonsils. Generally used in reference to the pharyngeal tonsils.

perléche (per-lĕsh′) A general term applied to superficial fissures occurring at the angles of the mouth. Lesions may result from a variety of causes but most often can be related to deep labial commissures, with associated drooling, licking of the lips, unhygienic conditions, and the overgrowth of bacteria, yeast, or fungi. The term has also been applied to angular cheilosis resulting from riboflavin deficiency but not to the split papule of syphilis or to herpetic lesions.

permanent Of a lasting or durable nature (opposite of temporary).

p. dentition *See* dentition, permanent.

permissible dose *See* dose, maximum permissible.

peroral Through or about the mouth.

personal Belonging to an individual; limited to the person; having the nature of the qualities of human beings or of movable property.

personality 1: The sum total of a patient's ideas, emotions, and behavior, including the rational and irrational, the conscious and unconscious, and the defensive and learned behavior patterns. Personality develops from both genetic factors and environmental factors. Thus the patient brings to a dental office an individual personality syndrome. It may be a well-adjusted, stable personality, a depressed, anxious, neurotic personality, or a manic, schizophrenic, psychotic personality. Patients have a broad spectrum of healthy and disordered personalities. **2:** The characteristics of a person by which other people evaluate him.

personnel The sum or aggregate of persons employed or engaged in an enterprise. In dentistry it refers to the staff employed by the dentist.

personnel monitoring *See* monitoring, personnel.

petazocine An analgesic approximately equivalent in analgesic effect to codeine. Brand name: Talwin.

petechiae (pē-tē′kē-ē) Capillary hemorrhages producing small red or purplish pinhead-sized discolorations of the mucous membrane and skin. Petechiae are typical of blood dyscrasias, vitamin C deficiency, positive

Rumpel-Leede test, liver disease, and subacute bacterial endocarditis.

petrolatum (pĕt″rō-lā′tŭm) **(petroleum jelly)** A mixture of hydrocarbons obtained from petroleum. In its semisolid form it is used as a protective covering to prevent gingival dehydration and inflammation during mouth breathing. A lubricant; protective covering for burns.

Peutz-Jeghers syndrome (pūtz-jĕg′erz) *See* syndrome, Peutz-Jeghers.

pH The concentration of hydrogen ions expressed as the negative logarithm of base 10.

phagocyte (făg′ō-sīt) Any cell that ingests microorganisms, cells, or other substances.

phagocytosis (făg″ō-cī-tō′sĭs) The engulfing of microorganisms, cells, and other substances by phagocytes. *See also* phagocyte.

phantom (făn′tom) A device that absorbs and scatters x radiation in approximately the same way as the tissues of the body.

pharmacodynamics (far″mah-kō-dī-năm′ĭks) The science of drug action.

pharmacology (far″mah-kol′ō-jē) The total science of drugs, including their use in therapeutics.

pharmacotherapy (fahr″mah-kō-ther″ă-pē) Treatment based upon the use of drugs or pharmaceuticals.

pharmacy (fahr′mah-sē) The art and science of preparing and dispensing drugs. Place where drugs are dispensed.

pharyngeal arch (fah-rin′jē-al) *See* arch, pharyngeal.

pharyngeal flap A pedicle flap usually raised on the posterior pharyngeal wall and attached to the soft palate to reduce the size of the velopharyngeal gap.

pharyngitis (far″ĭn-jī′tĭs) Inflammation of the pharynx.

pharyngoplasty (fah-rĭng′gō-plăs″tē) Reconstructive operation to alter the size and shape of the nasopharyngeal orifice.

pharyngospasm (fah-rĭng′gō-spăzm) Spasm of the pharyngeal muscles.

pharynx (făr′ĭngks) A funnel-shaped tube of muscle tissue between the mouth and nares and the esophagus, which is the common pathway for food and air. The nasopharynx lies above the level of the soft palate. The oropharynx lies between the upper edge of the epiglottis and the soft palate, whereas the laryngopharynx lies below the upper edge of the epiglottis and the openings into the esophagus and larynx.

p., activities of posterior and lateral pharyngeal wall The bulging of the posterior and lateral pharyngeal wall produced by the superior pharyngeal constrictors and palatopharyngeus during the acts of swallowing and phonation; seen in individuals with a congenitally short soft palate, operated soft palate, or unoperated cleft of the soft palate. These activities are rarely present in the individual with the normal soft palate.

p., implant surgical *First stage:* A major oral operation in which the mucoperiosteum is elevated, exposing the oral surface of the jawbone; the surgical jaw relations are established, and an impression is made of the exposed bone surfaces. *Second stage:* A major oral surgical operation in which the mucoperiosteum is reelevated, the prepared implant is placed on the bone surface, and the mucoperiosteum is coapted and sutured about the posts of the protruding implant abutments.

phase-contrast microscope A microscope with a special condenser and objective, which contains a phase-shifting ring by which small differences in the index of refraction become visible. The use of phase-contrast capabilities allows for direct viewing of transparent live cells and tissues. Phase-contrast microscopes are useful in educating a patient about the oral flora associated with dental plaque, dental caries, and periodontal disease.

phenacetin, caffeine, aspirin (fĕ-năs′ĕ-tĭn) *See* aspirin, phenacetin, caffeine.

phenol (fĕ′nol) **(carbolic acid)** An organic compound in which one or more hydroxyl groups are attached to a carbon atom in an aromatic ring that contains conjugated double bonds.

phenol coefficient A basis of comparison in determining the relative effectiveness of antiseptics. Phenol is used as the standard against which other agents are compared for their ability kill a well-dispersed suspension of salmonellae or staphylococci. It has little practical value.

phenomenon, Hamburger's (chloride shift) The exchange of a chloride ion for a bicarbonate ion across the erythrocyte membrane as part of the buffering system in blood. It accounts for the greater chloride content of venous erythrocytes than arterial erythrocytes.

phenotype (fĕ′nō-tĭp) Term referring to the expression of genotypes that can be directly distinguished (e.g., by clinical observation of external appearance or serologic tests).

phenylalanine (fen″il-al′ah-nēn) One of the essential amino acids. *See also* amino acid.

phenylephrine (fen″il-ef′rin) A vasoconstrictor and pressor drug chemically related to epinephrine and ephedrine. It is used as a decongestant; not recommended for prolonged use on patients with cardiovascular disease. Brand name: Neo-Synephrine.

phlebectasia (flĕb″ĕk-tā′zē-ah) Dilation of a vein.

phlebitis (flĕ-bī′tĭs) Inflammation of a vein. *See also* thrombophlebitis.

phlebolith (flĕb′ō-lĭth) A calcified thrombus in a vein.

phlegmon (flĕg′mŏn) An intense inflammation spreading through tissue spaces over a large area and without definite limits. Clinically, a hard, boardlike swelling without gross pus. *See also* cellulitis.

phobia (fō′bē-ah) A specific hysterical fear.

phonation (fō-nā′shŭn) The production of voiced sound by means of vocal cord vibrations.

p., speech Modification, by the vocal folds, of the airstream as it leaves the lungs and passes through the larynx, for the purpose of producing the various sounds that are the basis of speech. By opposing each other with different degrees of tension and space, the vocal folds create a slitlike aperture of varying size and contour, and by creating resistance to the stream of air, they set up a sequence of laryngeal sound waves with characteristic pitch and intensity.

phoneme (fō′nēm) A group or family of closely related speech sounds all of which have the same distinctive acoustic characteristics despite their differences; often used in place of the term *speech sound*.

phonetic values *See* values, phonetic.

phonetics (fō-net′iks) The study of the production and perception of speech sounds, including individual and group variations, and their use in speech.

phosphatase(s) (fŏs′fah-tā-sēz) A group of enzymes distributed throughout most cells and body fluids that are characterized by their ability to hydrolyze a wide variety of monophosphate esters to alcohols and inorganic phosphate.

p., acid A group of phosphatases (e.g., serum, liver, prostate) with optimal activity below a pH level of 7. Elevated serum levels have been observed in metastatic breast and prostatic cancer, Paget's, Gaucher's, and Niemann-Pick diseases, and myelocytic leukemia.

p., alkaline A group of phosphatases (e.g., serum, liver, bone) whose optimal activity ranges near a pH level of 9.8. Elevated blood levels occur in Paget's disease and pregnancy, whereas low levels are characteristic of dwarfism and a generalized nutritional protein deficiency.

phosphates (fos′fāts) The organic compounds of phosphorus. The blood phosphate level is normally 2.5 to 5 mg/100 ml. It is low in rickets and early hyperparathyroidism and high in tetany and nephritis.

phosphorus (fos′for-ŭs) A nonmetallic element; atomic weight, 30.98. It is essential, as is the phosphate, for the mineralization of the organic matrix of teeth and bone. It is also essential in the intermediary metabolism of carbohydrates as a vital constituent of the various intermediary compounds (e.g., glucose 6-phosphate) and of the enzyme systems (e.g., adenosine triphosphate [ATP]).

phossy jaw (fos′sē) *See* poisoning, phosphorus.

photon (fō′ton) A bullet or quantum of electromagnetic radiant energy emitted and propagated from various types of radiation sources. The term should not be used alone but should be qualified by terms that will clarify the type of energy (e.g., light photon, x-ray photon).

physical Relating to the body, as distinguished from the mind.

  p. plant The entire architectural and decorated suite of offices in which the dentist operates.

physical examination A diagnostic inspection of the body to determine its state of health using the means of palpation, auscultation, percussion, and smell.

physician A practitioner of medicine; one lawfully engaged in the practice of medicine.

physiologic occlusion See occlusion, physiologic.

physiologic rest position See position, rest, physiologic.

physiology (fĭz″ē-ol′ō-jē) Study of tissue and organism behavior. The physiologic process is a dynamic state of tissue as compared to the static state of descriptive morphology (anatomy). Physiology is differentiated from descriptive morphology by the following qualifying properties: rate, direction, and magnitude. Physiologic processes are thus morphologic alterations in the three dimensions of space associated with a temporary (time) sequence. Physiologic processes relate to a wide spectrum of life activities on three levels: biochemical and biophysical activity of a subcellular nature, the activity of cells and tissues aggregated into organ systems, and multiorgan system activity as expressed in human behavior. **p., oral** Physiology related to clinical manifestations in the normal and abnormal behavior of oral structures. The principal clinical functions in which the oral structures participate are deglutition, mastication, respiration, speech, and head posture.

physioprints (fĭz-ē-ō-prĭnts) Photographs obtained by projecting a grid on the subject's face and superimposing two exposures. The resultant picture gives a three-dimensional approach for the diagnosis of facial contours and swelling.

physiotherapy, oral (fĭz″ē-ō-ther′ah-pē) The collective procedures properly performed for the maintenance of personal hygiene of the mouth; those procedures necessary for cleanliness, tissue stimulation, tone, and preservation of the dentition. See also aid in physiotherapy.

pickling The process of cleansing from metallic surfaces the products of oxidation and other impurities by immersion in acid.

Pick's disease See disease, Niemann-Pick.

pickup impression See impression, pickup.

pier (pēr) An intermediate retaining or supporting abutment for a prosthesis. See also abutment.

Pierre Robin syndrome (pē-air′ rō′băn) See retrognathism; syndrome, Pierre Robin.

pigmentation, gingival See gingival pigmentation.

pigmentation, melanin The discoloration of tissues produced by the deposition of melanin. Seen normally in the oral mucous membranes (especially gingivae) of dark-complexioned individuals and abnormally in such conditions as adrenal hypofunction (Addison's disease).

pilocarpine (pī″lō-kar′pīn) An alkaloid that causes parasympathetic effects (e.g., secretion of salivary, bronchial, and gastrointestinal glands). It stimulates the sweat glands and also causes vasodilation and cardiac inhibition.

pilot program An experimental program designed to test administrative and operational procedures and to develop information on service demands and costs that will serve as a basis for operating programs efficiently.

pin A small cylindrical piece of metal.

  p., cemented A metal rod cemented into a hole drilled into dentin to enhance retention of a restoration.

  p., friction-retained A metal rod driven or forced into a hole drilled into dentin to enhance retention. It is retained solely by elasticity of dentin.

  p., incisal guide A metal rod that is attached to the upper member of an articulator and that touches the incisal guide table. It maintains the established vertical separation of the upper and lower arms of the articulator.

  p., retention The frictional grip of small metal projections extending from a metal casting into the dentin of the tooth.

  p., self-threading A pin screwed into a hole prepared in dentin to enhance retention.

  p., sprue A solid or hollow length of metal used to attach a pattern to the crucible former. A metal pin used to form the hole that provides the pathway through the refractory investment to permit the entry of metal into a mold.

  p., Steinmann A firm metal pin that is sharpened on one end; used for the fixation of fractures. It is sometimes passed through the maxillae or mandible to provide external points for attachment of upward-supporting devices.

pinna The external ear.

pit A small depression in enamel, usually located in a developmental groove where two or more enamel lobes are joined. A depression in a restoration resulting from nonuniform density.

  p. and fissure cavity See cavity, pit and fissure.

  p. and fissure sealant See sealant, pit and fissure.

Pituitrin (pĭ-tū′ĭ-trĭn) Trade name for an extract of the posterior lobe of the pituitary gland.

pityriasis rosea (pĭt″ĭ-rī′ah-sĭs rō′zē-ah) A noncontagious skin disease with reddish, scaly patches, and moderate fever.

pivot, occlusal An elevation artificially developed on the occlusal surface, usually in the molar region, and designed to induce sagittal mandibular rotation.

  p., adjustable occlusal An occlusal pivot that may be

adjusted vertically by means of a screw or by other means.

placebo (plah-sē′bō) A substance that resembles medicine superficially and is believed by the patient to be medicine but that has no intrinsic drug activity.

   p. effect The real or imagined effect of a placebo, which may actually be the same effect ordinarily associated with the administration of a therapeutically active agent.

placement The act of placing an object (e.g., removable denture in its planned location on the dental arch).

   p., choice of path of Determination of the direction of placement and removal of a removable partial denture on its supporting oral structures, which can be varied by altering the plane to which the guiding abutment surfaces are made parallel. The choice is a compromise to best fulfill five demands: to subject abutment teeth to a minimum or no torquing force, encounter the least interference, provide needed retention, establish adequate guiding-plane surfaces, and provide acceptable esthetics.

plaintiff A person who brings an action; the party who sues in a personal action and is so designated on the record.

plan, bank *See* bank plan.

plan, treatment The sequence of procedures planned for the treatment of a patient.

   p., provisional treatment Tentative treatment plan that is capable of modification or continuance after re-evaluation of periodontal status after initial therapeutic procedures.

plane An ideal flat surface that is supposed to intersect solid bodies, extend in various directions, or be determined by the position in space of three points.

   p., axial A hypothetical plane parallel to the long axis of an object.

      p., axial wall An instrument used to plane and true the axial wall of a Class 3 preparation.

   p., bite (bite plate) An appliance that covers the palate. It has an inclined or flat plane at its anterior border that offers resistance to the mandibular incisors when they come into contact with it.

   p., Broca's (brō′kahz) **(French plane)** A plane extending from the tip of the interalveolar septum between the upper central incisors to the lowermost point of the occipital condyle.

   p., Camper's A plane extending from the inferior border of the ala of the nose to the superior border of the tragus of the ear.

   p., eye-ear *See* plane, Frankfort horizontal.

   p., Frankfort horizontal A craniometric plane determined by the inferior borders of the bony orbits and the upper margin of the auditory meatus. It passes through the two orbitales and the two tragions.

   p., guide (guiding plane) 1: A mechanical device, part of an orthodontic appliance, having an established inclined plane that, when in use, causes a change in the occlusal relation of the maxillary and mandibular teeth and permits their movement to a normal position. **2:** A plane developed in the occlusal surfaces of occlusion rims to position the mandible in centric relation. **3:** Two or more vertically parallel surfaces of abutment teeth shaped to direct the path of placement and removal of a remarkable partial denture.

   p., guiding *See* plane, guide.

   p., Hamy's A plane extending from glabella to lambda.

   p., His' A plane extending from the anterior nasal spine to the opisthion.

   p., horizontal A plane that is parallel to the horizon and perpendicular to the vertical plane.

   p., Huxley's A plane extending from nasion to basion (basicranial axis).

   p., mandibular *See* border, mandibular.

   p., Martin's A plane extending from nasion to inion.

   p., mean foundation The mean of the inclination of the denture-supporting (basal seat) tissues. Since the tissues constituting the denture foundation are irregular in form and consistency, and since there is only one direction from which force may be applied if it is to comply with the law of statics, which requires the exertion of force at a right angle to maintain support, the mean foundation plane forms a right angle with the most favorable direction of force. The ideal condition for denture stability exists when the mean foundation plane is most nearly at right angles to the direction of force.

   p., median-raphe The median plane of the head.

   p., Montague's The plane extending from nasion to porion.

   p., occlusal 1: An imaginary surface that is related anatomically to the cranium and that theoretically touches the incisal edges of the incisors and tips of the occluding surfaces of the posterior teeth. It is not a plane in the true sense of the word but represents the mean of the curvature of the surface. *See also* curve of occlusion. **2:** A line drawn between points representing one half of the incisal overbite (vertical overlap) in front and one half of the cusp height of the last molars in back.

   p., orbital 1: A plane perpendicular to the eye-ear plane and passing through the orbitale. **2:** The plane that passes through the visual axis of each eye.

   p. of reference A plane that acts as a guide to the location of other planes.

   p., sagittal The anteroposterior median plane of the body.

      p., median sagittal A plane passing through the median raphe of the palate at right angles to the

Frankfort horizontal plane.

p., Schwalbe's (shvahl′behz) A plane that extends from glabella to inion.

p. of teeth For descriptive purposes, three planes are considered in the teeth proper: buccolingual, horizontal, and mesiodistal.

p., axial, of teeth Term that applies to the mesiodistal or the buccolingual plane.

p., axiobuccolingual, of teeth *See* plane of teeth, buccolingual.

p., axiomesiodistal, of teeth *See* plane of teeth, mesiodistal.

p., buccolingual, of teeth (axiobuccolingual plane) A plane that passes through the tooth buccolingually parallel with its long axis. In incisors and canines this is the labiolingual plane.

p., horizontal, of teeth A plane that is perpendicular to the long axis of the tooth and may be supposed to cut through the crown at any point in its length.

p., mesiodistal, of teeth (axiomesiodistal plane) A plane that passes through the tooth mesiodistally parallel with its long axis.

p., vertical, of teeth An upright plane that is perpendicular to the horizon.

p., Von Ihring's A plane extending from orbitale to the center of the bony external auditory meatus.

plaque (plăk) A flat plate or tablet.

p., mucin A sticky substance that accumulates on the teeth; composed of mucin derived from the saliva and of bacteria and their products; often responsible for the inception of caries and for gingival inflammation.

plasma (plăz′mah) The fluid portion of the blood that, after centrifugation, contains all the stable components except the cells. It is obtained from centrifuged whole blood that has been prevented from clotting by the addition of anticoagulants such as citrate, oxalate, or heparin.

p. accelerator globulin *See* proaccelerin; accelerator, prothrombin conversion, I.

p. ac-globulin *See* factor V; proaccelerin.

p., normal human Pooled sterile plasma from a number of persons to which a preservative has been added. It is stored under refrigeration or desiccated for later use as a substitute for whole blood.

p. proteolytic enzyme *See* plasmin.

p. thromboplastin antecedent (antihemophilic factor C, factor XI, PTA, plasma thromboplastin factor C) A factor required for the development of thromboplastic activity in plasma.

p. thromboplastin component (antihemophilic factor B, autoprothrombin II, Christmas factor, factor IX, platelet cofactor II, PTC) A clotting factor in normal blood necessary for the development of thrombo-

plastic activity in plasma. A deficiency results in Christmas disease. *See also* factor IX.

plasmacytoma (plăz″mah-sī-tō′mah) Term usually reserved to indicate the primary soft tissue plasma cell tumors of the oral, pharyngeal, and nasal mucous membranes. The lesion consists of typical and atypical plasma cells, and its behavior is unpredictable.

p., soft tissue A primary plasma cell tumor of the nasal, pharyngeal, and oral mucosa that has no apparent primary bone involvement. The lesions are sessile or polypoid sessile masses in the mucous membrane. The majority remain localized, but metastases have been reported.

plasmin (plăz′mĭn) **(fibrinolysin, lysin, plasma proteolytic enzyme, tryptase)** Collective term for one or more proteolytic enzymes found in the blood. The proteolytic enzymes are capable of digesting fibrin, fibrinogen, and proaccelerin. Plasminogen, the inactive form, may become active spontaneously in shed blood. An activator, fibrinokinase (fibrinolysokinase), is found in many animal tissues.

plasminogen (plăz-mĭn′ō-jĕn) **(profibrinolysin)** The precursor of plasmin found in plasma. It is probably activated by a tissue factor or by a blood activator, which first must be activated by a blood or tissue fibrinolysokinase.

plasmokinin (plăz-mō-kĭn′ĭn) *See* factor VIII.

plaster (plăs′ter) Colloquial term applied to dental plaster of paris.

p. headcap *See* headcap, plaster.

p., impression Plaster used for making impressions. Sets rapidly and is characterized by low setting expansion and strength.

p., model Plaster used for diagnostic casts and as an investing material.

p. of paris The hemihydrate of calcium sulfate that, when mixed with water, forms a paste that subsequently sets into a hard mass. *See also* beta-hemihydrate.

plastic Capable of being molded. A restorative material (e.g., amalgam, cement, gutta-percha, resin) that is soft at the time of insertion and may then be shaped or molded, after which it will harden or set.

p. base *See* base, plastic.

p. closure Suturing of tissues that involves their displacement by sliding or rotation to create a surgical closure.

p. strip A clear plastic strip of Celluloid or acrylic resin used as a matrix when silicate cement or acrylic is inserted into proximal prepared cavities in anterior teeth.

p. surgery Branch of medicine that deals with the surgical alteration, replacement, restoration, or reconstruction of a visible part of the body to correct a structural or cosmetic defect.

plasticity (plăs-tĭs′ĭ-tē) The quality of being moldable or workable. The degree of permanent deformation resulting from stress application; usually associated with substances that are classed as solids or semirigid liquids.

plate, lingual *See* connector, lingual plate, major

plate, occlusal plane A metal plate used in checking or establishing the occlusal plane of the teeth.

plate, palatal *See* connector, major.

platelet (plā″lĕt) A disk found in the blood of mammals that is concerned in the coagulation and clotting of blood.

    p. ac-globulin *See* factor, platelet, I.

    p. cofactor I *See* factor VIII.

    p. cofactor II *See* factor IX; plasma thromboplastin component.

    p. count The number of platelets found in 1 mm^3 of blood; the normal range is between 200,000 and 300,000 platelets.

    p. disorders *See* disorder, platelet.

platinocyanide crystals (plăt″ĭ-nō-sī′ah-nīd) *See* crystals, platinocyanide.

platinum matrix *See* matrix, platinum.

pleadings Written allegations of what is affirmed on the one side or denied on the other, disclosing the real matter to the court or jury having to try the cause.

pledget (plĕj′ĕt) A minute pellet of absorbent cotton used for accurately controlled placement of medication or base. *See also* cotton, absorbent.

pleomorphic adenoma (plē″ō-mor′fĭk ăd″ĕ-nō′mah) **(mixed salivary gland tumor)** A benign tumor of the salivary gland containing varying proportions of epithelial and mesenchymal elements. The intermediate type of epithelial cells are in sheets, cords, and acini. The mesenchymal tissue varies from myxomatous to cartilaginous to densely hyalinized connective tissue. The marked variations in histologic pattern are responsible for the designation of pleomorphic.

plethora (plĕth′or-ah) A nonspecific increase in blood bulk. Clinically, the patient is flushed and has a feeling of tenseness in the head; the blood vessels are full, and the pulse is firm.

pleurisy (ploo′rĭ-sē) Inflammation of the pleura, with exudation into its cavity and on its surface.

plexus (plĕk′sŭs) A network or tangle, especially of nerves, lymphatics, or veins.

    p., Haller′s A nerve plexus of sympathetic filaments and branches of the external laryngeal nerve on the surface of the inferior constrictor muscle of the larynx.

    p., intermediate The area of the periodontal membrane approximating in the midsection of the periodontal membrane, where the fiber bundles of the alveolar and cemental groups of periodontal fibers are woven together by small, thick strands of collagen fibers. The interweaving of fiber bundles of the intermediate plexus allows for tooth eruption and tooth movement between the cemental and alveolar periodontal fibers.

pliers (plural noun, but singular or plural in construction, as a pair of pliers) A tool of pincer design with jaws of varying shapes; used for holding, bending, stretching, contouring, cutting, etc.

    p., contouring Pliers with jaws curved to permit developing tooth contours in banding metal.

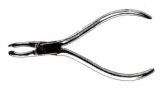

Contouring pliers

    p., cotton A slender, tweezerlike instrument used to hold cotton pellets or pledgets, apply medicaments, and carry small objects to and from the mouth.

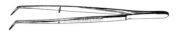

Cotton pliers (forceps)

    p., stretching Pliers whose jaws are designed as a hammer and anvil, with the handles sufficiently long to develop a high leverage ratio; used to enlarge metal bands (gold, aluminum, copper) or to thin the contact area of matrix bands.

plosive (plō′sĭv) Any speech sound made by impounding the airstream for a moment until considerable pressure has been developed and then suddenly releasing it (e.g., in the pronunciation of ″d,″ ″p,″ and ″g″).

plug A peg or any mass filling a hole or closing an orifice.

plugger An instrument used to compress the filling material in an apical and lateral direction when a root canal is being filled. *See also* condenser.

plugging Objectionable as a synonym for inserting or condensing.

plumbism (plŭm′bĭzm) **(lead poisoning, saturnism)** Acute or chronic intoxication resulting from the ingestion, inhalation, or skin absorption of lead. Manifestations of acute poisoning include abdominal pain, paralysis, metallic taste, and collapse. Chronic manifestations include gastrointestinal disturbances, headache, peripheral neuropathy (foot drop and wrist drop), lead in the urine and blood, basophilic granular

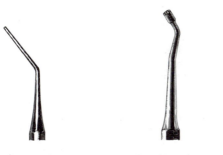

Endodontic plugger   Serrated amalgam plugger

degeneration, coproporphyrinuria, and stomatitis. *See also* stomatitis, lead.

Plummer-Vinson syndrome *See* syndrome, Plummer-Vinson.

plunger cusp A stamp cusp, the tip of which is made to occlude in an embrasure; its shoulder has not been restored to occlude in a fossa.

PMA (papillary-marginal-attached) A system of epidemiologic scoring of periodontal disease devised by Schour and Massler in which the symbols denote the areas involved in gingival inflammation.

pneumatic condenser (nū-măt′ĭk) *See* condenser, pneumatic.

pneumatodyspnea (nū″mah-tō-dĭsp′nē-ah) Difficulty in breathing result from emphysema.

Pneumocystis carinii (noo″mō-sĭs′tĭs kā-rī′nī-i) An opportunistic infection found in immunocompromised patients such as those with AIDS.

pneumonitis (nū″mō-nī′tĭs) Inflammation of the lungs of an acute, localized nature.

pneumothorax (nū″mō-thō′răks) An accumulation of air or gas in the pleural cavity. The air enters by way of an external wound, a lung perforation, a burrowing abscess, or rupture of a superficial lung cavity. Pneumothorax is accompanied by sudden, severe pain and rapidly increasing dyspnea.

pocket Diseased gingival attachment, characterized by gingival discoloration, retraction of gingivae from the tooth, bleeding, the presence of an exudate, loss of the presence of stippling, etc. A space bordered on one side by the tooth and on the opposite side by ulcerated crevicular epithelium and limited at its apex by the epithelial attachment.

   p., bleeding An occurrence that denotes ulcerations of the pocket epithelium, with hemorrhaging through the broken surface from exposed connective tissue capillaries.

   p. bottom The base of the pocket, marked or limited by the epithelial attachment to the cementum of the root (periodontal pocket) or the enamel of the crown (gingival pocket).

   p., calculus Calcified deposits that usually occupy the entire pocket. It is attached to the tooth structure, with the gingival tissues tightly adapted to the surface of the calculus.

   p., deepening Increase of the depth of the pocket, which is dependent on apical proliferation of the epithelial attachment alongside the cementum, with subsequent separation from the tooth, or on hyperplasia of the gingivae resulting from inflammation.

   p., depth of The measurement, usually expressed in millimeters, of the distance between the gingival crest and the base of the pocket.

   p., elimination The application of therapeutic measures to obtain a healthy gingival attachment and an intact, functioning attachment apparatus. The procedures employed include curettage (root and gingival), reattachment or new attachment operations, gingivectomy and gingivoplasty, and osseous and mucogingival surgical procedures.

   p., gingival A pseudopocket; gingival inflammation with edema, hyperplasia, and ulceration of the sulcular epithelium but without apical proliferation of the epithelial attachment.

   p., infrabony (infracrestal pocket, intra-alveolar pocket, intrabony pocket) A periodontal pocket, the base of which is apical to the crest of the alveolar bone. Consists basically of a vertical resorptive defect in alveolar and supporting bone, overlying which are a band of transseptal fibers connecting adjacent teeth, disintegrated fibers of gingival corium, inflammatory cellular infiltrate, and hyperplastic pocket epithelium, accompanied by apical migration of the epithelial attachment. Clinical signs are those of periodontitis, associated with radiographic evidence of vertical bone resorption. The infrabony pocket has been classified according to the number of remaining osseous walls supporting it for the purpose of therapeutic rationale.

   p., infracrestal *See* pocket, infrabony.

   p., intra-alveolar *See* pocket, infrabony.

   p., intrabony *See* pocket, infrabony.

   p. ionization chamber *See* chamber, ionization.

   p. in marginal periodontitis A condition in which the inflammatory process has progressed from the gingival tissues to the underlying alveolar process. The changes are those associated with gingivitis plus resorptive bone lesions. The base of the pocket is at the marginal point of the union of the epithelial attachment to the cementum of the root.

   p. marker, Crane-Kaplan An instrument used to delineate the depths of gingival and periodontal pockets prior to gingivectomy incision. The straight beak of the instrument is inserted to the limit of the pocket while the sharp angulated beak is pressed into the tissue until a small bleeding point is seen. The resultant series of bleeding points is used as a guide for the gingivectomy incision.

p., marking The accurate determination and delineation of pocket depth and topography as an aid to diagnosis and prognosis or to provide a guide for the gingivectomy incision.

p., periodontal A pathologic deepening of the gingival sulcus produced by destruction of the supporting tissues and apical proliferation of the epithelial attachment. Ulceration of the pocket epithelium lining is characteristic.

p. surgery A generic term referring to gingivectomy-gingivoplasty. *See also* gingivectomy, gingivoplasty.

pogonion (pō-gō′nē-on) **(Po)** The most anterior point on the chin. A cephalometric landmark in the lateral view.

poikilocytosis (poi″kĭ-lō-sī-tō′sĭs) Irregular shape of the red blood cells.

point A small spot; a minute area; a rotating instrument having a small cutting end or surface.

p. A The deepest point in the bony concavity in the midline at the base of the anterior nasal spine, in the region of the incisor roots. A landmark on the lateral cephalometric view.

p., abrasive, rotary Mounted carborundum, diamond, etc. Small abrasive instruments used in straight or contra-angle handpieces.

p. angle *See* angle, point.

p. B A mandibular point comparable to point A.

p., bleeding *See* bleeding points.

p., boiling The temperature at which the vapor pressure within a liquid equals atmospheric pressure.

p., Bolton The highest point of the curvature between the occipital condyle and the basilar part of the occipital bone; located behind the occipital condyle. The highest point of the curvature behind the occipital condyle. A substitute for the basion point when it cannot be ascertained on cephalometric headplates.

p., central-bearing The contact point of a central-bearing device.

p. of centricity If the point of the buccal cusp of the lower right molar, put in lateral position, is arced about the upright axis of the right condyle, it will reach a station where further muscular efforts leftward will change the cusp's direction so that it will arc about the left condyle. The station where the right arc ends and the left arc begins is a point of mandibular centricity. While the right cusp point was orbiting (arcing) about the near vertical axis, all other points in the jaw joined in orbiting (arcing). The left condyle arced rearward until it reached a cranial backstop; then the muscles started rotating it and carrying it leftward, and the right condyle be-

gan arcing forward, downward, and medially. In the right and left swings of the jaw, a condyle reciprocally alternates between being a rotator and an orbiter. The point of centricity of the mandible is demonstrated usually on a horizontal plane, but it can be demonstrated on all three planes of projection. The point of centricity is rearmost, midmost (between the arcs of motion), and uppermost. *See also* face-bow; relation, centric.

p., condenser The nib of a condensing instrument. A short instrument, for condensing foil or amalgam, that is inserted into a mechanical condenser or into a cone socket handle.

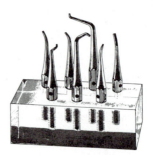

Assorted condenser points

p., contact (contact area) The area of contact of approximating surfaces of two adjacent teeth. The areas of contact are located at the line of junction between the occlusal and middle thirds of the posterior teeth and the incisal and middle thirds of the anterior teeth.

p., faulty contact Defective contact between the proximal surfaces of adjacent teeth, produced by wearing of the contact areas, dental caries, improper restoration, altered tooth position, etc.

p., loss of contact Failure of contact of convex proximal surfaces of adjacent teeth; produced by tooth migration, dental caries, improper restoration, etc.

p., convenience A small undercut in the cavity wall convenient for placing and retaining the first portion of a filling material. It is generally one of the retention points placed in a cavity preparation that provides the best access to the operator.

p. D The center of the body of the symphysis.

p., gutta-percha *See* gutta-percha points.

p., hinge axis A point placed on the skin corresponding with the opening axis of the mandible.

p., Hirschfeld's silver A calibrated silver rod used to record the clinical depth of periodontal pockets radiographically for the purpose of diagnosis.

p., incisor The intersection of the lower occlusal and midsagittal planes. The point at the mesioincisal angles of the two mandibular central incisors.

p., median mandibular A point on the anteroposterior center of the mandibular ridge in the median sagittal plane.

p., paper *See* paper point.

p., registration Any point considered as fixed for a particular pattern of analysis. Also, the midpoint of a perpendicular line from the sella turcica to the Bolton-nasion plane.

p., transition *See* Tg value.

p., treatment A piece of paper point, selected for the root canal being treated, that carries or holds the medication in place.

p., trial A cone of filling material placed in a canal and radiographed to check on the length and fit of the filling.

p., yield 1: The place on the stress-strain curve where marked permanent deformation occurs; it is just beyond the proportional limit. **2:** The point where permanent deformation starts in a metal.

pointing Term associated with fluctuation pertaining to the area where the purulent exudate is eroding through tissues to an external surface. It is at this point that an incision and drainage operation usually is performed.

poison A substance that, when ingested, inhaled, absorbed, injected into, or developed within the body, will cause damage to structures of the body and impair or destroy their function.

poisoning The morbid condition caused by poison.

p., arsenic Acute or chronic intoxication from the ingestion of insecticides or administration of organic arsenicals. Manifestations of acute poisoning include abdominal pain, nausea, vomiting, and collapse. Chronic manifestations include weakness, peripheral neuropathy, hyperkeratosis, skin rashes, and oral manifestations secondary to liver dysfunction and bone marrow depression. *See also* stomatitis, arsenical.

p., bismuth *See* bismuthosis.

p., chemical A form of poisoning caused by ingestion of a toxic chemical agent.

p., iodine *See* iodism.

p., lead *See* plumbism.

p., mercury *See* mercurialism.

p., metallic A toxic condition produced by excessive exposure to or intake of metals. In the oral cavity there may be definite signs of arsenic, bismuth, lead, phosphorus, radium, and other metals. Fluorides produce changes in developing teeth at levels far below those that are toxic for the rest of the human economy.

p., phosphorus The result of the ingestion of phosphorus, especially yellow phosphorus. Manifestations include burning of the mouth and throat, abdominal pain, vomiting, jaundice, liver damage, and death. In chronic poisoning, necrosis of the jaws (phossy jaw) occurs.

police power The authority of the state to enact laws to protect the public, such as a dental practice act. It is the police power reserved to the states under the United States Constitution.

policy The document embodying the insurance contract.

p. holder Under a group purchase plan, the employer, labor union, or trustee to whom a group contract is issued. In a plan providing for individual or family enrollment, the person to whom the contract is issued.

p. period The time during which an insurance contract affords protection.

p. year The year commencing with the effective date of the insurance contract or with an anniversary of that date.

poliomyelitis (pō″lē-ŏ-mī″ĕ-lī′tĭs) A disease produced by a small viral organism that enters the body via the alimentary tract and produces upper pharyngeal, pharyngeal, and intestinal inflammation in its mentor form. In the more severe variety, a subsequent viremia is produced, with extension of the infection to the anterior pulp horn cells and ganglia of the spinal cord, producing a flaccid paralysis. In bulbar poliomyelitis the viral infection involves the medulla, resulting in impairment of swallowing respiration, and/or circulation. It is now recognized that three types of viruses are responsible for the nonparalytic, paralytic, and bulbar varieties of poliomyelitis. Excellent immunization procedures have been provided by use of killed viruses (Salk) and attenuated mutant vaccines (Sabin).

polishing Making smooth and glossy, usually by friction; giving luster to.

p. brush *See* brush, polishing.

p., coronal Removal of mucinous film, superficial stain, deposits, etc., to provide a smooth enamel surface that will be more resistant to future accumulation of foreign substances (e.g., materia alba, calculus, mucinous plaque).

p. disk *See* disk, polishing.

pollakiuria (pol″ah-kē-ū′rē-ah) Unduly frequent urination. It may result from partial obstruction (e.g., in prostatic enlargement), or it may be of nervous origin.

pollen A fertilizing element of plants that travels in the air and produces seasonal allergic responses (e.g., hay fever, asthma) in sensitive individuals.

polyantibiotic (pol″ē-ān″tĭ-bī-ot′ĭk) A combination of two or more antibiotics used to eliminate bacteria from a root canal.

polychromatophilia (pol″ē-krŏ-măt″ŏ-fĭl′ē-ah) Irregular staining of cells, particularly red blood cells.

Polycillin (po″ē-cĭl-ĭn) Trade name for ampicillin, an

acid-stable semisynthetic pencillin effective against some gram-negative and gram-positive organisms.

polycythemia (pol″ē-sī-thē′mē-ah) Increase in blood volume as a result of an increase in the number of red blood cells, the erythrocytes. It may result from a blood-forming disease that increases cell production, or it may be a physiologic response to an increased need for oxygenation in high altitudes, cardiac disease, or respiratory disorders.

p., primary *See* erythremia.

p. rubra *See* erythremia.

p., secondary *See* erythrocytosis.

p. vera *See* erythremia.

polydactyly (pol″ē-dak′tĭ-lē) A congenital anomaly characterized by the presence of more than the normal number of fingers or toes. It may be a part of a complex genetic syndrome. Early surgical treatment is generally used to correct the problem.

polydipsia (pol″e -dĭp′sē-ah) Abnormally increased thirst.

polymer (pol′ĭ-mer) A long-chain hydrocarbon. In dentistry, the polymer is supplied as a powder to be mixed with the monomer for fabrication of appliances and restorations.

polymerization (pō-lĭm″er-ĭ-za ′shŭn) The chaining together of similar molecules to form a compound of high molecular weight.

p., addition A compound formed by a combination of simple molecules without the formation of any new products; e.g., methyl methacrylate $A + A = A - A - (A_n)$.

p., condensation Combination of simple, dissimilar molecules, with the formation of by-products such as water or ammonia (e.g., vulcanite).

p., cross (cross linkage, cross-linked polymerization) The formation of chemical bonds between linear molecules, resulting in a three-dimensional network. Used for artificial teeth and denture bases because of superior craze resistance.

p., cross-linked *See* polymerization, cross.

polymorphonuclear leukocytes (pol″ē-mor″fō-nūklē-ar loo′kō-sītz) A type of white blood cells with nuclei of varied forms.

polymyxin (pol″ē-mĭk′sĭn) An antibiotic substance derived from cultures of *Bacillus polymyxa*. Used topically, in troche form, in combination with bacitracin and neomycin in the treatment of various oral infections. Not used systemically; therefore sensitization is minimized. Systemic use may be attended by renal dysfunction and toxicity.

polyneuritis, endemic (pol″ē-nū-rī′tĭs) *See* beriberi.

polyostotic (pol″ē-os-tot′ĭk) Affecting more than one bone.

polyp (pol′ĭp) A smooth, pedunculated growth from a mucous surface such as from the nose, bladder, or rec-

tum.

p., pulp *See* pulpitis, hypertrophic.

polypharmacy The prescription or dispensation of unnecessarily numerous or complex medicines.

polypnea (pol″ĭp-nē′ah) A rapid or panting respiration.

polyposis, multiple (pol″ĭ-pō′sĭs) *See* syndrome, Peutz-Jeghers.

polystyrene (pol″e -sti ′rēn) A polymer of styrene, which is a derivative of ethylene; $[-CH(C_6H_5) CH_2-]n$. Often one of the resins present in materials designed for denture construction by the injection molding technique.

polysulfide polymer (pol″ē-sul′fīd pol′ĭ-mer) A rubber base impression material using a mercaptan bondage. Prepared by mixing a base material (mercaptan) with either an inorganic catalyst (lead peroxide) or an organic catalyst (benzoyl peroxide).

polyuria (pol″ē-ū′rē-ah) The passage of an abnormally increased volume of urine. It may result from increased intake of fluids, inadequate renal function, uncontrolled diabetes mellitus or diabetes insipidus, diuresis of edema fluid, or ascites.

pons (ponz) A structure dorsal to the medulla and intimately related to the pathways to the cerebrum. The cranial nerves whose nuclei lie in the pons are the trigeminal, abducens, and facial nerves, and part of the acoustic nerve. The pons is intimately related to the medulla, has the same blood vessel supply, and is involved in many lesions that affect the medulla. It is especially involved with the cerebellar manifestations of disease and may cause serious muscular incoordination in motor function of the head, neck, and facial structures.

pontic (pon′tĭk) The suspended member of a fixed partial denture; an artificial tooth on a fixed partial denture or an isolated tooth on a removable partial denture. It replaces a lost natural tooth, restores its function, and usually occupies the space previously occupied by the natural crown.

population All the instances about which a statement is made; all events, organisms, and items of a stated kind occurring or in existence in a specified time. In statistics, a hypothetical infinite supply or universe of events or objects like those being studied and from which a sample was drawn.

porcelain A material formed by the fusion of feldspar, silica, and other minor ingredients. Most dental porcelains are glasses and are used in the manufacture of artificial teeth, facings, jackets, and occasionally denture bases and inlays.

p., baked *See* porcelain, dental.

p., dental (baked porcelain, fired porcelain) A fused mixture that is glasslike and more or less transparent. Classification of the type of porcelain employed in inlays and crowns is based on the fusion temperature of the porcelain: high fusing, 2350° to 2500° F (1287.5° to 1371° C); medium fusing, 2000° to 2300° F (1093.5° to 1260° C); and low fusing, 1600° to 2000° F (871° to 1093.5° C).

p., fired *See* porcelain, dental.

p., synthetic *See* cement, silicate.

porion (po′rē-on) The superior surface of the external auditory meatus. In craniometry it is identified as the margin of the bony canal on the skull. In cephalometrics it may be identified from the earpost of the cephalostat (machine porion) or from bony landmarks on the film (anatomic porion).

porosity (pō-ros′ĭ-tē) Presence of pores or voids within a structure.

p., back-pressure Porosity produced in castings resulting from the inability of gases in the mold to escape through the investment.

p., occluded gas Porosity produced by improper use of the blowpipe (i.e., heating the metal in the oxidizing portion of the flame).

p., shrink-spot An area of porosity in cast metal that is caused by shrinkage of a portion of the metal as it solidifies from the molten state without flow of additional molten metal from surrounding areas.

p., solidification A porosity that may be produced by improper spruing or improper heating of the metal or the investment.

porphyria, congenital (por-fi′re-ah) *See* porphyria, erythropoietic.

porphyria, erythropoietic (congenital porphyria, photosensitive porphyria) An inborn error of metabolism (porphyrin synthesis) characterized clinically by skin photosensitivity, hypertrichosis, and reddish brown staining of the primary teeth.

porphyria, photosensitive *See* porphyria, erythropoietic.

port The opening through which x-ray photons or the useful beam of radiation exits from the head of a dental x-ray machine.

portfolio A list of stocks, bonds, and other commercial paper owned by an investor or holding company. In dentistry, it generally refers to the personal retirement investment package of the dentist or professional corporation created by the dentist.

position The placement of body members.

p., border, posterior The most posterior position of the mandible at any specific vertical relation of the maxillae.

p., centric 1: The position of the mandible in its most retruded relation to the maxillae at the established vertical relation. **2:** The constant position into which the patient will close the jaws; this relationship may be a convenience relationship or a true centric relationship.

p., eccentric (eccentric jaw position) Any position of the mandible other than that in centric relation. *See also* relation, jaw, eccentric.

p., eccentric jaw *See* position, eccentric; relation, jaw, eccentric.

p., finger *See* finger positions.

p., gingival *See* gingival position.

p., hinge The orientation of parts in a manner permitting hinge movements between them.

p., condylar hinge 1: Mandibular joints at which a hinge movement of the mandible is possible. **2:** The maxillomandibular relation from which a consciously stimulated true hinge movement can be executed.

p., mandibular hinge Any position of the mandible that exists when the condyles are so situated in the temporomandibular joints that opening or closing movements can be made on the hinge axis. *See* axis, hinge.

p., terminal hinge The mandibular hinge position from which further opening of the mandible would produce translatory rather than hinge movement. *See also* position, hinge.

p., intercuspal Term applied to the cuspal contacts of teeth when the mandible is in centric relation. Synonym: centric occlusion.

p., protrusive Occlusion of the teeth as the mandible and lower central incisors are moved straight forward toward the incisal edges of the upper central incisors; the normal anteroclusal relationship; the forward end position, with the upper and lower incisors in edge-to-edge contact.

p., rest 1: The position of the mandible when the jaws are in rest relation. *See also* position, rest, physiologic; relation, jaw, rest. **2:** The position that the mandible passively assumes when the mandibular musculature is relaxed.

p., physiologic rest The habitual postural position of the mandible when the patient is resting comfortably in the upright position and the condyles are in a neutral, unstrained position in the glenoid fossae. The mandibular musculature is in a state of minimum tonic contraction to maintain posture and to overcome its force of gravity. *See also* relation, jaw, rest.

p., tooth The placement or location of the tooth in the dental arch in relation to the bone of the alveolar process, its adjacent teeth, and the opposing dentition.

p., Trendelenburg A position in which the patient is on his back with the head and chest lowered and the leg elevated.

positioner A removable elastic orthodontic appliance molded to fit the teeth in a "setup" made by repositioning the teeth from a plaster cast. The material may be rubber or elastomeric plastic. It is typically used to achieve fine adjustments and retain corrected positions in the finishing stages of treatment.

positioning, surgical The surgical repositioning of a tooth or the tilting of a tooth without injuring its blood supply.

positions at the chair Posture and relative location of dentist or chairside assistant in respect to the dental chair and patient. Classified as standing or sitting and as right side behind, right side in front, left side behind, left side in front, and directly behind. The position used should permit the most efficient performance of the current procedure and also keep paramount the health and comfort of the dentist and the patient.

positive reinforcement A technique used to encourage a desirable behavior. Also called *positive feedback* in which the patient or subject receives encouraging and favorable communication from another person.

possession The control or custody of anything that may be the subject of property as owner or as one who has a qualified right in it.

post cibum (pŏst sī'bŭm) *See* p.c.

post, implant *See* substructure, implant, neck.

postcondensation (aftercondensation) The procedure of completing the condensation of the surface of a gold-foil restoration after all the gold has been placed.

postdam area *See* area, posterior palatal seal.

posterior Situated behind.

　p. nasal spine *See* spine, posterior nasal.

　p. palatal bar *See* connector, major, posterior palatal.

　p. palatal seal *See* seal, posterior palatal.

　　p. palatal seal area *See* area, posterior palatal seal.

posteroanterior extraoral radiographic examination *See* examination, radiographic, extraoral, posteroanterior.

postoperative care Care after surgery or other invasive procedures, usually of a supportive nature.

postpalatal seal *See* seal, posterior palatal.

　p. s. area *See* area, posterior palatal seal.

postperception (afterperception) The perception of a sensation after the stimulus producing it has ceased.

postsensation (aftersensation) A sensation lasting after the stimulus that produced it has been removed.

post-treatment review *See* audit.

posture, normal The configuration of the body in the upright position, which varies considerably among individuals. However, normal posture can be described as follows: the shoulder, pelvis, and eyes are level; the sagittal plane is between the feet, and the line of gravity passes through the center of gravity at the lumbosacral joint. When observed from the following positions, the line of gravity intersects the following structures: lateral position—anterior border of the ear, and the shoulder, hip, knee, and ankle joints; anterior position—nose, symphysis pubis, and between the knees and feet; posterior position—occiput, spinous

processes, gluteal crease, and between the knees and feet.

potassium oxalate (pŏtas'ē-um ok'sah-lāt) A dentin desensitizing agent that occludes the openings of the dentinal tubules and blocks the hydrodynamics that initiate the pain response. Brand name: Protect.

potassium sulfate (pŏtas'ē-um sul'fāt) An accelerator used to speed the setting of gypsum products. Hydrocolloid impressions are fixed in a 2% solution of potassium sulfate.

potency (po'ten-se) Power.

potential, action *See* action potential.

potentiation (pō-tĕn″shē-ā'shŭn) **(synergism)** 1: Increase in the action of a drug by the addition of another drug that does not necessarily possess similar properties. 2: Enhancement of action (e.g., of a drug).

Potter-Bucky diaphragm *See* grid, Potter-Bucky.

Potter-Bucky grid *See* grid, Potter-Bucky.

Pott's disease *See* disease, Pott's.

pour hole An aperture in a refractory investment or another mold material leading to the pattern space into which prosthetic material is deposited.

povidone-iodine (po'vĭ-dōn ī'ō-dīn) An antimicrobial agent with topical anesthetic properties used to irrigate periodontal pockets before debridement to control bleeding and pain.

powdered gold *See* gold, powdered.

power stroke *See* stroke, power.

pp *See* pauperissimus.

PPCF *See* factor V.

practice To follow or work at, as a profession, trade, or art.

　p. administration The organization, operation, and supervision of the business and professional aspects of a dental practice.

　p. building Increasing the number of patients and the number of services without sacrificing quality, by means of observing the principles of constantly improving professional care and maintaining effective human relations with patients.

　p. goal The planning of the objectives of a dental practice and the method of reaching those objectives. To be ascertained by the dental practitioner before or immediately on entering dental practice.

　p., group A large partnership formed for the purpose of practicing dentistry; may or may not include the services of the recognized specialties in dentistry.

　p., private The business and profession in which dental services are administered for a fee.

preanesthetic (prē″ăn-ĕs-thĕt'ĭk) A medicine for producing preliminary anesthesia (e.g., Avertin).

preauthorization 1: Approval of or concurrence with the treatment plan proposed by a participating dentist before the provision of service. Under some plans, preauthorization by the carrier is required before certain services can be provided. **2:** Statement by a third-party payer indicating that proposed treatment wlll be covered under the terms of the dental benefits contract. *See also* precertification, predetermination.

precertification Confirmation by a third-party payer of a patient's eligibility for coverage under a dental benefits program. *See also* preauthorization, predetermination.

precipitate (prē-sĭp′ĭ-tāt) An insoluble solid substance that forms from chemical reactions between solutions.

precision attachment *See* attachment, intracoronal.

precision rest *See* rest, precision.

precordial Pertaining to the region over the heart or stomach: the epigastrium and lower thorax.

precursor, fifth plasma thromboplastin *See* factor XII.

precursor of serum prothrombin conversion accelerator (cothromboplastin, factor VII, proSPCA) A clotting factor found in serum plasma and believed to be needed for the optimal action of tissue thromboplastin. Formerly, with the Stuart factor, it was known as *proconvertin* or *stable factor*. *See also* proconvertin.

predetermination An administrative procedure whereby a dentist submits a treatment plan to the carrier before treatment is initiated. Then the carrier returns the treatment plan, indicating the patient's eligibility, covered service amounts payable, application of appropriate deductibles, copayment factors, and maximums. Under some programs, predetermination by the carrier is required when covered charges are expected to exceed a certain amount, commonly $100. Synonyms: preauthorization, precertification, preestimate of cost, pretreatment estimate, prior.

prednisone (prĕd′nĭ-sōn) A steroid used systemically and topically as an anti-inflammatory agent. Useful also in the treatment of adrenal hypocorticism and the various collagen diseases.

preexisting condition Oral health condition of an enrollee that existed before his or her enrollment in a dental program.

preextraction cast *See* cast, diagnostic; cast, preextraction.

preextraction record *See* record, preoperative.

preferred provider organization (PPO) A formal agreement between a purchaser of a dental benefits program and a defined group of dentists for the delivery of dental services to a specific patient population as an adjunct to a traditional plan, using discounted fees for cost savings.

prefiling of fees The submission of a participating dentist's usual fees to a service corporation for the purpose of establishing, in advance, that dentist's usual fees and the customary ranges of fees in a geographic area to determine benefits under a usual, customary, and reasonable dental benefits program.

prematurities *See* contact, deflective occlusal; contact, interceptive occlusal.

premaxilla, floating *See* premaxilla, loose.

premaxilla, loose (floating premaxilla) 1: Nonunion of the premaxillary process with the lateral maxillary segments, so that the premaxilla is loose, or floating. The position of the loose premaxilla in relation to the lateral maxillary segments varies among patients. **2:** The administration of a tranquilizing drug, a drug that influences blood clotting time, or any other drug that produces a preplanned set of conditions and is administered preceding any dental procedures.

premium The amount charged by a dental benefits organization for coverage of a level of benefits for a specified time. **p., earned** That portion of a policy's premium payment for which the protection of the policy has already been given.

    p. rate The price per unit of insurance.

    p. tax An assessment levied by a state govemment, usually on the net premium income collected in that state by insurance companies.

    p. unearned That part of the premium applicable to the unexpired part of the policy period.

premolar (bicuspid) One of the eight teeth in humans, four in each jaw, between the canines and first molars; usually has two cusps; replaces the molars of the deciduous dentition.

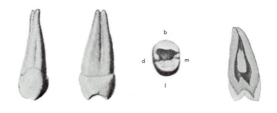

Right upper second premolar
Buccal surface   Mesial surface   Occlusal surface   Pulpal cross section

preoperative cast *See* cast, diagnostic.

preoperative record *See* record, preoperative.

prepaid dental plan A method of financing the cost of dental care for a defined population in advance of receipt of services.

prepaid group practice *See* closed panel.

preparation The selected form given to a natural tooth when it is reduced by instrumentation to receive a prosthesis (e.g., artificial crown or a retainer for a fixed or removable prosthesis). The selection of the form is guided by clinical circumstances and physical properties of the materials that make up the prosthesis. *See also* preparation, mouth.

    p., cavity One of the various operations in which carious material is removed from teeth and biomechanically correct forms are established in the teeth to receive and retain restorations. A constant requirement is provision for prevention of failure of the restoration through recurrence of decay or inadequate resistance to applied stresses.

p., initial One of a number of procedures aimed at preparing the patient for final treatment. The objectives consist of eliminating or reducing all the local etiologic factors and environmental influences prior to the operative procedures and establishing a sequence of therapy for the patient.

p., mouth One of the various necessary procedures applied to the oral structures preparatory to the making of a final impression for a prosthesis.

p., slice A type of cavity preparation for Class 2 cast restorations. The proximal portion is formed by removing a sufficient slice of the proximal convexity of the tooth to achieve cleansable margins and a line of draw; a tapered keyway or two keyed grooves or channels in the proximal surface provide retention form.

p., surgical Any modification using surgical procedures that may be required for preparing the oral structures for prosthodontic treatment.

prepubertal (prē-pū′ber-tal) Before the onset of puberty.

presbyopia (prĕs″bē-ō′pē—ah) **(farsightedness, hyperopia)** A form of optical distortion affecting the vision of patients, particularly those of advancing age. It is dependent on diminution of the power of the accommodation of the lens as a result of loss of elasticity of the crystalline lens, causing the near point of distinct vision to be removed farther from the eye.

prescription (prē-skrĭp′shŭn) A written direction for the preparation and use of medicine or an appliance; a medical recipe; a prescribed remedy. Also used in dentistry to describe the treatment plan.

p., extemporaneous (magistral prescription) 1: A prescription for a nonofficial drug. **2:** A prescription that directs the pharmacist to compound the specified medication, as contrasted with a prescription that specifies medication available in precompounded form.

p., magistral *See* prescription, extemporaneous.

p., official A prescription for an official drug.

preservation A neurologic phenomenon such as the involuntary repetition of motor response or the continuation of a sensation after the adequate external stimulus has ceased.

preservative A substance added to prevent deterioration.

pressure A stress or strain that may occur by compression, pull, thrust, etc.; an applied force.

p. area *See* area, pressure.

p. atrophy *See* atrophy, pressure.

p., biting The actual or potential power used in bring-

ing the teeth into contact. *See also* pressure, occlusal.

p., blood The pressure exerted on arterial walls by the blood when the heart is in systole (systolic pressure), and the pressure maintained by the elasticity of the arteries when the heart is in diastole (diastolic pressure). A consistent arterial pressure greater than 140/90 is considered abnormally high and suggestive of hypertensive vascular disease.

p., deeper Any pressure to the body—in excess of that which stimulates Meissner's corpuscles, Merkel's disks, or the hair receptors of light touch—that stimulates the deeper receptors such as Pacini's corpuscles. These latter deep-pressure perception organs lie in the inner layers of the dermis and in the muscle and tendon groups.

p., equalization of The act of distributing pressure evenly.

p., hand Force applied by an instrument held in the hand.

p., hydraulic Pressure transmitted by a liquid trapped between the tooth and a restoration being cemented.

p., hydrostatic The pressure in the circulatory system exerted by the volume of blood when it is confined in a blood vessel. The hydrostatic pressure, coupled with the osmotic pressure, within a capillary is opposed by the hydrostatic and osmotic pressure of the surrounding tissues. Fluids flow from the higher pressure areas to the lower pressure areas.

p., intrapleural Pressure within the pleura.

p., occlusal Any force exerted on the occlusal surfaces of teeth. *See also* force, occlusal; load, occlusal.

p., osmotic The stress that develops when solutions containing different concentrations of solute in a common solvent are separated by a membrane that is permeable to the solvent but not the solute.

p., partial The pressure exerted by each of the constituents of a mixture of gases.

p., pulse The difference between systolic and diastolic pressure.

p. sensibility The ability to detect light touch and deep pressure. *See also* corpuscle, Meissner's; corpuscle, Merkel's; corpuscle, Pacini's.

presumption An inference as to the existence of some fact, drawn from the existence of some other fact; an inference that common sense draws from circumstances usually occurring in such cases.

presurgical impression An overextended impression of the intact mandible before the first surgical stage. The cast made for this impression is altered so that the surgical tray may be fabricated on it.

pretreatment Before treatment; refers to the protocols required before beginning therapy, usually of a diagnostic nature.

p. estimate *See* predetermination.

prevailing fee Term used by some dental benefits organizations to refer to the fee most commonly charged for a dental service in a given area.

prevent To keep from happening or existing especially by precautionary measures.

preventive Avoiding occurrence.

   p. dentistry The procedures in dental practice and health programs that prevent the occurrence of oral diseases.

   p. orthodontic treatment Dental services intended to prevent the development of a malocclusion by maintaining the integrity of an otherwise normally developing dentition. Typical services include dental restorations, temporary prostheses (space maintainers) to replace prematurely lost deciduous teeth, and removal of deciduous teeth that fail to shed normally to allow the permanent successors to erupt satisfactorily.

prima facie (prī′mah fā′shē-ē″) On the face of it; so far as can be judged from the first appearance; presumably.

primary First in time; first in order in any series.

   p. beam *See* radiation, primary.

   p. fixation Immediate postoperative fastening of an implant to bone by means of wires, screws, or a superstructure until, through natural healing and adhesion, final fixation occur.

   p. intention healing The healing of a wound directly at the incision site.

   p. lymphoma of the brain A secondary neoplasm associated with AIDS.

   p. radiation *See* radiation, primary.

primate space (prī′māt) Space that occurs between the canine and first premolar teeth in adult primates but that is normally absent in man. However, spacing between the primary canine and primary first molar normally occurs in the anterior primary dentition in children. This spacing is referred to as a *primate space*.

principal Chief; highest in rank; the source of authority.

   p. in law of agency The employer; the person who gives authority to an agent to act for him.

prior authorization *See* predetermination.

p.r.n. *See* pro re nata.

pro forma A pro forma financial statement is one that shows how the actual statement will look if certain specified assumptions are realized. Pro forma statements are usually a future projection.

pro re nata (prō rē nē′tah) **(p.r.n.)** A Latin phrase meaning "occasionally as needed" or "according to circumstances."

proaccelerin (prō′ak-sel′er-in) **(factor V, labile factor, plasma accelerator globulin, plasma ac-globulin, proprothrombinase, prothrombin conversion accelerator I)** An unstable protein found in the blood; the precursor of accelerin.

proandrogens (prō-ăn′dro -jĕnz) Compounds that are not androgenic when applied locally but that have androgenic activity when metabolized in the organism. Included are cortisone and cortisol, which may be converted within the organism to androgens such as adrenosterone, 11-ketoandrosterone, and 11-hydroxyandrosterone.

probative (prō′bah-tĭv) In the law of evidence, tending to prove or actually proving.

probe A slender, flexible instrument designed for introduction into a wound or cavity for purposes of exploration.

   p., lacrimal An instrument useful in probing the lumen of duct structures, such as the nasolacrimal or salivary gland ducts.

   p., periodontal A fine calibrated instrument designed and used for measuring the depth and topography of gingival and periodontal pockets. Also used to determine the degree of attachment and adaptation of the gingival tissues to the tooth. procaine hydrochloride A local anesthetic agent; 2-diethylaminoethyl 4-aminobenzoate hydrochloride. procedure A series of steps, followed in a regular, orderly, definite way, by which a desired result is accomplished.

procaine hydrochloride (prō-kān hi″drō-klo′rīd) A local anesthetic agent; 2-diethylaminoethyl 4-aminobenzoate hydrochloride.

procedure (prō-sē′jur) A series of steps followed in a regular, orderly, definite way, by which a desired result is accomplished.

   p., dental prosthetic laboratory The steps in the fabrication of a dental prosthesis that do not require the presence of the patient for their accomplishment.

   p., Kazanjian's (kah-zan′gē-an) *See* operation, Kazanjian's.

   p., operating The technique or method of conducting or performing an operation or form of treatment.

   p., order of The sequence of steps made in performing an operation or following through a technique. In cavity preparation the sequence is as follows: (1) obtain the required outline form, (2) obtain the required resistance form, (3) obtain the required retention form, (4) retain the required convenience form, (5) remove any remaining carious dentin, (6) finish the enamel walls, and (7) make the désbridement.

   p., orthodontic Therapeutic measures employed to correct malalignment and malposition of the teeth and to immobilize and stabilize periodontally involved or previously moved teeth.

   p., restorative A method or mode of action that reestablishes or reforms a tooth or teeth or portions thereof to anatomic or functional form and health.

process (pros′es, prō′ses) In anatomy, a marked prominence or projection of a bone. In dentistry, a series of operations that convert a wax pattern, such as that of a denture base, into a solid denture base of another material. *See also* denture curing.

p., alveolar The portion of the maxillae or mandible that forms the dental arch and serves as a bony investment for the teeth. Its cortical covering is continuous with the compact bone of the body of the maxillae or mandible, whereas its trabecular portion is continuous with the spongiosa of the body of the jaws. *See also* ridge, alveolar.

p., dehiscence of alveolar *See* dehiscence.

p., fenestration of alveolar A circumscribed hole, located in the cortical plate over the root, that does not communicate with the crestal margin.

p., condyloid (kahn´dĭ-loid) **(capitulum mandibulae)** A projection of the mandible arising on the posterosuperior aspect of the mandibular ramus. It consists of a neck and an elliptically shaped head or condyle that enters into the formation of the temporomandibular joint in conjunction with the articular disk and the glenoid fossa of the temporal bone.

p., neck of condyloid The part of the condyloid process that connects the condyle to the main part of the ramus.

p., coronoid The thin triangular rounded eminence originating from the anterosuperior surface of the ramus of the mandible. Provides insertion for the various fiber bundles of the temporal muscle.

p., hamular (pterygoid process) The pterygoid process of the sphenoid bone; appears as a vertical projection distal to the maxillary tuberosity.

p., horizontal resorptive The pattern of bone resorption, occurring with periodontal disease, in which the resultant level of bone is more or less flat or level in nature.

p., pterygoid *See* process, hamular.

processing (prăh´sĕs-ĭng) Term that usually refers to the procedure of bringing about polymerization of appliances; processing of dentures. *See also* film processing.

p., denture The conversion of a wax pattern of a denture or trial denture into a denture with a base made of another material (e.g., acrylic resin). *See also* process.

p. tank *See* tank, processing.

procheilia (prō-kēl´ē-ah) A condition of protruding lips.

proconvertin (prō″kon-ver´tin) **(autoprothrombin I, cofactor V, cothromboplastin, factor VII, precursor of serum prothrombin conversion accelerator [pro-SPCA], stable factor)** Variously described as the inactive precursor of convertin. Recently proconvertin has been considered as a collective term for *pro-SPCA* and *Stuart factor*.

proconvertin-convertin *See* thromboplastin, extrinsic.

procumbency (prō-cŭm´bĕn-sē) Excessive labioaxial inclination of the incisor teeth.

production The amount of work that can be accomplished in a specific length of time.

products, fission *See* fission products.

profession A calling; vocation; a means of livelihood or gain.

professional ethics, codes of The rules of conduct governing the conduct, transactions, and relationships within a profession and among its publics.

professional liability insurance Insurance covering the insured against claims arising from injury, damage, or loss sustained by a patient during the course of professional services.

professional standards review organization (PSRO) A federal agency, established by Public Law 92-603, to determine the quality and appropriateness of health care services paid for, in whole or part, under the Social Security Act. Such determinations are to be made by local committees of providers.

profibrin (prō-fī´brĭn) *See* fibrinogen.

profibrinolysin (prō-fī″brĭ-nol´ĭ-sĭn) *See* plasminogen.

profile An outline or contour, especially one representing a side view of a human head.

p. extraoral radiographic examination *See* examination, radiographic, extraoral, profile.

p., facial The sagittal outline form of the face.

p. record *See* record, profile.

profit sharing A mechanism for funding a retirement plan for employees or members of a professional association. Members are eligible for a percentage of the net income based on predetermined formulae. Such plans, properly executed, are legal and ethical and are to be differentiated from fee-splitting, which is illegal and unethical, in which a referring professional shares in the fee-for-service income of another professional.

progeria (prō-jē´rē-ah) *See* syndrome, Hutchinson-Gilford.

progesterone (prō-jĕs´tĕ-rōn) The ovarian hormone produced by the corpus luteum and responsible for preparing the endometrium for nidation and nourishment of the ovum. It also suppresses the production of the pituitary luteinizing hormone, estrus, and ovulation and stimulates the mammary glands.

progestogen (prō-jes´tō-gen) An agent capable of producing effects similar to progestrone; used to correct abnormalities of the menstrual cycle.

prognathic (prŏg´năth´ĭk) Pertaining to a forward relationship of the jaws to the head (anterior to the skull); denoting a protrusive lower face.

prognathism (prŏg´nah-thĭzm) Facial disharmony in which one or both jaws project forward. Prognathism may be real or imaginary. Mandibular prognathism may exist when both the maxillae and the mandible increase in length or when the maxillae are of normal length but the mandible increases in length. Prognathism may be imaginary when the maxillae are underdeveloped and short and the mandible is of normal length or when the maxillary and mandibular dental relationships are normal but there is an increase in the mental prominence of the mandible.

prognathus (prŏg-năth'ŭs) The condition of having a marked projection of the mandible, usually resulting in a horizontal overlap of the lower anterior teeth in relation to the maxillary anterior teeth.

prognosis (prŏg-nō'sĭs) **1:** The foretelling of the probable course of a disease; a forecast of the outcome of a disease. **2:** A forecast of the probable result of a regimen of treatment.

program Instructions coded in a computer language to solve a problem.

programmer A person who writes applications in a computer language. It is usually the programmer (not the machine) who should be held responsible for satisfactory and efficient solution of the problem.

programming The process of describing in a computer language a problem or its method of solution. It includes planning, designing, writing, and debugging of programs.

projection, orthographic A projection made on the assumption that the projection lines from the object to the plane of projection are at right angles to the plane.

p., gnathic planes of orthographic The three planes of projection to which gnathologically mounted casts are oriented: the horizontal, vertical, (frontal), and profile planes. The horizontal plane is the axis-orbital plane. The hinge axis is the line of intersection for both the horizontal and frontal planes. The profile plane is the mechanical midsagittal plane of the articulator.

prolactin *See* hormone, lactogenic.

proliferation (prŏ-lĭf'ĕ-rā'shŭn) Growth by reproduction of similar cells.

p., epithelial A characteristic finding in inflammatory lesions affecting the gingival tissues; consists of hyperplasia of the pocket epithelium, with extension and elongation of epithelial rete pegs into the submucosa. Accompanying the hyperplastic changes in the crevicular epithelium, it is noticed that the epithelial attachment proliferates onto and alongside the cementum. Also, the multiplication of epithelial cells resulting either in increased thickness or new epithelial covering of a wound or an ulcer.

promissory (prom'ĭ-sŏr"ē) A promise; stipulation for a future act or course of conduct.

promotion The gaining and retaining of acceptance by others of the views, products, or services of the originator of the message. Components of promotion: personal selling, advertising, sales promotion, and publicity.

p., sales Sales promotion includes those marketing activities, other than personal selling, advertising, and publicity, which stimulate consumer purchasing and dealer effectiveness. They include point-of-purchase displays, shows and exhibit demonstrations, and other nonrecurrent selling efforts.

pronasion (prō-nā'zē-on) The most prominent point on the tip of the nose when the head is placed in the eye-ear (horizontal) plane.

proof The establishment of a fact by evidence; to find the truth.

p. beyond a reasonable doubt In criminal law, such proof as precludes every reasonable hypothesis except that which it tends to support and is wholly consistent with the defendant's guilt and inconsistent with any other rational conclusions.

p. of loss Contractual right of the carrier or service corporation to request verification of services rendered (expenses incurred) by the submission of claim forms, radiographs, study models, and/or other diagnostic material.

prop A device inserted between the jaws to maintain an open position of the mandible.

propagation (prop"ah-gā'shun) The reproduction or continuance of an impulse along a nerve fiber in an afferent or efferent direction.

property Rightful ownership; the exclusive right to a thing.

prophylactic (prō"fi-lak'tik) Preventing disease; relating to prophylaxis.

prophylaxis (prō"fi-lak'sis) The prevention of disease.

p., dental A series of procedures whereby calculus, stain, and other accretions are removed from the clinical crowns of the teeth, and the clinical crowns of the teeth are polished.

proportional limit *See* limit, elastic.

proprietary (prō-prī'ĕ-tă-rē) Controlled by a private interest; protected by patent, trademark, or copyright.

proprioceptive influence (prō"prē-ō-sĕp'tĭv) Influence of the muscle sense (kinesthetic sense) in guiding the jaw to close in such a way as not to be injurious to the teeth.

proprioceptors (prō"prē-ō-sĕp'torz) Sensory nerve receptors situated in the muscles, tendons, and joints that furnish information to the central nervous system concerning the movements and positions of the limbs, trunk, head and neck, and, more specifically for the dentist, the mandible, and its associated oral structures.

proprothrombinase (prō"prō-throm'bĭn-ās) *See* factor V.

proptosis (prop-tō'sĭs) Forward displacement or protrusion of the eyeball. *See also* exophthalmos.

prorating A clause in a contract with participating dentists wherein they agree to accept a percentage reduction in their billings to offset the amount by which the total cost of services provided exceeds the total premium received. A method of spreading a "loss" equitably among participating dentists.

pro-SPCA *See* precursor of serum prothrombin conversion accelerator.

prospective review Prior assessment by a payer or payer's agent that proposed services are appropriate for a particular patient, and/or the patient and the category of service are covered by a benefits plan. *See also* preauthorization, precertification predetermination, second-opinion program.

prostaglandins (pros′tah-glan′dinz) A group of potent hormonelike substances that produce a wide range of body responses such as changing capillary permeability, smooth muscle tone, clumping of platelets, and endocrine and exocrine functions. They may be used in some instances to terminate a pregnancy.

prosthesis (pros″the-sis pros-the′sis) The replacement of an absent part of the human body by an artificial part.

  p., cleft palate A restoration to correct congenital or acquired defects in the palate and related structures if they are involved.

  p., complete denture *See* denture, complete.

  p., cranial An artificial material (alloplast) used to replace a portion of the skull.

  p., dental An artificial replacement for one or more natural teeth and/or associated structures.

  p., definitive A permanent type of substitute for missing tissue.

  p., expansion A prosthesis used to expand the lateral segment of the maxilla in unilateral or bilateral cleft of the soft and hard palates and alveolar processes.

    p., fixed expansion A prosthesis that cannot be readily removed and stays in position for the required length of treatment.

    p., removable expansion A prosthesis that can be removed from the mouth and replaced when indicated.

  p., feeding A prosthesis worn by a young infant with a cleft palate to increase sucking power and to eliminate the escape of food through the nose.

  p., partial denture *See* denture, partial.

  p., periodontal Any restorative and replacement device that, by its intent and nature, is used as a therapeutic aid in the treatment of periodontal disease; it is an adjunct to other forms of periodontal therapy and does not cure periodontal disease by itself.

  p., postsurgical An artificial replacement for a missing part or parts after surgical intervention.

  p., surgical An appliance prepared to assist in surgical procedures and placed at the time of surgery.

  p., temporary A fixed or removable restoration for which a more permanent appliance is planned within a short period of time.

prosthetic appliance (pros-thĕt′ĭk) *See* appliance, prosthetic.

prosthetic restoration *See* prosthesis.

prosthetic speech aid *See* aid, speech, prosthetic.

prosthetics (pros-thĕt′ĭks) The art and science of supplying, fitting, and servicing artificial replacements for missing parts of the human body.

  p., complete denture 1: The restoration of the natural teeth and their associated parts in the dental arch by artificial replacements. **2:** The phase of dental prosthetics dealing with the restoration of function when one or both dental arches have been rendered edentulous.

  p., dental *See* prosthodontics.

  p., full denture *See* prosthetics, complete denture.

  p., maxillofacial The branch of prosthodontics concerned with the restoration of stomatognathic and associated facial structures that have been affected by disease, injury, surgery, or congenital defect.

  p., partial denture The dental service that, by replacing one or more but less than all the teeth of a dental arch, avoids the degenerative changes resulting from tooth movement and may thus achieve preventive measures of maximum benefit toward the maintenance of optimal oral health as well as reasonable restoration of dental functions.

prosthetist (pros′the-tĭst) The principal responsible individual involved in the construction of an artificial replacement for any part of the human body.

prosthion (pros′thē-on) The point of the upper alveolar process that projects most anteriorly in the midline.

prosthodontia (pros″thō-don′shē-ah) *See* prosthodontics.

prosthodontics (pros″tho-don′tĭks) **(prosthetic dentistry)** The part of dentistry pertaining to the restoration and maintenance of oral function, comfort, appearance, and health of the patient by the replacement of missing teeth and contiguous tissues with artificial substitutes. Prosthodontics has three main branches: removable prosthodontics, fixed prosthodontics, and maxillofacial prosthetics.

  p., fixed The branch of prosthodontics concerned with the replacement and/or restoration of teeth by artificial substitutes that are not readily removable.

prosthodontist (pros″thō-don′tĭst) A dentist engaged in the practice of prosthodontics. A specialist in the practice of prosthodontics.

protective apron *See* apron, lead.

protein(s) (prō′tĕ-ĭn) Any one of a group of complex organic nitrogenous compounds; the principal constituent of cell protoplasm. Polymers of amino acids that are joined by peptide or amide bonds.

  p., anabolic *See* steroid, C-19 cortico-.

  p., Bence Jones A special protein found in the blood and urine of patients with multiple myeloma and occasionally other diseases involving bone marrow, such as sarcoma and leukemia.

p., C-reactive A mucoprotein whose presence in serum is always abnormal. It may be present in a variety of inflammatory or necrotic disease processes. It is almost always present in the serum in acute rheumatic fever.

p. deficiency *See* deficiency, protein.

p., plasma Blood serum contains 6.5 to 8 Gm% of a complex mixture of proteins, including albumin, globulin, and fibrinogen.

p. specificity The arrangement of protein molecules in numerous spatial configurations to suit the special needs of the physical and chemical activity of the cell. The wide degree of variability of protein structures permits a high degree of specificity of tissue within one body. This characteristic of protein specificity is of great significance in blood transfusions, tissue grafts, and many allergic manifestations.

p., thromboplastic *See* factor III.

proteinuria (prō″tē-ĭ-nū′rē-ah) The presence of protein in the urine. An indication of kidney disease.

p., orthostatic (postural proteinuria) Proteinuria that occurs during daily activities but does not occur when the individual is recumbent.

p., physiologic *See* proteinuria, transient.

p., postural *See* proteinuria, orthostatic.

p., transient (physiologic proteinuria) Proteinuria that occurs in normal persons after a high-protein meal, violent exercise, severe emotional stress, or syncope. It may occur after an epileptic seizure or during pregnancy. It disappears after the cause subsides.

Prothero "cone" theory *See* retention.

prothrombase (prō-throm′bās) *See* factor II; prothrombin.

prothrombin (prō-throm′bĭn) **(factor II, prothrombase, thrombogen)** A glycoprotein precursor of thrombin that is produced in the liver and is necessary for the coagulation of blood. A prothrombin deficiency is uncommon but may occur in liver disease. Vitamin K is essential for the synthesis of prothrombin.

p. B *See* factor II.

p., component A of *See* factor V.

p., component B of *See* factor VII.

p. time A test for determining plasma coagulation defects caused by a lack of factor V, VII, or X. A prolonged clotting time indicates deficiency of one of the factors.

prothrombinase (prŏ-throm′bĭn-ās) **(complete thromboplastin, direct activator of prothrombin, extritsic prothrombin activator)** An inferred direct activator of prothrombin common to tissue and plasma coagulation systems. *See also* factor V.

prothrombinogen (prō″throm-bĭn′ō-jĕn) *See* factor VII.

prothrombokinase (prō-throm″bō-kī′nās) *See* factor VIII.

prothromboplastin, beta (prō-throm″bō-plăs′tĭn) *See* factor IX.

proton (prō′ton) An elementary particle having a positive charge equivalent to the negative charge of the electron but possessing a mass approximately 1845 times as great; the proton is a nuclear particle, whereas the electron is extranuclear.

protoplasm (prō′tō-plăzm) Living substance; composed mainly of five basic materials: carbohydrates, electrolytes, lipids, proteins, and water and having the properties of both a complex solution and a heterogeneous colloid. The cell nucleus and cytoplasm are two major subdivisions of protoplasm.

protraction (prō-trak′shŭn) A condition in which teeth or other maxillary or mandibular structures are situated anterior to their normal position.

protrusion (prō-troo′zhun) Teeth and/or jaws protruding farther forward than normal.

p., bimaxillary A relatively forward position, or prognathism, of the maxillary and mandibular teeth, alveolar processes, or jaws.

p., double A definite labioversion of the maxillary and mandibular anterior teeth.

p., forward A protrusion forward from the centric position.

p., mandibular Abnormal protrusion of the mandible, as in a Class III malocclusion.

p., maxillary Abnormal protrusion of the maxillae.

protrusive checkbite *See* record, interocclusal, protrusive.

protrusive occlusion *See* occlusion, protrusive.

protrusive position *See* position, protrusive.

protrusive record *See* record, protrusive.

protrusive relation *See* relation, jaw, protrusive.

provider A governmental term used to denote health care institutions; sometimes used as a synonym for *practitioner*.

provisional prosthesis An interim prosthesis worn for varying periods of time.

provisional splint *See* splint, provisional.

proximal surface *See* surface, proximal.

proximate cause One that directly produces an effect; that which in ordinary, natural sequence produces a specific result with no agencies intervening.

pruritus (proo-rī′tŭs) Itching.

pseudarthrosis (sū″dar-thrō′sĭs) A false joint; sometimes seen after a fracture.

pseudoepitheliomatous hyperplasia (PEH) (soo″dō-ep″ĭ-thē-lē-al hī″per-pla′zē-ah) A type of epithelial hyerplasia associated with chronic inflammatory response; distinguished from squamous cell carcinoma by the lack of dysplastic cytologic characteristics.

pseudohemophilia (sū″dō-hē″mō-fīl′ē-ah) Term used to describe several hemorrhagic states: (1) von Willebrand's disease, pseudohemophilia type B, vascular hemophilia; (2) a hereditary disease in which prolonged bleeding is the only consistent abnormality detected by currently available tests. *See also* **purpura, thrombocytopenic.**

pseudomembrane A loosely adherent, grayish false membrane typical of intracellular coagulation necrosis. It is formed by necrotic epithelium embedded in fibrin, leukocytes, and erythrocytes. It is seen in Vincent's infection and diphtheria. Removal leaves a raw, bleeding surface.

pseudopocket A pocket formed by gingival hyperplasia and edema without apical migration of the epithelial attachment. *See also* **pocket, gingival.**

psoriasis (sō-rī′ah-sĭs) A papulosquamous inflammatory skin disease of unknown etiology. Rare oral lesions consist of red patches with white, scaly surfaces.

PSP test *See* **test, phenolsulfonphthalein.**

psychoneurosis (sī″kō-nū-rō′sĭs) **1:** Abnormal reaction to the environment, including anxieties, phobias, hysteria, and hypochondria. **2:** Term that includes neurasthenia, hysteria, psychasthenia, and mental disorders short of insanity.

psychosedative (sī′kō-sĕd′ah-tĭv) A calming agent that reduces anxiety and tension without depressing mental or motor functions.

psychosis (sī-kō′sĭs) A functional or organic kind of mental derangement marked by a severe disturbance of personality involving autistic thinking, loss of contact with reality, delusions, and/or hallucinations.

p., manic-depressive (cyclothymia) A psychosis characterized by varying periods of depression and excitement. One state may predominate (e.g., manic-depressive reaction, manic type).

psychosomatic (sī″kō-sō-mat′-ik) Pertaining to the mind-body relationship; having bodily symptoms of a psychic, emotional, or mental origin. *See also* **disease, psychosomatic.**

p. factors *See* **factor, psychosomatic.**

PTA *See* **plasma thromboplastin antecedent.**

PTC *See* **plasma thromboplastic component.**

pterygoid process (ter′ĭ-goid) *See* **process, hamular.**

pterygomaxillary fissure (ter′ĭ-gō-mak′sĭ-ler″ē) *See* **fissure, pterygomaxillary.**

pterygomaxillary notch *See* **notch, pterygomaxillary.**

PTF *See* **factor, plasma thromboplastin.**

PTF-A (plasma thromboplastin factor A) *See* **factor VIII.**

PTF-B (plasma thromboplastin factor B) *See* **factor IX.**

PTF-C (plasma thromboplastin factor C) *See* **factor XI.**

ptosis (tō′sis) **(blepharoptosis)** A drooping of the upper eyelid.

PTT *See* **partial prothrombin time.**

ptyalectasis (tī″ah-lĕk′tah-sĭs) *See* **sialoangiectasis.**

ptyalism (tī′ah-lĭzm) *See* **sialorrhea.**

puberty (pū′ber-tē) The age at which the reproductive system becomes functional, with concurrent develop-

ment of secondary sex characteristics. Marked by increased estrogenic activity in the female and rise of androgenic activity in the male.

public health dentistry *See* **community dentistry.**

pulp (pulp) **(dental pulp, tooth pulp)** The organ, made up of blood vessels, nerves, and cellular elements, including odontoblasts, that forms dentin. It normally occupies the central portion of teeth.

p. amputation *See* **pulpotomy.**

p., anachoresis of Localization of microbes from the bloodstream in a damaged pulp.

p. canal *See* **canal, pulp.**

p. capping *See* **capping, pulp.**

p. cavity *See* **cavity, pulp.**

p. chamber *See* **chamber, pulp.**

p., dental *See* **pulp.**

p. extirpation *See* **pulpectomy.**

p. horn *See* **horn, pulp.**

p. involvement *See* **involvement, pulp.**

p., mummification of Dry gangrene of the dental pulp in which the pulp dries and shrivels.

p. removal *See* **pulpectomy.**

p. stone *See* **denticle.**

p. test The application of a physical stimulus (electrical, heat, or cold) to determine the degree of vitality of the pulp tissue.

p. tester (vitalometer) An electric instrument of high or low frequency designed to determine the response of a pulp to an electrical stimulus.

p., tooth *See* **pulp.**

p. vitality The health status of the pulp. When the pulp tissue of a tooth has undergone complete degeneration or has been removed, the tooth is termed *pulpless* or *nonvital.*

pulpal (pul′pal) Relating to the pulp or the pulp cavity.

pulpalgia (pul-păl′jē-ah) The sensitivity of the pulp to pain.

pulpectomy (pul-pĕk′tō-mē) **(pulp extirpation, pulp removal)** The complete removal of a pulp from the pulp chamber and root canal.

p., complete Surgical removal of the pulp to the dentinocemental junction at the apex of the root.

p., partial Surgical removal of only a part of the contents of the canal(s).

pulpitis (pul-pī′tĭs) Inflammation of the pulpal tissue of a tooth.

p., hypertrophic (pulp polyp) Formation and proliferation of granulation tissue from the surface of an exposed pulp.

pulpless (pulp′les) Having a nonfunctioning pulp (untreated), or a pulp that has been replaced with an inert material (treated).

p. tooth *See* **tooth, pulpless.**

pulpotomy (pul-pot′ō-mē) **(pulp amputation)** Surgical amputation of the dental pulp coronal to the dentinocemental junction.

p., partial Surgical removal of only a part of the tissue in the pulpal chamber.

p., total or complete Surgical removal of the entire contents of the pulpal chamber at the entrance of the root canal(s).

pulse (pŭls) Rhythmic expansion and contraction of arteries resulting from the surges of blood through the arteries. The pulse can be felt by the fingers in arteries that are close to the skin.

p., arterial Pulsation of an artery produced by the rise and fall in blood pressure as the heart goes into systole and diastole and observed clinically by palpation of the radial artery. The pulse rate at birth is approximately 130 beats/min., diminishing to approximately 70 beats/min. in the healthy adult. The range of normalcy is from 50 or 60 to 80 or 90 beats/min.

p. pressure *See* pressure, pulse.

p., venous Pulsation of a vein; most easily felt in the right jugular vein.

pumice (pŭm′ĭs) A type of volcanic glass used as an abrasive. Prepared in various grits and used for finishing and polishing in dentistry. Also used in the prophylaxis of natural teeth.

punch biopsy The removal of tissue for diagnostic purposes using a sharp, cylindrical, hollow instrument placed over the tissue to be excised and rotated with slight pressure until an incision of proper depth is achieved. The tissue within the incision is lifted, and the base is excised with a scissor or scalpel blade.

punch, rubber dam An instrument used to punch holes of varying sizes in a rubber dam so that it may be applied to the teeth.

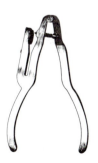

Rubber dam punch

pupil, Argyll Robertson Pupillary abnormalities associated with tabes dorsalis (neurosyphilis), manifested by miosis, the absence of a ciliospinal reflex, and a reaction to accommodation but not to light.

purchaser Program sponsor, often an employer or union, that contracts with the dental benefits organization to provide dental benefits to an enrolled population.

purchasing cooperative A group of dentists pooling their financial resources for the purchase of large quantities of supplies and equipment for the purpose of obtaining a discount.

purpura (pĕr′pŭ-rah) Extravasation of blood into the tissues, resulting in blue to black lesions of the skin or mucosa (petechiae and ecchymoses).

p., allergic (anaphylactoid purpura) Any thrombocytopenic or nonthrombocytopenic purpura related to an allergic reaction. Manifestations other than ecchymoses and petechiae associated with erythema and inflammation include the common symptoms of allergy.

p., anaphylactoid *See* purpura, allergic.

p., essential *See* purpura, thrombocytopenic, idiopathic.

p. hemorrhagica *See* purpura, thrombocytopenic; purpura, thrombocytopenic, idiopathic.

p., nonthrombocytopenic Purpura usually related to increased capillary permeability. Included are allergic purpuras and those resulting from vitamin C deficiency, bacterial toxins (scarlet fever, typhoid), drug intoxications, and metabolic toxins (nephritis, liver disease).

p., primary *See* purpura, thrombocytopenic, idiopathic.

p., secondary *See* purpura, thrombocytopenic, symptomatic.

p., thrombocytopathic Bleeding associated with qualitative abnormalities of the platelets.

p., thrombocytopenic (essential thrombopenia, pseudohemophilia, hemorrhagica, Werlhof's disease) Severe ecchymoses and petechiae associated with marked reduction in the numbers of blood platelets. There is prolonged bleeding time and poor clot retraction, but the coagulation and prothrombin times are normal. Hemorrhage may occur spontaneously from any area of the oral mu-cosa. This disease may be acute and fatal, whereas in other instances it may run a chronic course with intermittent attacks.

p., idiopathic thrombocytopenic (essential purpura, land scurvy, primary purpura, purpura hemorrhagica) A thrombocytopenic purpura of unknown cause.

p., symptomatic thrombocytopenic (secondary purpura) Purpura resulting from the effect of chemical, physical, vegetable, or animal agents, infections, or related blood disorders.

p., thrombotic thrombocytopenic A febrile disease of unknown cause characterized by hemolytic anemia, neurologic symptoms, hemorrhage into the skin and mucous membranes, icterus, hepatosplenomegaly, low platelet count, and platelet thrombi occluding capillaries and arterioles.

purulent discharge (pū′roo-lĕnt) *See* pus.

pus (pŭs) **(purulent discharge)** An inflammatory exudate formed within the tissues; consists of polymorphonuclear leukocytes, degenerated and liquefied tissue elements, microorganisms, tissue fluids, etc. It may form within the tissues in periodontitis and escape via the ulcerated pocket epithelium into the oral environment. The suppurative material may be retained within the tissues when the orifice of the periodontal pocket is blocked, thus creating a favorable circumstance for the formation of a periodontal abscess.

pustule (pus′tūl) A vesicular lesion containing pus rather than clear fluid.

pyknik (pĭk′nĭk) A constitution characterized by a short, squat appearance.

pyknosis (pĭk-nō′sĭs) Increased basophilia and shrinkage of the nucleus of a dying cell.

pyogenic (pī″ō-jĕn′ĭk) Pus producing.

pyorrhea (pī″ō-rē′ah) An antiquated term used to designate periodontal disease. Generally, it means "flow of pus," which previously was a feature of periodontal disease. Before the use of the term *pyorrhea, periodontitis* was designated as *Riggs' disease* and *Fauchard's disease.* Still retained in some communities as a lay term for *periodontal disease.*

pyrexia (pī-rĕk′sē-ah) *See* fever.

pyridoxine (pĭr″ĭ-dok′sēn) *See* vitamin B_6.

pyrometer (pī-rom′ĕ-ter) An instrument for measuring temperature by the change of electrical resistance within a thermocouple. It is a millivoltmeter calibrated in degrees of temperature.

pyuria (pī-ū′rē-ah) Abnormal numbers of white blood cells in the urine. Without proteinuria, it suggests infection of the urinary tract; with proteinuria, it suggests infection of the kidney (pyelonephritis).

q.i.d. (quater in die) Latin phrase used in prescription writing meaning four times a day.

p.4.h. (quaque 4 hora) Latin phrase used in prescription writing, meaning every 4 hours.

q.s. (quantum satis, quantum sufficiat) Latin phrase used in prescription writing meaning a sufficient quantity.

quack One who professes to have medical or dental skill that is not possessed; one who practices medicine or dentistry without adequate preparation or proper qualification.

quad helix appliance A fixed spring loaded orthodontic appliance, using four helix springs, used primarily to expand the maxillary dental arch.

qualified Having the required ability; fitted; entitled.

quality When applied to the voice, the acoustic characteristics of vowels resulting from their overtone structure or the relative intensities of their frequency component.

q. assessment 1: The measurement of quality; generally includes selecting an aspect of dental care or the dental care system to be evaluated; establishing criteria and standards for quality dental care and comparing what has actually been done with the criteria and standards. **2:** The measure of the quality of care provided in a particular setting.

q. assurance 1: Procedures for checking the quality of dental care provided by participating dentists and for correcting any irregularities discovered. Synonyms: quality control, quality evaluation. **2:** The asessment or measurement of the quality of care and the implementation of any necessary changes to maintain or improve the quality of care rendered.

q. assurance system A formally organized sequence of activities in dentistry that combines assessment of the existing situation; judgments about necessary changes; development of plans to effect such changes; implementation of these plans, and reassessment to determine that the desired changes have taken place.

q. of radiation *See* radiation quality.

q. review committee A committee established by a professional organization or institution to assess and/or ensure quality. Unlike peer review committees, it can function on its own initiative on a broad range of topics.

quantity of radiation *See* radiation quantity.

quantum A discrete unit of electromagnetic energy or of an x-ray. A quantity becomes quantized when its magnitude is restricted to a discrete set of values as opposed to a continuous set of values.

q. theory *See* theory, quantum.

quartz *See* silica.

q., fused A form of silica that is amorphous and exhibits no inversion at any temperature below its fusion point. Of little use in dentistry.

quasi contract An obligation similar in character to that of a contract, which arises not from an agreement of parties, but from some relation between them or from a voluntary act of one of them.

quaternary (kwah′tĕr-năr″ē) Having four elements. Quaternary ammonium salts are molecules containing four alkyl or aryl groups attached to a nitrogen atom and are used widely in medicine.

quench To cool a hot object rapidly by plunging it into water or oil.

question, hypothetical A combination of assumed or proved facts and circumstances stated so as to constitute a coherent and specific situation or state of facts, on which the opinion of an expert is asked by way of evidence at a trial.

questionnaire A form usually filled out by patients that provides data concerning their dental and general health.

q., health A list of key questions, answered by the patient, that permits an interpretation by the diagnostician of the general and oral health of the patient.

quick-cure resin See resin, autopolymer.

Quincke's disease (kwĭnk′ĕz) See edema, angioneurotic.

racemic (rā-sē′-mĭk) Referring to a mixture of equal quantities of the dextro and levo-isomers of a compound.

rachisensible (rā″-kē-sĕn′-sĭ-b'l) Abnormally sensitive to spinal anesthetics.

rad (r) A unit of absorbed dose of radiation: 1 r = 100 ergs/Gm. *See also* rem.

> **millirad (mr)** One one-thousandth of a rad. Normal background radiation in this country varies from about 50 to 200 mr per year, depending on geographic location.

radiate (rā′dē-āt) **1:** To diverge or spread from a common point; arranged in a radiating manner. **2:** To expose to radiation, as x radiation.

radiation (rā-dē-ā′shŭn) **1:** The process of emitting radiant energy in the form of waves or particles. **2:** The combined processes of emission, transmission, and absorption of radiant energy.

> **r., actinic** Radiation capable of producing chemical change (e.g., effect of light and x-rays on photographic emulsions).

> **r., background** Radiation arising from radioactive material other than the one directly under consideration. Background radiation resulting from cosmic rays and natural radioactivity is always present. There may also be background radiation because of radioactive substances in other parts of the building (e.g., building material).

> **r., backscatter** *See* radiation, scattered.

> **r., biologic effectiveness of** The ability of a particular type of ionizing radiation to produce biologic effects on an organism with small absorbed doses.

>> **r., relative biologic effectiveness of (RBE)** A comparison between one type of ionizing radiation and another with respect to the ability to produce biologic effects with small doses.

> **r., characteristic** Radiation that originates from an atom after removal of an electron or excitation of the nucleus. The wavelength of the emitted radiation is specific, depending only on the element concerned and the particular energy levels involved. Also, the specific type of secondary radiation resulting when rays from a radio ray tube strike another substance, such as copper.

> **r., corpuscular** Subatomic particles, such as electrons, protons, neutrons, or alpha particles, that travel in streams at various velocities. All the particles have definite masses, and they travel at various speeds. The properties are in opposition to electromagnetic radiations, which have no mass and travel in wave forms at the speed of light. *See also* radiation, electromagnetic.

> **r., cosmic** *See* ray, cosmic.

> **r., dermatitis** *See* dermatitis, radiation.

> **r. detector** Any device for converting radiant energy to a form more suitable for observation and/or recording. Examples include x-ray films and radiometers.

> **r., direct (primary radiation)** Radiation emanating from a tube aperture and comprising the useful beam, as compared with any stray radiation, such as that which comes from the tube container.

> **r., electromagnetic** Forms of energy propagated by wave motion, such as photons or discrete quanta. The radiations have no matter associated with them, as opposed to corpuscular radiations, which have definite masses. They differ widely in wavelength, frequency, and photon energy and have strikingly different properties. Covering an enormous range of wavelengths (from 10^{17} to 10^{-6} Å), they include radio waves, infrared waves, visible light, ultraviolet radiation, gamma rays, and cosmic radiation. *See also* radiation, corpuscular.

> **r. field** *See* x-ray beam, field size.

> **r., gamma** *See* ray, gamma.

> **r., genetic effects of** *See* genetic effects of radiation.

> **r., grenz** *See* ray, grenz.

> **r., hard** Radiation consisting of the short wavelengths (higher kilovolt peak equals greater penetration.

> **r. hazard** *See* hazard, radiation.

> **r., heterogeneous** A beam or "bundle" of radiation containing photons of many wavelengths.

> **r., homogeneous** A beam of radiation consisting of photons all of which have the same wavelength.

> **r. hygiene** *See* hygiene, radiation.

> **r. intensity** *See* intensity, radiation.

> **r., ionizing** Electromagnetic radiation such as x-rays and gamma rays; particulate radiation such as alpha particles, beta particles, protons, and neutrons; and

all other types of radiations that produce ionization directly or indirectly.

r. leakage (stray radiation) The escape of radiation through the protective shielding of the x-ray unit tube head. This radiation is detected at the sides, top, bottom, or back of the tube head; it does not include the useful beam.

r., monochromatic *See* radiation, homogeneous.

r. necrosis *See* necrosis, radiation.

r., neutron *See* ray, neutron.

r., primary All radiation produced directly from the target in an x-ray tube. *See also* radiation, direct.

r. protection Provision designed to reduce exposure of persons to radiation. For external radiation this provision consists of the use of protective barriers of radiation-absorbing material, ensuring adequate distances from the radiation sources, reducing exposure time, or combinations of these measures. For internal radiation it involves measures to restrict inhalation, ingestion, or other modes of entry of radioactive material into the body.

r. quality The ability of a beam of x-rays to allow the production of diagnostically useful radiographs. Usually measured in half-value layers of aluminum and controlled by the kilovolt peak.

r. quantity Amount of radiation. The amount of exposure is expressed in roentgens (R), whereas quantity of dose is expressed in rads.

r., remnant The radiation that passes through an object or part being examined and that is available either for recording on a radiographic film or for measurement.

r., scattered (backscatter radiation) Radiation whose direction has been altered. It may include secondary and/or stray radiation.

r., secondary The new radiation created by primary radiation acting on or passing through matter.

r. shield *See* shield, radiation.

r. sickness A self-limited syndrome characterized by varying degrees of nausea, vomiting, diarrhea, and psychic depression after exposure to very large doses of ionizing radiation, particularly doses to the abdominal region. Its mechanism is not completely understood. It usually occurs a few hours after treatment and may subside within a day. It may be sufficiently severe to necessitate interrupting the treatment series, or it may incapacitate the patient.

r., soft Radiation consisting of the long wavelengths (lower kilovolt peak = lesser penetrability).

r., speed of The speed of light, or approximately 186,000 miles per second.

r., stray *See* radiation leakage.

r. survey *See* survey, radiation.

r. therapy *See* therapy, radiation.

r., total body The exposure of the entire body to penetrating radiation. In theory, all cells in the body receive the same overall dose.

r., useful (useful beam) That part of the primary radiation that is permitted to pass from the tube housing through the tube head port, aperture, or collimating device.

radicular (răh-dĭk'-ū-lar) Pertaining to the root; in restorative dentistry, where the form of both the preparation and the restoration for the coronal portion of the natural tooth extends into the treated root canal of the pulpless tooth (e.g., radicular preparation, radicular restoration [dowel crown]).

radio- Prefix used to denote radiation from any source. radioactive decay *See* decay, radioactive.

radioactive decay *See* decay, radioactive.

radioactive isotope *See* radioisotope.

radioactivity (rặ"-dē-ō-ăk-tĭv'-ĭ-tē) Spontaneous nuclear disintegration with emission of corpuscular or electromagnetic radioations. The principal types of radioactivity are alpha disintegration, beta decay (negatron emission, positron emission, and electron capture), and isometric transition. Double beta decay is another type of radioactivity that has been postulated, and spontaneous fission and the spontaneous transformations of mesons are sometimes considered to be types of radioactivity. To be considered radioactive, a process must have a measurable lifetime between approximately 1 to 10 seconds and 1017 years, according to present experimental techniques. Radiations emitted within a time too short for measurement are called *prompt;* however, prompt radiations, including gamma rays, characteristic x-rays, conversion and auger electrons, delayed neutrons, and annihilation radiation, are often associated with radioactive disintegrations because their emission may follow the primary radioactive process.

radiogram (rā'dē-ō-gram") *See* radiograph.

radiograph(s) (rā'dē-ō-graf") An image or picture produced on a radiation-sensitive film emulsion, by exposure to ionizing radiation directed through an area, region, or substance of interest, followed by chemical processing of the film. It is basically dependent on the differential absorption of radiation directed through heterogeneous media.

r., bite-wing A form of dental radiograph that reveals approximately the coronal halves of the maxillary and mandibular teeth and portions of the interdental alveolar septa on the same film.

r., body-section Radiograph produced by rotation of the film and x-ray source around the region of interest in opposite directions during exposure, so as to blur interposed anatomic structures outside the region of interest.

r., cephalometric Extraoral radiographs produced under conditions ensuring maximum dimensional accuracy and reproducible film-object-beam relationship for purposes of cephalometric study.

r., composite Radiograph made by superimposing a radiograph of osseous tissue, whose exposed border has been cut away, on a radiograph of soft tissue for the purpose of detecting radiographic information concerning both the soft tissues and the osseous tissues of the head and face from a single radiographic view.

r., contrast media Radiograph that records the shadow images of the secretory apparatus of any of the salivary glands, body cavities, or fistulous tracts after the injection of a liquid radiopaque solution.

r., extraoral Radiograph produced on a film placed extraorally.

r., follow-up Radiographs made during and after therapy to follow the progress or regress of a disease, determine the course of healing, or ascertain the results of treatment.

r., intraoral Radiograph produced by placing a radiographic film within the oral cavity.

r., microscopic examination *See* microradiography.

r., occlusal A special type of intraoral radiograph made with the film held between the occluded teeth.

r., oral Radiographic representation of shadow images of all the tissues, structures, and regions of the oral cavity and its adjacent areas and associated parts.

r., panoramic A large radiograph depicting the curvatures of the maxillae and mandible and associated structures.

r., salivary gland *See* sialography.

r., stereoscopic A pair of radiographs of a structure made by shifting the position of the x-ray tube a few centimeters between each of two exposures. Such pairs provide a three-dimensional, or stereoscopic, presentation of the recorded images.

r., Towne projection 1: *n.* Radiographic view of the mandibular condyles and the midfacial skeleton. **2:** *v.* To produce a shadow image on a photographic emulsion.

radiographer (rā″dē-og-rah-fer) A specialist or technician in radiography.

r., oral A specialist or technician in oral radiography.

radiographic (rā″dē-ō-graf′ik) Relating to the process of radiography, the finished product, or its use.

r. anatomy *See* anatomy, radiographic.

r. contrast *See* contrast, radiographic.

r. density *See* density, radiographic.

r. diagnosis *See* diagnosis, radiographic.

r. examination *See* examination, radiographic.

r. grid A clear plastic device with the horizontal and vertical wires crossing one another at intervals of 1 mm; used in x-ray techniques for the purpose of measurement.

r. interpretation *See* interpretation, radiographic.

r. localization *See* localization, radiographic.

r. survey *See* survey, radiographic.

radiography (rā″dē-og′rah-fē) The making of shadow images on photographic emulsion by the action of ionizing radiation. The image is the result of the differential attenuation of the radiation in its passage through the object being radiographed. Roentgenography refers to production of film by the use of x-rays only.

r., bone in Radiography of bone and marrow tissue. Translucencies and opacities in bone in radiographs are dependent on the different densities that bone and marrow spaces present to the x-rays. The configuration of bone tissue represents the topography and arrangement of bone trabeculae, which register as opaque in contrast to the translucency of the marrow spaces.

r., oral The specialized operative and technical procedures and practices for making successful radiographic surveys, with the understanding that it involves the selection of the dental x-ray unit and its adjustments as well as the generation and application of x-rays to all phases of interest to the dental profession. It also takes into consideration all the processes necessary for the production of finished radiographs of the teeth and their supporting tissues, adjacent regions, and associated parts.

radioisotope (rā″dē-ō-ī′-sō-tōp) A chemical element that has been made radioactive through bombardment of neutrons in a cyclotron or atomic pile or found in a natural state.

radiologist (rā″dē-ol′ō-jist) A person who has special experience in the science of radiant energy and radiant substances (including roentgen rays); especially, a person engaged in the branch of medical science that deals with the use of radiant energy in the diagnosis and treatment of disease.

r., oral A specialist in the art and science of oral radiology.

radiology (rā″dē-ol′ō-jē) **1:** That branch of medicine dealing with the diagnostic and therapeutic applications of ionizing radiation. **2:** The science of radiant energy, its use toward the extension of present knowledge, and its diverse applications for the benefit of mankind.

r., oral All phases of the science and art of radiology that are of interest to the dental profession. It involves the generation and application of x-rays for the purpose of recording shadow images of teeth and their supporting tissues, adjacent regions, and associated parts. It also includes the interpretation of the radiographic findings.

radiolucence (rā-dē-ō-loo-sence) Relative term indicating the comparatively low attenuation of an x-ray beam produced by materials of relatively low atomic number. (The image on a radiograph of such materials will be relatively dark because of the greater amount of radiation that penetrates to reach the film.)

radiolucency (rā-dē-ō-loo-sen-sē) A radiographic representation of decreased density of hard and/or soft tissue structures.

radiolucent (rā-dē-ō-loo-sent) Permitting the passage of radiant energy, with relatively little attenuation by absorption. The image of radiolucent materials on a radiograph will range from shades of gray to black.

radionuclide (rā″dē-ō-nū-klīd) An unstable or radioactive type of atom characterized by the constitution of its nucleus and capable of existing for a measurable time. The nuclear constitution is specified by the number of protons (Z), number of neutrons (N), and energy content; or alternatively by the atomic number (Z), mass number (A − N + Z), and atomic mass.

radiopacity (rā″dē-o-păs′ĭ-tē) Relative term referring to the considerable attenuation of an x-ray beam produced by materials of relatively high atomic number. It should be noted that the image on a radiograph of such materials will be relatively light, since less radiation passes through, which prevents the exposure of the film in that area.

radiopaque (rā″dē-ō-pāk′) Permitting the passage of radiant energy but only with considerable or extreme attenuation of the radioation by absorption. The image of radiopaque materials on a radiograph will range from light gray to total white or clarity on the film. *See also* medium radiopaque.

radioparent (rā″dē-ō-par′ent) Made visible by means of roentgen rays or other means of radiation. Permitting the passage of x-rays or other radiation.

radioresistance (rā″dē-ō-rē-zĭs′tăns) The relative resistance of cells, tissues, organs, or organisms to the injurious effects of ionizing radiation. *See also* radiosensitivity.

radiosensitivity (rā″dē-ō-sen″sĭ-tiv′ĭ-tē) Relative susceptibility of cells, tissues, organs, organisms, or any substances to the injurious action of radiation.

radiotherapy *See* therapy, radiation.

radon seed (rā′don) A small sealed container or tube for carrying radon. It is made of gold or glass, is inserted into the tissues for the treatment of certain disease entities, and is visible radiographically.

rale (rāl) Abnormal sound that originates from the trachea, bronchi, or lungs.

ramify (răm′ĭ-fī) To branch; to diverge in various directions; to traverse in branches.

ramus (rā′mŭs) A branch, as of an artery, nerve, or vein. Any constant branch of a fissure, or sulcus, of the brain. In the *Basle Nomina Anatomica* terminology, the term *ramus* is given to a primary division of a nerve or blood vessel. The portions of the mandible that extend upward and backward from the horseshoe-shaped body and terminate in two processes: the artic-

ular condyloid process and the coronoid process.

r., mandibular The bilateral upturned angled bony process between the body and condylar process of the mandible.

range A crude measure of dispersion in a distribution; range is computed as in the distance from the highest score to the lowest score plus one unit.

r., melting The temperature range from the time an alloy begins to melt, until it is completely molten. It varies from 100° to 200° F (38° to 70° C) in gold-platinum-palladium alloys.

ranula (răn′ū-lah) **1:** A large mucocele in the floor of the mouth. It usually results from obstruction of the ducts of the sublingual salivary glands. Less frequently it results from obstruction of the ducts of the submandibular salivary glands. **2:** A large, mucus-containing pathologic space (mucocele) located in the floor of the mouth. It may be associated with submaxillary (submandibular) or sublingual gland secretions.

Ranvier, nodes of (rahn-vē-ă′) *See* node of Ranvier.

raphae, midpalatine (rā′fē) The ridge of mucous membrane that marks the median line of the hard palate.

rarefaction, bone *See* bone rarefaction.

rash, wandering *See* tongue, geographic.

ratchet wrench A wrench whose handle activates it through a hinged catch (pawl), thus rotating the wrench only in one direction (may be adjusted for either direction).

rate Measurement of a thing by its ratio or given in relation to some standard.

r., basal metabolic *See* basal metabolic rate.

r., DEF An expression of dental caries experience in deciduous teeth. The DEF rate is calculated by adding the number of decayed primary teeth requiring filling (D), decayed primary teeth requiring extraction (E), and primary teeth successfully filled (F). Missing primary teeth are not included in the count, since it is frequently impossible to determine whether they were extracted because of caries or were exfoliated normally.

r., DMF index A method of classifying the condition of the teeth based on the number of teeth in a given mouth that are decayed, missing, or indicated for removal and of those filled or bearing restorations. The DMF index rate is calculated by adding together the number of carious permanent teeth requiring filling (D), carious permanent teeth requiring extraction (Mr), permanent teeth previously extracted because of caries (Mp), and filled permanent teeth (F). Thus the number of DMF teeth per child of a specific age or age group can be calculated by using the following formula:

$$\frac{\text{D teeth} + \text{Mr teeth} + \text{Mp teeth} + \text{F teeth (in age or ages studied)}}{\text{Number of children examined (In specified age or ages)}} = \frac{\text{DMF rate per child in age groups}}{}$$

r., erythrocyte sedimentation The rate of settling of erythrocytes by gravity under conditions in which all factors affecting the rate are corrected, standardized, or eliminated, except for alterations in the physicochemical properties of the plasma proteins. These alterations are the basis for interpretation of the rate. There is an increase in the rate in most infections. Sedimentation velocity is useful in prognosis to determine recovery from infection. Normal values vary with the method used in the determination.

r., heart The rate of the heartbeat, expressed as the number of beats per minute. The heart rate is reflected in the pulse rate. The cardiac rate of contraction is described as normal (70 beats/min), rapid (above 100 beats/min), or slow (below 55 beats/min). Disturbances in heart rate and rhythm may be paroxysmal or persistent. Descriptive terms are *tachycardia* (increased, shallow heart rate to compensate for inadequate cardiac output) and *bradycardia* (slow, firm heart rate caused by cardiac sinus mechanisms and by the vagal effect over the sympathetic innervation of the heart).

ratification (rat-ĭ-fĭ-cā-shŭn) Confirmation of a previous act.

ratio Proportion; comparison.

r., A:G The ratio of the protein albumin to globulin in the blood serum. On the basis of differential solubility with neutral salt solution, the normal values are 3.5 to 5 Gm% for albumin and 2.5 to 4 Gm% for globulin.

r., clinical crown:clinical root The proportion of the length of the portion of the tooth lying coronal to the epithelial attachment to the length of the portion of the root lying apical to the epithelial attachment. Radiographically, the clinical crown is that portion of a tooth coronal to the alveolar crest; the clinical root is that part of the root apical to the alveolar crest. The radiographic crown: root ratio is useful in evaluation and prognosis of periodontal disease.

r., grid The relation of the height of the lead strips to the width of the nonopaque material between them. Common grid ratios are 2:8, 2:12, and 2:16.

r., water:powder Relative amounts of water and powder (usually gypsum products) in a mixture.

ray(s) A line of light, heat, or other form of radiant energy. A ray is a more or less distinct or isolated portion of radiant energy, whereas the word *rays* is a very general term for any form of radiant energy, whether vibratory or particulate.

r., alpha *See* particle, alpha.

r., beta *See* particle, beta.

r., cathode *See* electron stream.

r., central The center of an x-ray beam.

r., cosmic Radiation that has its origin outside the earth's atmosphere. Cosmic rays have extremely short wavelengths. They are able to produce ionization as they pass through the air and other matter and are capable of penetrating many feet of material such as lead and rock. The primary cosmic rays probably consist of atomic nuclei (mainly protons), some of which may have energies of the order of 1010 to 1015 eV. Secondary cosmic rays are produced when the primary cosmic rays interact with nuclei and electrons (e.g., in the earth's atmosphere). Secondary cosmic rays consist mainly of mesons, protons, neutrons, electrons, and photons that have less energy than the primary rays. Practically all the primary cosmic rays are absorbed in the upper atmosphere. Almost all cosmic radiation observed at the earth's surface is of the secondary type.

r., gamma Photons that have a shorter wavelength than those ordinarily used in diagnostic medical and dental radiography and that originate in the nuclei of atoms. A quantum of electromagnetic radiation emitted by a nucleus as a result of a quantum transition between two energy levels of the nucleus; e.g., as a radioisotope decays, it gives off energy, some of which may be in the form of gamma radiation.

r., grenz (grĕntz) Roentgen rays that are greater in length than 1 Å; used in radiography of soft tissues, insects, flowers, and microscopic sections of teeth and surrounding tissues. They are the result of using approximately 10 to 20 kV in a specially constructed radiation-generating device. They have a wavelength of about 2 Å.

r., neutron Particulate ionizing radiation consisting of neutrons. On impact with nuclei or atoms, neutrons possess enough kinetic energy to set the nuclei or atoms in motion with sufficient velocity to ionize matter or enter into nuclear reactions that result in the emission of ionizing radiation. The former variety is usually called the *fast neutron* and the latter the *thermoneutron*, with gradations of epithermal and slow neutrons between them.

r., roentgen (r) (rĕnt'gĕn) An international unit based on the ability of radiation to ionize air. The exposure to x or gamma radiation such that the associated corpuscular emission per 0.001293 Gm of air produces, in air, ions carrying 1 esu of quantity of electricity of either sign (2.083 billion ion pairs).

r.-equivalent-man (rem) The dose of any ionizing radiation that will produce the same biologic effect as that produced by 1 roentgen of high-voltage x radiation.

r.-equivalent-physical (rep) An unofficial unit of dose used with ionizing radiation other than x-rays or gamma rays. It is defined as that dose that produces an energy absorption of 93 ergs/Gm of tissue. For most purposes it can be considered equal to the rad; the latter is gradually replacing the use of rep.

rationale (rash′i-nal′) The fundamental reasons used as the basis for a decision or action.

Raynaud's phenomenon Spasm of the digital arteries with blanching and numbness of the extremities, induced by chilling, emotional states, or other diseases.

RBC *See* red blood cell count.

RBE *See* radiation, biologic effectiveness of, relative.

RDA The Recommended Dietary Allowances of the Food and Nutrition Board of the National Research Council.

reaction (rē-ăk′shŭn) Opposite action or counteraction; the response of a part to stimulation; a chemical process in which one substance is transformed into another substance or substances.

    r., alarm The first stage of the general adaptation syndrome of Hans Selye; occurs in response to severe physical and psychologic distress. Complete mobilization of body resources occurs in association with activity of the pituitary and adrenal glands and the sympathetic nervous system. *See also* syndrome, general adaptation.

    r., anaphylactoid A reaction that resembles anaphylactic shock. Probably caused by the liberation of histamine, serotonin, or other substances as a consequence of the injection of colloids or finely suspended material.

    r., Arthus′ *See* anaphylactic hypersensitivity.

    r., heterophil A heterophil agglutination test that measures the agglutination of the red blood cells of sheep by the serum of patients with infectious mononucleosis.

    r., -id Secondary skin eruptions occurring at a distance from the primary lesion (e.g., tuberculid).

    r., immune Altered reactivity of the tissues to a foreign substance that has previously been introduced into the body or was previously in contact with it.

    r., leukemoid An increase in normal and/or abnormal white blood cells in nonleukemic conditions. Simulates myelogenous, lymphatic, and, rarely, monocytic leukemia.

    r., Schwartzman An antigen AB local tissue response that occurs when an intravenous injection or challenge of a bacterial endotoxin that had previously been inoculated intradermally results in a hemorrhagic, often necrotic inflammatory lesion.

    r., tissue The response of tissues to altered conditions.

reactor (rē-ak′tar) An apparatus in which nuclear fission may be sustained in a self-supporting reaction at a controlled rate.

reagin(s) (rē′ah-jĭn) Noncommittal term used for antibodies or antibody-like substances that differ in several respects from ordinary antibodies. It refers to the antibodies of allergic conditions (atopy) and to the an-

tibody (reagin) concerned with the flocculation and complement fixation tests for syphilis.

reamer (rē′mer) An instrument with a tapered metal shaft, more loosely spiraled than a file; used to enlarge and clean root canals.

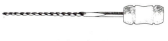

Endodontic reamer

reasonable and customary (R&C) plan A dental benefits plan that determines benefits based only on "reasonable and customary" fee criteria. *See also* usual fee; customary fee; reasonable fee.

reasonable fee The fee charged by a dentist for a specific dental procedure that has been modified by the nature and severity of the condition being treated and by any medical or dental complications or unusual circumstances and that therefore may differ from the dentist's "usual" fee or the benefit administrator's "customary" fee.

reattachment In dentistry the reattachment of the gingival ephithelium to the surface of the tooth.

rebase A process of refitting a denture by replacing the denture base material without changing the occlusal relations of the teeth.

rebound (rē′bownd) An outbreak of fresh reflex activity after withdrawal of a stimulus.

recall The procedure of advising or reminding a patient to have his oral health reviewed or reexamined; an important phase of preventive dentistry.

receipt A written acknowledgment by one person of having received money or something of value from another.

    r. book The book in which the dentist or one of the auxiliaries fills out forms verifying to the patient that a specific amount of money has been paid to the account.

reception room The area within the physical plant of the dental establishment through which patients enter the office. This is also the room in which patients await the attentions of the dentist and/or the receptionist.

receptor(s) (rē-sĕp′tŏr) A site or location within a cell or its membrane that combines with a haptophore group of a toxin, drug, enzyme, hormone, or other substance and that may elicit a specific or general response. A sensory nerve terminal that responds to stimuli of various kinds.

    r., adrenergic Alpha and beta "units" associated with sympathetic neuroeffectors that react with sympathomimetic drugs to elicit the response of the effector cells.

    r., sensory Receptor system built on the theoretic basis that receptor organs are specialized and respond to the law of specific nerve energies; i.e., each type of end-organ, no matter what stimulus is applied, will respond (if it responds) with only a single appropriate type of sensation. Common experience shows this to be true; e.g., when a person receives a blow in the eye, light is experienced as a consequence of the blow. Another factor is that the impulse will travel in only one direction, from the receptor organ back to the central nervous system. The receptor system is thus the summation in the brain of all the sensory stimuli that come from the special senses, general senses, mucous membrane, skin, and deeper tissues and is the basis for instruction sent to the musculoskeletal system for action, as in the masticatory phenomenon.

recess, rest *See* area, rest.

recession (rē-sesh'ŭn) A moving back or withdrawal.

  r., bone Apical progression of the level of the alveolar crest associated with inflammatory and/or dystrophic periodontal disease. A bone resorption process that results in decreased osseous support for the tooth.

  r., gingival Atrophy of the gingival margin associated with inflammation, apical migration (proliferation) of the epithelial attachment, and resorption of the alveolar crest.

recipient site The site into which a graft or transplant material is placed. *See also* donor site.

reciprocal arm *See* arm, reciprocal.

reciprocal forces The typical method of applying corrective orthodontic forces; each applied force is balanced by a reciprocal force elsewhere in the dentition or surrounding structures.

reciprocation (rē-sip″rō-ka′shun) The means by which one part of a removable partial denture framework is made to counter the effect created by another part of the framework.

  r., active Reciprocation in a clasp unit achieved by the use of two opposing and balanced retentive clasp arms. Reciprocation cannot be achieved unless there is a similar and balanced arrangement on the opposite side of the dental arch.

  r., passive Reciprocation in a clasp unit achieved by the use of a rigid part of the clasp, located on or above the height of contour line or on a guiding plane and opposite to the retentive arm. However, reciprocation cannot be achieved by a single clasp alone—there must be a similar action by another component of the removable partial denture located across the arch.

Recklinghausen's disease (rĕk′lĭng-how″zĕnz) *See* neurofibromatosis; osteitis fibrosa cystica.

reconstructive surgery Surgery to rebuild a structure for functional or esthetic reasons.

recontouring, occlusal The reshaping of an occlusal surface of a natural or artificial tooth.

record Information committed to, and preserved in, writing.

  r. base *See* baseplate.

  r., face-bow Registration, by means of a face-bow, of the position of the mandibular axis and/or the condyles. The face-bow record is used to orient the maxillary cast to the opening and closing axis of the articulator.

  r., functional chew-in 1: A record of the natural chewing movement of the mandible made on an occlusion rim by teeth or scribing studs. **2:** A record of the movements of the mandible made on the occluding surface of the opposing occlusion rim by teeth or scribing studs and produced by simulated chewing movements.

  r., interocclusal A record of the positional relation of the teeth or jaws to each other; made on occlusal surfaces of occlusal rims or teeth in a plastic material that hardens, such as plaster of paris, wax, zinc oxide–eugenol paste, or acrylic resin.

    r., centric interocclusal A record of the centric jaw position (relation).

    r., eccentric interocclusal A record of a jaw relation other than the centric relation.

    r., lateral interocclusal A record of a lateral eccentric jaw position.

    r., protrusive interocclusal A record of a protruded eccentric jaw position.

  r., jaw relation A registration of any positional relationship of the mandible in reference to the maxillae. The record may be of any of the many vertical, horizontal, or orientation relations.

  r., occluding centric relation A registration of centric relation made at the vertical dimension at which the teeth make contact or are to make contact.

  r., preoperative Any record or records made for the purpose of study, diagnosis, or use in treatment planning or for comparison of treatment results with the pretreatment status of the patient.

  r., profile A registration or record of the profile of a patient's face.

  r., protrusive A registration of the relation of the mandible to the maxillae when the mandible is anterior to its centric relation with the maxillae.

  r. rim *See* rim, occlusion.

  r., terminal jaw relation A record of the relationship of the mandible to the maxillae made at the vertical relation of the occlusion and at the centric position.

  r., three-dimensional (3-D record) A maxillomandibular interocclusal record.

recording The act of making a written record of the data collected during examination.

recovery In a suit at law, the obtaining or restoration of a right to something by a verdict, decree, or judgment of court.

recrystallization The return of a wrought metal to crystalline form because of excessive cold working or excessive application of heat.

rectification (rek″tĭ-fi-ka′shun) Conversion of electric current from alternating to direct (unidirectional).

rectifier (rek′tĭ-fī″er) A device used for converting an alternating current to a direct current; it also prevents or limits the flow of current in the opposite direction.

r., full-wave An apparatus for rectifying the entire wave of an alternating current in an x-ray machine by means of a mechanical rectifier or valve tube.

r., half-wave An apparatus used in the rectifying of half of the sine wave in x-ray units. red blood cell count The number of red blood cells (erythrocytes) in one cubic millimeter of blood; a useful diagnostic tool in the determination of several kinds of anemia. *See also* mean corpuscular hemoglobin.

red blood cell count The number of red blood cells (erthrocytes) in 1 mm^3 of blood; a useful diagnostic tool in the determination of several kinds of anemia. *See* mean corpuscular hemoglobin.

redressment (rē-drĕs′mĕnt) Replacement of a part or correction of a deformity.

reduced fee plan A program in which the fees established for some or all services are lower than those usually charged by dentists in the community. In some industrial plans, employers make lower fees possible by partially subsidizing the cost of providing care (e.g., furnishing rent-free facilities and paying costs of utilities). In welfare plans with limited funds, dentists may in effect subsidize the programs by accepting lower fees than they usually charge.

reducer A solution used to remove some silver from the image on a radiograph so as to produce a less intense image; an oxidizing agent used to remove excess density.

reduction in area A test to assess ductibility, whereby the cross-sectional area of the fractured end of a wire or rod is compared to the original area. A tensile test is used to break the wire.

referral The recommendation of another health professional to a patient for a specified reason.

reflection The act of elevating and folding back the mucoperiosteum, thereby exposing the underlying bone.

r., mucobuccal *See* fold, mucobuccal.

reflex(es) (rē′flĕks) A reflected action or movement; the sum total of any specific involuntary activity.

r., allied Reflexes that can join to effect a common purpose such as mastication. They may arise from diverse stimuli, such as smell, taste of food, and texture, shape, and resistance of the food bolus. Collectively, they encourage salivation and a se-

quence of masticatory closures of the mandible, followed by deglutition.

r., antagonistic Reflexes that cannot occupy the final pathway simultaneously. The weaker of these reflexes will give way to the stronger, especially if the latter is a protected reflex; e.g., a hot or nauseating food will cause involuntary retching or even vomiting rather than the pleasurable gustatory experience associated with chewing and swallowing tasty food.

r. arc *See* arc, reflex.

r., Breuer *See* reflex, Hering-Breuer.

r., Cheyne-Stokes *See* respiration, Cheyne-Stokes.

r., flexion-extension The reflexes based on the principle of reciprocal innervation. When a voluntary or reflex contraction of a muscle occurs, it is accompanied by the simultaneous relaxation of its antagonist. For example, when the jaw reflex is initiated by tapping the mandible downward, the masseter and other elevators of the mandible are stretched. Then reflex flexion-contraction of the elevators takes place, the mandible is elevated, and the depressor muscles of the mandible are stretched. There are many combinations, not only between the agonists and the antagonists about a given joint but also between reflexes that cross over to muscle groups of contralateral extremities, joints, and muscles.

r., Hering-Breuer The nervous mechanism that tends to limit the respiratory excursions. Stimuli from the sensory endings in the lungs (and perhaps in other parts) pass up the vagi and tend to limit both inspiration and expiration during ordinary breathing.

r., jaw An extension-flexion reflex that is initiated by tapping the mandible downward. The masseter and other elevators of the mandible are the first stretched; then the reflex flexion-contraction elevates the mandible by flexion of elevator muscles while there is a simultaneous stretching (extension) of the depressor muscles of the mandible.

r., pathologic Those reflexes observed in the abnormal or inappropriate motor responses of controlled stimuli initiated in the sensory organ that is appropriate to the reflex arc. They may be initiated in the superficial reflexes of the skin and mucous membrane; in the deep myotatic reflexes of the joints, tendons, and muscles; and in the visceral reflexes of the viscera and other organs of the body. The pathologic reflexes are thus syndromes of abnormal responses to otherwise normal stimuli.

r., pharyngeal Contraction of the constrictor muscles of the pharynx, elicited by touching the back of the pharynx.

r., stretch One of the most important features of tonic contraction of muscle. It is the reflex contraction of a healthy muscle that results from a pull. It has been found that stretching a muscle by as little as 0.8% of its original length is sufficient to evoke a reflex response. A stretch of constant degree causes a maintained steady contraction, muscle spindles and stretch receptors in the tendons show very slow adaptation, and the reflex ceases immediately on withdrawal of the stretching force. The stretch reflex ceases immediately on withdrawal of the stretching force. The stretch reflex is obtained predominantly from those muscles maintaining body posture, among which are the masticating muscles that maintain the position of the mandible and the neck muscles that hold the head erect. Together, the masticating muscles and neck muscles are responsible for the maintenance of the air and food passages.

r., vagovagal A reflex in which the afferent and efferent impulses travel via the vagus nerve. The afferent impulses travel centrally via the sensory nucleus of the vagus. The efferent impulses travel via the motor fibers of the vagus nerve.

refractory (re-frak′to-rē) Pertaining to the ability to withstand high temperatures used in certain dental laboratory procedures. *See also* **cast, refractory.**

refractory periodontitis (re-frak′to-rē per′ē-ō-don-tī′tis)) A progressive inflammatory destruction of the periodontal attachment that resists conventional mechanical treatment.

regeneration (rē-jen′er-ā′shun) The renewal or repair of lost tissue or parts.

r., muscle Repair of muscle tissue. When surgical intervention or inflammatory disease of dental structures injures the facial and masticatory muscles, two types of repair take place: repair by budding and repair by proliferation.

r., muscle, by budding Regeneration that takes place in destructive lesions of muscle, traumatic necrosis, hemorrhage, infarction, and suppurative myositis. The buds consist of undifferentiated plasmodial masses and certain sarcolemma nuclei. The rebuilt architecture is not classic and has bizarre and sometimes fibrous extensions that look like scarred defects.

r., muscle, by proliferation Regeneration in degenerating muscles by proliferation of bands of sarcoplasm in which the sarcolemma and its nuclei are preserved.

region, mylohyoid (mī′lō-hī′oid) The region on the lingual surface of the mandible marked by the mylohyoid ridge and the attachment of the mylohyoid muscle. A part of the alveololingual sulcus.

regional Pertaining to a region or regions.

registration The record of desired jaw relations that is made to transfer casts having these same relations to an articulator.

r. of functional form *See* **impression, functional.**

r., tissue The accurate record of the shape of tissues under any condition by means of suitable material.

regression analysis A method of correlation for computing the most probable value of one variable, y, from the known value of another variable, x; a method for computing the amount of change in one variable for a unit change in another. It is spoken of as the regression of x on y and notated r_{xy}.

regurgitation (rē-ger′jĭ-tā′shun) A backward flowing (e.g., casting up of undigested food, backward flowing of blood into the heart or between the chambers of the heart).

rehabilitation (rē″hă-bĭl″ĭ-tā′shun) Restoration of form and function.

r., mouth (oral rehabilitation) Restoration of the form and function of the masticatory apparatus condition to as near normal as possible.

rehalation Rebreathing.

reimbursement Payment made by a third party to a beneficiary or dentist on behalf of the beneficiary toward repayment of expenses incurred for a service covered by the contractual arrangement.

reimplant Replacement of a lost or extracted tooth back into its alveolus.

reimplantation *See* **replantation.**

reinforcement The increasing of force or strength.

reinsurance Insurance for third-party payers to spread their risk for losses (claims paid) over a specified dollar amount.

reintubation (rē″ĭn-tū-bā′shun) Intubation performed a second time.

Reiter's syndrome (rī′terz) *See* **syndrome, Reiter's.**

relapse To slip or fall back into a former state.

relation(s) The designation of the position of one object as oriented to another (e.g., centric relation of the mandible to the maxillae).

r., acentric *See* **relation, jaw, eccentric.**

r., centric (centric jaw relation) The relation of the mandible to the maxillae when the condyles are in their most posterosuperior unstrained positions in the glenoid fossae, from which lateral movements can be made at the occluding vertical relation normal for the individual. Centric relation is a relation that can exist at any degree of jaw separation.

r., acquired centric *See* **relation, jaw, eccentric.**

r., cusp-fossa *See* **cusp-fossa relations.**

r., dynamic Relations of two objects involving the element of relative movement of one object to another (relationship of the mandible to the maxillae).

r., eccentric *See* **relation, jaw, eccentric.**

r., intermaxillary The relation between the right and left maxilla. *See also* **relation, maxillomandibular.**

r., jaw Any relation of the mandible to the maxillae.

r., centric jaw *See* **relation, centric.**

r., eccentric jaw (convenience relationship, eccentric

relation, eccentric jaw position) Any jaw relation other than centric relation.

r., acquired eccentric jaw An eccentric relation that is assumed by habit to bring the teeth into a convenient occlusion.

r., median jaw Any jaw relation existing when the mandible is in the median sagittal plane.

r., posterior border jaw The most posterior relation of the mandible to the maxillae at any specific vertical dimension.

r., protrusive jaw (protrusive relation) A jaw relation resulting from a protrusion of the mandible.

r., rest jaw (rest) The postural relation of the mandible to the maxillae when the patient is resting comfortably in the upright position, the condyles are in a neutral unstrained position in the glenoid fossae, and the mandibular musculature is in a state of minimum tonic contraction to maintain posture.

r., unstrained jaw The relation of the mandible to the skull when a state of balanced tonus exists between all the muscles involved.

r., lateral The relation of the mandible to the maxillae when the lower jaw is in a position on either side of centric relation.

r., maxillomandibular (măk-sĭl″ō-măn-dĭb′ū-lar) Any one of the many relations of the mandible to the maxillae, such as the centric maxillomandibular relation or eccentric maxillomandibular relation.

r., median *See* relation, centric.

r., median retruded *See* relation, centric.

r., occluding The jaw relation at which the opposing teeth contact or occlude.

r., protrusive *See* relation, jaw, protrusive; position, rest, physiologic.

r., rest *See* position, physiologic rest.

r., ridge The positional relation of the mandibular ridge to the maxillary ridges.

r., static The relationship between two parts that are not in motion.

r., vertical The relative position of the mandible in a vertical direction. One of the basic jaw relations.

relationship The condition of being associated or interconnected.

r., buccolingual (bŭk″kō-lĭng′gwahl) The position of a space or tooth in relation to the tongue and cheek.

r., convenience, of teeth *See* occlusion, convenience.

r., normal A relationship in which structures conjoin as they should.

r., occlusal The individual and collective relationships of the mandibular teeth to the maxillary teeth and the relationship of the adjacent teeth in the same dental arch.

r., abnormal occlusal Occlusal relationships that deviate from the regular and established type in

such a manner as to produce esthetic disharmonies, interference with mastication, occlusal traumatism, and/or speech difficulties.

r., structure-activity (SAR) The relationship between the chemical structure of a drug and its activity.

r., tissue-base The relationship of the base of a removable prosthesis to the structures subjacent to it. There are three different possibilities: the base may be entirely tissue borne, it may be completely tooth borne, or support may be shared by both the tissue subjacent to its base and the abutment that bounds the edentulous space at one terminus.

relative value system Coded listing of professional services with unit values to indicate relative complexity as measured by time, skill, and overhead costs. Third-party payers typically assign a dollar value per unit to calculate provider reimbursement.

relaxant (rē-lăk′sănt) An antispasmodic; a drug that relaxes spasms of smooth or skeletal muscle. A drug used to eliminate muscle spasms, thus facilitating the establishment of centric relation, centric occlusion, rest position, etc. Also used in the treatment of painful muscle spasms associated with occlusal traumatism. Examples are mephenesin, the meprobamates, and methocarbamol (Robaxin).

r., muscle A drug that specifically aids in lessening muscle tension.

relaxation training A stress-reduction technique that uses a sequence of progressive exercises under the direction of a therapist to lower the level of anxiety and its neuromotor manifestations.

release To give up, as a legal claim; to discharge or relinquish a right to.

r., sustained *See* medication, sustained release.

reliability 1: In research, the reproducibility of an experimental result; the extent to which an experiment, test, or measuring procedure yields the same result during independent, repeated trials. **2:** The ability of two or more observers to examine the same data and arrive at a similar judgment within predefined bounds concerning the quality of care.

relicensure Being licensed to practice for a specific period of time with the license either being renewed at the end of that period or being forfeited. In some instances, evidence of continued competency must be submitted.

relief 1: The mitigation or removal of pain or distress. **2:** The reduction or elimination of pressure from a specific area under a denture base.

r. chamber *See* chamber, relief.

r., gingival Relief given to removable partial denture units at all gingival crossings to avoid impingement.

r. space *See* space, relief.

relieve 1: To mitigate or remove pain or distress. **2:** The procedure of placing hard wax in strategic areas on a master cast to be duplicated so that a refractory cast can be made. The purpose of relieving the master cast with wax is to provide space between certain components of the framework and the adjacent oral structures (e.g., minor connector to which the denture base will be attached, blockout or elimination of undesirable undercuts).

reline To resurface the tissue side (basal surface) of a denture with new base material so that it will fit more accurately. *See also* rebase.

rem (radiation-equivalent-man) A unit of absorbed radiation dose adjusted for biologic effects equivalent to 1 rad of 250 kV x-rays (dental and cephalometric x-rays require less than 100 kV).

millirem One one-thousandth of a rem.

remedial (re-me′de-al) Curative; acting as a remedy.

remit To send; to relinquish.

remineralization (rē-min″er-al-i-zā′shun) The reintroduction of complex mineral salts into bone, enamel, dentin, or cementum.

removable lingual arch *See* arch, removable lingual.

removable partial denture *See* denture, partial, removable.

removal, pulp *See* pulpectomy.

remuneration Pay; recompense; salary.

Rendu-Osler-Weber disease *See* telangiectasia, hereditary hemorrhagic.

rent A payment made by a tenant to an owner for the use of land or a building.

rental The fee paid by the dentist for the use of space in a building owned by someone else.

reoxidation (rē-ok″sĭ-dā′shun) The act of taking up oxygen again, as the hemoglobin of the blood.

repair 1: The process of reuniting or replacing broken parts of a denture. A means for extending the usefulness of a denture.   **2:** To make sound; to mend; restoration to former condition.   **3:** Formation of new tissues, by such processes as fibroplasia, osteogenesis, and endothelioplasia, to replace tissues damaged by disease or injury.

r., cemental Repair of areas of cemental resorption and/or cemental tears by apposition of cementum. Repair may be by formation of either cellular or acellular cementum.

replacement, prosthetic *See* prosthesis.

replantation (reimplantation) Replacement of a tooth or teeth that have been removed from the alveolus either intentionally or unintentionally, as in an accident.

replenisher A concentrated developing solution designed to maintain the active strength of developer through periodic addition to maintain original volume.

report generator A computer program for producing complete data processing reports giving only a description of the desired content and format of the out-

put reports, as well as certain information concerning the input file.

reposition, muscle Surgical replacement of a muscle attachment into a more acceptable functional position.

repositioning, jaw The changing of any relative position of the mandible to the maxillae, usually by altering the occlusion of the natural or artificial teeth.

repository Referring to long-acting drugs, usually when administered intramuscularly. *See also* medication, repository.

r., rapid Mixtures of rapid-acting and slow-acting drugs, usually administered intramuscularly.

reputation A person's credit, honor, and character; good moral estimation in which one is held.

res ipsa loquitur (rĕz ĭp′sah lōk′wĭ-ter) Latin phrase meaning the thing speaks for itself. Used in actions for injury by negligence where the happening itself is accepted as proof.

res judicata (rĕz joo′dĭ-kā″tah) Decided or determined by judicial power; a thing judicially decided.

resection Excision of a considerable portion of an organ.

r., root *See* amputation, root.

reserve Something kept in store for future use.

r., alkali *See* reserve, alkaline.

r., alkaline (alkali reserve) 1: The amount of buffer compounds (e.g., sodium bicarbonate, dipotassium phosphate, proteins) in the blood capable of neutralizing acids. One of the buffer systems of the blood than can neutralize the acid valences formed in the body. It is made up of the base of weak acid salts and usually is measured by determining the bicarbonate concentration of the plasma.   **2:** The concentration of bicarbonate ions (HCO_3) in the blood. These ions serve as a reserve in that they may be displaced by anions (e.g., CL^-, $SO_{4=}$, $PO_{4=}$). Displacement of bicarbonate ions occurs predominantly by means of the chloride shift (Hamburger's phenomenon). The role of the buffer system is such that a large influx of acid or base ions from either metabolic function or ingestion can be neutralized by the alkaline reserves from the mineral and protein salts in the blood and tissue fluids. A strong acid is transformed into a weak base. Consequently, the PH level of the blood fluctuates very little, and the tissue cells are constantly bathed in a continuously buffered solution.

r., cardiac The reserve strength or pumping ability of the heart, which may be called on in an emergency.

resident A graduate and licensed dentist or physician who has completed an internship and is serving and residing in the hospital while pursuing advanced didactic and clinical studies in special disciplines of knowledge.

residual ridge *See* ridge, residual.

residue Remainder; that which remains after the removal of other substances.

resilience (re-zil′ē-ens)   **1:** An act of springing back. **2:** Capability of a strained body to recover its size and shape after deformation.   **3:** The recoverable potential energy of an elastic solid body or stricture resulting from its having been subjected to stress not exceeding the elastic limit.

    r., modulus of The amount of energy stored up by a body when one unit volume is stressed to its proportional limit.

resin (rĕz′ĭn) Broad term used to indicate organic substances that are usually translucent or transparent and are soluble in ether, acetone, etc., but not in water. They are named according to their chemical composition, physical structure, and means for activation or curing. Examples are acrylic resin, autopolymer resin (cold-curing resin), synthetic resin, styrene resin, and vinyl resin. *See also* methyl methacrylate; varnish, cavity.

    r., acrylic 1: General term applied to a resinous material of the various esters of acrylic acid. It is used as a denture base material and also for trays and other dental restorations.   **2:** An ethylene derivative that contains a vinyl group (e.g., polymethacrylate [methyl methacrylate], the principal ingredient of many plastics used in dentistry).

    r., activated *See* resin, autopolymer.

    r., autopolymer (activated resin, autopolymerizing resin, cold-curing resin, direct restorative acrylic resin, self-curing resin) Any resin that can be polymerized by an activator and a catalyst without the use of external heat.

    r., composite A resin used for restorative purposes and usually formed by a reaction of an ether of bisphenol-A (an expoxy molecule) with acrylic resin monomers, initiated by a benzoyl peroxideamine system, to which is added as much as 75% inorganic filler (glass beads and rods, lithium aluminum silicate, quartz, and/or tricalcium phosphate).

    r., copolymer A synthetic resin that is the product of the concurrent and joint polymerization of two or more different monomers of polymers.

    r., direct restorative *See* resin, autopolymer.

    r., epoxy A resin molecule characterized by reactive epoxy, or ethoxyline, groups that serve as terminal polymerization points. Used in dentistry for denture bases.

    r., heat-curing Any resin that requires heat to activate its polymerization.

    r., quick cure *See* resin, autopolymer.

    r., self-curing *See* resin, autopolymer.

    r., thermoplastic A synthetic resin that may be softened by heat and hardened by cooling.

    r., vinyl An ethylene-derivative copolymer of vinyl

chloride and vinyl acetate. Used at one time for denture bases.

resin-filled Pertaining to a resin, usually poly (methyl methacrylate), to which has been added some inert material such as glass beads or glass rods.

resistance Ability of an individual to ward off the damaging effects of physical, chemical, or microbiologic injury. An immeasurable factor controlled and qualified by numerous local, systemic, and metabolic processes such as blood supply to tissues, nutritional status, age, and antibody formative ability.

    r., cross- A state in which an organism is insensitive to several drugs of similar chemical nature.

    r. form *See* form, resistance.

resolution The discernible separation of closely adjacent radiographic image details.

resonance (rĕz′ō-nǎns) The vibratory response of a body or air-filled cavity to a frequency imposed on it.

    r., speech The resonance of the body cavities and surfaces involved in the production of speech. The sound waves produced at the vocal folds are still far from the finished product heard in speech. The resonators give the characteristic quality to the voice. The resonating structures are the air sinuses; organ surfaces; cavities such as the pharynx, oral cavity, and nasal cavity, and chest wall. The resonating structures contribute no energy to the stream of air; they act to conserve and concentrate the energy already present in the laryngeal tone rather than to let it dissipate into the tissues. However, the resonated laryngeal tone still is not speech.

resorption (rē-sorp′shŭn)   **1:** Loss of substance (bone) by physiologic or pathologic means. The reduction of the volume and size of the residual alveolar portion of the mandible or maxillae.   **2:** The cementoclastic and dentinoclastic action that often takes place on the root of a replanted tooth.

    r. of bone 1: Destruction or solution of the elements of bone.   **2:** Loss of bone resulting from the activity of multinucleated giant cells, the osteoclasts, which are noted in irregular concavities on the periphery of the bone (Howship's lacunae).

    r., pressure, of bone Osteoclastic destruction of bone as a result of the application of sustained, excessive force on it. Remodeling of bone may occur to better adapt to these forces, or destruction may continue if the stresses are repeated and excessive.

    r., cemental Destruction of cementum by cementoclastic action. Noted as the presence of irregular concavities in the cemental surfaces.

    r., frontal Osteoclastic resorption of alveolar bone (lamina dura) by multinucleated cells on the osseous margin adjacent to the periodontal ligament.

    r., horizontal A pattern of bone resorption in marginal periodontitis in which the marginal crest of the alveolar bone between adjacent teeth remains level; in these instances the bases of the periodontal pockets are supracrestal. A pattern of bone loss in which the crestal margins of the alveolar bone are resorbed. A horizontal pattern, rather than vertical loss along the root, is the typical type of bone loss in periodontitis.

r., idiopathic Resorption that is not attributable to any known disease or is without an apparent cause.

r., internal (idiopathic internal resorption, pink tooth) A special form of idiopathic root resorption from within the pulp cavity; granulation tissue is present within the tooth, apparently with the resportion of the dentin occurring from the inside outward. The cause is unknown.

r., lacunar *See* osteoclast.

r., osteoclastic Loss of bone by cellular activity; osteoclasts are large, multinucleated cells Seen in irregular concavities in the margin of the bone (Howship's lacunae) and currently believed to be directly responsible for the active destruction of bone.

r., rear *See* resorption, undermining.

r., root Destruction of the cementum and/or dentin by cementoclastic or osteoclastic activity.

> **r., apical root** Dissolution of the apex of a tooth, resulting in a shortened, blunted root.
>
> **r., surface root** Localized resorptive areas on the cemental surface of the tooth root.

r., undermining Indirect, as opposed to frontal, removal of alveolar bone where pressure applied to a tooth has resulted in loss of vitality of localized areas of the periodontal membrane.

r., vertical A pattern of bone loss. Seen in occlusal traumatism, marginal periodontitis, periodontosis, etc. A pattern of bone loss in which the alveolar bone adjacent to a tooth is destroyed without simultaneous crestal loss, so that a vertical rather than a horizontal pattern of loss is observed.

respect To hold in high regard and to show consideration for another; mutual respect is the basis for a good doctor-patient relationship.

respiration (rĕs″pĭ-rā′shŭn) The gaseous exchange between cells of the body and the environment. There are four stages: pulmonary ventilation, diffusion of gases in the alveoli, transport of gases in the blood to and from cells, and regulation of the process.

r., artificial Maintenance of respiratory movements by artificial means. When respiration has been arrested and no mechanical device is available, resuscitation by means of artificial respiration is the only practical means of ventilating the lungs.

r., Cheyne-Stokes (chān stōks) **(Cheyne-Stokes reflex)** A type of breathing characterized by rhythmic variations in intensity that occur in cycles: rhythmic acceleration, deepening, and stopping of breathing movements.

r., controlled Maintenance of adequate pulmonary ventilation in apneic patients.

r., external Ventilation of the lungs and oxygenation of the blood.

r., internal The mechanism of gaseous exchange between blood and tissues.

r. in speech In normal speech, the action of the respiratory apparatus during exhalation, which provides a continuous stream of air with sufficient volume and pressure (under adequate voluntary control) to initiate phonation. The stream of air is modified in its course from the lungs by the facial and oral structures, giving rise to the sound symbols that are recognized as speech.

r., stertorous Snoring.

r., stridulous A high-pitched sound occurring during respiration resulting from adduction of the vocal cords.

respirator (rĕs′pĭ-rā″tor) An apparatus that qualifies the air that is breathed through it; a device for giving artificial respiration.

respirometer (res″pĭ-rom′ēter) An instrument for studying and determining the character and extent of respiration.

respondeat superior A legal doctrine that passes the legal responsibility for acts or omissions of an employee to the employer.

response Action or movement resulting from the application of a stimulus.

rest 1: Passive support. **2:** An extension from a prosthesis that affords vertical support for a restoration.

r. area *See* area, rest.

r., auxiliary The rest other than the one used as a component part of a primary direct retainer.

r., finger *See* finger rest.

r., incisal A metallic extension onto the incisal angle of an anterior tooth to supply support and/or indirect retention for a removable partial denture.

r., lingual A metallic extension onto the lingual surface of an anterior tooth to provide support or indirect retention for a removable partial denture.

r., occlusal (occlusal lug) A rest placed on the occlusal surface of a posterior tooth.

r. occlusion *See* position, rest, physiologic.

r. position *See* position, rest.

r., precision A unit consisting of two closely fitted parts, the insert of which rests firmly against the gingival portion of the tubelike receptacle.

r. relation *See* relation, jaw, rest.

r. seat *See* area, rest.

restoration (prosthetic restoration) Broad term applied to any filling, inlay, crown, bridge, partial denture, or complete denture that restores or replaces lost tooth structure, teeth, or oral tissues. A prosthesis.

r. of cusps (preferred to tipping, capping, or shoeing

cusps) Reduction and inclusion of cusps within a cavity preparation and their restoration to functional occlusion with restorative material.

r., dental prosthetic *See* prosthesis, dental.

r., faulty Restoration in which there are imperfections or incorrect attributes (e.g., overhanging or deficient fillings, incorrect anatomy of occlusal and marginal ridge areas, faulty clasps). Such faults may be present in individual tooth restorations, fixed bridges, removable partial dentures, etc., and are conducive to the initiation and perpetuation of inflammatory and dystrophic diseases of the teeth and/or periodontium.

r., implant The single-tooth implant crown or multiple-tooth implant, crown, or bridge that replaces a missing tooth or teeth.

r., prosthetic *See* prosthesis.

restorative 1: Promoting a return to health or to consciousness; a remedy that aids in restoring health, vigor, or consciousness. **2:** Pertaining to rebuilding, repairing, or reforming.

r. dentistry Branch of dentistry that deals with the reconstruction of the hard tissues of a tooth or group of teeth injured or destroyed by trauma or disease.

r. materials Materials used to reconstruct the hard tissues of teeth lost through trauma or disease.

restrainer A chemical ingredient (potassium bromide) of the photographic developing solution. Its function is to inhibit the fogging tendency of the solution. Like the activator, the restrainer also controls the rate of development.

restrictive covenant Common clause found in a contract for the sale of a dental practice. The seller contracts that he or she will not practice dentistry within a certain time and area. A junior partner may be asked to sign such a covenant to guarantee that he or she will not compete with the partnership for a period of time after leaving the partnership. Also used in an employment situation.

resuscitation (rē-sŭs″ĭ-tā′shŭn) Restoration of life or consciousness to one who appears to be dead.

resuscitator (rĕ-sŭs′ĭ-tā″tor) An apparatus for initiating respiration in asphyxia.

retail dentistry Fee for service dentistry practiced in an exclusively retail environment (e.g., shopping center, department store) and directed to the clientele of that retail center, using the marketing technique of the parent retailer.

retail store dentistry Dental services offered within a retail, department, or drug store operation. Typically, space is leased from the store by a separate administrative group that in turn, subleases to a dentist or dental group providing the actual dental services. The dental operation generally maintains the same hours of operation as the store, and appointments often are not necessary. Considered to be a type of practice, not a dental benefits plan model.

retainer (retaining appliance) 1: The part of a dental prosthesis that unites the abutment tooth with the suspended portion of the bridge. It may be an inlay, partial crown, or complete crown. **2:** An appliance for maintaining the positions of the teeth and jaws gained by orthodontic procedures. **3:** The portion of a fixed prosthesis attaching a pontic(s) to the abutment teeth (e.g., inlay, three-quarter crown). **4:** An form of clasp, attachment, or device used for the fixation or stabilization of a prosthetic appliance. **5:** Any orthodontic appliance, fixed or removable, used to maintain teeth in corrected positions during the period of functional adaptation following corrective treatment.

r., continuous bar A metal bar that is attached to a major connector and contacts lingual surfaces of anterior teeth, on or incisal to the cingula; it aids in the stabilization of a distal extension removable partial denture.

r., direct A clasp, attachment, or assembly applied to an abutment tooth for the purpose of maintain- ing a removable restoration in its planned position in relation to oral structures.

r., extracoronal 1: The type of retainer in which the preparation and its cast restoration lie largely external to the body of the coronal portion of the tooth and complement the contour of the crown. The retention or resistance to displacement is developed between the inner surfaces of the casting and the external walls of the prepared tooth. The extracoronal retainer may be a partial crown, a complete crown, etc. **2:** A direct retainer of the clasp type that engages an abutment tooth on its external surface in such a way as to afford retention and stabilization to a removable partial denture. A direct retainer of the manufactured type, the male portion of which is attached to the external surface of a cast crown on an abutment tooth (e.g., Dalbo and Crismani attachments).

r., Hawley A wire and acrylic resin removable appliance designed to stabilize teeth after tooth movement; to serve as a basis for tooth movement by providing an anchorage for wires, rubber dam elastics, etc., used in orthodontic tooth movement.

r., indirect That part of a removable partial denture that resists movement of a free end denture base away from its tissue support through lever action opposite the fulcrum line of the direct retention.

r., intracoronal 1: The type of retainer in which the prepared cavity and its cast restoration lie largely within the body of the coronal portion of the tooth and within the contour of the crown (e.g., inlay). The retention or resistance to displacement is developed between the casting and the internal walls of the prepared cavity.   **2:** The type of direct retainer used in the construction of removable partial dentures; it consists of a female portion within the coronal portion of the crown of an abutment and a fitted male portion attached to the denture proper. These retainers may be fabricated or machined in the dental office or obtained through commercial sources.

r., matrix (matrix holder) A mechanical device designed to engage the ends of a matrix around the tooth.

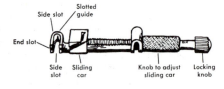

Tofflemire amalgam matrix retainer

r., radicular The type of retainer that lies within the body of the tooth and is usually confined to the root portion of the tooth (e.g., dowel crown). The retention or resistance to displacement and shear is developed by extending an attached dowel into the root canal of the tooth.

retaining ring A ring that holds the arch wire against the premolar bracket to allow free sliding and tipping.

retarder A chemical added to a certain substance to slow a chemical reaction, prolong the set of the material, and provide more working time.

rete pegs (rē-tē) *See* pegs, epithelial.

retention (rē-těn'shŭn)   **1:** Power to retain; capacity for retaining. The inherent property of a restoration to maintain its poiition without displacement under stress; results from close adaptation of the restoration to the prepared form of the tooth, usually aided by cement.   **2:** Term relating to the provision, in cavity preparation, for preventing displacement of a restoration. Retention supplements resistance form and is specifically created to resist any lateral or tipping force that may be brought against the restoration during and after its insertion.   **3:** Resistance of a denture to removal in a direction opposite that of its insertion. The quality inherent in the denture that resists the force of gravity, adhesiveness of foods, and forces associated with the opening of the jaws.   **4:** The period of treatment during which the individual is wearing an appliance to maintain the teeth in the position into which they have been moved.

r. arm *See* arm, retention.

r., circumferential Frictional resistance to displacement derived from completely veneering the exposed tooth surface.

r., denture 1: The means by which dentures are held in position in the mouth. The maintenance of a denture in its position in the mouth. The resistance to the movement of a denture from its basal seat in a direction opposite that in which it was inserted.   **2:** The resistance of a denture to vertical movement in the occlusal direction from its basal seat.

r., partial denture The fixation of a fixed partial denture by means of crowns, inlays, and/or other retainers.

r., removable partial denture The resistance to movement of a removable partial denture from its supporting structures, gained by the use of direct and indirect retainers and/or other attachments.

r., direct Retention obtained in a removable partial denture by the use of attachments or clasps that resist removal from abutment teeth.

r. form *See* form, retention.

r., indirect Retention obtained in a removable partial denture through the use of indirect retainers.

r. pin *See* pin, retention.

r., pinhole One or more small holes, 2 to 3 mm in depth, placed in suitable areas of a cavity preparation parallel with the general line of draft to provide or supplement resistance and retention form.

r., radicular Retention derived from projections of metal into the root canals of pulpless teeth.

r. terminal *See* clasp, circumferential arm; clasp, circumferential, arm, retentive.

reticulocytosis (rē-tĭk'ū-lō-sī-tō-sĭs) An increase in the normal number of reticulocytes in the circulating blood. Normal values range from 0.5% to 1.5% of the red blood cells.

reticuloendotheliosis, nonlipid (rē-tĭk"u-lō-ĕn"do-thē"lē-ō'sĭs) *See* disease, Letterer-Siwe.

retraction 1: A drawing or shrinking back; the laying back of tissues to expose a given part.   **2:** Distal movement of teeth. A distal or retrusive position of the teeth, dental arch, or jaw.

r., gingival Laying back of the free gingival tissue to expose the gingival margin area of a preparation by mechanical, chemical, or electrical means.

retractor An instrument for retracting tissues to assist in gaining access to an area of operation or observation.

r., beaver-tail A broad-bladed periosteal elevator.

r., rake A metallic instrument with prongs set transversely for engaging and retracting soft tissues.

r., vein hook A metallic instrument ending in a rounded flange set transversely for engaging and retracting soft tissues.

retroclination Posterior angulation (inclination) of anterior teeth.

retrofill Obturation of the apex of a tooth root by the direct surgical approach.

retrognathic (ret″rō-nath′ik) **1:** The condition of a mandible that is posterior to its normal relationship with other facial structures. May be a result of small mandibular size and/or posteriorly positioned temporomandibular fossae. **2:** Mandibular retrusion.

retrognathism (rĕt″rō-nǎth′ĭzm) Facial disharmony in which one or both jaws (usually the mandible) are posterior to normal facial relationships. This condition may be real or imaginary.

r., bird-face Typical facial profile associated with an underdeveloped mandible. A retrognathia and small mandible usually associated with interference of condylar growth because of trauma or infection affecting the condyles. Surgical intervention is necessary for improvement.

r., Pierre Robin *See* syndrome, Pierre Robin.

retromolar pad *See* pad, retromolar.

retromylohyoid eminence *See* eminence, retromylohyoid.

retromylohyoid space *See* space, retromylohyoid.

retrospective review A posttreatment assessment of services on a case-by-case or aggregate basis after the services have been performed.

retrosternal pain A pain behind the sternum usually on swallowing. If retrosternal pain is associated with oral or pharyngeal candidiasis, it may indicate candidiasis of the esophagus, which is an opportunistic infection indicative of AIDS.

retroversion (rĕt″rō-ver′zhŭn) A condition in which teeth or other maxillary and mandibular structures are located posterior to the normal or generally accepted standard.

Retrovir Brand name for zidovudine, a dideoxynucleoside used in the treatment of HIV-positive patients.

retrovirus (ret″rō-vī′rus) A virus containing RNA rather than DNA.

retruded contact position A tooth-to-tooth position at centric relation, sometimes referred to as *centric relation occlusion*.

retrusion (re-troo′zhun) Teeth and/or jaws posterior to their normal positions.

r., mandibular Abnormal retrusion of the mandible, as in a Class II malocclusion.

r., maxillary Abnormal retrusion of the maxillae.

reverse curve *See* curve, reverse.

reverse transcriptase An enzyme within a retrovirous that converts its RNA into DNA, which then penetrates the cell nucleus and joins the host's DNA.

reversible Capable of going through a series of changes in either direction, forward or backward (e.g., reversible chemical reaction).

r. hydrocolloid *See* hydrocolloid, reversible.

review coordinator A member of the staff of a PSRO or hospital generally responsible to a utilization review committee. Such persons perform or assist in concur-

rent review or audit studies, initiating or coordinating with discharge planning, recording and transmitting review decisions, or acting as liaison with persons and organizations participating in and affected by the review system.

rewards A motivation technique to improve patient compliance with oral hygiene protocols, generally used with young patients.

rhabdomyosarcoma (răb″dō-mī″ō-sar-kō′mah) A malignant tumor of striated, or voluntary, muscle.

rhagades (răg′ah-dēz) Fissures or cracks in the skin seen around body orifices and in regions subjected to frequent movement.

rheology (rē-ol′ō-jē) The study of blood flow, pressure, and velocity through the vascular system.

rheostat (rē′ō-stat) A resistor for regulating a current by means of variable resistances.

rheumatic fever *See* fever, rheumatic.

rheumatism (roo′mah-tĭzm) **(rheumatic disease)** Nonspecific term indicating any painful disorder related to joints, muscles, bone, or nerves; acute rheumatic fever; or, as used by lay persons, rheumatoid arthritis, bursitis, myositis, or degenerative joint disease.

rhinolalia (rī″nō-lā′lē-ah) Nasalized speech, of which there are two types: rhinolalia clausa (closed port) and rhinolalia aperta (open port).

rhinoplasty (rī′nō-plas″tē) Plastic or reconstructive surgery of the nose.

rhizotomy, retrogasserian (rī-zot′ō-mē, rĕt″rō-găs-sē′rē-ăn) Intracranial sectioning of the sensory root of the trigeminal nerve posterior to the semilunar ganglion. Used in the treatment of a severe trigeminal neuralgia.

rhythm (rĭth′m) A measured movement; the recurrence of an action or function at regular intervals.

r., heart The rhythm pattern in the sequence of heart beats that may be altered in the presence of cardiac disease.

riboflavin (rī″bō-flā′vĭn) *See* vitamin, riboflavin.

rickets (rĭk′ĕts) A condition caused by deficiency of vitamin D and/or calcium in infants and children with disturbance in the mineralization of osseous and dental tissues. Marked by bending and bowing of bones, nodular enlargements at the ends of bones, myalgia, delay in closure of fontanels, etc. *See also* osteomalacia.

r., adult *See* osteomalacia.

r., refractory *See* rickets, resistant.

r., renal A disturbance marked by excessive excretion of phosphorus and calcium resulting from a lowered renal threshold of excretion of these mineral elements. *See also* osteodystrophy, renal.

r., resistant (late rickets, refractory rickets) Rickets that responds only to extremely large amounts of vitamin D.

ridge The remainder of the alveolar process after the

teeth are removed.

r., alveolar The bony ridge of the maxillae or mandible that contains the alveoli (sockets of the teeth). *See also* process, alveolar.

r., center of The buccolingual midline of the residual ridge.

r., crest of The highest continuous surface of the ridge but not necessarily the center of the ridge. The top of a residual or alveolar ridge.

r. extension *See* extension, ridge.

r., key (zygomaxillare) The lowest point of the zygomaticomaxillary ridge.

r. lap The part of an artificial tooth that is adjacent to the residual ridge. The part of the artificial tooth that laps the ridge.

r., marginal A ridge or elevation of enamel that forms the boundary of the occlusal surface of a tooth.

r., mental A dense ridge extending from the symphysis to the premolar area on the anterolateral aspect of the body of the mandible.

r., mylohyoid A dense line or ridge of bone on the medial surface of the body of the mandible that extends obliquely upward and posteriorly from the symphysis, covers the cervical portion of the third molar, and then goes upward and backward onto the vertical ramus. The mylohyoid muscle is inserted into this ridge of bone.

r., Passavant's *See* pad, Passavant's.

r. relation *See* relation, ridge.

r., residual The portion of the alveolar ridge that remains after the alveoli have disappeared from the alveolar process after extraction of the teeth.

r. support *See* area, supporting.

Riga-Fede disease (rē′gah fā′dah) *See* disease, Riga-Fede.

right of action The right to sue; a legal right to maintain an action, based on a happening or state of fact.

right-angle technique *See* technique, parallel.

rigidity The characteristic of being nonflexible, which is essential in a connector, a reciprocal arm, or an indirect retaining unit of a removable partial denture.

Riley-Day syndrome *See* syndrome, Riley-Day.

rim The outer edge; often curved or circular.

r., occlusion (record rim) An occluding surface built on temporary or permanent denture bases for the purpose of making maxillomandibular relation records and for arranging teeth.

r., surgical occlusion A conventional occlusion rim, the base of which has been reduced until it is smaller than the surgical impression tray with which the surgical jaw relations are recorded.

r., record *See* rim, occlusion.

rinse bath A tank or container of water used in film processing to wash residual developer from the film prior to its being placed in the fixer.

Risdon wire *See* wire, Risdon.

Risdon's incision *See* incision, Risdon's.

risk factors Elements that may contribute to or increase risk to one's health, economic stability, or personal and professional liability.

risk management A program designed to identify, contain, reduce, or eliminate the potential for harm to patients, visitors, and employees and the potential financial loss to the facility if a compensable event occurs; usually concerned with the delivery system and/or site rather than practitioner performance.

risk pool A portion of provider fees or capitation payments withheld as financial reserves to cover unanticipated utilization of services in an alternative benefits plan.

RNA viruses *See* viruses.

Roach clasp *See* clasp, bar.

Rockwell test *See* test, Rockwell.

rod A straight, slim, cylindric form of material, usually metal.

r., analyzing The vertical part of a dental cast surveyor that is brought into contact with the surface contour of a tooth as a tangent related to a curve. It is used to determine the relative parallelism of one surface of a cast to other surfaces of the same cast. It is also used to estimate the cervical convergence of an infrabulge area of a tooth as it slopes from the contacting point of the surveying rod toward the cervical line, permitting evaluation of the retentiveness of the surface.

r., condyle The adjustable pointers of a face-bow, which are placed over the condyles or at points on the face, marking the opening axis of the mandible.

r., enamel A calcified column or prism, with an average diameter of 4 μ; extends in a wavy pattern through the entire thickness of the enamel and generally is perpendicular to the surface of the tooth.

roentgeno- (rĕnt′gĕn-ō) Prefix used to denote radiation originating only from an x-ray tube.

roentgenogram (rĕnt′gen-ō-grăm″) *See* radiograph and subentries.

roentgenograph (rĕnt′gĕn-ō-grăf) *See* radiograph.

roentgenographer (rĕnt″gĕ-nog′rah-fer) *See* radiographer.

roentgenographic detail *See* detail, radiographic.

roentgenography (rĕnt″gĕn-ŏgrah-fē) *See* radiography and subentries.

roentgenologist (rĕnt″gĕn-ol′ō-jĭst) *See* radiologist.

r., oral *See* radiologist, oral.

roentgenolucent (rĕnt″gĕn-ō-lū′sĕnt) *See* radiolucent.

roentgenopaque (rĕnt″gĕn-ō-pāk′) *See* radiopaque.

roentgenoparent (rĕnt″gĕn-ō-păr′ĕnt) *See* radioparent.

roentgenotherapy (rĕnt″gĕn-ō-thĕr′ah-pē) *See* therapy, radiation.

Roger's syndrome *See* syndrome, Roger's.

root 1: The part of a human tooth covered by cementum. **2:** A nerve root; the part of a nerve adjacent to the center with which it is connected; in spinal and cranial nerves, the part of the nerve between the cells of origin or termination and the ganglion.

r. amputation *See* amputation, root.

r. canal instrument stop A device placed on a root canal instrument to mark the measured depth of instrument penetration.

r. curettage *See* curettage, root.

r., intra-alveolar The portion of a tooth root enclosed in and supported by alveolar bone.

r. resection *See* apicoectomy.

r. retention Removal of the crown of a root canal-treated tooth, whose periodontium is not adequate to support a prosthesis, but with enough retention of the root and gingival attachment to give support to a removable prosthesis. *See also* overdenture.

r. submersion Root retention, in which the tooth structure is reduced below the level of the alveolar crest, and the soft tissue is allowed to heal over it. It is believed that residual ridge resorption can be minimized by this approach. *See also* root retention.

rosary, rachitic A beading of the ribs at the costochondral junction such as occurs in rickets.

Rosenthal's syndrome *See* hemophilia C.

rotary cutting instrument *See* instrument, cutting, rotary.

rotating anode *See* anode, rotating.

rotating condyle *See* condyle, rotating.

rotating spring An auxiliary wire used in conjunction with arch wire to rotate a tooth into proper position.

rotation 1: The act of turning about an axis or a center. **2:** Movement of a tooth around its longitudinal axis.

r. center *See* center, rotation.

Rothera's test *See* test, ketone bodies.

routine 1: A fixed pattern of procedures used in any phase of treatment. **2:** A set of instructions arranged in proper sequence to direct the computer to perform a desired operation or series of operations.

r., office A series of steps, to be followed in a carefully planned sequence, that provide a means of dealing with situations commonly developing in dental practice.

rubber dam *See* dam, rubber.

rubber dam clamp *See* clamp, rubber dam.

r. d. c. forceps An instrument used to place a clamp on a tooth or to adjust a clamp or remove it from a tooth. It engages the holes or notches of the flanges of the clamp.

rubber dam holder In endodontics, a rubber dam frame holder; in operative dentistry, a rubber dam frame.

rubella (roo-bĕl′ah) **(German measles, 3-day measles)** A highly contagious viral disease spread chiefly by direct contact and having an incubation period of about 18 days. Manifestations include pharyngitis, regional lymphadenopathy, mild constitutional symptoms, and a maculopapular rash that becomes scarlatiniform. Oral lesions are red macules.

rubeola (roo-bē-ō′lah) *See* measles.

Ruffini's corpuscles (roo-fē′nēz) *See* corpuscle, Ruffini's.

rugae (ru′gī; rū′jē) The irregular ridges in the mucous membrane covering the anterior part of the hard palate.

r. area *See* area, rugae.

rule, Clark's A formula used estimating the dosage of a drug for individuals whose weight varies from the arbitrarily selected official standard of 150 pounds (67.5 kg).

$$\frac{\text{Weight of patient}}{150} \times \text{Usual adult dose} = \text{Dose}$$

rule, Young's A mathematic expression used to determine a drug dosage for children.

$$\frac{\text{Age of child}}{\text{Age} + 12} \times \text{Usual adult dose} = \text{Child's dose}$$

Rumple-Leede test *See* test, capillary resistance.

run One performance of a program on a computer; performance of one routine or several routines automatically linked so that they form an operating unit, during which manual manipulating by the computer operator is usually not required.

Sabouraud's medium (sab'oo-roz) *See* medium, Sabouraud's.

saccharin The chemical sweetener benzosulfimide, which is 300 to 500 times as sweet as sucrose. Tests have demonstrated that large amounts of benzosulfimide can cause cancers in experimental animals. Saccharin is no longer in general use as a low-calorie sweetner.

saddle *See* base, denture.

s. connector *See* connector, major.

s., metal *See* base, metal.

safe-light A source of illumination in a darkroom of a color and intensity that will not fog a radiographic film.

safety measures Actions taken to protect patients and office personnel from known hazards (e.g., particles and aerosols from high-speed rotary instruments [glasses, face mask], mercury vapor, radiation exposure, anesthetic or sedative gases, falls, inadequate sterilization, cuts, puncture wounds, laboratory accidents).

sagittal (săj'ĭ-tăl) Shaped like or resembling an arrow; straight; situated in the direction of the sagittal suture. Said of an anteroposterior plane or section parallel to the long axis of the body.

s. plane *See* plane, sagittal.

s. splitting of mandible Intraoral osteotomy of the ascending ramus and posterior body of the mandible in the sagittal plane for the correction of prognathism, retrognathism, or apertognathia. An alternative procedure confines the split to the body of the mandible.

St. Vitus' dance (sānt vī'tŭs) *See* chorea.

Sainton's disease (săn'tōnz) *See* dysostosis, cleidocranial.

salary 1: A fixed regular compensation paid for service rendered involving professional knowledge or skill or employment above the degree of mechanical labor. **2:** The amount of take-home pay received by the dentist from the practice.

s. arrangements The clear understanding between the dentist and auxiliaries concerning the amount of money they will be paid, the increase in pay they may expect, and the time interval between pay increases.

salicylamide (sal'ĭ-sil-am'ĭd) An analgesic, antipyretic, and antiarthritic similar in action to aspirin.

salicylanilide (sal'ĭ-sil-an'ĭ-lid) An antifungal agent useful in the treatment of tinea capitus caused by *Microsporum audouinii*.

salicylates (sal'ĭ-sil"āts) Salts or esters of salicylic acid; salicylates are used as preservatives, antiseptics, fungicides, and keratolytic agents.

salicylism (săl'ĭ-sĭl"ĭzm) A toxic state resulting from excess ingestion of salicylates.

saline (sā'lēn) Salty; of the nature of a salt; containing a salt or salts.

saliva (sah-lī'vah) The clear, slightly acid mucoserous secretion formed in the parotid, submaxillary, sublingual, and smaller oral mucous glands. It has lubricative, cleansing, bactericidal, excretory, and digestive functions and is also an aid to deglutition. Its pH level is slightly acidic—6.3 to 6.9. Emotional disturbances affect the rate of salivary secretion either by stimulation of secretion or inhibition of activity, leading to xerostomia. A lowered rate of flow has been noted in depressed patients, whereas a higher degree of salivary activity has been exhibited in manic patients.

s., lingual Saliva secreted by Ebner's glands and other serous glands of the tongue.

s., loss of CO_2 in A theory of calculus formation in which the loss of CO_2 from saliva reduces the salivary carbonic acid content and causes the calcium phosphate in solution in the saliva to become supersaturated; calcium phosphate then precipitates in areas of stasis of the saliva.

s., parotid Saliva produced by the parotid gland. It is thinner and less viscous than the other varieties, containing no mucin.

s., supersaturated Saliva overladen with mineral elements associated with calculus formation. With a loss of CO_2 and a rise in the pH level of saliva, precipitation of calcium, phosphates, magnesium carbonate, etc., will occur, thus providing the mineral components of salivary calculus.

s. tests *See* tests, calorimetric caries susceptibility.

salivant (săl'ĭ-vănt) Provoking a flow of saliva.

salivary glands Three pairs of exocrine glands that produce saliva and empty it into the mouth. The parotid glands produce serous fluid, the sublingual glands produce mucous fluid, and the submandibular glands produce serous and mucous secretions.

salivary lactobacillus count Determination of the number of lactobacilli per milliliter of saliva; an indicator of caries susceptibility. High lactobacillus counts generally correlate with high caries activity.

salivation (săl″ĭ-vā′shŭn) Excessive discharge of saliva; ptyalism.

salt (săwlt) A compound of a base and an acid; a compound of an acid, some of whose replaceable hydrogen atoms have been substituted.

   s., basic A salt containing replaceable, or hydroxyl, groups.

   s. depletion *See* depletion, salt.

sample A selected part of a population that is taken to be representative of the whole population.

   s., random A sample drawn by chance; a sample drawn in such a way that every item in the population has an equal and independent chance of being included in the sample.

   s., stratified A sample derived by dividing the population into a number of nonoverlapping classes or categories from which cases are selected at random, the number of cases selected from each category being proportional to the number therein.

sanguinaria (sang″gwĭn-a′rē-ah) A benzophenanthridine alkaloid thought to be useful in reducing plaque and gingivitis. Although it has been marketed, test results have been equivocal, and untoward side effects have been reported.

SAR *See* relationship, structure-activity.

sarcoidosis (sar″koi-dō′sĭs) **(Besnier-Boeck-Schaumann disease, Boeck's sarcoid)** A chronic granulomatous disease of unknown etiology. Causes noncaseating granulomas in the skin, lymph nodes, salivary glands, eyes, lungs, and bones.

sarcoma (sar-kō′mah) **1:** A malignant neoplasm of connective tissue elements. **2:** A malignant neoplasm arising from mesenchyme or its derivatives.

   s., ameloblastic A rare mixed tumor of odontogenic origin in which the mesenchymal component has undergone malignant transformation.

   s., Ewing's *See* tumor, Ewing's.

   s., Kaposi's A condition affecting blood vessels believed to be of a neoplastic nature and of multicentric origin. Skin lesions appear as multiple red-brown nodules ranging from a few millimeters to 1 cm in size. Histologically, endothelial proliferation in sheets or small vessels, hemosiderin deposits, fibroblastic proliferation, and an inflammatory infiltrate of lymphocytes are seen.

   s., neurogenic (malignant schwannoma) The malignant form of neurilemoma.

   s., osteoblastic (osteogenic sarcoma) An osteosarcoma in which atypical bone formation is the most evident histopathologic feature. *See also* osteosarcoma.

   s., osteogenic A malignant connective tissue tumor that produces bone.

   s., reticulum cell A malignant tumor of reticulum cells. It may occur as a primary neoplasm in soft tissue or bone.

satin finish *See* finish, satin.

Sargenti technique *See* N2.

satisfaction Discharge of an obligation by actual payment of what is due or what is awarded by a court or otherwise.

saturated Having all the chemical affinities satisfied; unable to hold in solution any more of a given substance.

saturation, color The quality of color that distinguishes the degree of vividness of hue (e.g., differing in degree from gray).

saucerization (saw″ser-i-zā-shun) Excavation of the tissue of a wound, forming a shallow, saucerlike depression.

   s., pericervical The circular bone resorption that occurs about the necks of endosteal implants shortly after their insertion and that continues slowly during the time of the implant's biologic presence.

saw A cutting blade with a toothed edge used to cut material too hard to slice with a knife (e.g., plaster saw).

   s., Gigli's wire A flexible wire with teeth used for osteotomy procedures, frequently as a blind operation.

   s., gold An instrument with a thin sawlike blade used for removing surplus metal from the contact area of gold-foil restorations.

   s., Joseph's A nasal saw often used in a ramusotomy of the mandible.

   s., Koeber's A saw consisting of a thin, replaceable blade held in a frame; used to trim gross excess from the proximal portion of a Class 2 foil restoration in the preliminary stages of finishing and contouring.

   s., oscillating (Stryker-type saw) An oscillating blade in an electrical or compressed gas-driven unit used to cut bone.

   s., rotary A rotary blade on a shaft in an electrical or compressed gas-driven unit used to cut bone.

SBE *See* endocarditis, subacute bacterial.

scaffold A support, either natural or artificial, that maintains tissue contour.

scaler (skā′ler) An instrument used in the operation of removing calculus from teeth.

   s., sickle A hook-shaped instrument available in various sizes and shapes, designed to be used for the removal of tenacious supragingival deposits of calculus.

scaling The removal of calcareous deposits from the teeth by using suitable instruments.

   s., coronal The removal of deposits of calculus, heavy

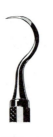

Sickle scaler

stains, materia alba, etc., from the crowns of the teeth by suitable instrumentation.

s., electrosurgical *See* electrosurgery; scalpel, electrosurgical.

s., root A technique of root surface cleansing designed to remove accretions of calculus and debris in the supragingival uninvested areas of a tooth.

s., subgingival The removal of accretions and debris from the surfaces of the tooth apical to the gingival margin. This process accomplishes the removal of primary irritants to the gingival tissues and permits the reduction of inflammation in these tissues.

s., supragingival The technique of meticulous cleansing of the surfaces of the teeth coronal to the gingival margin.

scalpel A delicate, razor-sharp, pointed knife, usually with a convex edge.

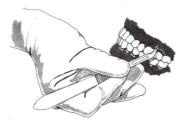

Scalpel

s., electrosurgical A scalpel that severs tissue by means of an electrically heated wire.

scar *See* cicatrix.

s., apical The end product of wound repair. A radiolucent area characterized histologically by dense fibrous connective tissue.

scarlatina *See* fever, scarlet.

scarlet fever *See* fever, scarlet.

scattered radiation *See* radiation, scattered.

Schaumann's body *See* body, Schaumann's.

Schaumann's disease *See* sarcoidosis.

schedule The division of the working day into segments of time to enable the dentist to render treatment.

s. of allowances (table of allowances) A list of specified amounts that will be paid toward the cost of dental services rendered; the patient pays the difference between the allowance and the actual cost of service.

s. of benefits A listing of the services for which payment will be made by a third-party payer without specification of the amount to be paid.

s. plan A plan that bases covered expenses on a schedule of allowances.

schema, Hamberger's (skē'mah) The bodily arrangement by which the external intercostal and intercartilaginous muscles are inspiratory muscles, and the internal intercostal muscles are expiratory muscles.

scheme, occlusal *See* system, occlusal.

Schick test (shĭk) *See* test, Schick.

schistometer (skĭs-tom'ĕ-ter) An instrument for measuring the aperture between the vocal cords.

schistosomiasis (skĭs"tō-sō-mī'ah-sĭs) **(biharziasis)** Infestation with blood flukes of the genus *Schistosoma*, causing cystitis, chronic dysentary, hepatosplenomegaly, and esophageal varices.

schizophrenia (skĭz'ō-frē'nē-ah) **(dementia precox)** A functional psychosis (split personality) characterized by emotional distortion, withdrawal from reality, and disturbances of thought processes. It includes such disorders as hebephrenia, catatonia, and paranoia.

Schüller-Christian disease *See* disease, Hand-Schüller-Christian.

Schüller' disease (shĭl'erz) *See* osteoporosis.

schwannoma (shwah-nō'mah) *See* neurilemoma.

s., malignant *See* sarcoma, neurogenic.

scissors, Fox Delicate, fine-pointed scissors designed to gain access to interproximal areas for the removal of small tissue tabs or slight soft issue deformities during gingivoplasty and/or gigivectomy. Can also be used to smooth the cut gingival surfaces.

scleroderma (sklĕ-rō-der'mah) **(dermatosclerosis, hidebound disease)** A collagen disease of unknown etiology; skin lesions are characterized by thickening, rigidity, and pigmentation in patches or diffuse areas. Dermal atrophy may also be seen. Periodontal lesions may simulate those of periodontosis, with widening of periodontal membrane space (vertified by radiographic evidence) resulting from bone resorption, loss of architectural arrangement, and degeneration of periodontal fibers, with absence of inflammatory change in the gingivae and remaining periodontium.

sclerosis (sklĕ-rō'sĭs) Hardening. As applied to the jaws, sclerosis usually indicates an increased calcification centrally, with radiopacity. Tracts of increased density in the dentin are referred to as areas of dentinal sclerosis. Sclerosis occurs beneath caries and with abrasion, attrition, or erosion.

s., multiple A remitting and relapsing disease of the central nervous system affecting principally the white matter. Manifestations include sensory and motor incoordination and paresthesias; ultimately there is often dementia, blindness, paraplegia, and death.

scoliosis (skō″lē-ō′sĭs) A lateral curvature of the spine.

scope of services The number, type, and intensity or complexity of services being provided.

scopolamine (sko-pol′ah-mēn) An alkaloid found in the leaves and seeds of *Atropa belladonna* and other solancaceous plants having an action similar to atropine and used when spasmolytic or antisecretory effects are desired.

scorbutus (skor-bū′tŭs) *See* scurvy.

screen, intensifying A layer of fluorescent crystals (usually calcium tungstate) supported on a flat base. Used in intimate contact with light-sensitive radiographic film in a cassette. The crystals fluoresce when exposed to x radiation and subsequently expose the film with light.

screen, oral A Plexiglas or acrylic resin appliance that fits into the vestibule of the mouth for the correction of mouth breathing.

screening 1: Any examination of individuals or their records to ascertain dental needs, assess treatment plans, or evaluate services rendered. Prescreening is the review by designated dentists of patients' examination records as a prerequisite to the authorization of some or all types of treatment. Postscreening is the examination by designated dentists, usually on a sample basis, to determine if services have been rendered adequately and in accordance with prescribed administrative procedures. **2:** A sample survey to determine initial treatment needs of a group seeking coverage under a dental plan; used in setting the initial premium.

screw, expansion An orthodontic mechanism for achieving movement of teeth or arch segments, consisting of a threaded shaft and sleeve arrangement that permits controlled separation of elements of the appliance.

screw, implant A small screw 3 to 5 mm long that is used as a means for primary retention of the implant.

screwdriver *See* instrument, screwdriver.

Screw-Vent A brand name of aa blade implant of solid design manufactured by Core-Vent of pure titanium and much smaller than the companion product, the Core-vent system.

scribe To write, trace, or mark by making a line or lines with a pointed instrument or carbon marker.

scrofula (skrof′ū-lah) A primary tuberculosis complex occurring in the orocervical region and consisting of tuberculous cervical lymphadenopathy and tuberculosis of adjacent skin (lupus vulgaris), with chronic draining sinuses below the angle of the jaw and cervical region.

scurvy (skŭr′vē) **(scorbutus)** A condition resulting from an ascorbic acid deficiency that is severe enough to desaturate the tissues. The development and manifestations depend on tissue storage of ascorbic acid and factors that influence the rate at which it is used in or released from the tissues. Manifestations of frank scurvy include weakness, poor wound healing, anemia, and hemorrhage under the skin and mucous membranes. Presence or severity of gingival changes is directly related to the presence of local irritants such as calculus. In a severe form and in infantile scurvy, painful subperiosteal hemorrhages occur.

s., infantile (Barlow's disease, Cheadle's disease, Moeller's disease) A nutritional disease of infants caused by a deficiency of vitamin C in the diet. It has the same symptoms as scurvy in adults.

s., land *See* purpura, thrombocytopenic, idiopathic.

seal 1: Something that firmly closes or secures. **2:** A tight and perfect closure. **3:** To keep shut, enclosed, or confined.

s., border *See* border seal.

s., double A seal consisting of gutta-percha underneath another material (e.g., temporary cement); used to close the coronal opening in a tooth during endodontic treatment.

s., hermetic Perfect and absolute obliteration of all space within a tooth.

s., peripheral *See* border seal.

s., posterior palatal The seal at the posterior border of a denture produced by displacing some of the soft tissue covering the palate by extra pressure developed in the impression or by scraping a groove along the posterior seal area in the cast on which the denture is to be processed.

s., postpalatal *See* seal, posterior palatal.

sealant, pit and fissure A resinous material designed for application to the occlusal surfaces of posterior teeth to seal the surface irregularities to prevent ingress of oral fluids, food, and debris.

sealer A substance used to fill the space around silver or gutta-percha points in a pulp canal. Most sealers contain some combination of zinc, barium, and bismuth salts and eugenol, Canadian balsam, and eucalyptol.

seat, basal *See* basal seat.

seat, rest *See* area, rest.

sebaceous glands (sĕ-bā′shus) Exocrine glands of the skin, many of which open into the hair follicles and secrete an oily substance that coats the hair and surrounding epithelium, helping to prevent evaporation of sweat and to retain body heat.

secobarbital (sē″kō-bar′bĭ-tal) A barbiturate capable of producing all levels of CNS mood alteration from excitation to sedation and finally to deep coma. Barbiturates are recommended only for short-time use as sedatives or hypnotics. Barbiturates are controlled substances. Brand name: Seconal.

secondary cancer An opportunistic neoplasm imposed on a host in whom there is reduced vitality and/or resistance resulting from a preceding neoplasm or infection.

secondary infectious disease An opportunistic infection imposed on a host in whom there is reduced vitality and/or resistance resulting from a preceding infection by a more virulent organism.

secondary radiation *See* radiation, secondary.

second-opinion program An opinion about the appropriateness of a proposed treatment provided by a practitioner other than the one making the original recommendation; some benefits plans require such opinions for selected services.

secretary-receptionist The auxiliary whose chief responsibilities are to receive patients into the office, handle the correspondence and bookkeeping, order supplies, supervise housekeeping, and answer the telephone.

secrete To discharge or empty a substance into the blood stream, into a cavity, or onto the surface of the body. The substance secreted is known as a *secretion*. Glands that secrete internally are endocrine or ductless glands; glands that secrete into a cavity or onto the surface are exocrine or duct glands.

sectional impression An impression made in two or more parts.

sectioning, surgical Dividing a tooth to facilitate its removal. A variety of instruments, including osteotomes and power-driven burs, are used.

sedation (se-dā′shŭn) The production of a sedative effect; the act or process of calming.

sedative (sĕd′ah-tĭv) **1:** Production of sedation. A drug that can produce sedation. **2:** Any one of the drugs that produces cortical depression of varying degrees. **3:** A remedy that allays excitement and slows down the basal metabolic rate without impairing the cerebral cortex.

seeds, radon *See* radon seed.

segment Any of the parts into which a body naturally separates or is divided, either actually or by an imaginary line.

seizure disorders *See* epilepsy.

selection Choosing among alternatives.
　s., shade (tooth color selection) The determination of the color (hue, brilliance, saturation, translucency) of the artificial tooth or set of teeth for a given patient.
　s., tooth The selection of a tooth or teeth (shape, size, color) to harmonize with the individual characteristics of a patient.
　s., tooth color *See* selection, shade.

selective grinding *See* grinding, selective.

selectivity, sensory The property of the specialized re-

ceptor end-organ by which it responds to one type of stimulus rather than another.

selenium (sĕ-le′nē-um) A trace element used as sulfide in the treatment of seborrhea or dandruff of the scalp. Selenium is toxic in large amounts.

Selenomonas (se″le-nō-mō′nas) A genus of gram-negative, anerobic, rod-shaped bacteria found in the oral cavity.

self-analysis Introspection on one's own behavior an actions in the total environment.

self-curing resin *See* resin, autopolymerizing.

self-funding The method of providing employee benefits in which the sponsor does not purchase conventional insurance but rather elects to pay for the claims directly, generally through the services of a TPA. Self-funded programs often have stop-loss insurance in place to cover abnormal risks.

self-insurance Setting aside of funds by an individual or organization to meet anticipated dental care expenses or its dental care claims and accumulation of a fund to absorb fluctuations in the amount of expenses or claims. The funds set aside or accumulated are used to provide dental benefits directly instead of purchasing coverage from an insurance carrier.

self-tapping implant An implant that cuts its own path into bone.

self-tapping screw A screw that cuts its own spiral threads into bone or tooth structure.

sella turcica (sella) (S) The pituitary fossa. The center is used as a cephalometric landmark.
　s. t., floor of Lowermost point on the internal contour of the sella turcica.

Selter's disease *See* erythredema polyneuropathy.

semicoma A mild coma from which the patient may be aroused.

seminarcosis *See* sleep, twilight.

semipermeable (sĕm″ē-per′mē-ah-bl) Permitting the passage of certain molecules and hindering that of others.

senescence, dental (se-nĕs′ĕns) A condition of the teeth and associated structures in which there is deterioration resulting from aging or premature aging processes.

senility (se-nil-ĭ-tē) Old age; generally used to describe the cognitive and physiologic signs of advancing age.

sensation(s) (sĕn-sā′shŭn) An impression conveyed by an afferent nerve to the sensorium commune.
　s., psychologic effects of Arousal, facilitation, and distortion of sensation by psychologic factors, the basis for which lies in the corticalization of the special senses.
　s., referred A group of vaguely classified sensations that are a consequence of cortical experience. They are the sensory hallucinations, paresthesias, and the phenomenon called *phantom limb*. Nonspecific and poorly localized pain in the alveolar ridges, which

have poor vascular supply, may be evidence of this phantom limb phenomenon associated with neurotic behavior.

s., specialized Sensations that are perceived by the specialized end organs associated with special senses, such as vision, hearing, and smell.

sense(s) (sĕns) A faculty by which the conditions or properties of things are perceived. Hunger, thirst, malaise, and pain are varieties of sense.

s., special One or all of the five senses: feeling, hearing, seeing, smell, and taste.

sensibility, deep (sĕn″sĭ-bĭl′ĭ-tē) Perception of pressure, tension, and pain from the deeper structures, as contrasted with sensations derived from the superficial layers of the skin.

sensitive (sĕn′sĭ-tĭv) Able to receive or transmit a sensation; capable of feeling or responding to a sensation.

sensitivity, tooth The state of responsiveness of teeth to external influences such as heat, sugar, and trauma. May result from occlusal traumatism, especially if the anatomic relation of the apical foramen to the traumatized tissue is such that the circulation of the pulp is disturbed.

sensitization (sĕn″sĭ-tĭ-zā′shŭn) The process of rendering a cell sensitive to the action of a complement by subjecting it to the action of a specific amboceptor; anaphylaxis.

sensorium (sĕn-so′rē-ŭm) Any sensory nerve center; more frequently, the whole sensory apparatus of the body.

sensory (sĕn′sō-rē) Pertaining to or subserving sensation.

separating medium *See* medium, separating.

separating spring Spring placed between adjacent teeth to obtain separation.

separating wire *See* wire, separating.

separator An instrument used to wedge teeth apart, out of normal contact by immediate separation; useful in the examination of proximal surfaces of teeth and in finishing proximal restorations. Must be used with care, and usually it should be stabilized against the teeth with modeling compound to prevent tissue damage.

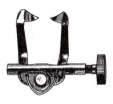

Mechanical separator

s., Ferrier's One of a set of balanced, double-bowed

adjustable separators designed by W.I. Ferrier.

s., noninterfering *See* separator, True's.

s., True's (noninterfering separator) A single-bowed separator designed to give greater access to the surface being operated on; designed by Harry A. True.

sepsis, oral (sĕp′sĭs) A condition occurring within the mouth and/or adjacent areas characterized by the presence of pathogens.

septicemia (sĕp″tĭ-sē′mē-ah) A condition in which pathogenic bacteria and bacterial toxins circulate in the blood. Manifestations include high temperature, leukocytosis, malaise, rapid pulse, and subsequent diffuse systemic degenerative disturbances.

septum, interdental (interdental alveolar septum) The portion of the alveolar process extending between the roots of adjacent teeth.

septum, nasal The thin, vertical bony septum separating the right and left nasal cavities.

sequence Order of occurrence or performance.

sequestrum (sē-kwĕs′trŭm) A piece of dead bone that has become separated from vital bone.

serial extraction A program of selective extraction of deciduous and sometimes permanent teeth over a period of time, with the objective of relieving crowding and facilitating the eruption of remaining teeth into improved positions. Close supervision of ensuing eruption is essential, because overclosure of the spaces and other sequelae can be expected in a significant number of cases. Comprehensive orthodontic treatment should almost always be initiated in the course of or after eruption, for space management, control of the autonomous tipping usually induced by the procedure, and other malrelationships that commonly accompany these conditions.

serology tests (se-rol′-ō-jē) Diagnostic tests of serum usually used to determine the immune or lytic properties of serum.

seronegative (se″ro-neg′ah-tiv) Serologic evidence of the lack of an antibody of a specific type in the serum; diagnostically useful in ruling out Lyme disease, syphilis, HIV, serum hepatitis B, and many other viral diseases.

seropositive (se″ro-poz′ĭ-tiv) Serologic evidence of the presence of an antibody of a specific type in the serum; diagnostically useful in identifying many types of viral diseases.

seroprevalence rates (se″ro-prev′ah-lens) A statistical measure of the rate of occurrence of seropositive status in a population or sample; used as a criterion of comparision between populations or samples.

serotonin (sē″rō-tō′nĭn) **(enteramine, thrombocytin)** A local vasoconstrictor (5-hydroxytryptamine) and general hypotensive agent synthesized from tryptophan and found in tissues, rather than being transferred by blood to sites of action. Most serotonin in mammals is found in the gastrointestinal tract, although the kidney, liver, and brain also produce it. It is absorbed by platelets from the site of tissue damage, where it aids hemostasis locally by vasoconstriction and systemically by reducing blood pressure.

serozyme (ser′ō-zīm) *See* factor VII.

serum (sē′rŭm) The fluid component of the blood containing all stable constituents except fibrinogen. When blood is allowed to clot and stand, a clear yellowish fluid, which is serum, separates.

  s. accelerator globulin *See* accelerator, prothrombin conversion, I.

  s. protein determination, electrophoretic Separation of serum protein fractions (albumin, alpha globulin, beta globulin, and gamma globulin) based on their different isoelectric points and thus their mobility in an electric field. Electrophoretic patterns and concentrations are of value in evaluating the hyperglobulinemias. Electrophoretic evaluation of serum protein abnormalities is usually related to moving-boundary or paper-strip separation patterns.

  s. prothrombin conversion accelerator (SPCA) *See* factor VII; thromboplastin, extrinsic.

  s. sickness Anaphylactoid or allergic reaction after injection of foreign serum; marked by urticarial rashes, edema, adenitis, arthralgia, high fever, and prostration.

servant One who is employed to perform personal services (other than those which would be rendered in an independent calling) for an employer and who, in that service, remains entirely under the control of the employer.

  s., loaned A person whose services have been granted by an employer to another person. service(s) Performance of labor for the benefit of another.

service(s) Performance of labor for the benefit of another.

  s., denture Diagnosis and treatment of edentulous and partially edentulous patients, including the diagnosis of existing and potential oral pathosis, planning of treatment for the preparation of the mouth for complete or partial dentures, fabrication and adjustment of the prostheses, and continuing observation of the changes in the oral conditions as the prostheses are in use.

  s., gratuitous A service that does not involve a return, compensation, or consideration.

  s., health Those services, including dentistry, which improve the general physical and mental wellbeing of the patient.

set Term applied to a state of a plastic material after it has hardened or jelled by chemical action, cooling, or saponification. It is used in connection with impression materials, waxes, and gypsum materials.

setting expansion *See* expansion, setting.

setting time *See* time, setting.

set-off *See* offset.

setup 1: The arrangement of teeth on a trial denture base. **2:** A laboratory procedure in which teeth are removed from a plaster cast and repositioned in wax. May be used as a diagnostic tool to evaluate alternatives, as when some teeth are missing; also used to produce the mold to make a positioner appliance.

sex Classification of an individual as a male or female on the basis of anatomic, functional, hormonal, and chromosomal characteristics.

  s., anatomic Classification of sex based on sexual differentiation of the primary gonads.

  s., chromosomal (genotype) Chromosomal characteristics involving normally 44 somatic and 2 sex chromosomes, the latter designated as XX for the normal female and XY for the normal male. The presence of the Y chromosome is associated with a male phenotype and its absence with a phenotypic female.

  s. chromosomes Chromosomes responsible for sex classification—XX for female, XY for male.

  s., functional (phenotype) Designation of sex based on the state of maturation and potential for use of the external genitalia.

  s., hormonal Contributory assignment of sex on the basis of adequate levels of estrogen and androgen for the development of typical phenotypic secondary sex characteristics.

  s., legal That sex assigned at birth or legally by a court of law.

  s. linkage *See* linkage, sex.

  s., nuclear Sex determination based on the presence or absence of the hyperchromatic nucleolar satellite in squamous cells from a buccal mucosa smear or of "drumsticks" in the polymorphonuclear neutrophil. Positives are normally seen in the female.

sexual harassment In 1986, the United States Supreme Court adopted the definition of *sexual harassment* formulated by the Equal Employment Opportunity Commission as follows: Unwelcome sexual advances, requests for sexual favors, and other verbal or physical conduct of a sexual nature when (1) submission to such conduct is made either explicitly or implicitly a term or condition of an individual's employment, (2) submission to or rejection of such conduct by an individual is used as a basis for employment decisions affecting such individual, (both quid pro quo harassment()or (3) such conduct has the purpose or effect of unreasonably interfering with an individual's work performance or creating an intimidating, hostile, or offensive working environment (condition of work harassment).

sexually transmitted diseases *See* venereal diseases.

sharpening, instrument Establishing or restoring of a keen edge on a cutting instrument.

Sharpey's fibers *See* fiber, Sharpey's.

shave biopsy The removal of a thin layer of tissue using a dermatome knife. *See also* biopsy, shave.

shear *See* strength, shear; strength, ultimate.

shearing cusps The upper buccal cusps, lower lingual cusps, upper canines, and upper incisors. Each of these cusps helps form the fossae that receive the stamp cusps. In the postcanine teeth, the tringular ridges of the shearing cusps are bold in arming the fossae with cutting ridges.

sheath, nucleated *See* neurilemma.

sheath, primitive *See* neurilemma.

sheath of Schwann *See* neurilemma.

shedding *See* exfoliation.

shelf, buccal The surface of the mandible from the residual alveolar ridge or alveolar ridge to the external oblique line in the region of the lower buccal vestibule. It is covered with cortical bone.

shelf life The length of time a material may be stored without deterioration; the length of time it remains usable.

shellac base *See* base, shellac.

shield, radiation A body of material used to prevent or reduce the passage of particles of radiation. A shield may be designated according to what it is intended to absorb (e.g., gamma ray, neutron shield) or according to the kind of protection it is intended to give (e.g., background, biologic, or thermal shield). The shield of a nuclear reactor is a body of material surrounding the reactor to limit the escape of neutrons and radiation into the protected area. Shields may be required to protect personnel or to reduce radiation sufficiently to allow use of counting instruments for research or for locating contamination or airborne radioactivity.

shift, axis *See* axis shift.

shift, chloride *See* phenomenon, Hamburger's.

shift to right or left An arbitrary description of an increase in the number per unit volume of immature (shift to left) or mature (shift to right) forms of neutrophils, in the differential counting system of Schilling.

shingles *See* herpes zoster.

shock 1: A state of collapse of the body after injury or trauma. Shock may be either primary or secondary. The principal effects of shock are the slowing of the peripheral blood flow and a reduction in cardiac output. **2:** Circulatory insufficiency caused by a disparity between the circulating blood volume and the vascular capacity.

    s., galvanic Pain produced as a result of galvanic currents caused by similar or dissimilar metallic restorations.

    s., hemorrhagic An ineffectual circulating volume of blood resulting from loss of whole blood.

    s., insulin Coma resulting from too much insulin or an inadequate intake of food. Symptoms include wet or moist skin, hypersalivation or drooling, normal blood pressure, tremors, dilated pupils, normal or bounding pulse, and firm eyeballs. Sugar and acetoacetic acid may be present in bladder urine but will be absent in the second specimen. The blood sugar will be low. *See also* coma, diabetic.

    s., neurogenic Shock caused by loss of nervous control of peripheral vessels, resulting in an increase in the vascular capacity. Onset is usually sudden but is quickly reversible if the cause is removed and treatment is instituted immediately.

    s., primary Shock that has a neurogenic basis in which pain and psychic factors affect the vascular system. Occurs immediately after an injury.

    s., secondary Shock that occurs some time after the injury (6 to 24 hours later). Secondary shock is associated with changes in capillary permeability and subsequent loss of plasma into the tissue spaces. Changes in capillary permeability are probably related to histamine release associated with tissue injury.

    s., traumatic Any shock produced by trauma, whether psychic or physical. In general usage, this term refers to shock following physical trauma, with hemorrhage, peripheral blood vessel dilation, and/or changes in capillary permeability.

shoeing cusps *See* restoration of cusps.

short-cone technique *See* technique, short-cone.

shoulder In extracoronal cavity preparations, the ledge formed by the meeting of the gingival wall and the axial wall at a right angle.

    s., linguogingival The portion of a prepared cavity in the proximal surface of an anterior tooth that is formed by the angular junction of the gingival and lingual walls. Developed to facilitate the dense compaction of the gold in this area.

shrinkage 1: Reduction or decrease in extent or quantity. **2:** Reduction in volume.

    s., casting Volume change (contraction) that occurs when the molten metal solidifies after being cast into the pattern mold. It is compensated for in three ways: by using the indicated water: powder ratio for the refractory investment to gain the maximum setting expansion of which that investment is capable; by exposing the investment to moisture as the refractory investment sets, causing some hydroscopic expansion; and by properly heating the mold to achieve thermal expansion. The total expansion must equal the contraction of the metal being cast.

shunt, arteriovenous (arteriovenous aneurysm, arteriovenous fistula) Abnormal communication between an artery and a vein; usually caused by trauma.

shut The part of an anterior artificial tooth between the ridge lap and the shoulder. The pins for retaining the tooth in the base material are located in the shut.

sialadenitis (sī″ăl-ăd″ĕ-nī′tĭs) Inflammation of the salivary gland, especially the accessory glands, because of trauma.

sialoadenectomy (sī″ah-lō-ăd″ĕnĕk′tō-mē) Excision of a salivary gland.

sialoangiectasis (sī″ah-lō-ăn′jē-ĕk′tah-sĭs) (ptyalectasis) **1:** Dilation of the salivary ducts. **2:** Operative dilation of the salivary ducts.

sialodochitis (sī″ah-lō-dō-kī′tĭs) Inflammation of salivary gland ducts.

sialodochoplasty (sī″ah-lō-dō′kō-plăs″tē) A surgical procedure for the repair of a defect and/or restoration of a portion of a salivary gland duct.

sialogogue (sī-ăl′ō-gog) A substance that increases the flow of saliva.

sialograph (sī-ăl′ō-grăf) A radiograph made to determine the presence or absence of calcareous deposits in a salivary gland or its ducts.

sialography (sī″ah-log′rah-fē) **1:** Inspection of the salivary ducts and glands by x-ray film after injection of a radiopaque medium. **2:** Production of a sialograph.

sialolith (sī-ăl′ō-lĭth) A salivary calculus. *See also* culus, dental.

sialolithiasis (sī″ah-lō-lĭ-thī′ah-sĭs) Presence of salivary gland or duct stones.

sialolithotomy (sī″ah-lō-lĭ-thot′ō-mē) Removal of calculus from a salivary gland or duct.

sialorrhea (sī″ah-lō-rē′ah) **(hypersalivation, ptyalism)** Excessive flow of saliva. It may be associated with acute inflammation of the mouth, mental retardation, neurologic disorders with lenticular involvement, mercurialism, pregnancy, ill-fitting dental appliances, dysautonomia, periodic diseases, cystic fibrosis of the pancreas, teething, alcoholism, and malnutrition.

   s., periodic Recurrent episodes of hypersalivation; of unknown cause but probably related to recurrent parotitis and other so-called periodic diseases.

sialoschesis (sī″ah-los′kĕ-sĭs) Suppression of salivary secretion (dry mouth). Usually this condition contraindicates the wearing of a dental prosthesis during sleep.

sialosemeiology (sī″ah-lō-sē″mī-ol′ō-jē) Analysis of the salivary secretion. The quantity and composition of saliva may be determined, although this procedure has not been used to any degree in oral diagnosis.

sib (sĭb) Abbreviated form for sibling, meaning brother or sister.

sibilant (sĭb′ĭ-lănt) Accompanied by a hissing sound; especially a type of fricative speech sound.

sickle (sĭk′l) *See* scaler, sickle.

sickle cell anemia *See* anemia, Sickle cell.

sicklemia (sĭk-lē′mē-ah) *See* anemia, sickle cell.

side effect An effect not sought in the case under treatment.

sideropenic dysphagia (sĭd″er-ō-pe′nĭk dĭs-fa′jē-ah) *See* syndrome, Plummer-Vinson.

side-shift Imprecise Anglo-Saxon–based term for lateral thrust of the rotating condyle. The Latin-based term for side-shift is laterotrusion.

sigh (sī) An audible and prolonged inspiration, followed by a shortened expiration.

sigmoid notch (sĭg′moid) *See* notch, mandibular.

sign(s) (sīn) An indication of the existence of something; any objective evidence of a disease.

   s., Battle's The ecchymosis that appears near the mastoid process of the temporal bone; indicative of a fracture of the base of the skull.

   s., Bell's The turning up of the eyeball on the affected side when a patient with Bell's palsy attempts to close the eyelid.

   s., Nikolsky's A diagnostic feature wherein apparently normal epithelium can be rubbed off with finger pressure.

   s. and symptoms, diagnostic The objective and subjective features of disease that are carefully evaluated to establish a diagnosis.

   s., Tinel's A paresthesia in the area served by a sensory nerve when the site of a lesion or injury to the nerve is percussed. Indicative of partial injury of a nerve or regeneration of an injured nerve.

signa (sĭg′nah) **(signature)** The portion of a prescription that contains a statement of the directions for use.

signature *See* signa.

silica (sĭl′ĭ-kah) **(quartz)** The purest of three major ingredients that make up dental procelain. It imparts stiffness and hardness to the product and is the framework around which the kaolin and feldspar contract.

silicate cement (sĭl′ĭ-kăt) *See* cement, silicate.

silicone (sĭl′ĭ-kōn) A compound of organic structural character in which all or some of the positions that could be occupied by carbon atoms are occupied by silicon. A plastic containing silicons.

silicophosphate cement *See* cement silicophosphate.

silver amalgam *See* amalgam, silver.

silver cones An endodontic filling material used in conjunction with gutta-percha points and sealing agents to effect a seal of the pulp chamber and canal. Synonym: master cones.

silver halide crystals *See* crystal, silver halide.

silver nitrate, ammoniacal (ăm″ō-nī′ah-kal) **(ammoniated silver nitrate, Howe's silver nitrate)** An ammonium compound of silver nitrate, introduced by Percy R. Howe in 1917, that is more readily reduced to silver and silver proteinates than the usual silver nitrate; formerly used to disclose carious tooth structure and to immunize incipient carious lesions of the enamel but is highly irritating to the pulp.

silver nitrate, Howe's *See* silver nitrate, ammoniacal.

Simmonds' disease *See* disease, Simmonds'.

silver points *See* silver cones.

Simon's classification of malocclusion A classification of malocclusion in which tooth malpositions are related to three craniofacial planes: midsagittal, orbital, and frankfort. Teeth too close to the midsagittal plane are in contraction, whereas those too far are in distraction. Teeth too anterior to the orbital plane are in protraction, whereas those too posterior to the orbital plane are in retraction. Teeth too close to the Frankfort plane are in attraction, whereas those too distance are in distraction.

sine curve The wave form of an alternating current characterized by a rise from zero to maximum positive potential, a descent back through zero to its maximum negative value, and then a rise back to zero.

single crystal sapphire A single crystal endosteal implant made of alpha alumina oxide with a Knoop Hardness Number of 1.750. The implants are threaded and supplied in three sizes: 3, 4, and 5.

single emulsion (film) *See* emulsion, single.

sinus (sī'nŭs) A cavity, recess, or hollow space.

  s., alveolar A passage connecting a pathologic cavity in the alveolus with the oral or nasal cavity and penetrating the mucous membrane. *See also* fistula, alveolar.

  s. balloon *See* balloon, sinus.

  s., carotid The dilated portion of the internal carotid artery.

  s., coronary The venous sinus in the groove between the left cardiac auricle and the left ventricle.

  s., maxillary (antrum of Highmore, maxillary antrum) A large pyramidal cavity within the body of the maxilla. Its walls are thin and correspond to the orbital, nasal anterior, and infratemporal surfaces of the body of the maxilla. On dental radiographs, the floor of the sinus is often observed approximating the root apices of the teeth and is seen to extend from the canine or premolar region posteriorly to the molar or tuberosity region.

  s., paranasal Accessory sinuses of the nose.

  s. tract *See* tract, sinus.

sinusitis Inflammation of the sinus.

Siwe's disease (se'vehz) *See* disease, Letterer-Siwe.

Sjögren's syndrome (syĕh'grĕnz) *See* syndrome, Sjögren's.

skeletal discrepancies An orthodontic term used to describe the nature of a malocclusion as being a malrelationship of the bony base rather than merely of the teeth.

skeletal relationships The orientation of bony parts one to the other; usually the lower to upper jaw or to the base with which they articulate.

skeleton of partial denture *See* framework.

skill Practical knowledge of an art, science, profession, or trade and the ability to apply it in practice in a proper manner.

  s., reasonable That which is ordinarily possessed and exercised by persons of similar qualifications engaged in the same employment or profession.

slander Oral defamation; the saying of false and malicious words about another, resulting in injury to the reputation of the other.

slant of occlusal plane The inclination measured by the angle the occlusal plane makes when extended to intersect with the axis-orbital plane.

sleep A period of rest for the body and mind, during which volition and consciousness are in partial or complete abeyance and the bodily functions partially suspended.

  s., twilight (seminarcosis) A state of amnesia and analgesia produced by an injection of scopolamine and morphine.

slice In cavity preparation, a straight-line (plane) cut that removes a thin layer from an axial convexity.

slim disease A constitutional disease of AIDS also called *HIV wasting syndrome* characterized by fever for more than 1 month, involuntary weight loss of greater than 10%, and diarrhea persisting for more than 1 month.

slope, lower ridge The slope of the mandibular residual ridge in the second and third molar region as seen from the buccal side.

slotted attachment *See* attachment, intracoronal.

Sluder's neuralgia *See* neuralgia, Sluder's.

Smallpox *See* variola.

smear, bacterial Bacteria taken from a lesion or area, spread on a slide, and stained for microscopic examination.

sneeze An involuntary, sudden, violent expulsion of air through the mouth and nose; may be elicited during thiopental (Pentothal) anesthesia by corneal stimulation.

snuff dipper's lesion A white or discolored lesion of the oral mucosa occurring at the site at which the powdered tobacco is retained. Malignant transformations are not common but do occur, usually as low-grade verrucous carcinomas.

Snyder's test *See* test, colorimetric caries susceptibility.

soap A salt or mixture of salts, of aliphatic acids, such as palmitic, stearic, or oleic acid, with sodium or potassium used for cleaning purposes.

sob A short, convulsive inspiration, attended by contraction of the diaphragm and spasmodic closure of the glottis.

social functioning Ability of the individual to interact in the normal or usual way in society; can be used as a measure of quality of care.

socket 1: The hollow part of a joint; the excavation in one bone of a joint that receives the articular end of another bone. **2:** Any hollow or concavity into which another part fits, as the eye(s).

  s., dry (alveolalgia, infected socket localized alveolar osteitis) An osteitis or periostitis associated with infection and disintegration of the clot after tooth extraction. Because of its painful nature, it also is called *alveolalgia*.

s., infected See socket, dry.

s., tooth Alveolus; the cavity in the alveolar process of the jaw in which the root of a tooth is fixed.

sodium aluminum fluoride See cryolite.

sodium fluoride (sō'dē-ŭm flor'īd) (NaF) A white, odorless powder used in 2% aqueous solution and applied topically to teeth as a caries-preventing agent; used as 33% NaF in kaolin and glycerin as a desensitizing agent for hypersensitive dentin. In drinking water, one part per million of NaF is used as a caries-prophylactic substance.

sodium perborate (sō'dē-ŭm per-bor'āt) ($NaBO_2 \cdot H_2O_2 \cdot 3H_2O$) An oxygen-liberating antiseptic that has been used in the treatment of necrotizing ulcerative gingivitis and other forms of gingival inflammation. Prolonged and/or indiscriminate use has produced burns of the oral mucosa and hyperplasia of the filiform papillae of the tongue (black hairy tongue). Also used to bleach pulpless teeth.

sodium thiosulfate (sō'dē-ŭm thī"ō-sŭl-'fāt) A powdered chemical, commonly called *hypo*, that is an ingredient of the fixing solution used in film processing. Its action is to clear the film of undeveloped silver halide crystals.

soft radiation See radiation, soft.

soft tissue All body tissue except bone, teeth, nails, hair, and cartilage.

soft tissue undercut See undercut, soft tissue.

software Various programming aids supplied by the manufacturer to facilitate the user's efficient operation of the equipment. The collection of programs, routines, and documents associated with a computer (e.g., compilers, library routines).

solder, *n.* (sod'er) A fusible alloy of metals used to unite the edges or surfaces of two pieces of metal.

soldering flux See flux, soldering.

soldering investment See investment, soldering; investment, refractory.

solubility (sŏl"ū-bĭl'ĭ-tē) The quality or fact of being soluble; susceptible to being dissolved.

solute (sō'lūt) The dissolved (usually the less abundant) constituent of a solution. **solution** (sŏ-lū'shŭn) The process of dissolving. In chemistry, a homogeneous dispersion of two or more compounds. In pharmacy, usually a nonalcoholic solution. Solutions containing alcohol are variously called *elixirs, tinctures, spirits, essences,* or *hydroalcoholic solutions.*

s., Carnoy's A sclerosing solution; mild; will not cauterize normal oral mucosa if used judiciously. A mild hemostatic.

s., cleansing A solution especially suited to the removal of adherent food particles by immersion of

the denture to avoid damaging the denture by brushing.

s., disclosing A topically applied dye used in aqueous solution to stain and reveal the extent of calcareous and mucinous deposition on the teeth.

s., hardening An aqueous solution (often of 2% potassium sulfate) in which a hydrocolloid impression may be immersed to reduce or retard syneresis of the impression material.

s., parenteral A sterile solution or substance prepared for injection.

s., pickling A solution of acid used for removing oxides and other impurities from dental castings (e.g., solutions of hydrochloric acid or sulfuric acid).

s., sclerosing An agent that will cause an intense inflammation, resulting in a fibrosis; used to treat subluxation of the temporomandibular joint, cauterize ulcers, arrest hemorrhage, treat hemangiomas, etc.

s., solid An alloy all of whose constituents are mutually soluble in the solid state.

solvent A substance capable of or used in dissolving or dispersing one or more other substances; a liquid component of a solution present in greater amount than the solute.

somatalgia (sō"mah-tăl'jē-ah) Bodily pain.

somatic (sō-măt'ĭk) Derived from *soma*, meaning the body, as distinguished from the mind. The adjective pertains to the framework of the body, as distinguished from the viscera; hence the term *somatic nerves* describes the nerves associated with the musculoskeletal function of the muscles of the body.

somatoprosthetics (sō-mah-tō-prŏs-thĕt'ĭks) The art and science of prosthetically replacing external parts of the body that are missing or deformed.

somatotropin (sō"mah-tō-trō'pĭn) See hormone, growth.

somnambulism (sŏm-năm'bū-lĭsm) Habitual walking in the sleep; a hypnotic state in which the subject has full possession of senses but no subsequent recollection.

somnifacient (sŏm"nĭ-fā'shĕnt) Causing sleep; hypnotic; a medicine that induces sleep.

somniferous (som-nĭf'er-ŭs) Inducing or causing sleep.

somnolence (sŏm'nō-lĕns) Sleepiness; also unnatural drowsiness.

somnolism (sŏm'nō-lĭsm) A state of mesmeric or hypnotic trance.

sonagram (sō'nah-grăm) The readily usable graph of the frequency bands (formants) produced by the sound spectrograph.

sonagraph (sō'nah-grăf) A wave analyzer that produces a permanent visual record showing the distri bution of energy in both freqquency and time.

sonant (sō'nănt) A speech sound that has in it a component of tone generated by laryngeal vibrations (e.g., "a-a-a," "z-z-z").

sonic devices See ultrasonics.

soporific (sop'ō-rĭf'ĭk) A sleep-producing drug.

sore, canker (aphthous ulcer, aphthous stomatis) A shallow ulcer of the oral mucosa; characterized by a grayish-yellow base, and erythematous halo; the result of local minor trauma or the rupture of vesicles produced by the herpes simplex virus.

sore, cold *See* sore, canker; herpes labialis.

sore, denture *See* ulcer, decubitus.

sort To arrange units of information according to rules dependent on a key or field contained in or with the information.

s. generator program A generalized program that can produce many different sorting programs in accordance with control information specified by the user.

source file A file containing information used as input to a computer run.

source language A language that is an input to a given translation process.

source program A program coded in other than machine language that must be translated into machine language before being executed.

source-collimator distance Distance from the focal spot to the diaphragm or collimator in an x-ray tube head.

source-film distance (SFD) Distance from the focal spot of an x-ray tube to the radiographic film. Synonym: to as TFD (target-film distance).

source-object distance (SOD) Distance from focal spot to object of which a radiographic image is to be obtained. Synonym: TOD (target-object distance).

space (spās) A delimited, three-dimensional region.

s., free-way The interocclusal distance or separation between the occlusal surfaces of the teeth when the mandible is in its physiologic rest position. *Interocclusal distance* is the preferred term. *See also* distance, interocclusal; clearance, interocclusal.

s., interalveolar *See* distance, interarch.

s., interocclusal rest *See* distance, interocclusal.

s., interproximal The space between adjacent teeth in a dental arch. It is divided into the embrasure (occlusal to the contact point) and the septal space (gingival to the contact point).

s., interradicular The area between the roots of a multirooted tooth; it is normally occupied by bony septum and the periodontal membrane.

s. lattice *See* lattice, space.

s. maintainer A fixed or removable appliance designed to preserve the space created by the premature loss of a tooth.

s. maintainer cast A space maintainer fabricated by a casting technique and cemented into place.

s. maintainer, fixed A space maintainer not intended to be removable by the patient.

s. maintainer, orthodontic A removable or fixed appliance fabricated to maintain space in the arch for erupting permanent teeth. The appliance may be designed to regain space needed to accommodate the erupting tooth or teeth.

s. maintainer, removable A space maintainer designed for easy removal for cleaning and/or adjustment.

s., marrow Spaces in the spongiosa of bone; in the mandible and maxilla, the marrow spaces are cupied by fatty and/or hematogenic (red) marrow. When inflammation progresses into the marrow in these spaces, a change is noted in which the marrow becomes fibrous. The spaces enlarge in atrophy of disuse because of resorption of surrounding trabeculae, and the marrow remains fatty in nature.

s. obtainer An appliance used to increase the space between two teeth.

s., occupied The space that might be occupied by persons or radiation-sensitive materials and vices during the time that x-ray equipment is in operation or radiation is being emitted.

s., physiologic dead The air passages up to, but not including, the alveoli of the lungs; equal to about 150 cc.

s. regainer A fixed or removable appliance capable of moving a displaced permanent tooth into its proper position in the dental arch.

s. relief Fabrication of a prosthesis so that certain predetermined, nonstress-bearing areas will not be contacted by the appliance.

s., retromylohyoid (rĕt"rō-mī"lō-hī'oid) The part of the alveololingual sulcus distal to the lingual tuberosity (the distal end of the mylohyoid ridge).

spasm (spăzm) A sudden involuntary contraction of a muscle or muscle group. It may cause a twitch or close a canal or passage, depending on its location.

s., muscle Increased muscular tension and shortness that cannot be released voluntarily and that prevent lengthening of the muscles involved. Caused by pain stimuli to the lower motor neuron.

spasmolysant (spăz-mol'ĭ-zănt) Relieving or relaxing spasms; any agent that relieves spasm.

spasmolytic (spăz"mō-lĭt'ĭk) Pertaining to a drug that reduces spasm in smooth or skeletal muscle.

spastic (spăs'tĭk) Characterized by a more or less constant state of hypertonic contraction of a muscle or group of muscles. The condition is regarded as an abnormally heightened muscular tonus present even in states of inactivity.

spatula A flat-bladed instrument without sharp edges used for mixing certain dental materials (e.g., cement, plaster of paris, impression pastes).

spatulate (spăt'ū-lāt) To manipulate or mix with a spatala.

spatulation (spăt"ū-lā'shŭn) Manipulation of material with a spatula to mix it into a homogeneous mass.

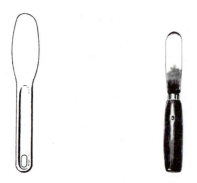

Cement spatula   Plaster spatula

spatulator (mechanical spatulator) A mechanical device that mixes ingredients to form a homogeneous mass.

s., mechanical *See* spatulator.

SPCA Abbreviation for serum prothrombin conversion accelerator. *See also* factor VIII; thromboplastin, extrinsic.

specialization The limiting of professional services to one isolated and distinct phase of dental practice.

specialty That particular field of attention and endeavor to which a therapist's efforts are devoted.

s., dental Organized dentistry recognizes eight specialties: endodontics, pedodontics, periodontics, prosthodontics, public health dentistry, oral pathology, and oral surgery.

specific gravity *See* gravity, specific.

spectograph, sound *See* sonagraph.

spectrum, antibacterial The range of antimicrobial activity of a drug.

spectrum, electromagnetic A family of radiant energies that travel in wave form, have neither mass nor charge, and travel at the speed of light. Radiations within the spectrum vary only in wavelength. X-ray photons and light rays are examples of electromagnetic radiation.

Spee, curve of *See* curve of Spee.

speech 1: Communication through conventional vocal and oral symbols. **2:** A basic biologic function of the maxillofacial structures. The essential characteristic of the speech function is the production and organization of sound into symbols.

s. aid *See* aid, speech.

s., delayed Failure of speech to develop at the expected age, usually resulting from slow maturation, hearing impairment, brain injury, mental retardation, or emotional disturbance.

s. device A prosthesis that assists in the management of speech disorders associated with a congenital or acquired defect of the palate.

s., infantile A speech defect characterized by substitu-

tion of speech sounds similar to those used by the child who speaks normally in the early stages of speech development.

s. phonation *See* phonation, speech.

s. resonance *See* resonance, speech.

s., retarded Slowness in speech development in which intelligibility in severely impaired; often preceded by late or delayed emergence of speech.

s., visible Audible speech patterns that have been transformed by electronic apparatus into visual patterns that may be read by the deaf.

speed Relative rapidity of action; rate of motion.

s., film *See* film speed.

s., high Relatively great rapidity of motion. In cavity preparations, rotary instruments are classified according to the number of revolutions per minute made by the cutting tool. Designation of each speed range presently varies with the author. In general, conventional speed is 10,000 to 60,000 rpm, high speed is 60,000 to 100,000 rpm, and ultrahigh speed is over 100,000 rpm.

s. of light A speed of 186,300 miles/sec.

s. of radiation *See* radiation, speed of.

sphenoid bone (sfē'noid) *See* bone, sphenoid.

spherocytosis, hereditary (sfēr"ō-sī-tō'sĭs) *See* jaundice, congenital hemolytic.

spheroiding (sfē'roid-ĭng) Assuming the form of a sphere, globe, or ball.

spicule (spik'ul) A small needle-shaped body.

s., cemental (cemental spike) A projection of cementum extending from the root surface into the periodontal membrane (usually along the path of the principal fibers). It represents calcification of the cemental fibers of the periodontal ligament and may not be true cementum. Hyperfunction is the etiologic agent for such spicules.

spike, cemental *See* spicule, cemental.

spillway A channel or passageway through which food escapes from the occlusal surfaces of the teeth during mastication. The occlusal, developmental, and supplemental grooves, as well as the incisal, occlusal, labial, buccal, and lingual embrasures, become spillways during function.

s., axial A groove that first crosses a cusp ridge or a marginal ridge and extends onto an axial (mesial or distal) surface of the tooth.

s., interdental A sluiceway formed by the interproximal contours of adjoining teeth and investing tissues.

s., occlusal A groove that crosses only a cusp ridge or a marginal ridge of the tooth; numerous on marginal ridges, thus increasing masticatory function.

spindle, muscle A fusiform body lying parallel to and between muscle fibers. It is composed of a conspicuously smaller modified muscle fiber that has its own motor end plate to cause it to contract and its own special sensory end organs (the flower spray ending and the anulospiral ending) that send information to the central nervous system regarding the state of contraction of the main muscle body.

spine, anterior nasal The small bony projection extending forward from the medial anterosuperior part of each maxilla. The tip of the anterior nasal spines may be seen on lateral radiographic head plates or cephalometric radiographs.

spine, posterior nasal The small, sharp, bony point projecting backward from the midline of the horizontal part of the palatine bone.

spirit (spĭr'ĭt) Any volatile or distilled liquid; also, a solution of a volatile material in alcohol.

spirograph (spī'rō-grăf) An instrument for registering the respiratory movements.

spirography (spī-rŏg'rah-fē) The graphic measurement of breathing, including breathing movements and breathing capacity.

spiroscope (spī'rō-skōp) An apparatus for respiration exercises by which the patient can see the amount of water displaced in a given time and thus gauge respiratory capacity.

splint(s) **1:** A rigid appliance for the fixation of displaced or movable parts. **2:** A support or brace used to fasten or to confine. **3:** Metal, acrylic resin, or modeling compound fashioned to retain in position teeth that may have been replanted or have fractured roots.

s., abutment Adjacent tooth restorations that have been rigidly united at their proximal contact areas to form a single abutment with multiple roots.

s., acrylic resin bite-guard An appliance, usually fabricated of resin, basically designed to cover the occlusal and/or incisal surfaces of the teeth to immobilize and stabilize the teeth and thus prevent them from being subjected to the effects of trauma from occlusal forces.

s., bridge *See* splint, fixed.

s., buccal A material (e.g., plaster) that can be placed on the buccal surfaces of assembled fixed partial denture units and onto which, after hardening, these components can be assembled and held in accurate relation.

s., cap Plastic or metallic fracture appliances that are designed to cover the crowns of the teeth; usually held in place by cementation. **s., cast bar (Friedman splint)** A provisional splint consisting of cast continuous clasps that follow the facial and lingual surfaces of the teeth at the height of contour. It is cemented onto the teeth to be splinted and simultaneously "wired closed" to bring the "clasps" into intimate contact with the teeth. May not be cemented in place to serve as a removable cast splint.

s., continuous clasp A cast splint used for the provisional immobilization of teeth.

s., copper band—acrylic A splint fabricated from copper bands and acrylic resin.

s., crib An appliance used for temporary tooth stabilization; constructed of gold, acrylic resin, chrome-cobalt alloys, or combinations thereof. It consists of a continuous crib clasp covering the facial and lingual surfaces of the teeth to be splinted.

s., cross arch bar A splint formed by a metal bar that unites one or more teeth of one side of the dental arch to one or more of the opposite side. Used to stabilize weakened teeth against lateral tilting forces. *See also* connector, cross arch bar splint.

s., cross arch bar, Bilson fixable-removable Type of cross arch bar splint.

s., fixed A fixed (nonremovable) restorative and replacement prosthesis used as a therapeutic aid in the treatment of periodontal disease. It serves to stabilize and immobilize the teeth and replace missing teeth.

s., Friedman *See* splint, cast bar.

s., Gunning's A maxillomandibular splint used to support the maxillae and mandible in mandibular and/or maxillofacial surgery.

s., implant surgical *See* superstructure, temporary.

s., inlay An inlay casting designed to give fixation or support to one or more approximating teeth. This may be accomplished by two inlays soldered together or a single casting made for prepared cavities in approximating teeth.

s., interdental An appliance made of plastic or metallic materials that is applied to the labial and/or lingual aspects of the teeth to provide points for applying mandibular and/or maxillofacial traction or fixation.

s., labial An appliance of plastic, metal, or combinations of plastic and metal made to conform to the labial aspect of the dental arch. Used in the management of mandibular and maxillofacial injuries.

s., lingual An appliance similar to a labial splint but conforming to the lingual aspect of the dental arch.

s., provisional A splint to be placed for a relatively short period. It is used to stabilize the teeth either during the healing period after accidental or deliberate tooth avulsion and replantation or in conjunction with periodontal therapy. It may also be used during a period of observation to determine the prognosis of the involved teeth.

s., Stader *See* appliance, fracture.

splinting The ligating, tying, or joining of periodontally involved teeth to one another to stabilize and immobilize the teeth, thus preventing them from being adversely affected by occlusal forces. Splinting includes acrylic resin bite guards, orthodontic band splints, wire ligation, provisional splints, and fixed prostheses.

s. of abutments The joining of two or more teeth into a rigid unit by means of fixed restorations.

s., cross arch The stabilizing of weakened teeth against tilting movements caused by laterally directed occlusal stress loads. This is accomplished by the use of a rigid connector that projects to the opposite side of the dental arch where attachment is made to one or more teeth, thus producing effective counterleverage.

s., Essig-type A method of stabilizing and repositioning injured teeth. Stainless steel fracture wire is passed labially and lingually around a segment of a dental arch, and the wire is held in position by individual ligatures around the contact areas of teeth.

split cast mounting *See* mounting, split cast.

split ring A casting ring made of three parts and designed to take advantage of the maximum expansion of the investment.

spongiosa *See* bone, cancellous.

spoon An instrument with a round or ovoid working end; designed to be used in a scraping or scooping manner.

spot(s) A small circular area.

s., café-au-lait Brown-pigmented areas of the skin occurring particularly in neurofibromatosis.

s., focal The specific area of the face of the anode or target that is bombarded by the focused electron stream when the x-ray tube is in action. It is usually an insert of tungsten.

s., effective focal (prolonged focus) The apparent size and shape of the focal spot when viewed from a position in the useful beam. With the use of a suitably inclined anode face, the area from which the useful beam stems is sharply concentrated, if seen from the perspective of the useful beam. *See also* line, focus.

s., Fordyce's (Fordyce's disease, ectopic sebaceous glands) The chamois-colored, slightly raised spots on the oral mucosa or lips produced by sebaceous glands in those tissues. The term *Fordyce's disease* is sometimes erroneously applied to these spots, which are present in 70% to 80% of the population.

s., Koplik's Oral lesions of measles (rubeola); usually occur on the buccal mucosa opposite the molar teeth as small white or bluish white spots surrounded by red zones.

s., pink *See* resorption, internal.

sprain An injury to a joint, with possible rupture of some of the ligaments or tendons but without dislocation or fracture. *See also* strain.

spray A liquid minutely divided, as by a jet of air or steam.

spreader *See* condensor.

spring A piece of metal having the physical characteristic that, when bent, it returns to its original shape.

s., auxiliary (finger spring) A short piece of wire, at-

tached to an orthodontic appliance at one end, that serves as a lever to apply force to a tooth or teeth.

s., coil A spiral winding of fine wire attached to an orthodontic appliance.

s., finger *See* spring, auxiliary.

sprue (sprū) In casting, the ingate through which melted metal passes into the heated mold. The waste piece of metal cast in the ingate.

s. base *See* sprue former; crucible former.

s. former (crucible former) A cone-shaped base made of metal or plastic to which the sprue is attached. Forms a crucible in the investment material.

s. pin *See* pin, sprue.

sputum (spū´tŭm) Matter ejected from the mouth; saliva mixed with mucus and other substances from the respiratory tract.

squamous cell C.A. (skwa´mus) *See* carcinoma, epidermoid.

stability The quality of being physically of emotionally predictable, orderly, not readily moved.

s. denture The characteristic of a removable denture that resists forces that tend to alter the relationship between the denture base and its supporting bony foundation.

s., dimensional The property of a material to retain its size and form.

s., emotional State of an individual that enables him or her to have appropriate feelings about common experiences and to act in a rational manner.

stabilization 1: The act or process of stabilizing; the state of being stabilized. 2: The seating or fixation of a fixed or removable denture so that it will not tilt or be displaced under pressure. 3: The control of induced stress loads and/or the development of measures to counteract these forces so effectively that the tilting of the teeth or the movement of a prosthesis is minimized to a point within tissue tolerance limits.

stabilized baseplate *See* baseplate, stabilized.

stabilizer An instrument used in an x-ray unit to render the milliamperage output of the tube constant.

stabilizing The process of fixing movable parts. Making firm and steady. The fixing of clamps, separators, or matrices to teeth by the application of tacky compound to the parts, then chilling the compound. In the case of clamps and separators, this also distributes the force of operating over adjacent teeth and the one being operated on.

s. circumferential clasp arm *See* clasp, circumferential, arm, stabilizing.

stable Term applied to a substance that has no tendency to decompose spontaneously. As applied to chemical compounds, it denotes their ability to resist chemical alterations.

s. isotope *See* isotope.

Stader splint (stā´der) *See* appliance, fracture.

staff *See* personnel.

stage, surgical A period or distinct phase in the course of anesthesia.

stain 1: To discolor with foreign matter.   **2:** A discoloration accumulating on the surface of a denture or teeth.

   s., Gram A staining method for microorganisms used to place them into two broad groups: gram positive, which retain crystal violet stain, and gram negative, which decolorize but counterstain with a red dye.

   s., methyl violet A dye used to color bacteria for microscopic examination.

staining Modification of the color of the teeth or denture base to achieve a more lifelike appearance.

stainless steel *See* steel, stainless.

stamp cusp A cusp made to work in a fossa. The maxillary lingual cusps are stamp cusps. In tooth-to-tooth occlusion, all lower buccal cusps may stamp into fossae. In tooth-to-two-tooth occlusion, the stamp cusps of the lower premolars may have their tips in embrasures and have only their shoulders in tiny fossae.

standard That which is established by authority, custom, or general acceptance as a model; criterion.

   s. deviation (SD or ς) A computed measure of the dispersion or variability of a distribution of scores around a given point or line. It measures how an individual score deviates from the most representative score (mean). A small SD indicates little in dividual deviation or a homogeneous group, and a large SD indicates much individual deviation or a heterogeneous group.

   s. error A measure or an estimate of the sampling errors affecting a statistic; a measure of the amount the statistic may be expected to differ by chance from the true value of the statistic.

      s.e. of estimate (ς est, ς xy) The standard deviation of the differences between the actual values of the dependent variable (results) and the predicted values. This statistic is associated with regression analysis.

      s.e. of the mean (SD$_M$, ς$_M$) An estimate of the amount that an obtained mean may be expected to differ by chance from the true mean. This value is reported as mean $(\bar{X}) \pm$ ς$_M$; i.e., a mean $(\bar{X})$ of 38 with a standard error of 4.5 would be reported as $(\bar{X}) = 38 \pm 4.5$.

   s. score Any derived score indicating the degree of deviation of an individual score from the mean using the standard deviation as the unit of measure.

stanine A unit consisting of one ninth of the total range of the standard scores of a normal distribution. The term is a condensation of *standard nine*. The mean falls at 5, the SD at ± 2. The stanine was developed by the Air Force and is used to report scores on the Dental Aptitude Test.

stannous fluoride (stan'us floo'o-rīd) A fluoride salt of tin, used in tooth paste and mouth rinses to reduce dental caries incidence and as an antiplaque agent.

Staphcillin *See* methicillin.

Staphylococcus albus (stăf'ĭ-lō-kok'ŭs ăl'bŭs) (***Staphylococcus pyogenes* var. *albus***) A species of spherical, gram-positive bacteria growing in grapelike clusters; of low pathogenicity, although occasional strains may be coagulase positive and produce hemolysis. Normally present as part of the oral flora and mucosa-lined cavities, such as the mouth and the nasal cavity. Can be isolated, along with *S. aureus*, streptococci, pneumococci, fusiform bacilli, *Borrelia vincentii*, molds, yeasts, etc., from the gingival crevice by cultural examination.

Staphylococcus aureus (stăf'ĭ-lō-kok'ŭs awr'ē-us) (***Staphylococcus pyogenes* var. *aureus***) A pathogenic variety of staphylococci capable of producing suppurative lesions; cultured colonies are golden yellow. Produces hemolysis on blood agar, is coagulase positive, and may be resistant to commonly used antibiotics. Has been isolated along with other microorganisms (e.g., *S. albus*) from the gingival crevice.

Staphylococcus pyogenes* var. *albus *See* Staphylococcus albus.

Staphylococcus pyogenes* var. *aureus *See* Staphylococcus aureus.

stare decisis (stăr'ē dĭ-sī'sĭs) Latin phrase meaning to stand by decisions and not disturb settled matters; to follow rules or principles laid down in previous judicial decisions.

statement 1: A printed form stating the balance of the account due the dentist.   **2:** In computer programming, a meaningful expression or generalized instruction in a source language.

static electricity *See* film fault, static electricity.

static relation *See* relation, static.

stationary grid *See* grid, stationary.

statistic Any value or number that describes a series of quantitative observations or measures; a value calculated from a sample.

statistical significance A difference of such magnitude between two statistics, computed from separate samples, that the probability of the value obtained will not occur by chance alone with significant frequency and hence can be attributed to something other than chance. In modern investigation, the generally accepted value for significance must have a probability of occurrence by chance factors equal to or less than five times in 100 ($p < .05$). Other significance levels commonly used are as follows: less than one chance in 100 ($p < .01$), less than five chances in 1000 ($p < .005$), and less than one chance in 1000 ($p < .001$).

statistically based utilization review A system that examines the distribution of treatment procedures based on claims information and, to be reasonably reliable, the application of such claims. Analyses of specific dentists should include data on type of practice, dentist's experience, socioeconomic characteristics, and geographic location.

statistics The branch of mathematics that gathers, arranges, condenses, coordinates, and mathematically manipulates obtained facts so that the numerical relationships between those facts may be seen clearly and freed from anomalies resulting from chance factors.

    s., descriptive Statistics used only to describe the observed group or sample from which they were derived; summary statistics such as percent, averages, or measures of variability that are computed on a particular group of individuals.

    s., inference Allows inferences to be made regarding characteristics or general principles about an unseen population based on the characteristics of the observed sample. Statistical findings from a sample are generalized to pertain to the entire population. The process of drawing inferences, making predictions, and testing significance are examples of inferential statistics.

    s., nonparametric Statistical methods used when it is not possible to assume that the variable being studied in normally distributed in a population. Synonym: distribution-free statistics.

status (stā′tŭs) State or condition.

    s. lymphaticus Enlargement of lymphoid tissue, particularly the thymus, in children. It may lead to sudden death in inhalation anesthesia.

    s. thymicolymphaticus A constitutional disturbance of controversial existence believed to be responsible in some way for sudden and unexplained deaths from trivial causes such as the extraction of teeth. There is enlargement of the thymus and lymphoid tissue and underdevelopment of the adrenal glands, gonads, and cardiovascular system.

statute A law enacted and established by a legislative department of government.

    s. of frauds A requirement that, for legal validity, contracts for conveying real property or contracts for the performance of personal services requiring a year or more to perform must be in writing.

    s. of limitations A statute that sets a time limit within which legal action on certain causes of action must be brought.

    s., wrongful death A statute that provides for the recovery of damages by one other than the party who received the fatal injuries.

steel crown *See* crown, stainless steel.

steel, stainless A steel that contains a minimum of 12% chromium and approximately 0.5% carbon that resists corrosion.

Stellite (stĕl′ĭt)   **1:** Any of various cobalt-chromium alloys.   **2:** A very hard, noncorrosive alloy of cobalt, chromium, and sometimes tungsten used for special instruments, particularly surgical instruments.

stem, brain *See* brainstem.

stenosis (stĕ-nō′sĭs) Narrowing or stricture of a duct, canal, or vessel.

Stensen's duct *See* duct, Stensen's.

stent 1: A device used to hold a skin graft placed to maintain a body orifice, cavity, or space. An acrylic resin appliance used as a positioning guide or support. **2:** An appliance that maintains tissue, (e.g., skin transplant in a predetermined position).

step wedge *See* penetrometer.

step-up transformer *See* transformer, step-up.

stereoisomer *See* isomers.

stereoscope An optical instrument for viewing photographs or radiographs; it produces binocular vision, or a blending of images, so that new perspectives can be seen with an appearance of depth. It operates on the same principle as the eyes; i.e., two views are registered on the retinas of the eyes, and the brain merges them into one.

stereoscopic radiograph *See* radiograph, stereoscopic.

sterile Free from viable microorganisms.

sterilization The act or process of rendering sterile; the process of freeing from germ life.

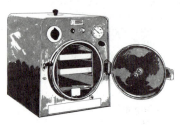

Steam heat sterilizer (autoclave)

sterilizer for root canal instruments A special device for heat sterilization of root canal instruments and dressings that depends on molten metal, glass beads, salt, or fine sand for the conduction of the heat.

Sternberg-Reed cell *See* cell, Sternberg-Reed.

steroid(s) (stēr′oid) **(sterid)** A group name for compounds that resemble cholesterol chemically and that contain also a hydrogenated cyclopentanophenanthrene ring system. Included are cholesterol, ergosterol, bile acids, vitamin D, sex hormones, adrenocortical hormones, and cardiac glycosides.

    s., adrenocortical (adrenal corticosteroid) 1: A hormone extracted from the adrenal cortex or a synthetic substance siirilar in chemical structure and biologic activity to such a hormone. **2:** The biologically active steroids of the adrenal cortex, which include 11-dehydrocorticosterone (compound A), corticosterone (compound B), cortisone (compound E), 17α-hydroxycorticosterone (compound F, hydroxycortisone, or cortisol), and aldosterone. The effects of the corticosteroids include increased resorption of sodium and chloride by the renal tubules and metabolic effects on protein, carbohydrate, and fat.

s., 17 alpha-hydroxycortico- (17-OHCS) Term used for cortisol and other 21-carbon steroids possessing a dihydroxyacetone group at carbon 17. Serum and urinary determinations give a direct measurement of adrenocortical activity.

s., C-19 cortico- (anabolic protein, N hormone) Adrenocortical hormones similar in action to the male and female sex hormones. They cause nitrogen retention and, in excessive amounts, masculinization in the female.

s., C-21 cortico- (glycogenic steroid, sugar hormone) 21-Carbon adrenocortical hormones that are oxygenated at carbon 11 or at both carbon 11 and 17. They affect protein, carbohydrate, and fat metabolism; e.g., they elevate blood sugar, increase glyconeogenesis, decrease hepatic lipogenesis, mobilize depot fat, and increase protein metabolism.

s., glycogenic *See* steroid, C-21 cortico-.

s., 17-keto- (17-KS) Steroidal compounds with a ketone (carbonyl) group at carbon 17. Derived from cortisol and from adrenal and testicular androgen. Urinary neutral 17-ketosteroids represent the catabolic end products of the endocrine glands. Produced by the adrenal cortex and testes. Increased values occur in the adrenogenital syndromes, adrenocortical carcinoma, bilateral hyperplasia of the adrenal cortex, and Leydig's cell tumors. Normal adult values for a 24-hour urine sample are 10 to 20 mg for men and 5 to 15 mg for women.

s., 11-oxy Term that refers collectively to the C-21 corticosteroids, all of which are oxygenated at carbon 11.

sterols (stē′rolz) Steroids having one or more hydroxyl groups and no carbonyl or carboxyl groups (e.g., cholesterol).

stethospasm Spasm of the chest muscles.

Stevens-Johnson syndrome *See* syndrome, Stevens-Johnson.

Stillman's cleft *See* cleft, Stillman's.

stimulant (stĭm′ū-lănt) An agent that causes an increase in functional activity, usually of the central nervous system.

s., psychomotor A drug that increases psychic activity.

stimulation 1: Increased functioning of protoplasm induced by some extracellular substance or agent. **2:** The act of energizing or activating.

stimulus (stĭm′ū-lŭs) A chemical, thermal, electrical, or mechanical influence that changes the normal environment of irritable tissue and creates an impulse.

stippling (stip′ling) **1:** An orange-peel appearance of the attached gingiva believed to result from the bundles of collagen fibers that enter the connective tissue papillae. **2:** A roughening of the labial and buccal surfaces of denture bases to imitate the stippling of natural gingiva.

s., basophilic *See* basophilia.

s., gingival *See* gingiva, stippling.

stipulation A material; an article in an agreement; an agreement in writing to do a certain thing.

stock A security certificate that represents an equity ownership in a corporation.

Stokes' disease *See* disease, Adams-Stokes.

stomatitides (stō″mah-tī-tĭ-dēs) The oral lesions associated with various forms of stomatitis.

stomatitis (stō″mah-tī′tĭs) Inflammation of the soft tissues of the mouth occurring as a result of mechanical, chemical, thermal, bacterial, viral, electrical, or radiation injury, reactions to allergens, or as secondary manifestation of systemic disease.

s., aphthous (aphthae, canker sore) Refers to recurrent ulcers of the mouth that appear to be the same clinically as herpetic ulcers and for that reason have been considered to be a manifestation of recurrent herpes simplex, although the herpesvirus has never been conclusively isolated from recurrent aphthae. *See also* gingivostomatitis, herpetic; stomatitis, herpetic; ulcer, aphthous.

s., arsenical Oral manifestations of arsenical poisoning. The oral mucosa is dry, red, and painful. Ulceration, purpura, and mobility of teeth may also occur.

s., Atabrine A stomatitis considered by some to be associated with the use of the antimalarial and anthelmintic drug quinacrine hydrochloride (Atabrine) and characterized by oral changes simulating lichen planus.

s., bismuth A stomatitis resulting from systemic use of bismuth compounds over prolonged periods. Sulfides of bismuth are deposited in the gingival tissue, resulting in bluish black pigmentation known as a bismuth line. Oral manifestations of bismuth poisoning include gingivostomatitis like that of Vincent's infection, a blue-black line on the inner aspect of the gingival sulcus or pigmentation of the buccal mucosa, a sore tongue, metallic taste, and a burning sensation of the mouth.

s., epidemic *See* disease, foot-and-mouth.

s., epizootic *See* disease, foot-and-mouth.

s., gangrenous (cancrum oris, noma) Destruction of

large masses of the oral tissues, particularly the cheek. It usually is found in weakened patients with very low resistance to infection because of lowered white blood cell count or other causes. In advanced states a large segment of the cheek may be lost, leaving the teeth visible through the defect. *See also* noma.

s., gonococcal Inflammation of the oral mucosa caused by gonococci.

s., herpetic 1: Oral manifestations of primary herpes simplex infection. The term is also used by some for herpetiform ulcers considered to be oral manifestations of secondary or recurrent herpes simplex. *See also* ulcer, aphthous, recurrent. **2:** Inflammation of the oral mucosa caused by herpesvirus. *See also* gingivostomatitis, herpetic.

s., acute herpetic (acute herpetic gingivostomatitis) The manifestations of clinically apparent primary herpes simplex characterized by regional lymphadenopathy, sore throat, and high temperature, followed by localized itching and burning, with the formation of small vesicles of an erythematous base that give way to plaques and then painful herpetic ulcers. The gingivae are swollen and erythematous and bleed easily. Manifestations subside in 7 to 10 days, and recovery usually occurs within 2 weeks.

s., iodine *See* iodism. **s., lead** Oral manifestations of lead poisoning. Included are a bluish line along the free gingival margin, pigmentation of the mucosa in contact with the teeth, metallic taste, excessive salivation, and swelling of the salivary glands.

s. medicamentosa An allergic response of the oral mucosa to a systemically administered drug. Possible manifestations include asthma, skin rashes, urticaria, pruritus, leukopenia, lymphadenopathy, thrombocytopenic purpura, and oral lesions (erythema, ulcerative lesions, vesicles, bullae, and angioneurotic edema).

s., membranous Inflammation of the oral cavity, accompanied by the formation of a false membrane.

s., mercurial Oral manifestations of mercury poisoning consisting of hypersalivation, metallic taste, ulceration and necrosis of the gingivae with a tendency to spread posteriorly and to the buccal mucosa and palate, glossodynia, and periodontitis with loosening of the teeth in severe cases of chronic intoxication.

s., mycotic Infection of the oral mucosa by a fungus, most commonly *Candida albicans,* which produces moniliasis (thrush). *See also* moniliasis.

s. nicotina *See* stomatitis, nicotinic.

s., nicotinic (stomatitis nicotina) An inflammation of the palate caused by irritation of tobacco smoke and characterized by raised small palatal lesions with red centers and white borders. The palatal mucosa usually has a generalized leukoplakia accompanying the smaller lesions.

s., recurrent Recurrent manifestations of herpes simplex involving the lips and labial and buccal mucosa (fever blisters, cold sores). Considered by many to include also recurrent aphthae (canker sores). Episodes may result from fever, sunlight, menses, trauma, and gastrointestinal upset. Lesions begin as clear vesicles with an erythematous base that give way to ulcers and superficial crusts if the outer surfaces of the lip and skin are involved.

s., uremic Oral manifestations of uremia, consisting of varying degrees of erythema, exudation, ulceration, pseudomembrane formation, foul breath, and burning sensations. *See also* gingivitis, nephritic.

s. venenata Inflammation of the oral mucosa as the result of contact allergy. The most common causative agents are volatile oils, iodides, dentifrices, mouthwashes, denture powders, and topical anesthetics. Possible manifestations include erythema, angioneurotic edema, burning sensations, ulcerations, and vesicles.

stomatodynia (stō″mah-tō-dīn′ē-ah) Sore mouth.

stomatoglossitis (stō″mah-tō-glŏs-sī′tĭs) Inflammation involving oral mucous membranes and the tongue. May be seen in nutritional disorders such as pellagra, beriberi, vitamin B complex deficiency, and infections.

stomatognathic system (stō″mah-tō-năth′ĭk) *See* system, stomatognathic.

stomatology (stō″mah-tol′ō-jē) The study of the morphology, structure, function, and diseases of the contents and linings of the oral cavity.

stomion (stō′mē-ahn) The median point of the oral slit (orifice) when the mouth is closed.

stone An abrading instrument or tool.

s., Arkansas A fine-grained stone, novaculite, used to make hones for the final sharpening of instruments.

s., artificial (dental stone) A specially calcined gypsum derivative similar to plaster of paris; because its grains are nonporous, the product is stronger than plaster of paris. **s., carborundum 1:** A stone made of silicon carbide. **2:** An abrasive, handpiece-mounted rotary instrument of various sizes, shapes, and degrees of abrasiveness.

s., dental (Hydrocal) 1: Alpha-hemihydrate of calcium sulfate. **2:** A gypsum product that, when combined with water in proper proportions, hardens in a plasterlike form. Used for making casts and dies.

s., diamond Rotary instruments containing diamond chips as the abrasive. Available in various sizes, shapes, and abrasive consistency. Used for tooth reduction in operative dentistry and crown and bridge prostheses, tooth contouring in the occlusal adjustment procedure, osseous and gingival contouring in periodontal surgery, etc.

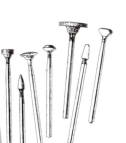

Diamond stones

s. die *See* die, stone.

s., lathe (lathe wheel) A grindstone mounted on a chuck and used on a lathe.

s., mounted point A small abrasive tooth of various shapes and sizes bonded or cemented onto a shaft or mandrel.

s., pulp *See* denticle.

s., sharpening A hand stone, or a stone driven mechanically, that is used to sharpen instruments.

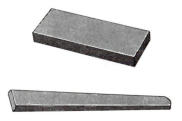

Sharpening stones

s., wheel A small grindstone of carborundum or corundum of various grits, mounted on a mandrel; of various thicknesses, ranging in diameter from ½ to 1 inch (1.3 to 2.5 cm).

stop *See* rest.

s., occlusal *See* rest, occlusal.

stop-loss A general term referring to that category of coverage that provides insurance protection (reinsurance) to an employer for a self-funded plan.

stopping, temporary Gutta-percha mixed with zinc oxide, white wax, and coloring. Softens on heating and rehardens at room temperature. Used for temporary sealing of dressings in cavities. Lack of strength makes it ineffective in areas under occlusal stress. It has poor sealing properties.

storage, computer A device or portion of a device that is capable of receiving data, retaining them for an indefinite time, and supplying them on command. Synonym: memory.

Stout's method *See* wiring, continuous loop.

straightening of teeth *See* orthodontics.

strain **1:** Deformation induced by an external force. **2:** Deformation expressed as a pure number or ratio resulting from the application of a load. **3:** A traumatic stretching or compression of such tissues as the ligaments, capsule, or musculature associated with a joint. *See also* sprain.

s. hardening *See* hardening, strain.

strangulation Choking or throttling. The arrest of respiration resulting from occlusion of the air passage or arrest of the circulation in part because of compression.

stray radiation *See* radiation leakage.

strength Toughness; ability to withstand or apply force.

s., biting **1:** The force available for application against food or other material placed between the teeth. *See also* force, masticatory. **2:** The amount of force the muscles of mastication are capable of exerting. *See also* force, masticatory.

s., compressive (crushing strength) The amount of resistance of a material to fracture under compression. *See also* strength, ultimate.

s., crushing *See* strength, compressive.

s., dry Term generally used in conjunction with materials whose strengths vary markedly in the wet and dry states. The strength of gypsum products is usually reported in both wet and dry states.

s., edge Term indicative of the ability of fine margins to resist fracture or abrasion. There is no specific test for this property; it is a composite of ductility and shear, tensile, and other strength characteristics.

s., gel Usually, the ability of the material to withstand a load without rupture.

s., impact The ability of a material to withstand a striking force.

s., shear (shear) **1:** Resistance to a tangential force. **2:** Resistance to a twisting motion.

s., tensile **1:** Resistance to a pulling force. **2:** The amount of stress a material is able to withstand when being pulled lengthwise before permanent deformation results.

s., ultimate (shear) The greatest stress that may be induced in a material or object before or during rupture; may be compressive, tensile, or shear strength. *See also* strength, tensile.

s., wet Term that refers to compressive strength while water in excess of that required for hydration of the hemihydrate is present in the specimen. Used in connection with gypsum products.

s., yield A definite proportionality obtained by drawing a line parallel to the proportional limit line. Yield strength is reported in terms of the degree of strain.

Streptococcus, alpha hemolytic (strĕp″tō-kok′ŭs, ăl′fah hē″mō-lĭt′ĭk) A spherical, gram-positive bacterium, occurring in chains of bacterial cells. Produces a zone of greenish discoloration around the colony in blood-agar medium. Part of an individual's normal oral flora; has been isolated from the gingival crevice. Capable of producing bacteremia and subsequent subacute bacterial endocarditis in patients with a history of rheumatic fever; thus prophylactic antibiotic therapy is necessary prior, during, and after periodontal, operative, and surgical therapy.

Streptococcus mutans A cariogenic bacteria found in dental plaque and one of two the index organisms (lactobacillus) used to assess caries susceptibility.

Streptococcus salivaius A bacteria found in dental plaque that may cause endocarditis and dental caries.

Streptococcus sanguis A bacteria found in dental plaque that may cause endocarditis and dental caries.

Streptococcus viridans (vī′rĭ-dănz) See Streptococcus, alpha hemolytic.

streptothricosis (strĕp-tō-thrĭ-kō′sĭs) See actinomycosis.

stress 1: A force induced by or resisting an external force; measured in terms of force per unit area. **2:** The force of energy directed against a tissue structure or against the function of tissue as the result of injury and trauma associated with fracture, burn, infection, surgical procedure, pharmacologic action, or anxiety states. The response to stress involves local metabolic function, the hormonal activity of the endocrine system regulated by the pituitary gland, and the autonomic and central nervous systems. The stress phenomenon is frequently associated with the general adaptation syndrome. **3:** In prosthetic dentistry, forcibly exerted pressure (e.g., the pressure of the upper teeth against the mandibular teeth or the pressure contact of a distorted removable partial denture on the supporting teeth or ridge structures).

s., axial Excessive force applied vertically to the teeth and their attachment apparatus.

s., bone in Responses of bony structures to applied force. With application of excessive pressure stimuli to bone, adaptation may occur by the formation of thicker and more numerous trabeculae; or if tissue components cannot compensate for excessive stress, bone resorption will occur.

s., buccolingual Excessive pressure exerted against teeth and their attachment apparatus from a buccal and/or lingual aspect.

s., compressive The internal induced force that opposes shortening of the material in a direction parallel to the direction of the stress.

s. control See control, stress.

s., shearing The internal induced force that opposes the sliding of one plane of the material on the adjacent plane in a direction parallel to stress.

s. tensile The internal induced force that opposes elongation of a material in a direction parallel to the direction of stress.

stress-bearing area See area, basal seat.

stressbreaker (stress equalizer, stress divider) A device or system that is incorporated in a removable partial dentare to relieve the abutment teeth of occlusal loads that may exceed their physiologic tolerance. See also connector, nonrigid.

stress-breaking action of clasp See clasp, stress-breaking action of.

stretch reflex See reflex, stretch.

stretching, longitudinal The vertical elongations of gutta-percha that occur because of packing forces during the filling of large root canals. The material returns to the original form when force is released.

stretching pliers See pliers, stretching.

striations, muscle (strī-ā′shŭnz) The transverse alternating light and dark bands of skeletal muscles that result from differences in light absorption. The light bands contain actin and are called "I" bands because they are isotropic to polarized light. The dark areas contain myosin filaments and are called "A" bands because they are anisotropic to polarized light.

stridor (strī′dor) A peculiar, harsh, vibrating sound produced during respiration.

s., inspiratory The sound heard in inspiration through a spasmodically closed glottis.

s., laryngeal Stridor resulting from laryngeal stenosis.

strip A thin, narrow, comparatively long piece of material.

s., abrasive (linen strip) A ribbonlike piece of linen of varying lengths and widths on one side of which are bonded abrasive particles of selected grit; used for contouring and polishing proximal surfaces of restorations.

s., boxing A metal or wax strip used for making an enclosure to regulate the size and form of a cast. **s., Celluloid** See strip, plastic.

s., lightning (separating strip) A strip of steel with abrasive bonded on one side; used to open rough or improper contacts of proximal restorations or to begin the reduction of proximal excess of a foil restoration.

s., linen See strip, abrasive.

s., plastic A clear plastic strip of Celluloid or acrylic resin that is used as a matrix when silicate cement or acrylic resin cement is inserted into proximal prepared cavities in anterior teeth.

s., polishing A strip with a very fine abrasive such as crocus powder.

s., separating See strip, lightning.

stripping 1: The mechanical removal of a very small amount of enamel from the mesial or distal surfaces of teeth to alleviate crowding. **2: (electrochemical)** The process of subjecting the surface of a gold casting, attached to an anode from a rectifier and transformer unit, to the dissolving action of a heated cyanide solution, the metal container for which is the cathode of the unit. A microscopic amount of the surface of the alloy is removed by the reverse electrolysis. The electrochemical stripping or milling is in contrast to electropolishing, wherein sharp edges are dissolved more rapidly than broader areas.

stroke A single, unbroken movement made by an instrument or the mandible.

 s., circumferential One of the basic strokes used for root and gingival curettage; the blade of the periodontal curet is negotiated mesiodistally while it is in contact with either the root or the inner aspect of the soft tissue wall of the gingival or periodontal pocket.

 s., exploratory A phase of subgingival root scaling in which the curet is held in featherlike grasp to tactilely ascertain the amount and extent of the accretions on the root surface; the ingress stroke into the pocket area.

 s., power The phase of the working stroke that is designed to split or dislodge calculus from the root surface. It is prefaced by the exploratory stroke and followed by the shaving stroke.

 s., shaving The phase of the working stroke of a periodontal curet that is designed to smooth or plane the root surface. It follows the power stroke, which is designed to dislodge calculus from the root surface.

 s. volume The volume of blood put out by the heart per heartbeat. Stroke volume is directly proportional to the volume of blood filling the heart during diastole.

structure(s) The architectural arrangement of the component parts of a tissue, part, organ, or body. Also the individual components of the body.

 s., border *See* border structures.

 s., cored In metallurgy, a grain structure with composition gradients resulting from the progressive freezing of the components in different proportions. Nonmetals used in dentistry (e.g., zinc phosphate and silicate cements) are also cored structures in that they have a nucleus of undissolved powder particles surrounded by a matrix of reacted material.

 s., denture-supporting The tissues, either teeth and/or residual ridges, that serve as the foundation or basal seat for removable partial dentures.

 s., histologic The minute structure of organic tissues.

 s., radiolucent The structures or substances that permit the penetration of x radiation and are thus registered as relatively dark areas on the radiograph.

 s., radiopaque The structures that prevent the x rays from penetrating them because of their density, which causes them to appear as light areas on the radiograph.

 s., supporting The tissues that maintain or assist in maintaining the teeth in position in the alveolus (i.e., gingivae, cementum of the tooth, periodontal ligament, alveolar and trabecular bone).

  s., functional form of supporting Term that refers to the state of denture-supporting structures when they have been placed in such a position as to be able to begin resisting occlusal forces.

Stuart factor *See* factor X.

study Pursuance of education; analysis.

 s. cast *See* cast, diagnostic.

 s., graduate Baccalaureate educational efforts pursued for credit toward an advanced degree in institutions of higher learning.

 s. model *See* cast, diagnostic.

 s., postgraduate Postdoctoral educational endeavors that may or may not earn credits for advanced degrees.

 s., time The technique of random sampling used for analysis of the time spent for rendering each phase of each of the various professional services performed by the dentist.

stupor The condition of being only partly conscious or sensible; also, a condition of insensibility.

Sturge-Weber-Dimitri disease *See* disease, Sturge-Weber-Dimitri.

stylet A wire inserted into a soft catheter or cannula to secure rigidity; a fine wire inserted into a hollow needle to maintain patency.

stylus Ancient form of writing instrument. It is still used much as it was used when the Egyptians were figuring out geometry with a stylus and sand sprinkled on a polished stone. It has assumed importance in gnathology, since a well-pointed stylus can be slid on dust-covered glass with a minimun of friction, thereby making the jaw-writing data more accurate.

 s., surgical indicator A small pointed instrument devised to mark the spot in the tissue where the intramucosal inserts will be placed. Styluses are seated in prepared depressions in the denture base and mark the mucosal tissue by puncturing it.

 s. tracer *See* tracer, needle point.

 s. tracing *See* tracing, needle point.

styptic A hemostatic astringent.

sub- Prefix signifying under, beneath, deficient, near, almost.

subconscious The state in which mental processes take place without the mind's being distinctly conscious of its own activity.

subgingival (sŭb-jĭn′jĭ-val) At a level apical to the gingival margin.

subgingival curettage *See* curettage, subgingival.

subjacent tissue (sŭb-jā´sĕnt) *See* tissue, subjacent.

sublabial adhesion (sŭb-lā´bē-al) *See* adhesion, sublabial.

sublease A lease executed by the lessee of an estate to a third person, conveying the same estate for a shorter term than that for which the lessee holds it.

sublingual (sŭb-lĭng´gwal) Pertaining to the region of structures located beneath the tongue.

　s. administration *See* administration, sublingual.

　s. crescent *See* crescent, sublingual.

　s. fold *See* fold, sublingual.

　s. gland *See* salivary glands.

subluxation (sŭb˝lŭk-sā´shŭn) **1:** Incomplete dislocation of a joint. **2:** Term applied loosely to the temporomandibular joint, indicating relaxation of the capsular ligaments and improper relationship of the joint components, resulting in cracking and popping of the joint during movement.

submandibular Below the mandible.

submarginal Pertaining to a deficiency of contour at the margin of a restoration or pattern.

submaxillary Situated beneath a maxilla.

　s. caruncle *See* caruncle, submaxillary.

　s. ganglion *See* ganglion, submaxillary.

submental Situated below the chin.

submucosa (sub˝mū-kō´sah) The tissue layer beneath the oral mucosa. It contains connective tissues, vessels, and accessory salivary glands.

submucous cleft (occult cleft) A congenital anomaly of the soft and/or hard palate, in which the midportion of the soft and/or hard palate lacks proper mesodermal development. Nonunion of bone and muscle tissues of the soft and hard palates and concealment by the superficial intact mucoperiosteum.

subnasion (sŭb-nā´zē-ŏn) The point of the angle between the septum and the surface of the upper lip. It is sought at the point where a tangent applied to the septum meets the upper lip.

subocclusal connector *See* connector, subocclusal.

subpoena (sŭ-pē´nah) The process or writ issued by the court by which the attendance of a witness at a certain time and place is required so that he may testify. It may also order him or her to bring any books, records, or other things under his control that he is bound by law to produce in evidence.

subroutine The set of instructions necessary to direct the computer to carry out a well-defined mathematical or logical operation; a subunit of a routine.

subscriber The person, usually the employee, who represents the family unit in relation to the prepayment plan. Other family members are "dependents." Synonym: certificate holder or enrollee.

subspinale (sŭb˝spĭ-nā´lē) The deepest midline point on the premaxilla between the anterior nasal spine and the prosthion.

substance P One of several endogenous inflammatory substances thought to mediate or cause pain.

substitute One acting for or taking the place of another.

　s., tinfoil Alginate separating material painted on gypsum molds to serve as a liner in preventing both the penetration of monomers into the surrounding investing medium and the leakage of water into acrylic resin.

substitution A standard or nonstandard speech sound used for another consonant speech sound (e.g., "w" for "l" [wady for lady]).

substructure A structure built to serve as a base or foundation for another structure.

　s., implant (implant denture substructure) 1: A skeletal frame of inert material that fits on the bone under the mucoperiosteum. **2:** The metal framework that is embedded beneath the soft tissues in contact with the bone for the purpose of supporting an implant superstructure.

　s., implant, abutment The portion of the implant that extends from the surface of the mucosa into the oral cavity for the retention of crowns, bridges, or superstructure bearing the teeth of the denture.

　s., implant, auxiliary rest A small metal protrusion through the mucosa connected to the labial or buccal and lingual (peripheral) frame to furnish additional support for the superstructure between the abutments.

　s., implant, interspaces Any one of the spaces between the primary and secondary struts that allows infiltration of tissue.

　s., implant, neck (implant post, implant substructure, post) The constriction that connects the implant frame with the implant abutment.

　s., implant, part The root section shaped in the form of a wire loop. This part of the substructure sinks into the alveolar socket or sockets after the extraction of one or two remaining anterior teeth. Newly formed bone tissue will grow through the loop and firmly affix the implant.

　s., implant, peripheral frame The labial, buccal, lingual, and distal outline of the frame.

　s., implant, post *See* substructure, implant, neck.

　s., implant, primary struts The main traverse struts that connect the implant necks or posts with the peripheral frame.

　s., implant, secondary struts The additional smaller transverse, diagonal, and longitudinal struts that are added when necessary to give additional strength and rigidity to the implant, increase the area of bone support, and afford additional intermeshing of the mucoperiosteal tissue.

suffocate Asphyxiate.

suffocation Interference with the entrance of air into the lungs.

suit Any proceeding in court in which the plaintiff pursues the remedy that the law gives for the redress of an injury or the enforcement of a right.

sulcus (sŭl′kŭs) **1:** A furrow, trench, or groove, as on the surface of the brain or in folds of mucous membrane. **2:** A groove or depression on the surface of a tooth. **3:** A groove in a portion of the oral cavity.

   s., alveololingual The space existing between the alveolar or residual alveolar ridge and the tongue. It extends from the lingual frenum to the retromylohyoid curtain and is a part of the floor of the mouth.

   s., gingival The shallow groove between the free gingiva and the surface of a tooth and extending around its circumference.

     s., implant gingival A sulcus around the implant abutment post that resembles the sulcus around a healthy natural tooth.

   s., occlusal A groove or spillway on the occlusal surface of a tooth.

sugar One of a number of water-soluble carbohydrates. Sugars are divided into two major categories; monosaccharides and disaccharides. Table sugar or sucrose is the principal disaccharide; glucose or blood sugar is the principal monosaccharide.

sulfa (sŭl′fah) *See* sulfonamide.

sulfhemoglobinemia (sŭlf″hē-mō-glō′bĭ-nē′mē-ah) An abnormality of the heme moiety of the hemoglobin molecule resulting from inorganic sulfides (e.g., acetanilide).

sulfonamide (sŭl-fon′ah-mīd) A derivative of sulfanilamide that is effective against microorganisms.

sulfur granules A yellow-white particle found in actinomycosis and diagnostic of actinomycosis infection.

Sulkowitch's test (sŭl′kō-wĭch-ĕz) *See* test, Sulkowitch's.

summary plan description *See* benefit plan summary.

summation The phenomenon in which similar actions of more than one drug result in a total action that may be expressed as the arithmetic sum of the effects of the individual drugs.

summons A writ directed to the sheriff or other proper officer, requiring him or her to notify the person that an action has been begun against him or her in the court from which the writ was issued and that he is required to appear on a certain day to answer the complaint.

superexcitation Excessive excitement.

superoxol A 30% solution of hydrogen peroxide used to bleach endodontically treated teeth.

superplant A bayonet-shaped bar used as a subperiosteal implant whose purpose it is to serve as an abutment for a free end fixed prosthesis.

supersaturation The addition to or presence of an ingredient in a solution in greater quantity than the solvent can permanently take up.

superstructure A structure that is constructed on or over another structure.

   s. casting In the subperiosteal implant, a surgical alloy bar designed with clasps to telescope over the four abutments. To this casting is processed the final denture superstructure.

   s., implant (implant denture superstructure) 1: A removable denture that fits snugly onto the protruding implant abutments. Sometimes called the *implant denture*. **2:** The denture that is retained, supported, and stabilized by the implant denture substructure.

   s., implant, attaching material The denture resin by which the superstructure teeth are attached to the superstructure frame.

   s., implant, attachment Any part of the superstructure that fits onto the implant abutments. May be a precision attachment coping, a conventional clasping, or a combination of preci-sion attachment with clasps.

   s., implant, connectors The rigid bars that unite the superstructure attachments into one strong element.

   s., implant, denture *See* superstructure, implant.

   s., implant, frame The metal skeleton of the superstructure, consisting of attachments and connectors.

  s., temporary (implant surgical splint) An acrylic resin immediate appliance with six anterior teeth; has no metal clasps, precision coping, or frame; fitted closely over the implant abutments immediately after the surgical insertion of the substructure.

supervision The active administering and overseeing of all the functionings of the dental practice and the auxiliaries employed therein.

supplemental tooth A type of supernumerary tooth that is so well formed that it mimics a fully formed tooth. A supplemental tooth usually appears distal to a lateral incisor. Its detection requires the careful counting and identification of each tooth in the dental arch.

supplements Usually, dietary substances used to augment, enhance or enrich the nutritional status of a patient.

support Resistance to vertical components of masticatory force in a direction toward the basal seat.

   s., ridge *See* area, supporting.

supporting area *See* area, supporting.

supporting bone *See* bone, cancellous.

supportive periodontal therapy *See* periodontal therapy.

suppuration The formation and discharge of pus.

suprabulge The portion of the crown of a tooth that converges toward the occlusal surface from the height of contour of survey line.

supraclusion (sū″prah-klū′zhŭn) A position occupied by a tooth that is too high in the line of occlusion.

supramentale (sū″prah-mĕn-tā′lē) The most posterior oint in the concavity between the infradentale and the pogonion.

supraversion (sū″prah-ver′zhŭn) A condition in which teeth or other maxillary structures are situated above or below their normal vertical relationships.

surcharge A stated dollar amount paid to the dentist by the beneficiary, in addition to other reimbursement received by third-party payer(s).

surface(s) The outer portion of a mass or object.

s., **basal** *See* denture, basal surface of.

s., **buccal** Any surface adjacent to and facing the cheek.

s., **foundation** *See* denture, basal surface of.

s., **implant-bearing** The area of bone that has been selected from the surgical bone impression to be in direct contact with the implant frame.

s., **impression** *See* denture, basal surface of.

s., **occlusal** The anatomic superior surface of the mandibular posterior teeth and the inferior surface of the maxillary posterior teeth. These surfaces are limited mesially and distally by marginal ridges and buccally and lingually by the buccal and lingual boundaries of the cusp enrinences.

s., **balancing occlusal** The surfaces of the teeth or denture bases that make contact to provide balancing contacts.

s., **working occlusal** The surface or surfaces of the teeth on which chewing can occur.

s., **proximal** The surface of a tooth or the portion of a cavity that is nearest to the adjacent tooth; the mesial or distal surface of a tooth.

s., **smooth** A surface of a tooth on which pits and fissures are not found normally.

surfactant (sŭr-făk′tănt) A surface-active agent.

surgeon One whose profession is to cure diseases or injuries by manual operation or by medication.

surgery, mucogingival Surgical procedures designed to retain a functionally adequate zone of gingiva after surgical pocket elimination, to create a functionally adequate zone of attached gingiva, to alter the position of, or eliminate, a frenum, or to deepen the vestibule.

s., **apically repositioned flap in mucogingival** A surgically created flap of gingival tissue that is repositioned apically to maintain or create a functionally adequate zone of attached gingiva. In the surgical procedure, the existing attached and free gingiva is detached by employing a reverse bevel incision and apically repositioning the flap.

s., **full flap in mucogingival** A flap in which all the soft tissue elements are raised and repositioned, as opposed to the split-thickness flap.

s., **oblique flap in mucogingival** An increased band of attached gingiva created by preparing a narrow papillary flap (to avoid donor site radicular recession), which is then rotated 90 degrees and sutured into the prepared recipient site.

s., **pedicle flap in mucogingival** An increased band of attached gingiva created to repair a cleft by using proximal gingiva situated mesial and distal to the cleft, since gingiva in either location alone is not wide enough to cover the cleft if repositioned. The pedicles are repositioned laterally and sutured. Synonym: double papilla procedure.

surgery, osseous The therapeutic surgical measures used and designed to eliminate osseous deformities by means of ostectomy and/or osteoplasty or create a favorable environment by means of meticulous removal of the soft tissue contents of the infrabony osseous defect for the formation of new bone, periodontal membrane, and cementum to fill in the area of bone resorption.

s., **access flap in osseous** A full-thickness or split-thickness flap created for the purpose of gaining access to the alveolar bone when surgical remodeling is indicated.

surgical preparation *See* preparation, surgical.

surgical prosthesis *See* prosthesis, surgical.

surgical template *See* template, surgical.

surgical tray A prefabricated appliance constructed in advance of the first surgical stage and used for making an impression of the exposed mandibular bone. *See also* stage, surgical.

survey The study and/or examination of an area of consideration, a diagnostic cast, or a radiograph.

s. **line** *See* line, survey.

s., **radiation** Evaluation of the radiation hazards incidental to the production, use, or existence of radioactive materials or other sources of radiation under a specific set of conditions.

s., **radiographic** The production of the minimum number of radiographic examinations necessary for a radiographic interpretation.

s., **roentgenographic** *See* survey, radiographic.

s., **x-ray** *See* survey, radiographic.

surveying The procedure of studying the relative parallelism or lack of parallelism of the teeth and associated structures so as to select a path of placement for a restoration that will encounter the least tooth or tissue interference and that will provide adequate and balanced retention; locating guiding plane surfaces to direct placement and removal of the restoration, as well as to achieve the best appearance possible.

surveyor An instrument used to determine the relative parallelism of two or more surfaces of teeth or other portions of a cast of the dental arch.

s., Ney The paralleling instrument that was the first cast surveyor made available commercially.

susceptible The opposite of immune; having little resistance to disease.

suspension (sŭs-pĕn′shŭn) A mixture of two or more immiscible phases, such as a solid in a liquid or a liquid in a liquid. Suspensions differ from emulsions in that the former usually have to be shaken before each use.

Sutton's disease *See* periadenitis mucosa necrotica recurrens.

suture 1: A synarthrosis between two bones formed in a membrane, the uniting medium (which tends to disappear eventually) being a fibrous membrane continuous with the periosteum.   **2:** A surgical stitch or seam. **3:** Materials with which body structures are sewn, as after an operation or injury.   **4:** To sew up a wound.

s., absorbable A suture that becomes dissolved in body fluids and disappears (e.g., catgut).

s., approximation A suture made to bring about apposition of the deeper tissues of an incision or laceration.

s., button A suture passed through buttonlike disks on the skin to prevent the suture from cutting through the soft tissue.

s., chromic A chromatized sheepgut suture.

s., continuous A suture in which an uninterrupted length of suture material is used to close an incision or a laceration.

s., frontomalar Most lateral point of the suture between the frontal and malar bones.

s., intermaxillary (median palatine suture) The line of fusion of the two maxillae, starting between the central incisors and extending posteriorly across the palate, ″separating″ it into two nearly equal parts.

s., interrupted Individual stitches, each tied separately.

s., mattress A continuous suture that is applied back and forth through the tissues in the same vertical plane but at a different depth, or in the same horizontal plane but at the same depth.

s., median palatine *See* suture, intermaxillary.

s., nonabsorbable A suture that does not dissolve in body fluids (e.g., silk, tantalum, Nylon).

s., purse-string A horizontal mattress suture used generally about an implant cervix.

s., shoelace A continuous surgical suture for depression of the tongue and for retaining and holding the lingual flap out of the field of operation during the surgical impression.

swage (swāj) To shape metal by adapting or hammering it onto a die. Usually completed by forcing a counterdie into position on a die with the metal sheet interposed.

swager A laboratory instrument used for swaging.

s., wax An instrument used to swage wax to a die.

swallowing *See* deglutition.

s. threshold *See* threshold, swallowing.

swear To take an oath; to become legally obligated by an oath properly administered.**sweat** (swĕt) Perspiration. A clear liquid exuded or excreted from the sudoriferous glands. It possesses a characteristic odor, is slightly alkaline, is salty to the taste, and, when mixed with sebaceous secretion, is acid. Sweating is under the control of the sympathetic nervous system, although it can be stimulated by parasympathetic drugs. Thermoregulatory sweating is influenced by the blood temperature's affecting the nervous centers and by reflexes associated with heat receptors in the skin.

sweating, gustatory *See* syndrome, auriculotemporal.

swelling One of the cardinal signs of acute inflammation caused by the exudation of fluid from the capillary vessels into the tissue.

s., familial intraosseous *See* cherubism.

Swift's disease *See* erythredema polyneuropathy.

symbiotic relationship (sĭm″bī-ŏt′ĭk) In implantology, that relationship assumed by an implant and the natural teeth to which it has been splinted; the continuing existence of their relationship is based on their interdependence.

symbolic coding Instructions written in nonmachine language.

symmetric Evenly balanced or uniformly developed.

sympathetic (sĭm″păh-thĕt′ĭk) The sympathetic nervous system.

sympatholytic (sĭm″pah-thō-lĭt′ĭk) Pertaining to a drug that blocks the effects of stimulation of the sympathetic nervous system. *See also* adrenolytic.

sympathomimetic (sĭm″pah-thō-mĭ-mĕt′ĭk) Resembling the effect produced by stimulation of the sympathetic nervous system. *See also* adrenergic.

sympathy The kind understanding of a patient.

symptom Any morbid phenomenon or departure from the normal in function, appearance, or sensation, experienced by the patient and indicative of disease.

s., constitutional Symptoms related to the systemic effects of a disease (e.g., fever, malaise, anorexia, loss of weight).

s., diagnostic signs and *See* signs and symptoms, diagnostic.

synalgia (sĭ-năl′jē-ah) **1:** Pain felt in a distant part from an injury or stimulation of another part.   **2:** Reflex or referred pain.

Synalgos DC *See* dihydrocodeine.

synapse (sĭn′ăps) The region of contact between the processes of two adjacent neurons forming the place where a nervous impulse is transmitted from the axon of one neuron to the dendrites of another. It is called the *synaptic junction.*

synarthrosis (sĭn″ar-thrō′sĭs) A joint formed by thin intervening layers of cartilage, connective tissue, or direct contact of bone to bone. It results in a rigid union, and there is little movement of the bones except during growth. Suture lines may be obliterated in adults with a synarthrodial joint when the bones joined together become fused as one bone.

synchronous Having constant time intervals between events or occurrences.

s. device A term applied to a device in which the performance of a sequence of operations in controlled by equally spaced clock signals or pulses.

syncope (sĭng'kō-pē) Swooning or fainting; temporary suspension of consciousness caused by cerebral anemia. *See also* shock.

syndactyly (sin-dak'tĭ-lē) A congenital anomaly characterized by the fusion of fingers and/or toes, usually as a finding of a more complex cogenital syndrome.

syndrome (sĭn'drōm) A group of signs and symptoms that occur together and characterize a disease.

s., Adams-Stokes *See* disease, Adams-Stokes.

s., adaptation *See* disease, adaptation; syndrome, general adaptation.

s., adrenogenital Disorders of sexual development or function associated with abnormal adrenocortical function resulting from bilateral adrenal hyperplasia, carcinoma, or adenoma. Pseudohermaphroditism occurs congenitally, and masculinization occurs later in females. Precocious sexual development and occasionally feminization occur in males.

s., AHOP Adiposity, hyperthermia, oligomenorrhea, and parotitis appearing in females. Parotid gland enlargement begins at puberty and is followed by obesity, oligomenorrhea, and psychic disturbances.

s., Albright's A polyostotic form of fibrous dysplasia, usually associated with precocious puberty in females, endocrine disturbance influencing growth, and brown pigmentation of the skin.

s., Apert's (acrocephalosyndactyly) Craniostenosis characterized by oxycephaly and syndactyly of the hands and feet. Facies manifestations include exophthalmos, high prominent forehead, small nose, and malformation of the mandible and mouth.

s., Ascher's Syndrome consisting of double lip, a redundance of the skin of the eyelids (blepharochalasis), and nontoxic thyroid enlargement. The sagging eyelids are obvious when the eyes are open and the double lip is seen when the patient smiles.

s., auriculotemporal (Bogarad's syndrome, Frey's syndrome, gustatory hyperhidrosis syndrome, gustatory lacrimation, gustatory sweating syndrome) Sweating and flushing in the preauricular and temporal areas when certain foods are eaten. May be related to parotid trauma or a complication of parotidectomy.

s., autoimmunization *See* disease, autoimmune.

s., Behçet's (bā'sĕts) **(Behçet's disease)** Recurrent iritis and aphthous ulcers of the mouth and genitalia. Other manifestations include arthralgia, hydrarthrosis, swelling of the salivary glands, cutaneous eruptions, and central nervous system disorders.

s., Bloch-Sulzberger (incontinentia pigmenti) Syndrome in which there are pigmented skin lesions, defects of the eyes and central nervous system, skeletal anomalies, and hypoplasia of the teeth.

s., Bogarad *See* syndrome, auriculotemporal.

s., Böök's (bŭks) Syndrome characterized by premature graying of the hair, hyperhidrosis, and premolar hypodontia.

s., Bourneville-Pringle (epiloia) Neurocutaneous complex consisting of adenoma sebaceum, mental deficiency, and epilepsy.

s., Caffey-Silverman *See* hyperostosis, infantile cortical.

s., Christ-Siemens-Touraine *See* hypohidrotic ectodermal dysplasia.

s., Costen's Various symptoms of discomfort, pain, or jaw pathosis claimed by Costen to be caused by lack of posterior occlusion, loss of vertical dimension, malocclusion, trismus, or muscle tremor.

s., cri-du-chat Clinical syndrome associated with the deletion of the short arm of a B chromosome. Manifestations include mental retardation, various congenital abnormalities, and an infant cry resembling the mewing of a cat.

s., crocodile tears A syndrome in which a spontaneous lacrimation occurs with the normal salivation of eating. It follows facial paralysis and seems to result from straying of the regenerating nerve fibers, some of those destined for the salivary glands going to the lacrimal glands.

s., Crouzon's *See* dysostosis, craniofacial.

s., Cushing's (Cushing's disease) A symptom complex associated with an excess of adrenal steroids of all types resulting from hyperplasia of the adrenal cortex, malignant neoplasms, pituitary basophilia, or prolonged administration of ACTH. Manifestions include hypertension, buffalo obesity, diabetes mellitus, osteoporosis, purple striae of the skin in areas of tension, and disorders of glucose tolerance.

s., Down *See* mongolism.

s., Ehlers-Danlos A congenital or familial disorder characterized by fragility of the skin and blood vessels, hyperlaxity of the joints, hyperelasticity of the skin, subcutaneous pseudotumors, and tendency to hemorrhage postoperatively.

s., Ekman's *See* osteogenesis imperfecta.

s., Ellis–van Creveld *See* chondroectodermal dysplasia.

s., Feer's *See* acrodynia.

s., Frey *See* syndrome, auriculotemporal.

s., Fröhlich's Adiposity and genital hypoplasia resulting from hypopituitarism or hypothalamohypophys-dystrophy.

s., Gardner's Multiple osteomas, multiple polyposis of the large bowel, multiple epidermoid or sebaceous cysts, and multiple cutaneous fibromas.

s., general adaptation (adaptation syndrome, GAS) A three-stage physiologic response to physical or psychologic stress. The first stage is the alarm reaction, consisting of bodily changes typical of emotion. A second stage is resistance to stress, wherein an attempt is made to adapt to the physiologic changes. Certain hormones of the anterior pituitary gland and the adrenal cortex hypersecrete to increase resistance. Such resistance leads to diseases of adaptation, such as hypertension. Continual stress results in the third stage, exhaustion.

s., Goldscheider's Dystrophic form of epidermolysis bullosa, leading to scars. The disturbance is inherited on an autosomal dominant or recessive basis. This form of epidermolysis bullosa leads to retardation of mental and physical growth. *See also* syndrome, Weber-Cockayne.

s., Greig's A condition manifested by ocular hyper-telorism, often mental retardation, ectodermal and mesodermal abnormalities, and dental and oral anomalies.

s., Gunn's *See* syndrome, jaw-winking.

s., gustatory hyperhidrosis *See* syndrome, auriculotemporal.

s., gustatory sweating *See* syndrome, auriculotemporal.

s., Heerfordt's *See* fever, uveoparotid.

s., Horner's A tetrad of symptoms resulting from paralysis of the cervical sympathetic trunk: pupillary constriction, ptosis of upper eyelid, dilation of orbital blood vessels (redness of conjunctiva), and blushing and anhidrosis of side of face.

s., Hunt's Herpetic inflammation of the geniculate ganglion, with herpes zoster of the soft palate, anterior tonsillar pillar, and auricular area. *See also* herpes zoster.

s., Hurler's (mucopolysaccharidosis i, gargoylism, dysostosis multiplex) A heritable disorder of mucopolysaccharide metabolism in which excessive acid mucopolysaccharides—dermatan sulfate and heparitin sulfate—are made and stored in the tiasues. Clinical manifestations include hypertelorism, open mouth with large-appearing tongue, thick eyelids and lips, anomalies of the teeth, and short, broad neck. The skeletal and facial deformities resemble the gargoyles of Gothic architecture. Mental retardation, corneal clouding, hepatosplenomegaly, deafness, and cardiac defects are present.

s., Hutchinson-Gilford (progeria) Syndrome of dwarfism, immaturity, and pseudosenility. Patient appears to be bald and elderly at an early age. There is hypoplasia of the mandible, and the face is small in relation to the neurocranium.

s., jaw-winking (winking-jaw syndrome) Congenital unilateral ptosis and elevation of the lid on opening of the jaw or moving of the mandible to the contralateral side.

s., Klinefelter's (XXY syndrome, chromatin-positive syndrome, medullary gonadal dysgenesis) Presence in men of an abnormal sex-chromosome constitution. Persons with XXY constitution show the clincal signs of sterility, aspermatogenesis, variable gynecomastia, and often mental retardation. About 50% of subjects with XXXXY variant have cleft palate.

s., Klippel-Feil Fusions of cervical vertebrae, short neck with limited head movement, and extension of the posterior hairline.

s., Lobstein's *See* osteogenesis imperfecta.

s., Marfan's Tall, thin stature, long, tapered fingers and toes (arachnodactyly), dislocation of the lens of the eye (ectopia lentis), and aneurysm leading to rupture of the aorta.

s., Melkersson-Rosenthal Transient facial edema, especially swelling of the upper lip, facial paralysis, and lingua plicata. Plicated swelling of the mucosa of the tongue, palate, and buccal mucosa may not be present, or the paralysis may be incomplete.

s., Mikulicz' A condition characterized by swelling of the parotid, submandibular, sublingual, and lacrimal glands; associated with lymphosarcoma, leukemia, tuberculosis, sarcoidosis, or syphilis.

s., Möbius' Congenital facial diplegia consisting of facial paralysis as well as lingual and masticatory muscle paralysis, inability to abduct the eyes, and anomalies of the extremities.

s., myeloproliferative Extramedullary myelopoiesis in adults. It may follow contact with benzol compounds or polycythemia, or it may precede leukemia.

s., nephrotic (ne-frot'ik) Syndrome that includes proteinuria, hyperlipemia, hypoproteinemia, and edema. It occurs in a variety of conditions in which there is increased glomerular permeability and urinary loss of protein.

s., nonarticular pain One of several painful disorders that limit joint motion and affect the periarticular structures: the tendons, tendon sheaths, bursae, connective tissue, and muscles. Patients commonly call this syndrome *muscular aches and pains*. The pains are chronic and nagging and may occur in acute exacerbations. The neck, shoulder, back, thighs, hands, and legs are common sites of irritation. The nonarticular disorders are associated with fibrositis, tenonitis, tenosynovitis, and periarticular muscle spasm. The precipitating agents are frequently obscure and may be associated with postural or personality disorders. When the acute symptoms of pain, stiffness, and restricted motion are reduced, the tissues resume their normal function. The common temporomandibular joint syndrome is believed to be caused by a postural occlusal imbalance associated with the muscular tension induced by psychologic stress. The combination precipitates an acute muscle spasm in the muscles associated with the protection and movement of the joint.

s., Papillon-Lefevre Extensive periodontal disease in young patients (juvenile periodontosis) accompanied by keratotic lesions of the palmar and plantar surfaces. In some patients changes similar to hereditary ectodermal dysplasia are also present.

s., paratrigeminal Trigeminal neuralgia, sensory loss, weakness and atrophy of the masticatory muscles, miosis, and ptosis of the upper eyelid on the affected side of the face resulting from a lesion of the semilunar ganglion and fibers of the carotid plexus.

s., Patau's See trisomy-D.

s., Paterson-Kelly See syndrome, Plummer-Vinson.

s., Peutz-Jeghers Generalized multiple polyposis of the intestinal tract, consistently involving the jejunum, and associated with melanin spots of the lips, buccal mucosa, and fingers; autosomal doriinant inheritance.

s., PHC See syndrome, Böök's.

s., Pierre Robin Micrognathia of the newborn. Congenital retrognathism associated with cleft palate, glossoptosia, difficult in swallowing, respiratory obstruction, and cyanosis. This congenital micrognathia will correct itself during the growth of the child if proper care is provided.

s., Plummer-Vinson A symptom complex that includes fissures at the corners of the mouth, sore tongue, dysphagia, achlorhydria, and iron-deficiency anemia. Most commonly seen in females in the fourth and fifth decades of life and associated with a predisposition to carcinoma of the oral cavity and esophagus.

s., Reiter's A syndrome that consists of arthritis (often of the rheumatoid type), conjunctivitis, nonspecific urethritis, and occasionally aphthous ulcers of the oral mucosa.

s., Rieger's Characteristics include hypodontia, conical crowns, enamel hypoplasia, dysgenesis of the iris and cornea, and myotonic dystrophy.

s., Riley-Day (familial dysautonomia) Disturbances of the autonomic and central nervous systems consisting of hypersalivation, defective lacrimation, excessive sweating, erythematous blotching after emotional upset, relative indifference to pain, and hyporeflexia. Normal growth and motor development are retarded.

s., Robin's See syndrome, Pierre Robin.

s., Roger's Continuous excessive secretion of saliva as the result of cancer of the esophagus or other esophageal irritation.

s., Rosenthal's See hemophilia C.

s., rubella Enamel defects of the primary teeth at-tributed to prolonged effect of the rubella virus on ameloblasts during fetal life and in the postnatal period.

s., Scheuthauer-Marie-Sainton See cleidocranial dysostosis.

s., sicca See syndrome, Sjögren's.

s., Sjögren's (sicca syndrome, xerodermostecisis) Condition related to deficient secretion of salivary, sweat, lacrimal, and mucous glands (xerostomia, keratoconjunctivitis, rhinitis, dysphagia), increased size of salivary glands, and polyarthritis.

s., Smyth's See hyperostosis, infantile cortical.

s., Stevens-Johnson An acute inflammatory disease characterized by oral, ocular, and genital lesions with severe generalized symptoms. The oral lesions are irregularly shaped, painful ulcers. See also erythema multiforme.

s., Sturge-Weber An encephalofacial angiomatosis characterized by cutaneous facial cerebral angiomatosis, ipsilateral gyriform calcifications of the brain, mental retardation, seizures (epilepsy), contralateral hemiplegia, and ocular involvement. Facial lesions (port-wine stain) may join intraoral angiomas on the buccal mucosa and gingiva.

s., Swift's See acrodynia.

s., temporomandibular joint An acute muscle spasm in the muscles associated with the protection and movement of the joint. It is believed to be caused by a postural (occlusal) imbalance associated with the muscular tension induced by psychologic stress. The principal symptoms are pain in the region of the joint, limitation of mobility of the mandible, crepitus, clicking sounds in the joint, and frequently tinnitus.

s., thalassemia (Cooley's anemia, Mediterranean anemia, hereditary leptocytosis) Any of a group of closely related and genetically determined disorders in which there is a specific decrease in one of the polypeptide chains comprising hemoglobin. The defect results in hypochromic microcytic erythrocytes. There are alpha, beta, and delta variants as well as several subtypes based on biochemical techniques. See also thalassemia.

s., Treacher Collins An incomplete mandibulofacial dysostosis in which there are congenital deformities of the eyelids, mandible, and malar bones, and malocclusion, cleft lip and palate, and nasal deformities.

s., Turner's (XO syndrome, gonadal dysgenesis, genital dwarfism) Absence of one of the X chromosomes, with affected females being sterile and short of stature and having various congenital anomalies such as webbing of the neck, low-set ears, wide-set eyes, shieldlike chest, absence of breasts, and cubitus valgus. Common orofacial findings are hypoplastic mandible, high palatal vault, and dental anomalies.

s., Ullrich-Feichtiger Micrognathia, polydactyly, and genital malformations.

s., Urbach-Wiethe Hyalinosis of the skin and mucous membranes and hoarseness. The skin is infiltrated with yellowish, waxy nodules, and the oral tissues with similar plaques beginning before puberty and becoming increasingly severe. The teeth may be hypoplastic or may fail to develop.

s., vestibular disorder One of several syndromes involving the vestibule of the ear. The two most common syndromes of vestibular disorders are seasickness, which results from the continuous movement of the endolymph in susceptible individuals (probably related to a disturbance in the reflex control of the eyeball movements), and Menière's syndrome, in which paroxysmal vertigo is the principal sign, but there are other associated vascular and metabolic disorders.

s., Waardenburg-Klein A syndrome consisting of congenital deafness, white forelock, increased distance between the inner canthi, the iris of the same eye or of the two eyes having different color (heterochromic irides), and prognathism. Inherited as an autosomal dominant disorder.

s., Weber-Cockayne Simple nonscarring form of epidermolysis bullosa; transmitted as an autosomal dominant trait. *See also* syndrome, Goldscheider's.

s., Weech's *See* hypohidrotic ectodermal dysplasia.

s., Witkop–von Sallman Hereditary benign intraepithelial dyskeratosis with gelatinous plaques on hyperemic bulbar conjunctiva and white folds and plaques involving the oral mucosa.

s., Zinsser-Engman-Cole Syndrome consisting of reticular atrophy of the skin, with pigmentation, dystrophic fingernails and toenails, and oral leukoplakia. Hyperhidrosis of the palms and soles is present, as well as acrocyanosis of the hands and feet.

syneresis (sĭ-nĕr′ĕ-sĭs) A process by which a fluid exudate forms on the surface of a hydrocolloid gel, even when the gel is in water or in a humid atmosphere. It is accompanied by shrinkage of the gel.

synergism (sĭn′er-jĭzm) Joint action of two drugs in such a manner that one supplements or enhances the action of the other to produce an effect greater than that which can be obtained with either one of the drugs in equivalent quantity or to produce effects that could not be obtained with any safe quantity of either drug or both. *See also* potentiation.

synthetic porcelain *See* cement, silicate.

syphilid (sĭf′ĭ-lĭd) A cutaneous lesion of syphilis.

syphilis (sĭf′ĭ-lĭs) **(lues)** A contagious venereal disease caused by *Treponema pallidum* and usually transmitted by direct contact. Oral lesions include the primary chancre, secondary mucous patches and split papule, and tertiary gumma. Congenital syphilis may lead to Hutchinson's incisors, mulberry molars, or rhagades. *See also* chancre; gumma; incisors, Hutchinson's; molar, mulberry; patch, mucous; *Treponema pal-lidum*.

s., latent A stage of syphilis in which there are no clinical signs or symptoms of the disease. It is usually discovered by serologic tests.

Synthodont A brand name for a prefabricated ceramic implant.

Syrette (sĭ-rĕt′) Trade name for a small hypodermic syringe containing a dose of the drug to be administered.

syringe (sĭ-rĭnj′; sĭr′ĭnj) An apparatus of metal, glass, or plastic material consisting of a nozzle, or needle, barrel, and plunger or rubber bulb; used to inject a liquid into a cavity or under the skin.

s., air A device by which air may be applied to a given area. An instrument supplied as part of the dental unit, consisting of a hand grip, nozzle, pressure-regulating valve, and hose connected to the compressed air supply.

s., hand air An air syringe consisting of a metal tube bent at one end, terminating in a reduced diameter, and enlarged at the other end to engage a rubber bulb. The bulb is compressed by hand to supply a controlled spurt of air to a given area.

s., warm air An air syringe equipped with an electric heating element to heat the air to any desired temperature.

s., combination A syringe that is usually part of the dental unit through which air, water, or a combination of the two may be delivered under pressure to the desired area.

s., water A device, usually part of the dental unit, permitting controlled application of water to a given area. It has a flow control, pressure regulator, and heating element.

system A set or series of organs or parts that unite in a common function.

s., acid-base buffer The system by which a virtually constant pH level of the blood and body fluids is maintained. The base and acid electrolytes associated with normal metabolism are continuously introduced into the bloodstream. Notwithstanding the marked amounts of base or acid or both introduced into the bloodstream during exercise, rest, hunger, or the ingestion of fluid and solid foods, the pH level of the blood remains rather constant between the range 7.3 and 7.5. There are four means by which this relatively narrow but constant pH level is maintained: the buffer system of the blood, tissue and cell fluids, and mineral salts of the bone matrix; excretion and retention of cabon dioxide by the lungs; excretion of an acid or alkaline urine; and the formation or excretion of ammonia and/or organic compounds.

s., apothecaries' A nondecimal system of weights and measures traditionally used by druggists. *See also* system, avoirdupois.

s., autonomic nervous The part of the nervous system that regulates the reflex control of bodily functions. It controls the functioning of glands, smooth muscle, and the heart.

s., avoirdupois A commercial nondecimal system of weights and measures. *See also* system, apothecaries'.

s., central nervous The brain and spinal cord, including their nerves and end organs; controls all voluntary acts.

s., circulatory The heart and blood vessels. There are three major groups of blood vessels: arteries, capillaries, and veins. The system transports metabolites to and from the tissue cells.

s., computer An assembly of procedures, processes, methods, routines, techniques, or equipment united by some form of regulated interaction to form an organized whole. It is an approach to a complex problem.

s., flowchart A pictorial diagram illustrating the flow of information into, through, and out of a system of programs.

s., hematopoietic Term used to describe collectively the blood, bone marrow, lymph nodes, spleen, and reticuloendothelial cells.

s., masticatory The organs and structures primarily functioning in mastication: the jaws, teeth and their supporting structures, temporomandibular articulation, mandibular musculature, tongue, lips, cheeks, and oral mucosa and their nerve supplies.

s., metric A decimal system of weights and measures almost universally used in scientific and professional work, including the writing of prescriptions. The individual units are based on an international set of standards, notably the meter, liter, and kilogram. See Appendix H.

s., musculoskeletal The system of body structures that provides the energy and movement necessary for the functions of life. The muscles, bones, and connective tissues of the body are grouped together into one system, and they are intimately connected in their individual and combined functions; e.g., for muscle to accomplish its ultimate purpose of movement by contraction, bone, leverage, and connective

tissue are required to transmit the force that the contraction generates. In the oral cavity and its related structures the musculoskeletal tissues fulfill the mechanical and structural requirements for movement of the mandible and for some related visceral functions such as respiration and digestion.

s., neurohormonal The system by which the hormone secretions of the endocrine glands function, in part as the regulator of both visceral and somatic function and have intimate anatomic and functional relationships with the nervous system by the union of the pituitary gland and the hypothalamus of the cerebrum. The pituitary gland has a pars nervosa, which is an extension of the anterior part of the hypothalamus, and a pars intermedia, which is an epithelial evagination of the secretory tissue from the stomodeum of the embryo. From its position in the cranial structures in the sella turcica, the pituitary gland regulates, by its union with the nervous system, the whole endocrine system with its many glands; these glands, in turn, partially regulate the viscera and somatic muscle organs.

s., occlusal (occlusal scheme) The form or design and arrangement of the occlusal and incisal units of a dentition or of the teeth on a denture. *See* system, masticatory.

s., parasympathetic nervous One of the motor divisions of the autonomic nervous system. It is described as the craniosacral division and does not have the simplified structural apparatus of the strong sympathetic adrenal axis about which to function. The parasympathetic system inhibits the heart, contracts the pupils, and, in emotional states, produces a vagus-insulin axis of activity. The several parts function rather independently. The ocular division relates to the midbrain, and the bulbar division relates to the hindbrain. The bulbar division supplies the facial, glossopharyngeal, and vagus nerves. It also supplies the secretory and vasodilator fibers of the salivary glands and mucous membranes of the mouth and pharynx. In conditions of very loud noise or unusual anxiety states, the parasympathetic system will cause unaccounted-for spontaneous urination, excessive salivary and gastric juices, and either nausea or vomiting.

s., proaccelerin-accelerin *See* factor V.

s., proconvertin-convertin *See* factor VII.

s., stomatognathic The combination of all the structures involved in speech, and the reception, mastication, and deglutition of food. The system is composed of the teeth, jaws, muscles of mastication, epithelium, and temporomandibular joints and nerves that control these structures.

s., sympathetic nervous One of the two opposing motor systems in the autonomic nervous system that mediate the activity of the viscera. (That other is the parasympathetic system.) The sympathetic system is composed of 21 or 22 ganglia in chains on each side of the spinal cord. The fibers connect with the spinal cord through these ganglia. The actions of the sympathetic division of the autonomic nervous system are closely allied to the action of the medulla of the adrenal gland; thus a sympathetic-adrenal axis that functions as a unit to protect and regulate the body environment may be conceived. The sympathetic control is modified by the volitional somatic control of the patient. The volitional control, superimposed on the autonomic control, gives rise to great variations in motor patterns, as seen in the face in the presence of emotional changes, such as in the blushing of shame and pallor of fear.

s., vascular, closed tube The type of vascular system, as in humans, in which the blood circulates through the vessels (or tubes) and is not dissipated into the tissues. The closed vascular tube system offers resistance to the pumping action of the heart because the pressures are cumulative with each pumping action. The elastic walls in the arterial vessels, particularly in the aorta, absorb the additional energy and release its slowly, thus creating the possibility of maintaining a fairly steady and safe pressure head throughout the vascular system. The high-pressure point at the height of cardiac contraction is the systole, and the low point before the ventricular contraction is the diastole.

s., vascular, open tube In some vertebrates, a vascular system with an open end that causes the blood fluid to dissipate into the tissues. This system starts with a maximum head pressure that diminishes until inertia in the blood is overcome. The blood is returned to the heart by muscle function, gravity, and diffusion. The blood pressure in this system fluctuates from a maximum at the heart to a minimum at the tissue cell.

s., venous A system of interconnected blood vessels that returns blood to the heart from the tissue and capillary bed through progressively larger vessels. The following affect the return of blood to the heart: thoracic pressure, associated with respiration; gravity, associated with body posture; the valves, diameter of the lumen, and muscle structure of the veins; muscle contraction of the somatic structures; the pressures in the arteriole system and capillary bed; and the nervous and hormonal system controls that regulate cardiomuscular activity. The influences over the venous system circulation are collectively termed *venopressor mechanisms*.

systematically Done in a well-organized, carefully followed pattern of procedure.

systemic lupus erythematosus (SLE) (sis-tem′ik loo′pus er″ĭ-thēm′ah-tō-sus) An autoimmune disease that can be life threatening. Patients may have a distinctive pattern of facial redness and oral lesions. Endothelial damage to heart valves can occur similar to those caused by rheumatic fever.

systole (sĭs′tō-lē) The period of contraction of the heart. The term specifically designates the contraction of the ventricles as distinguished from auricular contraction. It occurs with the first heart sound. The pressure from the systolic contractions is taken up and stored as potential energy by the elastic properties of the aorta and other great vessels of the arterial system. This storage of energy protects the smaller, more fragile vessels from undue pressure. The even flow and steady pressure of the blood are sustained by the controlled release of the potential energy stored in the arterial walls into kinetic energy for movement of the blood during the diastolic phase of heart function. The pressure recorded at the height of the ventricular contraction is the systolic pressure. In the adult, the normal blood pressure is 120/80 mm Hg (systolic/diastolic). It rises with advancing age to 135/89 at 60 years of age.

t-test An inferential statistic used to test for differences between two means (groups) only. It is used for small samples (N <30). Synonyms: t-ratio, student's t.

tabes dorsalis (tā′bēz dor-sā′lĭs) **(locomotor ataxia)** A form of neurosyphilis in which there is degeneration in the posterior roots of the spinal nerves and posterior column of the spinal cord. Manifestations include pains and paresthesias of the trunk, hands, and feet, abdominal pain crises, ataxia, Argyll Robertson pupil, atrophy of the optic nerve, and Charcot's joint.

table, occlusal The occlusal surfaces of the premolarsa and molars; the basic collective topography, including the form of the cusps, inclined planes, marginal ridges, and central fossae and grooves of the teeth. tachycardia (tak″e-kar′de-ah) Excessively rapid action of the heart; the pulse rate is usually above 100 beats/min.

table of allowances A list of covered services with an assigned dollar amount that represents the total obligation of the plan with respect to payment for such service but does not necessarily represent the dentist's full fee for that service. Synonyms: schedule of allowances, indemnity schedule.

tachycardia (tăk″ē-kar′dē-ah) Excessively rapid action of the heart; the pulse rate is usually above 100 beats/min.

tachyphylaxis (tăk″ē-fĭ-lăk′sĭs) **1:** The rapid development of tolerance on administration of closely spaced successive doses of a drug or poison. **2:** A decreasing response that follows consecutive injections at short intervals.

tachypnea (tăk-ĭp-nē′ah) Excessively rapid respiration. A respiratory neurosis marked by quick, shallow breathing.

tailpiece *See* aid, speech, prosthetic, velar section.

Takahara'a disease *See* disease, Takahara's.

Talwin Brand name for pentazocine lacatate, a potent analgesic, as effective as morphine. Talwin is a controlled substance.

tang *See* connector, minor.

tank, processing A receptacle used in the photographic or radiographic darkroom for the chemical solutions used in the processing of films.

tannic acid A vegetable tanning agent that attaches itself to collagen by hydrogen bonds. It is used in dentistry as a cavity conditioner before placing a restoration.

tantalum (tăn′tah-lŭm) A noncorrosive, malleable metal used for plates and devices to bridge bony defects, or as a wire mesh for sutures.

tape, dental A ribbon of waxed nylon or silk used to aid the prophylaxis of interproximal spaces and the proximal surfaces of the teeth. The flattened, wide form of dental floss.

tapering A process of shaping a clasp arm to better distribute flexure throughout its length, thus reducing fatigue, strain hardening, and resultant fracture.

t., arch *See* arch, tapering.

target The small tungsten block, embedded in the face of the anode, that is bombarded by electrons from the cathode in an x-ray tube.

target-film distance (TFD) *See* distance, target-film; source-film distance.

target-object distance (TOD) *See* source-object distance.

tarnish 1: Surface discoloration or loss of luster by metals. Under oral conditions, it often results from hard and soft deposits. **2:** A chemical process by which a metal surface is discolored or its luster destroyed.

tartar *See* calculus, dental.

taste enhancers Food additives that have little or no flavor of their own but when added to food bring out the taste of certain foods. Monosodium glutamate (MSG) is the most common flavor or taste enhancer.

tattoo, amalgam *See* amalgam tattoo.

taurodontism (taw″rō-don′tĭzm) A tooth in which the pulp chamber is elongated, enlarged, and extends deeply into the region of the roots. A similar condition is seen in the teeth of cud-chewing animals.

tax A ratable portion of the proceeds or value of theroperty and labor of the citizen; any contribution imposed by government for the use and service of the state.

tax brackets The income intervals of the graduated income tax law that establishes the rate of tax for each level of income.

Tax Equity and Fiscal Responsibility Act of 1982 (TEFRA) Legislation (Public Law 97-248) affecting health maintenance organizations and the Medicare and Medicaid programs. Provides regulations for the development of HMO risk contracting with the Medicare program and, through amendment, established new provisions for the foundation and operation of peer review organizations.

tax planning Basing business and investment decisions on estimated income and current and projected tax laws.

tax shelter investments Investments that reduce, remove, or defer income from state and federal income tax liability.

taxes The sum of monies collected by the various branches of a government.

technic (tĕk′nĭk) *See* technique.

technician A person skilled in the performance of technical procedures.

　　t., dental *See* technician, dental laboratory.

　　t., dental laboratory (dental technique) One skilled in the art of executing the dentist's prescription for the mechanical fabrication of dental appliances

technical competence Ability of the practitioner, during the treatment phase of dental care and with respect to those procedures combining psychomotor and cognitive skills, to consistently provide services at a professionally acceptable level.

technical quality The degree to which the physically measurable attributes of procedures in dental care meet professionally acceptable standards.

technique (tĕk-nēk′) **1:** A skillful and detailed method of executing procedures to accomplish a desired result. **2:** The method of performance of manipulation in any art; the terms *technique* and *technic* are used synonymously, but the word technique pertains more to the artistic skill involved.

　　t., bisection of the angle An intraoral radiographic technique whereby an angle formed by the mean plane of the tooth and the mean plane of the film is bisected, and the central ray is directed through the tooth perpendicular to the bisection. This is the application of Cieszynski's rule of isometry. *See also* rule of isometry, Cieszynski's.

　　t., calibrated angle An intraoral radiographic technique using a specified degree in vertical angulation from the horizontal plane. It is a variation of the bisection of the angle technique and assumed to be the correct angulation for the majority of patients.

　　t., chew-in *See* chew-in technique.

　　t., double investing A method of investing wax patterns, whereby the pattern is covered with a primary layer of investment; this core is then invested, before or after the primary investment has set, in an outer, thinner mix of the same or a different type of investing material.

　　t., Eames' In dental amalgam, a procedure using mercury and alloy in approximately a 1:1 ratio, thus not having residual mercury in the plastic mix.

　　t., filling The method used to obliterate the space in

the root of the tooth once occupied by the dental pulp.

　　t., Fones' *See* method, Fones'.

　　t., hydroflow *See* dentistry, washed-field.

　　t., impression A method and manner used in making a negative likeness. The series of operations or procedures used for making an impression.

　　　t., dual impression A technique by which the anatomic form of the teeth and immediately adjacent structures is recorded and by which the free-end denture foundation areas are registered in their functional form.

　　t., long cone The use of an extended cone distance, generally 14 inches (35 cm) or more, in oral radiography. It is generally used with, but not confined to, parallel film placement.

　　t., Nealon's A technique for the insertion of resin restorations whereby the monomer and polymer are applied incrementally with a brush.

　　t., parallel (right-angle technique) A technique in intraoral radiography in which the film is positioned parallel to the long axes of the teeth, and the central ray is directed perpendicular to both the film and the teeth.

　　t., short cone The use of a short cone distance, usually 8 inches (20 cm) or less, that is supplied by the manufacturer as short cone. It is generally used with, but not confined to, the bisection of the angle technique.

　　t., telephone The friendly but businesslike conveying of ideas over the telephone.

　　t., thermal expansion A casting procedure whereby compensation is made for metal shrinkage by thermal expansion of the refractory investment mold.

　　t., wax expansion A casting procedure whereby compensation is made for metal shrinkage by thermal expansion of the wax pattern prior to setting of the investment.

teeth *See* tooth.

teething Eruption of primary teeth that is preceded by increased salivation. Young children may become restless during this period. Inflammation of the gingival tissues prior to complete emergence of the crown may cause a temporary painful condition.

Teflon A proprietary plastic material used in surgery as an implant.

Tegopen Brand name for cloxacillin, an antistaphylococcal penicillin.

Tegretol *See* carbamazepine.

telangiectasia (tĕl-ăn″gē-ĕk-tā′zē-ah) **1:** Dilation of the capillaries and small arteries of a region. A hereditary form (hereditary hemorrhagic telangiectasia) may appear intraorally. **2:** A disorder characterized by cutaneous and mucosal vascular macules, nodules, and arterial spiders that tend to bleed sporadically.

t., hereditary hemorrhagic Rendu-Osler-Weber disease) Dilation of small vessels and capillaries resulting from a genetic factor, with a tendency to bleed.
Lesions may occur on the tongue as small, raised,
red to bluish red elevations.

teleradiography (tĕl″ĕ-rā″dē-ŏg′rah-fē) Radiography at a
longer distance than is usually used (6 feet; 1.8 m).

telic (tel-ik) **(teleologic)** Assigning purpose to functions
as if they were provided by a creative planner.

temperature The degree of sensible heat or cold.

t., body The measurable temperature of the body (normal range of variation, 98° to 99° F [35.5° to 37° C]
orally and 99° to 100° F [37° to 38° C] rectally, with
much wider ranges for skin).

t., body, regulation Homeostasis of body temperature. Results from a balance of heat production
(external heat plus heat from muscle contraction
and other chemical processes) and heat loss
(through lungs, sweating, surface radiation, and
excretions).

t., casting The required degree of heat necessary to
bring a metal to proper fluidity for introduction into
a refractory mold.

t., recrystallization The lowest temperature at which
the distorted grain structure of a cold-worked metal
is replaced by a new, strain-free grain structure during prolonged annealing. Time, purity of metal, and
prior deformation are important factors.

tempering (hardening heat treatment) Hardening or
toughening of steels by heating. Treatment of an alloy
in such a manner that solid-solid transformation occurs. Precipitation of intermetallic substances occurs,
increasing the proportional limit and hardness of the
alloy.

t., gold The hardening of gold alloys by cold working
or by heating and then cooling slowly.

t., hydrocolloid Storing of the material after liquefac-
tion at a temperature that will increase the viscosity
to the optimal manipulative degree of sol.

t., steel Counteracting of the hardening heat treatment
to the extent needed for the particular tool or structure. It is heated to a predetermined temperature and
then quenched in water or oil.

template (tĕm′plāt) A pattern or mold forming an accurate copy of an object or shape.

t., prosthetic A curved or flat plate used as an aid in
setting denture teeth.

t., implant An early type of subperiosteal implant that
was fabricated from a cast carved to simulate the
host bone. Measurements made from radiographs
taken with a template or wire mold resting on the
soft tissues determined the carving of the cast.

t., occlusal A stone or metal (electroformed) occlusal
table made from a wax occlusal path registration of
jaw movements and against which the opposing

supplied teeth are occluded.

t., orthodontics A cephalometric tracing of an age-
and sex-normed facial and dental profile used in the
analysis of facial and dentition variations in malocclusion.

t., surgical A thin transparent resin base shaped to duplicate the form of the impression surface of an immediate denture and used as a guide for surgically
shaping the alveolar process and its soft tissue covering to fit an immediate denture.

t., wax A wax recording of the occlusion of the teeth.

t., viral The process of RNA/DNA replication associated with retrovirus activity. **temporal eminential
angle** The degree of slope between the axis-orbital
plane and the discluding slope of the eminence.

temporary Pertaining to the interim treatment used to
protect a patient between appointments.

t., base See baseplate.

t., prosthesis See prosthesis, temporary.

t., stopping See stopping, temporary.

t., superstructure A prosthodontic appliance (removable or fixed) that is used, often immediately postoperatively, as a transitional appliance either for
cosmetics or splinting or both.

temporomandibular articulation (tĕm″pō-rō-măn″dĭb′ū-
lar) See articulation, temporomandibular.

**temporomandibular extraoral radiographic examina-
tion** See examination, radiographic, extraoral, temporomandibular.

temporomandibular joint See articulation, temporomandibular.

temporomandibular pain-dysfunction syndrome A triad
of signs and symptoms consisting of pain in the muscles of mastication and jaw joints, clicking in the jaw
joints, and limitation in jaw movements. Lesser findings may include dislocation and/or locking of the jaw
joints and sensory changes in hearing. Synonyms:
Costen's syndrome, mandibular pain-syndrome
(MDS), TMJ pain-dysfunction syndrome (PDS), and
myofacial pain-dysfunction syndrome (MPD).

tenant One who has the temporary use and occupation of
real property owned by another, the length and terms
of the tenancy being usually fixed by a lease.

tender, legal The kind of coin or money that the law
compels a creditor to accept in payment of a debt,
when offered by the debtor in the right amount.

tendonitis Inflamation of a tendon, usually stress or
strain related.

tensile strength (ten-sīl) See strength, tensile.

tension (tĕn′shŭn) The state of being stretched, strained,
or extended.

t., interfacial surface The tension or resistance to separation possessed by the film of liquid between two
well-adapted surfaces (e.g., the thin film of saliva
between the denture base and the tissues).

teratogens (ter′ah-tō-jenz) Agents that form monsters; drugs or substances that cause congenital deformities.

teratoma (tĕr″ah-tō′mah) A tumor arising from cells that retain their embryonic totipotentiality (ovary, embryonic rest, testis) and can differentiate into any of the three primary germ layers.

terminal, computer A device in a system or communications network at which data can either enter or leave.

terminal hinge position *See* position, hinge, terminal.

terminal jaw relation record *See* record, terminal jaw relation.

termination date *See* expiration date.

terminology, technical The use of terms that are descriptive and meaningful to the dentist but that are not a part of the vocabulary of the patient.

terra alba (ter′ah al′bah) Gypsum added to plaster or stone to accelerate the setting reaction.

test(s) Any clinical or laboratory procedure designed to evaluate constituents or functions of the body.

  t., acetone *See* test, ketone bodies.

  t., ACTH-stimulation (Thorn's test) A test of adrenocortical reserve based on changes in the eosinophil count and urinary levels of 17-ketosteroids and 17-hydroxycorticoids as a result of intravenous infusion or intramuscular injection of ACTH.

  t., Addis' A test to estimate the number of formed elements in urine collected under standard conditions (restricted food intake, minimal patient activity, night collection).

  t., allergy, intradermal A test for allergy performed by injecting a preparation containing the suspected allergen into the dermis.

  t., amylase (ăm′ĭ-lās) Determination of serum amylase, which is useful in the diagnosis of acute pancreatitis and after operations in which the pancreas might have been injured. The Somogyi sarcogenic method is often used, and the results are given in Somogyi units, defined as the amount of amylase needed to digest 1.5 Gm of starch in 8 minutes at 37° C. The normal range is 60 to 200 units/100 ml. The serum amylase is also elevated in mumps and other diseases of the salivary glands.

  t., amyloid (ăm′ĭ-loid) *See* test, Congo red.

  t., antiviral antibody Antibody tests in viral diseases. Included are complement-fixation tests for poliomyelitis, psittacosis, and Coxsackie infections; hemagglutination-inhibition tests for mumps, influenza, and encephalitides; and neutralization tests.

  t., Aschheim-Zondek (ăsh′hīm tson′dĕk) *See* test, pregnancy.

  t., ascorbic acid, intradermal A test for ascorbic acid deficiency based on the decoloration of an intradermal injection of a purple dye (2,6-dichlorphenol-indophenol). Normally with a wheal of 4 mm, using a dye concentration of N/300, decoloration occurs in 10 to 15 minutes.

  t., basophilic aggregation (bā″sō-fīl′ĭk) A test for lead poisoning based on increased stippling of erythrocytes. More than 2% stippled cells is seen in lead poisoning. *See also* test, lead.

  t., Bell's palsy Simple clinical tests such as motor function tests, in which the patient is asked to whistle, pucker the lips, smile, or wrinkle the forehead, and sensory function tests, in which the patient is asked to taste sweet with sugar, sour with citric acid, bitter with quinine, and salt with sodium chloride.

  t., Benedict's A nonspecific copper reduction test for glucose in the urine. Cupric sulfate in the Benedict's reagent is reduced by glucose during the reaction to cuprous oxide, a reddish orange precipitate.

  t., bilirubin (bĭl″ĭ-roo′bĭn) Qualitative, presumptive, quantitative, or specific determinations for bilirubin in the urine and blood serum. Included are Gmelin's test and van den Bergh's test.

  t., bleeding time Techniques for determining the time interval required for hemostasis to occur after a standardized wound has been made in the capillary bed. *See also* test, Duke's; test, Ivy's.

  t., Brinell hardness (brin-el′) A means of determining surface hardness by measuring the amount of resistance to the indentation of a steel ball. Recorded as the Brinell hardness number (BHN); the higher the number, the harder the material. Generally indicative of abrasion resistance.

  t., Bromsulphalein (BSP) A test of liver function based on the removal of a known quantity of Bromsulphalein from the blood in a measured period of time. Normal values are less than 5% retention at the end of 45 minutes with an intravenous dose of 5 mg/kg body weight. It is a useful test of hepatocellular disease and detoxifying ability but is not applicable in the presence of extrahepatic or intrahepatic obstructive jaundice.

  t., Bunnell *See* test, Paul-Bunnell.

  t., capillary resistance (Rumple-Leede-Hess test, Gothlin's test) A test of capillary fragility based on the number of petechiae that develop when a standardized intraluminal positive pressure is applied to the capillaries either by a blood pressure cuff or a suction cup applied to the skin. *See also* test, tourniquet.

  t., CO$_2$ capacity (CO$_2$ combining power test) A general measure of the alkalinity or acidity of the blood. Various normal adult ranges are given (e.g., 23 to 30 mEq/L of serum or 55 to 70 vol/100 ml of serum). A low value is found in diabetic acidosis, hyperventilation, certain kidney diseases, and severe diarrhea. A high value is found in excessive administration of ACTH or cortisone, intake of sodium bicarbonate, and persistent vomiting.

t., CO₂ combining power *See* test, CO_2 capacity.

t., cold bends A mechanical test used for assessing ductility.

t., colorimetric caries susceptibility (Snyder's test) A method of determining the concentration of acid-producing bacteria in the saliva by use of bromcresol green in a culture medium. The reliability of this and other salivary bacterial tests for dental caries susceptibility is questionable.

t., Congo red A test for amyloidosis based on the more rapid disappearance (excess of 60% injected dye in 1 hour) of Congo red from the serum of affected patients than from that of normal individuals. Gingival biopsy and positive staining with methyl violet or crystal violet also indicate amyloidosis.

t., creatinine clearance (krē-ăt'ĭ-nĭn) A renal function test of exogenous creatinine clearance. It is a convenient clinical test of glomerular infiltration rate. It is calculated as the quotient of the product of urine creatinine (mg/L) and urine volume (L/24 hr) divided by the serum creatinine concentration (mg/L). The normal value for young healthy adults of average size (1.73 M² body surface area) is 115 to 155 L/24 hr (±15%).

t., dermal *See* test, skin.

t., Dick's (scarlet fever test) A skin test to determine susceptibility or immunity to scarlet fever. A positive test is indicated when an area of erythema and edema measuring more than 10 mm in diameter occurs 8 to 24 hours after an intradermal injection of a standardized erythrogenic toxin.

t., Duke's A test of bleeding time as indicated by the time that elapses before a puncture wound of the earlobe ceases to bleed. Normal range is 2 to 4½ minutes.

t., electric A test to determine whether a pulp is vital.

t., erythrocyte sedimentation A macroscopic test of the blood used to detect certain pathologic conditions, particularly inflammation. The blood cells are allowed to settle in the presence of an anticoagulant and the time (sedimentation time) determined. The greater the time or rate, the more severe the condition. Pregnancy and menstruation affect the sedimentation.

t., flow Used in the ADA specification for dental amalgam; measured as the percentage shortening of a cylinder of the material.

t., fluorescent treponemal antibody, absorbed (FTA-APS) A modification of the original FTA test for syphilis that employs a protein preparation from the Reiter treponeme.

t., Foshay's A skin test for tularemia using the Foshay antigen.

t., Frei's (frīz) An intradermal skin test for lymphogranuloma venereum employing an antigen called *Lygranum*. It gives a specific dermal reaction in patients infected with lymphogranuloma venereum. A false positive test may occur with psittacosis.

t., Friedman's (frēd'mănz) *See* test, pregnancy.

t., glucose paper A test in which paper is impregnated with glucose oxidase and other reagents (TesTape, Clinistix). When the paper is moistened with fresh urine, the presence of glucose will cause a change in color of the paper.

t., glucose tolerance (GTT) A test for abnormalities of carbohydrate tolerance by glucose loading and subsequent serial measurements of the concentration of glucose in the blood. Graphic representation of the concentration and the elapsed time make up the glucose tolerance curve. Abnormal curves occur in diabetes mellitus, thyrotoxicosis, Cushing's syndrome, acromegaly, and pheochromocytoma.

t., Göthlin's *See* test, capillary resistance.

t., hardness *See* hardness, Mohs; test, Brinell hardness; test, Knoop hardness; test, Vickers hardness.

t., Henderson's Test for acidosis. A normal person can hold his breath without preliminary deep inspiration for 30 seconds or more; the inability to hold it for more than 15 or 20 seconds in a person free from cardiorenal or pulmonary disease indicates the presence of acidosis.

t., Hess' *See* test, capillary resistance.

t., Hinton's A precipitation test for syphilis.

t., histoplasmin (his"tō-plaz'min) A skin test to determine sensitization to *Histoplasma capsulatum*. A positive test indicates past or present infection (histoplasmosis).

t., infectious mononucleosis One of several tests for the diagnosis of infectious mononucleosis (e.g., Paul-Bunnell test).

t., intracutaneous *See* test, skin.

t., intradermal *See* test, skin.

t., ivy's A test of bleeding time performed by making a standard wound and touching the blood with filter pap every 30 seconds until no blood appears on the paper. Normal range is 3 to 7 minutes.

t., Janet's A test to differentiate between functional and organic anesthesia. With the eyes closed, a patient is instructed to say "yes" or "no" as he feels or does not feel the examiner's touch. In functional anesthesia, he will say "no," whereas in organic anesthesia, he will say nothing.

t., Kahn's A precipitation test for the diagnosis of syphilis. *See also* test, serologic.

t., ketone bodies (acetone test, Rothera's test) Nitroprusside reaction tests for acetone and acetoacetic acid and the ferric chloride test for acetoacetic acid. Commercially prepared nitroprusside test tablets (Acetest) and powder (Acetone Test Denco) are available.

t., Kline's A flocculation test for syphilis based on the combination of the cardiolipin antigen with reagin to form grossly visible aggregates.

t., Knoop hardness A means of measuring surface hardness by resistance to the penetration of an indenting tool made of diamond. Produces an indentation that has a diamond or rhombic shape. Especially preferred for testing hardness of tooth structure.

t., laboratory Investigative procedures performed in the laboratory that are useful in the diagnosis of disease, including biopsy examination of tissue specimens, determination of type and characteristics of associated microorganisms, serology, blood and urine chemistry, hemogram (red cell count, hemoglobin content, white cell count, differential white cell count, etc.), metabolic studies (e.g., basal metabolic rate), etc.

t., LE A test for lupus erythematosus based on the presence of a single (or multiple) homogenous basophilic inclusion in polymorphonuclear leukocytes. Such LE cells have also been found in cases of rheumatoid arthritis, allergic reactions to penicillin, hydrolazine toxicity, and "lupoid cirrhosis."

t., lead Any of several tests used to detect clinical lead poisoning or exposure to lead (e.g., coproporphyrinuria test, trace element analysis, urinary lead content test, and basophilic aggregation test).

t., Leede's *See* test, capillary resistance.

t., liver function Tests to measure the severity of liver disease, aid in the differential diagnosis of the various types of disease of the hepatobiliary system, and follow the course of liver disease. Screening test include urine bile, urine urobilinogen, Bromsulphalein (BSP) excretion, serum transaminases, thymol turbidity, cephalin-cholesterol flocculation, and van den Bergh's reaction (1 minute direct and total).

t., Mann-Whitney U- A powerful nonparametric statistical test of significance between two means with unequal sample size.

t., Mantoux (mahn-too′) An intracutaneous tuberculin test using either old tuberculin (OT) or purified protein derivative (PPD). A positive reaction read 24 and 48 hours after injection shows erythema and edema greater than 5 mm in diameter and indicates past or present tuberculosis.

t., Mazzini's (mah-zē′nēz) A flocculation test for syphilis.

t., Mohs *See* hardness, Mohs.

t., nontreponemal antigen Serologic tests for syphilis using nontreponemal antigens. Such tests are not absolutely specific or sensitive for syphilis. Included are the Kline, Kahn, and Kolmer tests, and the VDRL slide test.

t., one-stage *See* time, prothrombin.

t., pancreatic function Tests of enzyme levels in blood and urine (amylase, lipase), fecal fat content, trypsin activity, nitrogen content, alteration of digestive capacity, and alteration of pancreatic secretion via duodenal intubation.

t., patch (percutaneous test) A test for allergy performed by placing the suspected allergen in direct contact with the skin or mucosa. *See also* test, skin.

t., Paul-Bunnell A test for infectious mononucleosis based on increased agglutination of sheep red blood cells resulting from heterophil antibodies in the serum. Considered positive if dilution of serum of 1:80 or higher agglutinates the sheep cells. Elevated agglutinin titers are more likely to be found during the second or third week of the disease but the serum may not become positive until 7 weeks have elapsed.

t., percussion A method of examination executed by striking the tissues of the area being examined with the fingers or an instrument, listening for resulting sounds, and observing the response of the patient.

t., percutaneous (per″kū-tā′nē-ŭs) *See* test, patch.

t., phenolsulfonphthalein (PSP) (fē″nol-sŭl″fōn-thal′ē-n) A renal test that roughly estimates glomerular function by measuring the rate of excretion of the dye after intravenous injection. Normally, after 15 minutes 25% or more of the dye should be excreted in the urine.

t., plasma ketone A test using nitroprusside for the detection of high levels of ketone bodies in the blood. The test is read 0 to 4+. A strongly positive reaction is seen in diabetic ketoacidosis.

t., pregnancy (Aschheim-Zondek test, Friedman's test) Biologic or chemical tests to determine pregnancy; usually based on changes in the ovaries of an animal injected with the urine of a pregnant woman. Included are the Aschheim-Zondek test (using mice or rats) and the Friedman test (using virgin rabbits). Male frogs and female and male toads are also used. A saliva test has also been used.

t., prothrombin consumption (serum prothrombin time) A convenient screening test of the first stage of blood coagulation as determined by the quantity of prothrombin remaining after coagulation. The test reflects the formation of plasma thromboplastin, provided the one-stage prothrombin time of plasma is normal. *See also* time, prothrombin.

t., pulmonary function Tests used to evaluate respiratory function (e.g., tests of vital capacity, tidal volume, maximal breathing capacity, timed vital capacity, arterial blood gases).

t., pulp A diagnostic test to determine clinical pulp vitality and/or abnormality.

t., rapid reagin Serologic tests for syphilis that permit rapid and economical screening in the field. Included are the rapid plasma reagin (RPR) test and the unheated serum reagin (USR) test.

t., Reiter protein complement-fixation (RPCF) (re'ter) Treponemal antigen test for syphilis using extracts from the nonpathogenic Reiter treponeme.

t., renal function Quantitative tests including inulin or mannitol clearance for the glomerular filtration rate (GFR), para-aminohippurate (PAH) clearance for renal plasma flow, and the maximum rate of tubular excretion of para-aminohippurate and the maximum rate of reabsorption of glucose for the measurement of excretory and reabsorptive functions of the renal tubules. Clinical renal tests are used to assess the extent of renal impairment. They include blood urea nitrogen (BUN), nonprotein nitrogen (NPN), urea clearance, endogenous creatinine clearance, filtration fraction, phenolsulfonphthalein (PSP), and concentration tests.

t., Rockwell An indentation test for hardness of a material. A static load is placed on a steel ball or diamond point, and the depth of the indentation is measured on the instrument. The depth of the indentation is remeasured after the load is increased. The hardness number is related to the type of point used and to the depth of the indentation.

t., Rothera's *See* test, ketone bodies.

t., routine A test or group of tests performed on most or all patients to detect relatively common disorders or to establish a base for further evaluation of a patient.

t., Rumple-Leede-Hess *See* test, capillary resistance.

t., scarlet fever *See* test, Dick's.

t., Schick A skin test to demonstrate the presence or absence of an immunity to diphtheria.

t., scratch (skin test) A test for allergy performed by placing a preparation containing the allergen on the skin and scratching the skin. A positive reaction is indicated by the formation of a wheal and flare.

t., screening A group of tests especially chosen to detect specific abnormalities.

t., serologic (sē″rō-loj′ĭk) Tests of blood serum for the diagnosis of infectious diseases.

t., skin Tests to determine the sensitivity or susceptibility to infections by a specific agent, the presence of an allergy, or the presence of a nutritional deficiency. Included are the Mantoux, Schick, Dick, Frei, histoplasmin, and Foshay tests for infectious diseases (tests in which allergens are placed onto or into the skin) and the intradermal ascorbic acid, dermal, intradermal (intracutaneous), patch (percutaneous), scratch, and subcutaneous tests.

t., tuberculin skin (tū-ber′kū-lin) Intradermal injection of old tuberculin (OT) or purified protein derivative (PPD) to determine a specific sensitivity or susceptibility to tuberculosis.

t., Snyder's *See* test, colorimetric caries susceptibility.

t., sterilizer Periodic use of spore strip, color strip, or other microbial test to ensure that a sterilizer (autoclave, oven, etc.) is killing all microbes predictably.

t., subcutaneous *See* test, skin.

t., Sulkowitch's A simple but rough qualitative evaluation of calcium in the urine based on the degree of precipitation following addition of oxalate.

t., syphilis Refers to any serologic test for syphilis based on the presence of a reagin, appearing during the second or third week of infection. Included are the Hinton, Kahn, Kline, Mazzini, Wassermann, and *Treponema pallidum* immobilization tests.

t., thermal The use of heat or cold as an aid in diagnosis (e.g., the use of heat or cold in testing the pulp).

t., Thorn's *See* test, ACTH-stimulation.

t., thromboplastin generation A test of the integrity of the first stage of blood coagulation and the nature of the defect. A patient's serum, plasma, or platelets are substituted in a system that is complete except for one of the factors to be tested for (antihemophilic factor, plasma thromboplastin antecedent, plasma thromboplastin component, or platelets), and the rate of thromboplastin generation is determined.

t., thyroid function Tests for thyroid function (e.g., radioactive iodine uptake, protein-bound iodine, basal metabolic rate, serum cholesterol, triiodothyronine suppression, thyroid-stimulating hormone tests).

t., tourniquet (toor′nĭ-kĕt) A test for capillary fragility based on counting petechiae in a given area of the arm after application of the rubber cuff of a sphygmomanometer for 15 minutes.

t., transaminase (trăns-ăm′ĭ-nās) Tests for serum glutamic oxaloacetic transaminase (SGOT) and serum glutamic pyruvic transaminase (SGPT). The normal value for serum glutamic oxaloacetic transaminase is 40 units or less; that for serum glutamic pyruvic transaminase is 35 units or less. The serum glutamic oxaloacetic transaminase value in myocardial infarction is 3 to 20 times the normal.

t., transillumination A test for a pulpless tooth in which the use of transmitted light shows a shadow of the root when the pulp is necrotic or has been replaced by a filling (not always reliable).

t., treponemal antigen Tests for syphilis using *Treponema pallidum* or extracts from a treponeme as antigen. Included are *T. pallidum* immobilization (TPI), *T. pallidum* agglutination (TPA), fluorescent treponemal antibody (FTA), Reiter protein complement-fixation (RPCF), and *T. pallidum* complement-fixation (TPCF) tests.

t., *Treponema pallidum* immobilization (TPI) A test to confirm syphilis by demonstrating the immobilization of *Treponema pallidum* by specific antibodies in the serum of an infected individual; not widely used.

t. for trigeminal nerve function Three simple clinical tests for trigeminal nerve function: sensation, apply gentle touch, pinpricks, or warm or cold objects to areas supplied by the nerve and note responses; reflex, try the jaw jerk, eye, and sneeze reflexes; motor function, test the patient's ability to chew and work against resistance and observe contraction of the masseter and temporal muscles by visual examination and digital palpation.

t., tuberculin A test for past or present infection with tubercle bacilli. *See also* test, Mantoux.

t., tularemia *See* test, Foshay's.

t., Tzanck's A supplemental test for pemphigus based on the presence of degenerative changes in epithelial cells (Tzanck's cells) in the bullous lesions of pemphigus. Degenerative changes include swelling of the nuclei and hyperchromic staining.

t., U-, Mann-Whitney *See* test, Mann-Whitney U-.

t., urea clearance A clinical test of renal function determined by the clearance of urea from the plasma by the kidney each minute. Average normal value is 75 ml/min (75% to 125% of normal).

t., urine, routine Routine examination of the urine, including amount, appearance, pH level, specific gravity, qualitative tests for sugar and protein, and microscopic examination of sediment.

t., van den Bergh's A test of hepatic function by measuring serum conjugated ("direct-reacting") 1 minute bilirubin, total serum bilirubin, and, by difference, unconjugated (indirect) biliiubin. Obstructive jaundice and hemolytic jaundice give abnormal values.

t., VDRL (Venereal Disease Research Laboratory) A serologic nontreponemal antigen test for the detection of syphilitic reagin by means of a reaction between the reagin and a standard antigen.

t., Vickers hardness A penetration type of hardness test using a square-based pyramid made of diamond.

t., viscosity of saliva A dental caries susceptibility test on freshly secreted saliva. An Oswald pipette is used in the determination of viscosity.

t., vitality The procedure using thermal, electrical, or mechanical stimuli to determine the response of the pulp in a tooth.

t., Wassermann A complement-fixation test for syphilis.

t., Zondek's *See* test, pregnancy.

testimony Evidence of a witness, given orally under oath or affirmation.

tetany, hyperventilation (tĕt′ah-nē hī″per-ve″n″tĭ-lā′shŭn) The neuromuscular irritability and tonic carpopedal muscle spasm resulting from the alklosis that

may be caused by forced respiration over an extended length of time.

tetracycline (tĕ″trah-sī′klēn) An antibiotic produced by certain strains of *Streptomyces*. Its administration during tooth formation may lead to enamel discoloration.

Tg value Transition point of glass. In dentistry, the temperature at which resin becomes soft.

thalamus (thăl′ah-mŭs) An ovoid mass in the brain immediately lateral to the third ventricle, which serves as the principal relay and integration station for the sensory systems in the body.

thalassemia (thăl″ah-sē′mē-ah) **(hereditary leptocytosis, hereditary microcytosis)** A hereditary, chronic, hemolytic anemia with erythroblastosis. A complex of hereditary disorders characterized by microcytosis and increased red blood cell destruction and frequently associated with abnormal hemoglobins and increased normal trace hemoglobins. These disorders are prevalent in people of Mediterranean, African, and Asian ancestry. Disorders include Cooley's anemia, Cooley's trait, hemoglobin H disease, Hb S—thalassemia, Hb C—thalassemia, and Hb E—thalassemia.

t., major (Cooley's anemia, erythroblastic anemia, familial erythroblastic anemia, hereditary microcytosis, Mediterranean anemia, Mediterranean disease) The severe homozygous form of thalassemia characterized by a marked microcytic hypochromic anemia, atypical nucleated red blood cells, marked increase in hemoglobin F, and skeletal changes (underdevelopment, mongoloid facies, anterior open bite).

t., minor (Cooley's trait) A heterozygous form of thalassemia that is a carried state with relatively mild manifestations. A_2 hemoglobin is elevated.

theory (thē′ō-rē) An opinion or hypothesis not based on actual knowledge.

t., Prothero "cone" *See* retention.

t., quantum The theory that in emission or absorption of energy by atoms or molecules, the process is not continuous but takes place by steps, each step being the emission or absorption of an amount of energy called a *quantum*.

t., somatotype The theory of W.H. Sheldon, suggesting that body structure is correlated with certain temperaments and predisposes to mental disorders.

therapeutic index (thĕr″ah-pū′tĭk) *See* index, therapeutic.

therapeutic vehicle A device used to transport and retain some agent for therapeutic purposes (e.g., radium carrier).

therapeutics (thĕr″ah-pū′tĭĸs) The art and science of treatment of disease.

therapy (thĕr′ah-pē) The treatment of disease.

t., antibiotic The treatment of disease states by the local or systemic administration of antibodies.

t., indirect pulpal Application of a drug that heals the pulpal cells beneath a layer of sound or carious dentin, as in a moderately deep preparation for a restoration.

t., myofunctional (myotherapeutic exercises) Use of muscle exercises as an adjunct to mechanical correction of malocclusion.

t., periodontal Treatment of the periodontal lesion. Such therapy has two principal objectives: the eradication or arrest of the periodontal lesion with correction or cure of the deformity created by it, and the alteration in the mouth of the periodontal climate that was conducive or contributory to the periodontal breakdown.

t., periodontal, maintenance phase The part of periodontal therapy that is necessary for the preservation of the results obtained during active therapy and for the prevention of further periodontal disease; an extension of active periodontal therapy, requiring the combined efforts of both the periodontist and the patient.

t., pulp canal See endodontology.

t., radiation (radiotherapy) Treatment of disease with any type of radiation.

t., replacement The administration, as a therapeutic agent, of an essential constituent in which the body is deficient (e.g., insulin in diabetes mellitus).

t., root canal See endodontology.

t., speech The science that deals with the use of procedures, training, and remedies for the cure, alleviation, or prevention of speech disorders.

thermal conductivity See conductivity, thermal.

thermal expansion See expansion, thermal.

thermal sensitivity See sensitivity, tooth.

thermionic emission The release of electrons when a material is heated (e.g., electron emmission when the tungsten cathode filament of an x-ray tube is heated to incandescence by means of its low-voltage heating circuit).

thermocouple The joining of two dissimilar metals. The unequal thermal expansion of the two metals is used to indicate temperature changes.

thermoluminescence (ther″mō-lū″mĭ-nĕs′ĕns) The capability of certain crystalline compounds, such as lithium fluoride, to release stored energy as luminescent energy when heated.

thermoluminescent dosimetry (ther″mō-lū-mĭ-nĕs′ĕnt dō-sĭm′ĕ-trē) Determination of the amount of radiation to which a thermoluminescent material has been exposed. This is accomplished by heating the material in a specially designed instrument that relates the amount of luminescence emitted from the material to the amount of radiation exposure.

thermoplastic (ther′mō-plăs′tĭk) The property of becoming soft with the application of heat, rigid at normal temperature, and again soft with the reapplication of heat. A reversible physical phenomenon.

thermosetting Having the property of becoming rigid or hardened with the application of heat. Not reversible. In dentistry, the term is used in connection with resins.

thermostat An automatic temperature control device.

thiamine (thī′ah-mĭn) See vitamin, thiamine.

Thiersch's skin graft (tērsh′ēz) See graft, Thiersch's skin.

thimble See coping.

t., ionization chamber See chamber, ionization, thimble.

Thiokol (thī′ō-kol) Trade name for polysulfide polymer using a mercaptan bond. The basic ingredient of rubber base impression materials. See also mercaptan.

third party The party to a dental benefits contract that may collect premiums, assume financial risk, pay claims, and/or provide other administrative services. Synonyms: administrative agent carrier, insurer, underwriter.

third-party administrator (TPA) Claims payer who assumes responsibility for administering health benefit plans without assuming any financial risk. Some commercial insurance carriers and Blue Cross/Blue Shield plans also have TPA operations to accommodate self-funded employers seeking administrative services only (ASO) contracts.

third-party payer An organization other than the patient (first party) or health care provider (second party) involved in the financing of personal health services.

third party payment Payment for services by someone other than the beneficiary (e.g., when an employer or union makes such payment).

threat A menace; a statement of one's intention to harm or injure the person, property, or rights of another.

threshold (thrĕsh′ōld) The lowest limit of stimulus capable of producing an impression of the consciousness or of evoking a response in an irritable tissue.

t. dose See dose, threshold.

t., swallowing The minimum stimulation required to initiate the reflex action of deglutition.

threonine (thre′ō-nĭn) One of the essential amino acids See also amino acid.

thrill 1: A vibration felt on the chest wall over the heart. It is caused by eddy flow of the blood, which is produced by a structural defect in the heart. **2:** Palpable high-frequency vibration that may accompany cardiac murmurs or vascular disease.

thrombasthenia (thrŏm″băs-thē′nē-ah) A hemorrhagic diathesis associated with qualitative abnormalities of the platelets.

thrombin (throm′bĭn) A proteolytic enzyme formed from prothrombin by the action of thromboplastin. Ca^{++}, and other factors. Thrombin forms fibrin from fibrinogen, speeds up the disruption of platelets, and activates factor V.

thrombocatalysin (thrŏm″bō-kă-tăl′ĭ-sĭn) *See* factor VIII.

thrombocythemia (thrŏm″bō-sī-thē′mē-ah) An increase in the number of circulating blood platelets.

thrombocytin (throm″bo-si′tin) *See* serotonin.

thrombocytolysin (thrŏm″bō-sī-tol′ĭ-sĭn) *See* factor VIII.

thrombocytosis (throm″bō-sī-tō′sĭs) Unusually large numbers of platelets in the circulating blood. It may occur after surgical procedures, parturition, and injury, or with thrombocythemia.

thrombogen (thrŏm′bō-jĕn) Prothrombin. *See also* factor V.

thrombogene *See* factor V.

thrombokatilysin (thrŏm″bō-kă-tĭl′ĭ-sĭn) *See* factor VIII.

thrombokinase (throm″bō-kī′nās) *See* factor III.

thrombokinin (throm″bō-kĭn′ĭn) *See* factor III.

thrombopenia, essential (throm″bō′nē-ah) *See* purpura, thrombocytopenic.

thrombophlebitis (throm″bō-fle-bī′tis) An inflammation of the vein in which the vein becomes closed or occluded resulting from the development of a clot or thrombus.

thromboplastic plasma component (TPC) *See* factor VIII.

thromboplastin (throm″bō-plăs′tĭn) A substance necessary to the coagulant activity of tissue extracts; also has been referred to as the direct activator of prothrombin and as a substance from plasma, platelets, and tissues that initiates thromboplastic activity in blood coagulation. *See also* thromboplastin, extrinsic.

t., activated *See* thromboplastin, extrinsic.

t., cofactor of *See* factor V.

t., extrinsic (prothrombinase, extrinsic prothrom-bin activator, proconvertin-convertin, cothromboplastin, activated thromboplastin) A direct prothrombin activator formed by the interaction of brain extracts, factors V and VH, and Ca^{++}.

t., incomplete Tissue thromboplastin.

t., intrinsic (plasma thromboplastin, intrinsic prothrombin activator) A prothrombin activator formed from interaction of blood coagulation factors V, VHI, IX, and X and Ca^{++} with a foreign surface.

t., tissue A factor in tissue extract responsible for coagulation of blood.

thromboplastinogen (throm″bō-plăs-tĭn′ō-jĕn) *See* factor VIII.

thromboplastinogenase (throm″bō-plăs-tĭn′ō-jĕn-ās) *See* factor, platelet, 3.

thrombosis (thrŏm-bō′sĭs) Presence of a clot or deposit in a blood vessel, formed in situ and remaining in place.

t., cavernous sinus A blood clot in the cavernous sinus occasionally arising from maxillary periapical infection. The prognosis is poor but not so grave as be-

fore antibiotic therapy.

t., coronary Thrombosis of the coronary artery; Synonyms: heart attack and coronary occlusion.

thrombotonin *See* serotonin.

thrombozyme (throm′bō-zīm) *See* factor II.

thrombus (throm′bŭs) A blood clot in a vessel or in one of the chambers of the heart that remains at the point of its formation.

thrush (candidiasis, moniliasis) A disease caused by *Candida albicans* and characterized by white patches that scrape off with some difficulty, leaving bleeding bases. This term usually is used for the intraoral disease, whereas *moniliasis* is the term applied to the condition in other areas of infection by the yeast, as well as the oral cavity. *See also* candidiasis; moniliasis.

thumb sucking *See* finger sucking.

thyroid, lingual (thī′roid) Presence of thyroid tissue in the tongue, which is related to abnormal embryonic activity of the thyroglossal duct.

thyroxine (thī-rŏk′sĕn) The hormone secretion of the thyroid gland, 3,5,3′,5′-tetraiodothyronine.

tic An involuntary purposeless movement of muscle, usually occurring under emotional stress. It is a survival in stereotyped form of a movement or muscle set once used voluntarily and purposefully.

t. douloureux Spontaneous trigeminal neuralgia associated with a "trigger zone" and causing spasmodic contraction of the facial muscles. *See also* neuralgia, trigeminal.

ticaricillin (ti″kar-sil′in) An anti-*Psuedomonas* penicillin.

t.i.d. Abbreviation for *ter in die*, a Latin phrase meaning "three times day."

time A measure of duration.

t., clot retaction The time required for a given quantity of blood to separate in the tube in which it has been placed. For 3 ml of blood at room temperature, 1 hour is normal. It is very slow in thrombocytopenia.

t., coagulation The time required for blood clotting to begin in a capillary tube, normally 2 to 8 minutes. A coagulation time three times normal is a definite danger sign.

t., gel (gelation time) The interval of time required for a colloidal solution to become a solid or semisolid jelly or gel. Usually refers to the working time of a hydrocolloid or alginate impression material.

t., gelation *See* time, gel.

t. limits The periods of time within which a notice of claim must be filed.

t., median lethal (LD$_{50}$ time, MLT) The time required for 50% of a large group of animals or organisms to die after administration of a specified dose of radiation.

t., prothrombin (one-stage test) A gross but useful screening test of the completeness of the second and third stages of blood coagulation. Normal prothrombin time by the Quick method is 12 to 15 seconds. The time will be affected by deficiencies of factor V or factor VH as well as of prothrombin. *See also* test, prothrombin consumption.

t., serum prothrombin *See* test, prothrombin consumption.

t., setting The length of time for a mixed preparation of materials to reach a state of hardness, measured from the start of the mixing. The end point for dental materials is usually determined by a penetration test.

timer Radiographic timing device that functions as an automatic exposure timer and as a switch to control the current to the high-tension transformer and filament transformer. The face of the timer is calibrated in seconds and fractions of seconds. The timer controls the total time that the current passes through the x-ray tube and thus the time during which the x rays are emitted. The timer activates a switch or contractor that closes and opens the low-voltage circuit of the high voltage.

t., electronic An electronic vacuum tube device, with no moving parts, that covers a time range of $\frac{1}{20}$ to 10 seconds. It automatically sets itself, it more accurate than mechanical timers, and meets all the needs of modern high-speed dental techniques.

t., foot A timer with an attachment that permits the timing device to be activated by foot pressure. This is the preferred type of timer.

t., hand An attachment to or part of a timer that requires thumb or finger pressure to activate the timing device.

t., mechanical A timer using a spring mechanism for determination of length of expsoure. Accuracy of timing is not assumed in exposure of less than 1 second with a mechanical timer.

tinfoil *See* foil, tin.

t. substitute *See* substitute, tinfoil.

tin octoate (ŏk′tō-āt) Substance used to accomplish vulcanization of silicone rubber impression materials. It is not a true catalyst because it becomes part of the final polymer.

tincture (tĭngk′tūr) An alcoholic, hydroalcoholic, or ethereal solution of a drug.

Tinel's sign (tĭn-ĕlz′) *See* sign, Tinel's.

tinnitus (tĭ-nī′tŭs) Noises or unpleasant sounds in the ears, such as ringing, buzzing, roaring, or clicking; is usually high pitched and heard by many persons with auditory impairment. Clicking tinnitus may be heard by others.

tinted denture base *See* base, denture, tinted.

tipping of cusps *See* restoration of cusps.

tissue (tĭsh′ū) An aggregation of similarly specialized cells united in the performance of a particular function.

t. adhesives Agents or materials that can seal two cut tissue surfaces together or that can cover a surgically exposed surface such as butyl cyanoacrylate, which is used to cover palatal donor sites in periodontal surgery.

t.-borne partial denture *See* denture, partial, tissue-borne.

t., compression of *See* tissue displaceability.

t., connective The binding and supportive tissue of the body; derived from the mesoderm; depending on its location and function, it is composed of fibroblasts, primitive mesenchymal cells, collagen fibers, and elastic fibers, with associated blood and lymphatic vessels, nerve fibers, etc.

t., critical Tissue that reacts most unfavorably to radiation or, by its nature, attracts and absorbs specific radiochemicals.

t. displaceability The quality of oral tissues that permits them to be placed in, or to assume, other than their relaxed position.

t. displacement Change in the form or position of tissues as a result of pressure.

t., flabby *See* tissue, hyperplastic.

t., hyperplastic In dentistry, excessively movable tissue about the mandible or maxillae resulting from increase in the number of normal cells.

t., interdental The gingivae, cementum of the teeth, free gingival and transseptal fibers of the periodontal membrane (ligament), and alveolar and supporting bone.

t. molding *See* border molding.

t., peripheral *See* border structures.

t., redundant *See* epulis fissuratum.

t., subjacent The structures that underlie or are in border contact with a denture base; they may or may not have a supporting relationship to the overlying base.

titanium (tĭ-tā′nē-ūm) A metallic element used extensively in implant dentistry and in orthodontic arch wires.

titer (tī′tĕr) The standard amount by volume of a material required to produce a desired reaction with another material.

title Evidence of the right of a person to the possession of property.

titration (tī-trā′shŭn) Incremental increase in drug dosage to that level which provides the optimal therapeutic effect.

TMJ facebow *See* facebow, kinematic.

TMJ pain-dysfunction syndrome *See* temporomandibular pain-dysfunction syndrome.

TMP-SMZ Abbreviation for trimethroprim-sulfamethroxazole.

TNF An abbreviation for tumor necrosis factor, a genetic triggered, tumor-killing agent produced by the body in small amounts to counteract neoplastic growth. An experimental agent used in the treatment of cancers.

toilet of cavity *See* cavity, toilet.

tolerance (tŏl'ĕ-rănce) The ability to endure the influence of a drug or poison, particularly acquired by continued use of the substance. *See also* resistance.

t., acquired Tolerance that develops with successive doses of a drug. If it develops within a short span of time, such as 24 hours, it is called *tachyphylaxis*. Slowly acquired tolerance is sometimes called *mithridatism*.

t., carbohydrate The ability of the body to use carbohydrates. A decrease in tolerance is seen in diabetes mellitus, liver damage, and some infections and in the presence of hyperactivity of the adrenal cortex or pituitary gland.

t., cross Tolerance to a number of drugs of similar mode of action or chemical structure.

t., individual Tolerance characteristic of an individual.

t., pseudo- A state of apparent tolerance because the drug does not reach its usual receptor sites.

t., species Tolerance characteristic of a species of animal.

t., tissue The ability of structures to endure environtmental change without ill effect.

tomogram *See* examination, radiographic, extraoral body section.

tomograph A radiograph produced while rotating the film and x-ray source in opposite directions around an axis located in the region of interest. This movement blurs outside structures while maintaining sharpness in the region of interest.

tongue (tŭng) The muscular organ that is the main articulatory element in the production of speech and accounts for the clarity and fluidity of speech. There are two groups of tongue muscles, the intrinsic and extrinsic, which are united into one organ. Each group, however, has separate structural and functional characteristics.

t., amyloid (amyloid macroglossia) Enlargement of the tongue resulting from amyloidosis.

t., antibiotic A glossitis caused by sensitivity to an antibiotic, vitamin B complex deficiency associated with antibiotic therapy.

t., bald *See* glossitis, atrophic.

t., Sandwith's bald A condition in which the tongue is very smooth because of a loss of fusiform papillae and is fiery red and enlarged because of severe inflammation; seen in pellagra.

t., beefy Erythematous and/or atrophic glossitis *See also* glossitis, atrophic; glossitis, Moeller's.

t., bifid (cleft tongue) A tongue divided by a midline cleft.

t., cleft *See* tongue, bifid.

t., coated Nonspecific term used to describe the condition of the tongue resulting from whitish or otherwise discolored accumulations of food debris, bacterial plaques, and hyperplastic filiform papillae. Reduced function, as in general illness or laryngitis, is a primary cause.

t. crib An appliance used to limit undesirable tongue movements, usually constructed to prevent its protrusion between the anterior teeth.

t., cobblestone Hyperplasia and hyperemia of fungiform and filiform papillae of the tongue in riboflavin deficiency. Formerly used to describe syphilitic glossitis with leukoplakia.

t., fissured (furrowed tongue) A tongue traversed by clefts that may be arranged like the veins of a leaf or that may be such as to give the tongue a "pavement block" appearance. It is seen in 5% of all dental patients but in 13% of those past 50 years of age.

t., flat Paralysis of the transverse lingual muscles such that the borders of the tongue cannot be rolled resulting from congenital syphilis.

t., furrowed *See* tongue, fissured.

t., geographic (benign migratory glossitis, glossitis areata exfoliativa, glossitis migrans, wandering rash) A condition characterized by a chronic, circumscribed, more or less circinate desquamation of the superficial epithelium of the dorsum of the tongue. The spots of desquamation migrate continuously, usually passing from the region near the vallate papillae toward the tip of the tongue.

t., hairy Hyperplasia of the filiform papillae of the tongue, frequently associated with oral moniliasis and the use of antibiotics or tobacco.

t., black hairy (lingua nigra) A black appearance of the dorsal surface of the tongue; caused by elongated filiform papillae and an accumulation of dark pigments, microorganisms, and food debris.

t., white hairy (lingua alba, lingua villosa alba) Hairy tongue characterized by elongation of the filiform papillae but without the dark staining seen in lingua nigra (black hairy tongue). *See also* tongue, black hairy.

t., lobulated A congenital defect with a secondary lobe of the tongue arising from its surface.

t., magenta The reddish purple tongue of riboflavin deficiency.

t. room *See* tongue space.

t., smooth *See* glossitis, atrophic.

t. space The space available for functioning of the tongue.

t., strawberry The red, inflamed tongue with prominent fungiform papillae characteristic of scarlet fever.

t. thrust Thrusting of the tongue between the anterior teeth, especially in the initial stage of swallowing.

This action, often combined with a resting position also between the teeth, can inhibit normal eruption and so produce an open bite.

tonofibril (tŏn-ŏ-fī′brĭl) A fibril emanating from epithelial cells. Recent electron microscopy has shown such fibrils to be irregular formations of the cell membrane.

tonsil (tŏn′sĭl) A rounded mass of tissue, usually of a lymphoid nature (especially the palatine tonsil).

tonsillitis (ton″sĭ-lī′tĭs) Inflammation of the tonsils.

    t., lingual A form of tonsillitis at the posterior part of the base of the tongue in the lymphoid masses (lingual tonsils) located there.

tonus, muscle (tō′nŭs) The steady reflex contraction that resides in the muscles concerned in maintaining erect posture. Tonus has its basis in the positional interactions of the muscle and its accompanying nerve structure; e.g., a muscle holds the body (mandible) in a given position, and the awareness of this position is constantly being relayed by the sensory approaches to the cortex. Any change in position or contractility of the muscle that affects its tonus is immediately relayed by the sensory apparatus for readjustment.

    t., facial muscle The tone of the facial musculature, which is a major factor in providing the esthetic values of the human face. The configurations of the face, which are maintained by good muscle tonus, are the modiolus, philtrum, nasolabial sulcus, and mentolabial sulcus. These functional contours are present when the nerve tissue is intact. They are altered by the loss of teeth or impaired nerve function. Their presence is an indication of the good state of health of the nerve and possibly of the dental arch.

tooth, teeth One of the hard bodies or processes usually protruding from and attached to the alveolar process of the maxillae and the mandible; designed for the mastication of food.

    t., abutment A tooth or teeth selected to support a prosthesis on the basis of the total surface areas of a healthy attachment apparatus.

    t., accessory (ăk-sĕs′ō-rē) Supernumerary teeth that do not resemble normal teeth in size, shape, or location. *See also* distomolar; mesiodens; paramolar; tooth supernumerary.

    t., acrylic resin (ah-krĭl′ĭk) A tooth made of acrylic resin.

    t., anatomic An artificial tooth that closely resembles the anatomic form of a natural unabraded tooth.

    t., ankylosed Abnormal calcification of the periodontal ligament resulting in abnormal fixation of a tooth.

    t., anterior One of the incisor or canine teeth.

    t., artificial A tooth fabricated for use as a substitute for a natural tooth in a prosthesis; usually made of porcelain or plastics.

    t., canine The four canines; the third tooth located distal to the midline in any one of the four quadrants of the dentition.

    t., conical (peg-shaped tooth) Failure of morphologic development of the tooth germ found in ectodermal dysplasia and other disorders and occasionally found in normal children.

    t., cross-bite Posterior teeth designed to permit the modified buccal cusps of the upper teeth to be positioned in the central fossae of the lower teeth.

    t., cuspless Teeth designed without cuspal prominences on the masticatory surfaces.

    t., deciduous *See* deciduous; tooth, primary.

    t., devital *See* tooth, pulpless.

    t., drifting The migration of teeth from their normal positions in the dental arches as a result of such factors as loss of proximal support, loss of funtional antagonists, occlusal traumatic tooth relationships, inflammatory and retrograde changes in the attachment apparatus, and oral habits.

    t., embedded An unerupted tooth, usually one completely covered with bone; also spelled imbedded. *See also* tooth, impacted.

    t., evulsed (avulsed tooth) A tooth that has been abnormally luxated from its alveolar support, commonly as a sequela to trauma.

    t. form *See* form, tooth.

    t., fulcrum The axis of movement of a tooth when lateral forces are applied to the tooth. The fulcrum is considered to be at the middle third of the portion of root embedded in the alveolus and thus moves apically as the bone resorbs in periodontal disease.

    t., fused Two teeth united during development by the union of their tooth germs. The teeth may be joined by the enamel of their crowns, root dentin, or both. Usually consists of a single large crown.

    t., geminated (jĕm′ĭ-nā-tĕd) Teeth with bifid crowns and confluent root canals resulting from the division of the enamel organ during the developmental period.

    t., grinding of The selective modification of tooth form and contour in the occlusal adjustment operation to eliminate occlusal interferences and establish tooth contours conducive to the health of the periodontium. *See also* bruxism.

    t., hereditary brown *See* hypoplasia, enamel, hereditary.

    t., Hutchinson's After Sir Jonathan Hutchinson, who reported the typical defects of the permanent incisors associated with congenital syphilis. Dental hypoplasia affects primarily the incisors, canines, and first permanent molars. The incisors have a screwdriver or peg-shaped appearance. *See also* triad, Hutchinson.

    t., hypoplasia of (hī″pō-plā′zē-ah) A reduction in the amount of enamel formed, resulting in irregular pits and grooves of the enamel.

t., impacted A condition in which the unerupted or partially erupted tooth is positioned against another tooth, bone, or soft tissue so that complete eruption is unlikely. An impacted third molar tooth may be further described according to its position: buccoangular, distoangular, vertical, etc. An impacted maxillary canine tooth may also be further described according to its position: palatal (maxillary canine), lingual (mandibular canine), labial, vertical, etc.

t., inclination of The angle of slope of teeth from the vertical planes of reference. Thus a tooth may be mesially, distally, lingually, buccally, or labially inclined.

t., loss of The separation of a tooth from its investing and supporting structures as a result of normal exfoliation attending loss of deciduous dentition, exfoliation as a sequela to excessive bone resorption and periapical migration of the epithelial attachment in periodontal disease, and instrumentation for extraction necessitated by pathologic involvement of the dental pulp, periodontium, periapical tissues, etc.

t., mesial movement of Migration of teeth toward the midline, occurring as a phenomenon associated with the action of the anterior component of force. Mesial migration of teeth occurs with the wear of their proximal surfaces resulting from the buccolingual movements of the teeth.

t., metal insert An artificial tooth, usually of acrylic resin, containing an inserted ribbon of metal, or a cutting blade, in its occlusal surface, with one edge of the blade exposed; sometimes used in removable dentures.

t., migration of The movement of teeth into altered positions in relationship to the basal bone of the alveolar process and to adjoining and opposing teeth as a result of loss of approximating or opposing teeth, occlusal interferences, habits, inflammatory and dystrophic disease of the attaching and supporting structures of the teeth, etc.

t., missing The absence of teeth from the dentition because of congenital factors, exfoliation, extraction, etc.

t., mobility The movability of a tooth resulting from loss of all or a portion of its attachment and supportive apparatus. Seen in periodontitis, occlusal traumatism, and periodontosis.

t. morphology The anatomic topography of the teeth.

t. movement *See* movement, tooth.

t., natal Primary teeth found in the oral cavity at birth.

t., neonatal A primary tooth that erupts into the oral cavity during the neonatal period (from birth to 30 days).

t., nonanatomic Artificial teeth so designed that the occlusal surfaces are not copies from natural forms,

but rather are given forms which, in the opinion of the designer, seem more nearly to fulfill the requirements of mastication, tissue tolerance, etc.

t., peg-shaped *See* tooth, conical.

t., permanent *See* dentition, permanent.

t., pink *See* resorption, internal.

t., plastic Artificial teeth constructed of synthetic resins.

t., polishing of The removal of film, plaque, soft deposits, etc. from the teeth by appropriate hand- and/or engine-driven instrumentation. Abrasive cups, wheels, or disks are often used in conjunction with abrasive pastes such as pumice and water.

t. position *See* position, tooth.

t., posterior The maxillary and mandibular premolars and molars of the permanent dentition, or the premolars and molars of prostheses.

t., primary 1: Term used by some in preference to deciduous teeth; however, it has not received the approval of preference by the American Dental Association. *See also* deciduous. **2:** As a result of a survey of the terminology used to name the teeth of the first dentition, the College Committee Report of Dentistry for Children recommended in 1942 the use of *primary teeth* as the term preferred to *deciduous, first, milk, temporary, baby, or foundation teeth.* The term *primary* was suggested as a word "which may be acceptable to the dental profession, significant in its meaning, with no connotations of impermanence, and readily understood by nonprofessional people."

t., pulpless A tooth from which the dental pulp has been removed or is necrotic.

t., replaced *See* tooth, supplied.

t., rotated An altered position of the tooth in relation to the adjacent and opposing teeth and to its basal alveolar process; in such an altered position the tooth has been turned on its long axis and is in a state of torsiversion. The result is an altered contact with adjacent teeth that produces a possible locus for food impaction between the teeth, with consequent gingival damage.

t. selection *See* selection, tooth.

t., sensitivity of A painful pulpal response to external stimuli such as heat, cold, and sweet substances. The most common clinical findings is a hyperesthetic state of the root surface resulting from loss of a portion of the cemental covering with exposure of the dentin.

t., drugs for sensitivity of The medicaments used to treat hypersensitivity of the teeth; they should cause relatively little pain when applied; should be easily applied, rapid in action, and permanently effective; and should not discolor the teeth or unduly irritate the pulp. Substances used include 33% sodium fluoride in kaolin and glycerin, a 25% aqueous solution of strontium chloride, hot medicinal olive oil, 0.9% solution of sodium silicofluoride, etc.

t., separation of The action of moving a tooth mesially or distally out of contact with its neighboring tooth.

t., immediate separation of Separation of teeth accomplished rapidly by the wedging action of an appliance during restorative procedures.

t., slow separation of Separation of teeth accomplished over a long period of time, usually by the wedging action of a material such as guttapercha, orthodontic wire, thread, or fibers in orthodontic therapy.

t., set of Term that usually refers to a full complement of maxillary and/or mandibular artificial teeth, as they are carded by the manufacturer.

t., setting up of The arranging of teeth on a trial denture base; includes proper relation with occluding teeth.

t. size discrepancy Lack of proportional harmony in the width of various teeth, causing relative spacing and crowding in different parts of the dentition.

t., shell A form of dentinal dysplasia characterized by large pulp chambers, meager coronal dentin, and, usually, no roots.

t., supernumerary Extra erupted or unerupted teeth that resemble teeth of normal shape.

t., supplied (replaced teeth) Artificial replacements for natural teeth.

t., supportive mechanisms of The anatomic structures that function to maintain or to aid in maintaining the teeth in position in their alveoli: the gingivae, cementum of the tooth, periodontal membrane, and alveolar and supporting bone. *See also* structures, supporting.

t., tube Artificial teeth constructed with a vertical, cylindric aperture extending from the center of the base up into the body of the tooth into which a pin or cast post for the attachment of the tooth to a denture base may be placed.

t., Turner's A permanent tooth showing hypoplasia resulting from injury or inflammation of the precedent deciduous tooth.

t., vital staining of The staining of enamel and dentin of primary and permanent teeth during development with vital stains (e.g., with bile pigment in Rh incompatibility or with tetracyclines).

t., zero degree Prosthetic teeth having no cusp angles in relation to the horizontal plane; cuspless teeth.

toothache Dental pain.

tooth-borne Term used to describe a prosthesis or a part of a prosthesis that depends entirely on the abutment teeth for support.

t.-b. base The denture base restoring an edentulous

area that has abutment teeth at each end for support. The tissue that it covers is not used for support of the base.

toothbrushing The use of a brush of varying design to brush the teeth and gingivae for cleanliness and to massage for oral hygiene.

t., faulty The improper performance of toothbrushing, resulting in defective cleansing, inadequate stimulation of the gingival tissues, or destructive effects on the teeth and marginal gingivae resulting from overzealous brushing.

tooth eruption The process by which the tooth moves from its site of formation to its position of function.

toothpaste *See* dentifrice.

toothpick A wood sliver used to cleanse the interdental space.

t., balsa wood A triangular wedge of balsa wood used to clean the teeth interproximally and to stimulate the interdental gingival tissues.

topographic intraoral radiographic examination *See* examination, true occlusal topographic intraoral radiographic.

torque (tork)   **1:** A force that produces or tends to produce rotation in a body. Such force applied to a tooth tends to cause rotation around its long axis.   **2:** Force applied to a tooth to produce rotation of a tooth on a mesiodistal or buccolingual (labiolingual) axis.   **3:** A rotary force applied to a denture base.

t. wire An auxiliary wire used to torque the roots of the anterior teeth.

torsion In dentistry, the twisting of a tooth on its long axis.

t., clasp The twisting of the retentive clasp arm on its long axis. It has been suggested that a retentive clasp be formed so that it traverses a vertical distance before encircling the abutment to increase the torsion component of the clasp opening as compared to the flexure that it undergoes.

torsiversion An axially rotated tooth position.

tort A legal wrong perpetrated on a person or property independent of contract.

torus A bulging projection of bone.

t. mandibularis A bony enlargement (hyperostosis) appearing unilaterally or bilaterally on the lingual aspect of the mandible in the canine-premolar region of about 7% of the population.

t. palatinus A bony enlargement (hyperostosis) occurring in the midline of the hard palate in about 20% of the population.

total filtration *See* filtration, total.

touch The sense by which contact with an object provides evidence of its properties.

t., light Tactile sense. The principal organs of light touch are Meissner's corpuscles, which are large in size and oval in shape. Each capsule receives several nerve fibers that shed their myelin sheath and coil into a spiral complex network. Associated with Meissner's corpuscles in the perception of light touch are both Merkel's disks and a basketlike arrangement of nerve fibers around the hair follicles.

t., screen A type of screen on some video terminals that may be touched with the finger to specify the selection of an item from a displayed list.

toxic (tŏk′sĭc) Poisonous; produced by a poison.

toxicity (tŏks-ĭs′ĭ-tē) Poisonous; produced by a poison; the ability of a drug or poison to produce harm, especially to cause permanent injury or death. Usually distinguished from allergenic properties.

t., acute A condition produced after short-term use of a toxic agent. *See also* dose, lethal, median; dose, lethal, minimum.

t., chronic A condition produced after long-term use of a toxic agent.

toxicologist (tŏk′sĭ-kol′ō-jĭst) One versed in toxicology.

toxicology (tŏk″sĭ-kŏl′ō-jē) The scientific study of the nature and effects of poisons, their detection, and the treatment of their effects.

toxiods Toxins that have been treated to destroy their toxic properties but to retain their ability to induce antibody production, thus creating an active immunity.

toxoplasmosis (tŏk″sō-plăz-mō′sĭs) A disease caused by protozoa in the bloodstream and body tissues.

TPC (thromboplastic plasma component) *See* factor VIII.

TPI *See* test, *Treponema pallidum* immobilization.

tracer 1: A mechanical device used to trace a Pattern of mandibular movements. **2:** A foreign substance mixed with or attached to a given substance to enable the distribution or location of the latter to be determined subsequently. A radioactive tracer is a physical or chemical tracer having radioactivity as its distinctive property.

t., Gothic arch *See* tracer, needle point.

t., needle point A mechanical device consisting of a weighted or a spring-loaded needle that is attached to one jaw and a coated plate that is attached to the other jaw. Movement of the mandible causes a tracing to be formed on the horizontally placed plate. When the needle point is in the apex of the tracing, the mandible is said to be in the horizontal position of centric relation.

trachea (trā′kē-ah) The windpipe; a cartilaginous and membranous tube extending from the lower end of the larynx to its division into two bronchi.

tracheal tugging (trā′kē-ăl) The downward tugging movement of the larynx.

tracheo- (trā′kē-ō) Combining form denoting connection with or relation to the trachea.

tracheobronchial (trā″kē-ō-brŏng′kē-al) Pertaining to the trachea and a bronchus or bronchi.

tracheobronchoscopy (trā″kē-ō-brong-kŏs′kō-pē) Inspection of the interior of the trachea and bronchus.

tracheolaryngeal (trā″kē-ō-lah-rĭn′jē-al) Pertaining to the trachea and larynx.

tracheolaryngotomy (trā″kē-ō-lar″ĭng-got′ō-mē) Incision into the larynx and the trachea; tracheotomy and laryngotomy.

tracheoscopy (trā″ke-os′kō-pē) Inspection of the interior of the trachea by means of a laryngoscopic mirror and reflected light or through a bronchoscope.

tracheostenosis (trā″kē-ō-stĕ-nō′sĭs) Abnormal constriction or narrowing of the trachea.

tracheostomy (trā″kē-os′tō-mē) **1:** The formation of an opening into the trachea and the suturing of the edges of the opening to an opening in the skin of the neck. **2:** Surgical formation of an opening into the trachea, usually through the tracheal rings below the cricoid cartilage, to give the patient an airway.

tracheotome (trā′kē-ō-tōm″) **1:** A cutting instrument used in tracheotomy; a tracheotomy knife. **2:** An instrument for use in creating an airway through the skin into the trachea below the cricoid cartilage.

tracheotomy (trā″kē-ot′ō-mē) The operation of cutting into the trachea to give the patient an airway.

tracing A line or lines or a pattern scribed by a pointed instrument or stylus on a tracing plate or tracing paper.

t., arrow point *See* tracing, needle point.

t., cephalometric A line drawing of pertinent features of a cephalometric radiograph made on a piece of transparent paper placed over the radiogaph.

t., extraoral A tracing of mandibular movements made outside the oral cavity.

t., Gothic arch *See* tracing, needle point.

t., intraoral A tracing of mandibular movements made within the oral cavity.

t., needle point (arrow point tracer, Gothic arch tracer) A tracing made by a mechanical device, consisting of a weighted or spring-loaded stylus that is attached to one jaw and contacts a coated plate attached to the other jaw. Movement of the mandible causes a tracing to be formed on the horizontally placed coated plate. When the stylus point is in the apex of the tracing, the mandible is said to be in the horizontal position of centric relation. The shape of the tracing depends on the relative location of the marking point and the tracing table. The various tracing shapes have been called *Gothic arch, arrow point*, and *sea gull tracings*. The apex of a properly made tracing indicates the most retruded unstrained relation of the mandible to the maxillae (i.e., the centric relation). The tracings are made by a stylus (or needle point) by the movement of the mandible. Unless otherwise designated, stylus tracings are made by lateral movements registered on a horizontal plate.

t., sea gull *See* tracing, needle point.

t., stylus *See* tracing, needle point.

tracings, pantographic Mandibular tracings, made on maxillary held planes, that record simultaneously the movements made by the mandible about its axes.

tract, sinus A communication between a pathologic space and an anatomic body cavity or between a pathologic space and the skin. A sinus tract may or may not be lined with epithelium.

traction The act of drawing (pulling).

t., external A fracture reduction appliance principally used in the management of midfacial fractures. Points of fixation are located in the oral cavity and over the cranial area, with elastic or rigid connectors between the cranial and oral points of fixation.

t., intermaxillary *See* traction, maxillomandibular.

t., internal A pulling force created by using one of the cranial bones, above the point of fracture, for anchorage.

t., maxillomandibular (intermaxillary traction) The technique for reducing fractures of the maxillae or mandible into functional relations with the opposing dental arch through the use of elastic or wire ligatures and interdental wiring and/or splints.

tragion (trā′jē-on) The notch just above the tragus of the ear. It lies 1 to 2 mm below the spina helicis, which may be easily palpated.

tragus (trā′gŭs) A prominence in front of the opening of the external ear.

trait (trāt) An inherited set of mental or bodily characteristics.

t., Cooley's *See* thalassemia minor.

t., sickle cell A form of sickle cell disease in which patients are asymptomatic, but their erythrocytes can be caused to assume a sickle shape under certain conditions. The trait is present when one parent has the gene (heterozygous condition) for sickle cell disease. *See also* disease, sickle cell.

tranquilizer (trăn′kwĭ-lī″zer) One of a poorly defined group of drugs designed to control anxiety and reduce tension or stress. Tranquilizers tend to induce drowsiness and can cause physical and psychologic dependence. Most tranquilizers are controlled substances.

transaminase (trăns-ăm′ĭ-nās) One of several enzymes involved in the reversible transfer of an amino group (NH_2) from an alpha-amino acid to an alpha-ketoacid, especially alpha-ketoglutaric acid. Characteristic high values are seen in myocardial infarction and viral hepatitis.

transformer An electrical device that increases or reduces the voltage of an alternating current by mutual induction between primary and secondary coils or windings.

t., auto- *See* autotransformer.

t., Coolidge filament A step-down transformer that reduces the line voltage of 110 volts to one of 12 volts, which in turn heats the tungsten filament of the Coolidge tube for the production of electrons.

t., step-down A transformer in which the secondary voltage is less than the primary voltage.

t., step-up A transformer in which the secondary voltage is greater than the primary voltage.

transillumination (trăns′ĭ-lū″mĭ-nā′shŭn) **1:** Examination of an organ, cavity, or tissue (e.g., tooth or gingival tissue) by transmitted light. A valuable aid in detecting carious lesions, disclosing carious or demineralized dentin during cavity preparation, checking the finish or gingival margins of restorations, and revealing cement, debris, or calculus subgingivally. **2:** A test in which the use of transmitted light may disclose a discoloration of the coronal aspect, indicating dentinal tubular hemorrhage as a result of trauma and/or pulpal necrosis or a fracture. **3:** Examination of tissues by means of a light placed so that the region under study is between the light source and the observer.

transition point *See* Tg value.

transitional dentition The final phase of the transition from deciduous to permanent teeth, in which most deciduous teeth have been lost or are in the process of shedding, and the permanent successors are not yet in function.

transitional denture *See* denture, transitional.

translation Movement of a rigid body in which all parts move in the same direction at the same speed.

translatory movement *See* movement, translatory.

transosteal implant jig An instrument designed to guide a bone drill from inferior border through alveolar ridge to create a path for the seating of a transosteal implant.

transpirable Capable of passing in a gaseous state through the respiratory epithelium or skin.

transplant **1:** *v.* To remove and plant in another place, as from one body or part of a body to another. **2:** *n.* Implantation of living or nonliving tissue or bone into another part of the body; it then serves as a scaffold in the healing process and is progressively resorbed and replaced by newly formed bone. **3:** *v.* To move a tooth or tissue from one site to another, often but not always autogenously.

transplantation, tooth The transfer of a tooth from one alveolus to another.

t., autogenous tooth Transplantation of a tooth from one position to another in the same individual.

t., homogenous tooth Transplantation of a tooth from one human to another.

transseptal fiber *See* fiber, transseptal.

transtrusion, magnitude of The amplitude of condylar transtrusion, which varies among persons as determined clinically by measuring it in the jaw tracings at the levels of the tragi from a few millimeters to 7 mm.

The side shifts of many condyles equal the fore shifts. The transtrusion increases the capacity of the person to manage larger boluses by lengthening the lateral stroke of the lower cusps. This evidence is recordable in the horizontal and frontal craniofacial space planes.

transudate (trăn′sū-dāt) Any fluid substance that has passed through a membrane which may or may not be associated with inflammation. It is low in proteins and colloids and has a low specific gravity.

transversion Eruption of a tooth in the wrong position

trauma (traw′mah) A hurt; a wound; an injury damage; impairment; external violence producing bodily injury or degeneration.

t., occlusal Abnormal occlusal relationships of the teeth, causing injury to the periodontium.

t., injury in occlusal The damaging effects of occlusal trauma, which are of a dystrophic nature and affect the tooth and its attachment apparatus. Lesions include wear facets on the tooth, root resorption, cemental tears, thrombosis of blood vessels of the periodontal membrane, necrosis and hyalinization of the periodontal membrane on the pressure side, resorption of alveolar and supporting bone, etc. Clinically, tooth mobility and migration may be evident; radiographically, evidence is the widening of the periodontal membrane space and fraying or fuzziness of the lamina dura, formation of infrabony resorptive defects, etc. Pocket formation is not a sequela to occlusal traumatism.

traumatic (traw-măt′ĭk) Of, or pertaining to, or caused by an injury.

t. occlusion See occlusion, traumatic.

t. shock See shock, traumatic.

traumatism 1: An injury. 2: A wound produced by an injury; trauma.

t. by food Impingement of the gingival margin by coarse foodstuff caused by improper contour of the tooth or faulty position of the tooth.

t., occlusal Lesions of the attachment apparatus; caused by force placed on the tooth in excess of that which the supporting structures can withstand.

t., primary occlusal The force, or forces, that are caused by mandibular movement and resultant tooth percussion and that are capable of producing pathologic changes in the periodontium.

t., secondary occlusal Destruction of the attachment apparatus by factors other than those of occlusion (e.g., periodontitis). In secondary occlusal traumatism, even the forces of mastication become pathologic in nature.

t., periodontal The application of stress to the structures comprising the attachment apparatus, which exceeds the adaptive capacities of the tissues, with resultant tissue destruction.

traumatogenic (traw″mah-tō-jĕn′ĭk) Capable of producing a wound or injury.

t. occlusion See occlusion, traumatic.

tray A receptacle or device that holds or carries.

t., acrylic resin A tray made of acrylic resin.

t., impression A receptacle or device that is used to carry the impression material to the mouth, confine the material in apposition to the surfaces to be recorded, and control the impression material while it sets to form the impression.

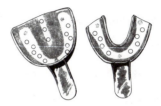

Casts for orthodontic impression trays

Treacher Collins syndrome See syndrome, Treacher Collins.

treatment The mode or course pursued for remedial ends.

t., heat 1: Subjecting a metal to a given controlled heat, followed by controlled sudden or gradual cooling to develop the desired qualities of the metal to the maximum degree. 2: A process of giving a metal predetermined physical properties by controlled temperature changes.

t., hardening heat See tempering.

t., homogenizing heat See anneal. **t., softening heat** See anneal.

t., indirect pulp capping See capping, indirect pulp.

t., prescription The formal outline of the projected treatment of a patient (e.g., blueprint from which the dentist projects treatment).

t., rest (sedative treatment) Use of a drug sealed into a root canal to relieve pain or discomfort; not used primarily for its antiseptic value.

t., root canal The techniques and pharmaceuticals used in removing pulp tissue, sterilizing the root canal, and preparing the root canal for filling.

t., sedative See treatment, rest.

tremolo (trĕm′ō-lō″) An irregular and exaggerated speech pattern that may be the symptom of an emotional disturbance or of various diseases affecting the nervous control of the organs of respiration and phonation.

trench mouth See gingivitis, acute necrotizing ulcerative.

Trendelenburg position (trĕn-dĕl'ĕn-bĕrg) *See* position, Trendelenburg.

trepanation (trephination) The act of surgically cutting a round hole.

trephine (trĕ-fīn') A circle-cutting surgical instrument designed to remove a circumscribed portion of tissue. It permits the insertion of the heads of the intramucosal inserts into the tissue.

Treponema (trĕp″ō-nē'mah) A genus of schizomycetes composed of parasitic and pathogenic spiral microorganisms.

  T. microdentium A species found in the normal oral cavity.

  T. mucosum A species found in periodontal infections in man.

  T. pallidum The spirochete that causes syphilis in humans.

  T. vincenti A spirochete associated with acute necrotizing ulcerative gingivitis.

triad, Hutchinson (trī'ăd) Interstitial keratitis, deafness, and hutchinsonian teeth resulting from congenital syphilis.

trial An examination before a competent tribunal of the facts or law in issue in a cause of action for the purpose of determining the issue.

  t. base *See* baseplate.

Triamcinolone A synthetic adreocorticosteroid that has a potent antiinflammatory effect and is used topically in the treatment of angular cheilosis.

triangle A three-cornered area.

  t., Bolton A triangle formed by drawing a line from the nasion to the sella turcica and from there to the Bolton point.

  t., Bonwill's An equilateral triangle with 4-inch (10-cm) sides bounded by lines from the contact points of the lower central incisors (or the median line of the residual ridge of the mandible) to the condyle on either side and from one condyle to the other. It is the basis for Bonwill's theory of occlusion.

  t., Lesser's A surgical landmark for locating the lingual artery; the triangle is located above the hyoid bone and is formed by the posterior belly of the digastric muscle and the posterior edge of the mylohyoid muscle below and the hypoglossal nerve above. The floor of the triangle is the hypoglossus muscle, and directly below the hyoglossus muscle is the lingual artery.

  t., Tweed A triangle formed by the mandibular plane, frankfort plane, and long axis of the lower central incisor. Proposed as a diagnostic aid by C.H. Tweed.

trichoepithelioma (trĭk″ō-ĕp″ĭ-thē″lē-ō'mah) *See* epithelioma adenoides cysticum.

tridymite (trĭd'ĭ-mīt) A physical form of silica used in combination with cristobalite to limit thermal expansion.

trifurcation Division into three parts or branches, as the three roots of a maxillary first molar.

trigeminal nerve The fifth cranial nerve, which provides motor innervation to the muscles of mastication and sensory innervation to the face, jaws, and teeth.

trigger point The point from which referred pain initiates. In the myofascial pain syndrome, usually a localized, deep tenderness in a taut bundle of muscle fibers from which pain is referred to other sites.

trimethoprim-sulfamethoxazole A synthetic antibacterial combination effective in urinary tract infections; it is the drug of choice in the treatment of *Pneumocystis carinii* pneumonia, one of the opportunistic infections associated with AIDS.

trimmer, gingival margin (margin trimmer) A binangled, double-paired, chisel-shaped, single-beveled, double-planed, lateral cutting instrument. The blade is curved left or right like a spoon excavator; the cutting edge is straight and not perpendicular to the axis of the blade. The pair with the end of the cutting edge farthest from the shaft forming an acute angle is termed *distal* and is used to bevel a distal gingival margin or accentuate a mesial axiogingival angle; the pair with the acute angle of the cutting edge closest to the shaft is called *mesial* and is used to bevel a mesial gingival margin or accentuate a distal axiogingival angle. When one of these trimmers is used, all four must be used.

trimmer, margin *See* trimmer, gingival margin.

trimming, tissue *See* border molding.

tripoding (trī'pŏd-ĭng) The marking of a cast at three points in the same plane as a means of repositioning the cast in that plane during subsequent procedures.

tripodism A widely used principle to gain instant stability on uneven terrains in all landings. It is referred to as a *three-point landing*. Stamp cusps in well-organized occlusion have only three-point contacts with their fossa brims (none with their tips).

trismus (trĭz'mŭs) Spasms of the muscles of mastication, resulting in the inability to open the mouth; often symptomatic of pericoronitis.

trisomy (trī'sō-mē) An additional chromosome in the normal complement, so that in each nucleus a chromosome is represented three times rather than twice. *See also* mongolism.

trisomy-D (trisomy 13-15, Patau's syndrome) Clinical syndrome associated with an autosomal abnormality in which the extra chromosome occurs in the 13 to 15 group. Numerous anatomic defects are present, including hemangiomas, hernia, arrhinencephaly, eye anomalies, cleft lip and palate, and characteristic changes in the footprint and palm print.

trituration (trĭt″ū-rā'shŭn) The process of mixing together silver alloy fillings with mercury to produce amalgam.

t., hand The mixing of ingredients by hand in a mortar and pestle.

t., mechanical The mixing of constituents in a mechanical device or amalgamator.

troche (trō'kē) *See* lozenge.

Trousseau's twitching *See* twitching, Trousseau's.

True's separator *See* separator, True's.

truss arm *See* connector, minor.

trust A relationship in which one person or entity holds fiduciary responsibility for another's property or enterprise.

try-in A preliminary placement of trial dentures (complete or removable partial), a partial denture casting, or a finished restoration to evaluate fit, appearance, maxillomandibular relations, etc.

tryptase (trĭp'tās) *See* plasmin.

TSH *See* hormone, thyrotropic.

tub and tray system A system of instrument and supply management in which the instruments for a particular task are prearranged on a tray and the accompanying disposables are prearranged in an accompanying tub. The prepared trays and tubs are appropriately sterilized, stored, and delivered to the dental operatory at the proper time.

tube A hollow cylindrical structure.

t., buccal A section of tubing attached to the buccal side of a molar band in a horizontal position, serving as an attachment for the labial arch wire, which slides into the tube.

t., Coolidge An x-ray tube in which the gas pressure is purposely made so low that it plays no role in the operation of the tube, the operation depending on the emission of electrons by the heated filament of the cathode. *See also* x-ray tube, Coolidge.

t., discharge Any vacuum tube in which a high-voltage electric current is discharged (e.g., an x-ray tube).

t., horizontal A metal tube attachment that is placed in a horizontal position on the buccal surface of each anchor molar tooth to allow for the insertion of the labial arch wire.

t., intubation A tube for insertion into the larynx through the mouth.

t., line focus An x-ray tube in which the target face is about 20 inches (50 cm) from the cathode face. The focal spot is rectangular, with the length approximately three times the width. The acute angle provides an effective focal spot area approximately square and a fraction of the actual area.

t., protective, housing An x-ray tube enclosure that provides radiation protection.

t., protective, housing, diagnostic A tube housing that reduces the leakage radiation to, at most, 0.10 r/hr at a distance of 1 mm from the tube target when the tube is operating at its maximum continuous rated voltage.

t., protective, housing, therapeutic A tube housing that reduces the leakage radiation to, at most, 1 r/hr at a distance of 1 meter from the tube target when the tube is operating at its maximum continuous rated current for the maximum rated voltage.

t., right-angle An x-ray tube in which the target is at right angles to the cathode.

t. tooth *See* tooth, tube.

t., vertical An attachment that is usually placed on the lingual surface of the anchor band to allow for the insertion of the lingual wire.

t., x-ray *See* x-ray tube.

tubercle (tū'bĕr-kl) A small rounded nodule or elevation on the surface of the skin, bone, or other tissue.

t., genial (jē'nē-ăl) **(geniohyoid tubercle)** A small rounded elevation on the lingual surface of the mandible on either side of the midline near the inferior border of the body of the mandible, serving as a point of insertion for the geniohyoid muscles.

t., superior genial The small spines on the lingual surface of the mandible that serve as the attachment for the genioglossus muscles. On resorbed mandibles, these tubercles may be at or above the crest of the residual ridge.

t., geniohyoid (jē"nē-ō-hī'oid) *See* tubercle, genial.

tuberculin skin test *See* test, tuberculin.

tuberculosis (tū-bĕr'kū-lō'sĭs) An infectious disease caused by *Mycobacterium tuberculosis* and characterized by the formation of tubercles in the tissues.

tuberosity (tū'bĕr-ŏs'ĭ-tē) A protuberance or elevation from the surface, usually of a bone.

t., maxillary The most distal aspect of the maxillary alveolar process with its posterior border curving upward and distally.

t., reduction Surgical excision of excessive fibrous or bony tissue in the area of the maxillary tuberosity prior to the construction of prosthetic appliances.

tumor(s) A swelling. Through usage the term is now used synonymously with *neoplasm*. *See also* neoplasm.

t., Brooke's *See* epithelioma adenoides cysticum.

t., brown A central giant cell tumor of the bone; associated with parathyroidism.

t., carotid body A tumor formed about the carotid artery.

t., collision A rare condition in which two neoplasms, both growing in the same general area, collide with the tumor elements and become intermingled.

t., Ewing's (endothelioma, Ewing's sarcoma) A rare malignant tumor of disputed histogenetic origin in bone. It is characterized by pain, a radiographic appearance called *onionskinning*, and a histologic picture consisting of solid sheets of small round cells that appear on the many small blood vessels present.

t., giant cell A benign neoplasm of bone, producing resorption and characterized by giant cells.

t., hormonal Localized enlargements of the gingivae that have the appearance of neoplasms and are associated with hormonal imbalance during pregnancy.

t., mixed 1: One of a group of neoplasms of the salivary glands whose histologic appearance suggests both epithelial and connective tissue origin, although they presently are considered of epithelial origin only. There are benign and malignant types. **2:** Any tumor arising from cells derived from more than one germ layer.

t., basaloid mixed *See* carcinoma, adenocystic.

t., mucoepidermoid A tumor of the salivary glands composed of mucous cells, epidermoid cells, and clear cells. Benign and malignant forms are recognized.

t., odontogenic (ō-don″tō-jĕn′ĭk)   **1:** A neoplasm produced from tooth-forming tissues (e.g., odontogenic fibroma, odontogenic myxoma, ameloblastoma). *See also* calcifying epithelial odontogenic tumor. **2:** A gingival enlargement seen during pregnancy, the microscopic examination of which reveals the features of a pyogenic granuloma.

t., turban *See* carcinoma, basal cell.

t., Warthin's *See* cystadenoma, papillary, lymphomatosum.

turbulence Casting term used to denote irregular flow of the metal into the mold. May result in porosity.

Turner's tooth *See* tooth, Turner's.

Tweed triangle *See* triangle, Tweed.

twilight sleep *See* sleep, twilight.

twins Two siblings produced in the same pregnancy and developed from one egg (identical, monozygotic) or from two eggs fertilized at the same time (fraternal, dizygotic).

twin-wire *See* appliance, twin-wire.

twist drill 1: A drill having one or two deep helical grooves, extending from the point to the smooth portion of the shank.   **2:** A spiral bone bur.

twitch A short, sudden pull or jerk.

twitching An irregular spasm of a minor extent.

t., Trousseau's A twitching of the face that the patient can exhibit at will and occurs obsessively to relieve tension.

Tylenol *See* acetaminophen.

type A hepatitis *See* hepatitis, infectious.

type B hepatitis *See* hepatitis, homologous serum.

typewriter ribbon as a marking medium Typewriter ribbon is more desirable than carbon paper when setting teeth because the porcelain tooth that is being adjusted will not perforate the ribbon and abrade the surface of the stone template record of jaw movement.

typical implant connective tissue The tendonlike condensed elongated avascular tissue formed in direct contact with implant infrastructure metal underlaid by normal collagenous fibrous connective tissue.

typodont (tī′pō-dont) An artificial model containing artificial or natural teeth used for teaching technique exercises.

tryptophan One of the essential amino acids *See also* amino acid.

Tzank cell (tsănk) *See* cell, Tzank.

Tzank's test *See* test, Tzank's.

ugly duckling stage A stage of dental development preceding the eruption of the permanent canines in which the lateral incisors may be tipped laterally because of crowding by the unerupted canine crowns. Incisor crowns may be spaced because of the tipping despite the crowding of the roots. The condition may be transitory in an otherwise normal dentition. First described and named by B.H. Broadbent.

ulcer (ŭl'sĕr) A loss of covering epithelium from the skin or mucous membranes, causing gradual disintegration and necrosis of the tissues.

u., aphthous, recurrent (ăf'thŭs) **(RAU, canker sore, recurrent aphthae)** Periodic episodes of aphthous lesions ranging from 1 week to several months. Trauma, menses, immunologic factors, upper respiratory tract infections, herpes simplex, and other exciting causes have been suggested. The single or multiple discrete or confluent ulcers have a well-defined marginal erythema and central area of necrosis with sloughing. The herpetic appearance suggests a common mechanism with herpes simplex, but no known infectious agents have been demonstrated.

ulcerative stomatitis, recurrent (ul'ser-a"tiv stō-mah-tī-'tis) *See* ulcer, aphthous, recurrent.

u., autochthonous (ăw-tok'thō-nŭs) *See* chancre.

u., decubitus (dē-kū'bĭ-tŭs) **(traumatic ulcer)** A bedsore. Loosely used to refer to a traumatic ulcer of the oral mucosa.

u., diabetic (dī"ah-bĕt'ĭk) An ulcer, usually of the lower extremities, associated with diabetes mellitus.

u., herpetic (her-peqt'ĭk) An ulcer that is secondary to the vesicle of herpes simplex. A shallow ulcer with an irregular, erythematous border and a yellow-gray base.

u., Mikulicz' (mĭk'ū-lĭch) *See* periadenitis mucosa necrotica recurrens.

u., peptic (pĕp'tĭk) An ulcer of the stomach or duodenum probably resulting in large part to an increased secretion of hydrochloric acid. Nervous, emotional, and endocrine factors have been implicated.

u., pterygoid (tĕr'ĭ-goid) *See* aphtha, Bednar's.

u., rodent *See* carcinoma, basal cell.

u., traumatic *See* ulcer, decubitus.

ulceration (ŭl"sĕr-ā'shŭn) The process of forming an ulcer or of becoming ulcerous.

ultimate strength *See* strength, ultimate.

ultra (ul'trah) Beyond; in addition; in excess of.

u., damages Damages beyond those paid in court.

ultrasonic (ŭl"trah-son'ĭks) Instrument that functions by the physical principle of magnetostriction and aids in calculus removal, especially large and hard deposits, and instrument cleaning.

u. cleaner An electronic generator that transmits high-energy and high-frequency vibrations to a fluid-filled container used to remove particulate matter from dental instruments and appliances.

u. scaler An electronic generator that transmits high-frequency vibrations to a handpiece used to remove heavy calcified deposits from the surface of a tooth.

unbundling of procedures The separating of a dental procedure into component parts with each part having a charge so that the cumulative charge of the components is greater than the total charge to patients who are not beneficiaries of a dental benefits plan for the same procedure.

unconscious (ŭn-kŏn'shŭs) Insensible; not receiving any sensory impression and not having any subjective experiences.

undercut 1: The portions of a tooth that lies between its height of contour and the gingivae, only if that portion is of less circumference than the height of contour. **2:** The contour of a cross section of a residual ridge of dental arch that would prevent the placement of a denture or other prostheses. **3:** The contour of flasking stone that interlocks in such a way as to prevent the separation of parts. **4:** The portion of a prepared cavity that creates a mechanical lock or area of retention; may be desirable in a cavity to be filled with gold foil or amalgam but undesirable in a cavity prepared for a restoration to be cemented.

u., gauge *See* gauge, undercut.

u., retentive An area of the abutment surface suitable for the location of a retentive clasp terminal which, to escape the undercut, would be forced to flex and thus generate retention.

u., soft tissue An undercut in a residual ridge or soft tissue covering of a dental arch that would prevent or influence the placement of a removable denture.

u., unusable The area of an abutment tooth or soft tissue across which a unit of the removable partial denture must pass without interference and hence must be blocked out (filled with wax or clay) before the master cast is duplicated. A surveyor can be used to produce a surface that is parallel to the proposed path of a placement and removal.

undermine To surgically separate the skin or mucosa from its underlying stroma so that it can be stretched or moved to cover a defect or wound.

unerupted Not having perforated the oral mucosa. In dentistry, used with reference to a normal developing tooth, an embedded tooth, or an impacted tooth.

unification The act of uniting or the condition of being united (e.g., the result of joining the components of a removable partial denture by connectors).

unilateral One-sided.

union-sponsored plan A program of dental benefits developed through a union's initiative. May be operated directly by the union or the union may contract for provision of the benefits. Funds to finance the benefits are usually paid out of a trust fund that receives its income from employer contributions, employer and union member contributions, or union members alone.

Unipen *See* nafcillin.

unit One of the components of a whole.

u., Ångstrom (ăng′strom) **(Å, Au)** The unit of measure of wavelengths; one one-hundred millionth of a centimeter.

u., dental 1: Basically, the tooth, attachment apparatus, and gingival unit—all of which are necessary for proper masticatory activity. **2:** An article of equipment in which are assembled numerous items used in dental operations, such as a dental engine, cuspidor, or operatory light, bracket, working table, saliva ejector, water supply, electric outlets, compressed air, and miscellaneous instruments.

u., dentoperiodontal Referring to the tooth and periodontium together.

u., gingival The tough collagenous and epithelial covering of the neck of the tooth and the underlying attachment apparatus.

u., partial denture The individual parts of the partial denture, each contributing some particular function.

u., x-ray A device designed to produce x rays.

u., x-ray, calibration The determination of the kilovoltage peak (KVP) value of each autotransformer tap at various milliamperages, checking these values by means of a sphere gap or a prereading voltmeter.

United States Pharmacopeia (USP) A compendium officially recognized by the Federal Food, Drug, and Cosmetic Act that contains the descriptions, uses, strengths, and standards of purity for selected drugs.

United States dietary goals The recommendation of a Senate committee in 1977 outlining the levels of consumption of complex carbohydrates, sugar, protein, fat, cholesterol, and salt for diets necessary to enhance the health status of Americans.

universal precautions The protocols used to maintain an aseptic field and to prevent cross contamination and cross infection between health care providers, between health care providers and patients, and between patients. These include but are not limited to the sterilization of instruments and goods; the isolation and disinfection of the immediate clinical environment; the use of sterile disposables; scrubbing, masking, gowning and gloving; and the proper disposal of contaminated wastes.

universal tooth coding system A tooth numbering system in which each tooth carries a number from 1 to 32 beginning with the maxillary right third molar and ending with the mandibular left third molar. The primary teeth are similarly numbered preceded by a *D* for deciduous. The ADA numbering system is similar to the universal system except the primary teeth are identified by letters from A to T. See Appendix D.

unmedullated (ŭn-měd′ŭ-lāt′ĕd) Not possessing a medulla or medullary substance.

unpolarized Not polarized.

unsharpness, geometric *See* geometric unsharpness.

unstable 1: Not firm or fixed in one place; likely to move. **2:** Capable of undergoing spontaneous change. **3:** A nuclide in an unstable state is called *radioactive*. **4:** An atom in an unstable state is called *excited*.

upcode Using a procedure code that reflects a higher-intensity service than would normally be used for the services delivered.

upright arm *See* connector, minor.

uprighting spring An auxiliary wire used to torque roots mesially or distally.

uremia (ū-rē′mē-ah) The presence of urinary components in the circulating blood and the resultant symptoms. Manifestations include weakness, headache, confusion, vomiting, and coma, and in terminal chronic renal disease, purpura and epistaxis may be present. Caused by insufficient urinary excretion of any cause. *See also* stomatitis, uremic.

uric acid (u′rik) A product of protein metabolism and present in the blood and urine.

urinalysis (u″rĭ-nal′ĭ-sis) A physical, microscopic, and chemical diagnostic examination of urine. Abnormal constituents indicate disease and can include ketone bodies, protein, bacteria, blood, glucose, pus, and certain types of crystals.

urine The fluid exceted by the kidneys. Normal urine is clear, straw-colored, and slightly acidic and has the characteristic odor of urea.

urticaria (ur″tĭ-kā′rē-ah) **(hives)** A vascular reaction pattern of the skin marked by the transient appearance of smooth, slightly elevated patches that are more red or more pale than the surrounding skin and attended by severe itching.

u., giant *See* edema, angioneurotic.

USAN Council The United States Adopted Names Council, which is responsible for the selection of appropriate nonproprietary names for drugs used in the United States.

useful beam *See* beam, useful.

U.S.P. The Pharmacopeia of the United States.

usual, customary and reasonable (UCR) plans A dental benefits plan that determines benefits based on usual, customary, and reasonable fee criteria. *See* usual fee; customary fee; and reasonable fee.

usual fee The fee that an individual dentist most frequently charges for a given dental services. *See also* customary fee; reasonable fee.

ut dict. Abbreviation for *ut dictum,* a Latin phrase meaning "as directed."

utilization 1: The extent to which a given group uses a specified service in a specified period of time. Usually expressed as the number of services used per year per 100 or per 1000 persons eligible for the service, but utilization rates may be expressed in other ratios. **2:** The extent to which the members of a covered group use a program over a stated time; specifically measured as a percentage determined by dividing the number of covered individuals who submitted one or more claims by the total number of covered individuals.

u. review (UR) 1: Analysis of the necessity, appropriateness, and efficiency of medical and dental services, procedures and facilities, and practitioners; in a hospital, this includes review of the appropriateness of admissions, services ordered and provided, length of stay and discharge practices, on concurrent and retrospective bases. **2.** Statistically based: A system that examines the distribution of treatment procedures based on claims information and, to be reasonably reliable, the application of such claims. Analyses of specific dentists should include data on type of practice, dentist's experience, socioeconomic characteristics, and geographic location.

utilization management A set of techniques used by or on behalf of purchasers of health care benefits to manage the cost of health care before its provision by influencing patient-care decision making through case-by-case assessments of the appropriateness of care based on accepted dental practices.

uveoparotitis (ū″vē-ō-păr″ō-tī′tĭs) *See* fever, uveoparotid.

uvula (ū-vū-lah) A general term indicating a pendent fleshy mass.

u., bifid A congenital cleft resulting in a split uvula.

u., palatine A small fleshy mass hanging from the posterior of the soft palate.

vaccine (vak′sēn) Agent prepared to produce active immunity that usually kills microbes, attenuated live microbes, or variant strains of microbes and that can induce antibody production without producing disease.

Vacudent (vak′ū-dĕnt) Trade name for a high-volume suction apparatus designed to remove strongly but gently any fluids and debris from an operating field.

vacuum *See* oral evacuator.

vacuum mixing *See* mixing, vacuum.

vagomimetic (vā″gō-mī-mĕt′ĭk) Pertaining to a drug with actions similar to those produced by stimulation of the vagus nerve.

validity The degree to which data or results of a study are correct or true.

valine (val′in) One of the essential amino acids. *See also* amino acid.

Valium *See* diazepam.

values, normal laboratory Generally, statistically and biologically significant qualitative and/or quantitative measurements of cellular and clinical components of the body. The values derived from such measurements are based on averages of a survey of presumably healthy persons. The concept of individual normal values is based on an acceptable response (comparable with known evidence of health or disease) of the individual to a known alteration of cellular and/or chemical components or systems.

values, phonetic (fō-nĕt′ĭk) The character or quality of vocal sounds.

valve A structure that controls flow of the contents of a canal or passage.

    v., exhalation A valve that permits escape of exhaled gases into the atmosphere and prevents them from being rebreathed.

van den Bergh's test *See* test, van den Bergh's.

vapor 1: The gaseous form assumed by a solid or liquid when sufficiently heated. **2:** A visible emanation of fine particles of a liquid.

Vaquez' disease (vah-kāz′) *See* erythremia.

variable Changing; able to vary in quantity or magnitude; a characteristic that may take several values.

    v., continuous A variable that between any two values it is possible to find an intermediate value. Continuous variables can be refined by smaller, more pre-

cise values. Length, weight, and time, and the points on a line are continuous variables.

    v., control Those variables not being studied which are held constant so as not to influence the experimental outcome. Environmental conditions, in telligence quotients, social and psychologic variables are examples of variables that must be controlled.

    v. costs Costs, such as dental service claims, that generally increase or decrease as the size and composition of the enrollment fluctuates.

    v., dependent A variable whose value is consequent on change in the independent variable. The dependent variable is always the response or reaction to the independent variable. Synonym: criterion variable.

    v., discrete A variable that is expressed in whole units or mutually exclusive categories. Whole numbers and category designations such as sex and marital status are examples of discrete data.

    v., independent The variable being studied that is manipulated or controlled by an experimenter. In a drug study an experiment may give several dosages of a drug (independent variable) to determine the most effective, symptom-reducing (dependent variable) level.

variance A measure of dispersion; standard deviation squared; in some statistical computations the squared value of standard deviation, variance, is preferred.

varicella (vār″ĭ-sĕl′ah) **(chickenpox)** An acute communicable disease with an incubation period of 2 or 3 weeks and caused by herpesvirus, usually found in children. Manifestations include coryza, fever, malaise, and headache, followed in 2 or 3 days by the eruption of macular vesicles.

varicosity (var″ĭ-kos′ĭ-tē) An abnormal condition characterized by the presence of tortuous, abnormally dilated veins, usually in the legs or the lower trunk; may also appear in the esophagus.

variola (vah-rī′ō-lah) **(smallpox)** An acute, viral contagious disease transmitted by the respiratory route and direct contact. The incubation period is 1 to 2 weeks. Manifestations include headache, chills, and temperature up to 106° F, followed by macules on the third and fourth day, which then become papules, and then constitutional symptoms abate. On the sixth day the papules become vesicles and then pustules, with desquamation occurring in about 2 weeks.

varnish (cavity liner, cavity varnish) A clear solution of resinous material or natural gum, such as copal or rosin dissolved in acetone, ether, or chloroform, that is capable of hardening without losing its transparency. Used in cavity preparations to seal out dentinal tubules, reduce microleakage, and insulate the pulp against shock from thermal changes.

vascular reactions The response of the blood vessels to injury or introduction of chemical agents, particularly certain chemical mediators such as histamine and bradykinin.

vascular spasm A sudden constriction of the blood vessels causing reduction or stoppage in blood flow. A vascular spasm in vessels of the brain can result in stroke and in the vessels of the heart can result in a "heart attack."

vasoconstrictor (vas″ō-kon-strik′tor) **(vasopressor)** An agent that causes a rise in blood pressure by constricting the blood vessels. In local areas, it causes constriction of the arterioles and capillaries.

vasodepressor (vas″ō-de-pres′or) An agent that depresses circulation and causes vasomotor depression.

vasodilator (vas″ō-dī-lāt-or) An agent that causes dilation of the blood vessels. Also, a drug that relaxes the smooth muscle walls of the blood vessels and increases their diameter.

vasomotor (văs″ō-mō′tor) Pertaining to any agent or nerve that causes expansion or contraction of the walls of blood vessels.

vasopressin (vas″ō-pres′in) See hormone, antidiuretic.

vasopressor (vas″ō-pres′or) See vasoconstrictor.

vault 1: An anatomic part resembling an arched roof or dome, as the vault of a denture. **2:** A cavity or specially prepared area within the jawbone for placement of an implant magnet.

VDRL test Abbreviation for Venereal Disease Research Laboratory test, a serologic flocculation test for syphilis or yaws.

vehicle (vē′h-īk-ĕl) A pharmaceutic ingredient, usually a liquid, employed as a medium for dissolving or dispersing the active drug in a mass suitable for its administration.

Veillonella alcalescens (vā″yon-ĕl′ah ăl-kah-lĕs′ĕnz) An organism of the genus *Veillonella*. A schizomycete that has been found in the flora of the periodontal pocket and, by association, has been implicated in the origin and perpetuation of periodontitis in human beings.

vein (vān) A blood vessel that conducts blood from the capillary bed to the heart. Size may range from the venules, to small veins, to large veins.

velopharyngeal adequacy (vĕl″ō-fah-ri″n′jē-ăl) See closure, velopharyngeal.

velopharyngeal closure See closure, velopharyngeal.

velopharyngeal inadequacy See inadequacy, velopharyngeal.

veneer (vĕ-nēr′) In the construction of crowns or pontics, a layer of tooth-colored material, usually porcelain or acrylic resin, attached to the surface by direct fusion, cementation, or mechanical retention.

venereal disease (ve-ne′rē-al) Any contagious condition acquired by sexual intercourse or genital contact. Venereal diseases include chancroid, gonorrhea, granuloma inguinale, herpes simplex type II, HIV, lymphogranuloma venereum, and syphilis.

venereal wart (condylomatum acuminatum) A soft wartlike growth found on the warm and moist skin and mucous membranes of the genitalia caused by a virus and transmitted by sexual contact. Synonym: acuminate wart.

venipuncture (vĕn′i-pŭng′tŭr) Surgical or therapeutic puncture of a vein.

ventilation (ven″tĭ-lā′shun) The constant supplying of oxygen through the lungs.

v., air The process of supplying alveoli with air or oxygen.

v., respiratory The process of getting air into and out of the lungs. The air enters the mouth and nose and must go through the conduction system (the pharynx, larynx, trachea, and bronchial tree) into the lungs. This ventilating process involves many other structures as well, including the abdomen, thorax, and maxillofacial tissues. The latter structures make two significant contributions to the respiratory process; they provide the portal of entry and egress for the air to and from the lungs, and they alter the physical properties of inspired air for protection of the very sensitive lung tissues.

venting A exit passage constructed in a casting mold to allow gases to escape during the casting process.

venue (vĕn′ū) The neighborhood, place, or county in which an injury is declared to have occurred or fact is declared to have happened; also designates the county in which an action or prosecution is presented for trial.

venule (vĕn′ūl) The smallest of the venous blood vessels. Consists of an endothelial tube enclosed in a variable amount of elastic and collagenous tissue. Smooth muscle is introduced in the media as the caliber of the vessel increases. The muscle fibers are distributed sparsely in the smaller vessels and coalesce into circumferential bands in the larger vessels.

verbal By word of mouth; oral, as a verbal agreement.

verdict The formal decision or finding of a jury on the matters or questions duly submitted to them at the trial.

vermilion border The junction between lip and the facial skin.

vernier (ver'nē-er) *See* gauge, Boley.

Verocay body (ver'ō-kā) *See* body, Verocay.

verruca (vĕ-roo'kah) A wartlike lesion.

v. senilis (sĕ-nĭl'ĭs) *See* keratosis, seborrheic.

v. vulgaris (wart) A common wart of the skin or mucosa.

verrucous carcinoma (ver'oo-kus kar"sĭ-nō'mah) A squamous cell carcinoma, usually intraoral, that is exophytic and has a papillary appearance.

vertical Perpendicular to the horizontal plane in an up and down direction.

v. angulation *See* angulation, vertical.

v. dimension *See* dimension, vertical.

v. lug *See* connector, minor.

v. opening *See* dimension, vertical.

v. overlap *See* overlap, vertical.

v. relation *See* relation, vertical.

vertigo (ver'tĭ-gō) **1:** A sensation described as dizziness. **2:** A sensation of the room revolving about the patient or the patient revolving in space. It is a form of dizziness, but the terms are not synonymous.

vesicant (vĕs'ĭ-kănt) A chemically active substance that can produce blistering on direct contact with the skin or mucous membrane.

vesicle (vĕs'ĭ-kl) **1:** A small, blisterlike elevation of the skin or mucous membrane resulting from an intraepithelial collection of fluid. It is a primary type of lesion and may be seen in herpes simplex, recurrent herpes, recurrent aphthae, stomatitis medicamentosa, stomatitis venenata, erythema multiforme, Reiter's syndrome, Behçet's syndrome, Stevens-Johnson syndrome, herpangina, varicella, and many others. **2:** A circumscribed, elevated lesion of the skin containing fluid and having a diameter up to 5 mm.

vessels, blood, visualization of Any one of various methods by which the blood vessels are seen by the examiner. Direct visualization of blood vessels is possible only to a limited extent. The blood vessels in the retina can be directly visualized; the capillary loops in the fingernail can be seen by microscopy, and the blood vessels in the oral mucosa and gingivae can be visualized by infrared photography. More recently, radiopaque substances can be visualized by radiography and cineradiography. The methods can reveal the actual blood column, its width, variation in contour, and tortuosity. Arteriograms and venograms are useful in revealing spasms, obstructions, congenital defects, and collateral circulation of the deeper tissues.

vested A nonforfeitable interest of a participant in a pension plan.

vestibule of oral cavity The part of the oral cavity that lies between the teeth and gingivae and lips and cheeks or between the residual ridges and lips and cheeks.

v., buccal The space between the alveolar ridge and teeth or residual ridge and the cheek distal to the buccal frenum.

v., lower buccal The space between the mandibular alveolar ridge and teeth and the cheek; bounded anteriorly by the lower buccal frenum and posteriorly by the distobuccal end of the retromolar pad.

v., upper buccal The space between the maxillary alveolar ridge and teeth or the residual ridge and the cheek; bounded anteriorly by the upper buccal frenum and posteriorly by the hamular notch.

v., labial The space between the alveolar ridge and the teeth or the residual ridge and lips anterior to the buccal frenum.

vestibuloplasty (vĕs-tiqb'ū-lō-plăs"tē) Any of a series of surgical procedures designed to restore alveolar ridge height by lowering muscles attaching to the buccal, labial, and lingual aspects of the jaws.

viable (vī'ah-bl) Capable of life; able to live.

Viadent Brand name for an antiplaque mouthrinse containing sanguinarine, an alkaloid, as the active ingredient. *See* sanguinarine.

vibrating line *See* line, vibrating.

Vicat needle (vē-kah') *See* needle, Vicat.

Vickers hardness number *See* number, Vickers hardness.

Vickers hardness test *See* test, Vickers hardness.

Vicodin Brand name for hyrocodone, a ketone derivative of codeine that is about 6 times more potent than codiene. Vicodin is a controlled substance.

Vincent's angina *See* angina, Vincent's.

Vincent's bacillus *See* Fusobacterium fusiforme.

Vincent's gingivitis *See* gingivitis, necrotizing ulcerative.

Vincent's infection *See* gingivitis, necrotizing ulcerative.

Vincent's organism *See* organism, Vincent's.

vinegar as a solvent A warm dilute solution of household vinegar; used, as a substitute for acetic acid, to dissolve accumulated dental calculus from a removable dental prosthesis.

Vinethene (vĭn'ē-thēn) Trade name for vinyl ether.

violence Severe physical force; the assault of a person with great force.

violation Injury; encroachment; breach of right, obligation, or law.

violet, gentian (vī'ō-lĕt, jĕn'shŭn) A rosaniline dye, useful as a protective covering and an antiseptic in the treatment of minor lesions of the oral mucosa. It is an effective fungicide and is therefore of value in the treatment of moniliasis.

violet stain *See* stain, methyl violet.

vinyl resin (vī'nĭl) *See* resin, vinyl.

viral hepatitis *See* hepatitis.

viral infection An infection by any of the more than 200 pathogenic viruses. A virus acts on the cell nucleus, taking over the genetic material within the nucleus and replicating itself.

virus (vī′rŭs) One of a group of heterogeneous infective agents characterized by the lack of independent metabolism or the ability to replicate outside the host cell.

   v., herpes simplex *See* herpes simplex.

vision (vizh′ŭn) Sight; the faculty of seeing.

   v., field of The portion of space that the fixed eye can see.

   v., stereoscopic Vision in which the visual fields of the two eyes are unified. Sensations from a common object received by the two eyes are superimposed, and as a result of the slight differences in the fields and the superimposition of the fields, the effects of depth and shape of the object are attained.

visual acuity *See* acuity, visual.

visual disorders *See* disorders, visual.

visual treatment objective (VTO) A diagnostic and communication aid, consisting of a cephalometric tracing, modified to show changes anticipated in the course of growth and treatment.

vital Necessary to or pertaining to life.

   v. capacity *See* capacity, vital.

vitalometer (vī″tăl-om′ĕ-ter) An electric-powered instrument for delivering and measuring an electrical stimulus to a tooth. *See also* pulp tester.

vitalometry (vī″tăl-ōm′ē-trē) The use of high-frequency pulp-testing equipment to establish the vital condition of the pulp of a tooth.

vitamin (vī″ah-mĭn) One of a number of unrelated organic substances that occur in small amounts in food and are required for normal metabolic activity. The vitamins may be water or fat soluble.

   v. A (retinal, retinol, retinoic acid) A fat-soluble substance, occurring in several chemical forms in food and function: retinal, an aldehyde; retinol, an alcohol; and retinoic acid, an acid. All three function in calcified and epithelial tissue growth. The aldehyde (retinal)-alcohol (retinol) interconversion allows regeneration of rhodopsin (visual purple) in the rod cells of the retina. A deficiency results in hyperkeratinization of nonsecretory protective epithelium, deranged secretory function of the mucous membrane, dark dysadaptation (night blindness) and possibly, enamel hypoplasia. Dietary sources include liver, kidney, and lung as well as carotenes (provitamins A) from the plant kingdom.

   v., ascorbic acid (ă′skŏr-bĭk) **(vitamin C, antiscorbutic factor)** A water-soluble vitamin resembling glucose in structure that is found in citrus fruits, tomatoes, cabbage, and other fresh fruits and vegetables. Necessary for hydroxylation of peptide-bound lysine and proline to hydroxylysine and hydroxyproline during collagen synthesis. A deficiency leads to scurvy, in which pathologic signs are confined mainly to the connective tissues with hemorrhages, loosening of teeth, gingivitis, and poor wound healing.

   v. B complex Collectively, the various B vitamins; thiamine, riboflavin, nicotinic acid, pyridoxine, biotin, para-aminobenzoic acid, folic acid, pantothenic acid, cyanocobalamin, pteroylglutamic acid, and others that are unknown.

   v. B₁ *See* vitamin, thiamine.

   v. B₂ *See* vitamin, riboflavin.

   v. B₆ *See* vitamin, pyridoxine.

   v. B₁₂ *See* vitamin, cobalamin.

   v., biotin (bī′ō-tĭn) **(vitamin H, antieggwhite injury factor)** One of the B complex vitamins found in organ meats (e.g., liver, heart, kidney) egg yolk, cauliflower, chocolate, and mushrooms. Its synthesis by intestinal bacteria makes human deficiency states rare unless the diet contains significant raw egg white protein (avidin), which complexes the vitamin to prevent intestinal absorption. Dermatitis, retarded growth, and loss of hair and muscular control occur in experimental animals. Biotin functions as a coenzyme for carboxylase enzymes that catalyze fixation of carbon dioxide (e.g., in fatty acid synthesis).

   v. C *See* vitamin, ascorbic acid.

   v., calciferol *See* vitamin D.

   v., cholecalciferol *See* vitamin D.

   v., choline (kō′lēn) **(trimethylaminoethanol)** Not truly a vitamin, since it can be synthesized in the body if sufficient precursors are available. Prevents the accumulation of fat in the liver of certain animal species. Occurs as a constituent of lecithin, sphingomyelin, and acetylcholine.

   v., cobalamin (kō-băl′ah-mĭn) **(antipernicious factor, vitamin B₁₂, cyanocobalamin, erythrocyte maturing factor [EMF], extrinsic factor)** A vitamin that contains cobalt and is essential for the maturation of erythrocytes. Inability of the body to produce intrinsic factor, which is necessary for vitamin B₁₂ absorption, results in pernicious anemia. Liver, kidney, muscle, and milk are good sources.

   v. D (antirichitic factor, calciferol, cholecalciferol ergosterol ergocalciferol) The group of lipid-soluble sterol compounds capable of preventing occuring rickets. Of primary importance are D_2, or ergosterol, from plants and D_3, or cholecalciferol, from animal sources, especially fish liver oils. The latter is also formed in the skin from 7-dehydrocholesterol on exposure to ultraviolet light. Liver mitochondria further activate vitamin D to 25-(OH)-D, which in turn is metabolized to 1,25-$(OH)_2$-D by the kidney. The dihydroxy metabolites significantly increase dietary calcium absorption and bone resorption to maintain proper blood calcium and phosphorus levels. A primary vitamin D deficiency results from inadequate exposure to sunlight and low dietary intake. Secondary deficiencies occur from abnormalities of intestinal resorption and interference with vitamin D hydroxylation. The manifestations of rickets include enamel hypoplasia, poorly calcified bones, bowed legs, and a deformed rib cage with beadlike swellings of the ribs (rachitic rosary) in infants and children and osteomalacia in adults. Vitamin D intake in excess is toxic.

v. E (tocopherol, tocotrienol antisterility factor) The tocopherol and tocotrienols have varying degrees of vitamin E activity but alpha-tocopherol is the most active. These fat-soluble compounds are found in eggs, muscle meats, liver, fish, chicken, oatmeal, and the oils of corn, soya, and cottonseed. In rats, the lack of vitamin E leads to fetus resorption in the female and atrophy of spermatogenic tissue with permanent sterility in the male. Vitaimin E deficiency in humans is correlated with increased hemolysis of erythrocytes. The tocopherols prevent peroxidation of unsaturated fatty acids, and vitamin E requirements appear directly related to the dietary intake of unsaturated fatty acids. Although animals develop symptoms of muscular dystrophy on deficient diets, the vitamin has no effect on the human disease.

v., ergocalciferol *See* vitamin D.

v., folacin (adermine, folic acid, citrovorum factor, pteroylglutamic acid, vitamin N, vitamin B$_c$) Occurs in many tissues as the free acid or conjugated with one to seven glutamic acid molecules. Green leafy vegetables, kidney, liver, and yeast are good sources and bacterial synthesis in humans occurs readily. As a coenzyme, the vitamin serves as a carrier of one-carbon units (formyl, hydroxymethyl, formimino groups) especially in the synthesis of nucleoproteins. Inadequate folate levels produce a variety of species-dependent symptoms that include megaloblastic anemia in humans.

v. G *See* vitamin, riboflavin.

v. H *See* vitamin, biotin.

v., inositol (ĭn-ō′sĭ-tŏl) **(myoinositol, mesoinositol)** A six-carbon alcohol closely related to the hexoses, which is not truly a vitamin, since the body can synthesize significant amounts from glucose. Its biologic role remains to be established, but it is essential to the growth of liver and bone marrow cells and helps alleviate fatty livers.

v. K (farnoquinone, phytylquinone antihemorrhagic factor) One of the many fat-soluble naphthoquinone compounds with vitamin D activity. Vitamin K$_1$ is found chiefly in leafy vegetables, K$_2$ is synthesized by human intestinal bacteria, and K$_3$ (menadione, N.F.) is a synthetic compound. Vitamin K is essential for the synthesis of prothrombin by the liver. A dietary deficiency of vitamin K is rare, however. The vitamin has been used in conjunction with extensive oral antibiotic therapy to treat hemorrhagic disease of the newborn, hemorrhage of obstructive jaundice, sprue, and during anticoagulant therapy. Prothrombin, Stuart factor, Christmas factor, and serum prothrombin conversion accelerator require vitamin K for their synthesis.

v., niacin (nī′ah-sĭn) **(nicotinic acid, nicotinamide, niacinamide, pellagra preventive factor)** A deficiency of niacin or its amide derivative, niacinamide, results in acute pellagra that is characterized by dermatitis, diarrhea, dementia, stomatitis, and glossitis. Dietary sources include liver, kidney, lean meats, wheat germ, yeast, soybeans, and peanuts. There is some intestinal synthesis by bacteria. Although the amino acid tryptophan contributes to the body supply of niacin, sufficient vitamin B$_6$ must be present for its metabolism. Niacin and niacinamide are interconvertible in the body, and the latter functions as a constituent of two coenzymes, NAD and NADP, which operate as hydrogen and electron transfer agents by virtue of their reversible oxidation and reduction in several enzyme systems.

v., pantothenic acid (păn-tō′thĕn-ĭc) **(pantothen, panthenol)** This vitamin is a component of coenzyme A and thereby functions in the metabolism of lipids, carbohydrates, and proteins. A deficiency is unusual because of its wide distribution, but a "burning feet syndrome" has been reported in people suffering from acute malnutrition.

v., pyridoxine (pĭr′ĭ-dŏk′sēn) **(vitamin B$_6$, pyridoxal, pyridoxol, pyridoxamine)** Part of the B-complex vitamins, the group includes three chemically related substances: pyridoxol, pyridoxal, and pyridoxamine, all of which serve as substrate in the formation of pyridoxal phosphate, the prosthetic group for several enzymes that decarboxylate, deaminate, transaminate, or desulfurate specific amino acids. It further functions in porphyrin, fatty acids, and cholesterol metabolism. Deficiency signs include an acrodynia-like syndrome, convulsive seizures, arteriosclerotic-like lesions, hypochromic microcytic anemia, and impaired antibody formation. Dietary sources include wheat, corn, liver, milk, eggs, and green leafy vegetables.

v., retinal *See* vitamin A.

v., retinol *See* vitamin A.

v., retinoic acid *See* vitamin A.

v., riboflavin (rī″bō-flā′vĭn) **(vitamin B$_2$, vitamin G, lactoflavin)** A heat-stable B complex vitamin that functions as a component of FAD and FMN for the reversible transfer of hydrogen and electrons in several enzyme systems. It is found in green leafy vegetables, whole grains, eggs, liver, milk, and legumes, and small amounts are synthesized in the intestinal tract by microorganisms. Signs of aribo-flavinosis include angular stomatitis, seborrheic dermatitis of the face, and glossitis (magenta tongue).

v., thiamine (thī'-ăh-mīn) **(vitamin B₁, aneurine, antiberiberi factor, antineuritic factor)** A B complex vitamin found chiefly in plants, especially legumes, whole grains, and green leafy vegetables; it is also synthesized by bacteria in the large intestine, which is not a reliable source. Thiamine diphosphate (TPP, cocarboxylase) is a coenzyme in the oxidative decarboxylation of pyruvate and alpha-ketoglutarate, in the transketolase reaction of glucose metabolism and in the metabolism of branched chained amino acids. A deficiency results in beriberi.

v., tocopherol *See* vitamin E.

v., tocotrienol *See* vitamin E.

vitiate (vĭsh'ē-āt) To weaken; to make void or voidable.

vitiligo (vĭt-ĭ-lī'gō) A skin condition characterized by spotty areas of depigmentation.

vitrification (vĭ"trĭ-fĭ-kā'shŭn) The act, instance, art, or process of converting dental porcelain (frit) to a glassy substance; the process of becoming vitreous by heat and fusion.

VLDL Abbreviation for very low density lipids.

vocal cords *See* cords, vocal.

voice Sound produced primarily by the vibration of the vocal bands.

void 1: Empty or unfilled space. **2:** Space not filled with anything solid. **3:** Ineffectual; having no legal binding effect.

volatile (vol'ah-tĭl) Having a tendency to evaporate rapidly.

v. oil *See* oil, essential.

volt The unit of electromotive force. It is the unit that s used to measure the tendency of a charge to move from one place to another. The unit of electrical pressure or electromotive force; the force necessary to cause 1 amp of current to flow against 1 ohm of resistance.

v., electron The kinetic energy gained by an electron in falling through a potential difference of 1 volt. It is equivalent to 1.6×10^{-12} ergs. One thousand and one million electron volts are referred to as *keV* and *meV*.

voltage The potential of electromotive force of an electric charge, measured in volts.

volume Measure of the quantity of space occupied by a substance, such as air.

v., blood The total amount of blood in the body.

v., expiratory reserve (reserve air, supplemental air, supplemental volume) The maximum volume that can be expired from the resting expiratory level.

v. index of blood *See* blood, volume index of.

v., inspiratory reserve (complemental air) The maximum volume that can be inspired from the end of tidal inspiration.

v., packed-cell *See* hematocrit.

v., residual (residual air) The volume of air in the lungs at the end of maximal expiration.

v., stroke *See* stroke volume.

v., supplemental *See* volume, expiratory reserve.

v., tidal (tidal air) The volume of gas inspired or expired during each respiratory cycle.

von Recklinghausen's disease of bone (von rĕk'lĭng-how"zĕnz) *See* hyperparathyroidism; osteitis fibrosa cystica, generalized.

von Recklinghausen's disease of skin *See* neurofibromatosis.

voucher A receipt or release that may serve as notice of payment of a debt or may prove the accuracy of accounts.

vowel A conventional vocal sound in the production of which the speech organs offer little obstruction to the airstream and form a series of resonators above the level of the larynx.

vs Abbreviation for versus (against); commonly used in legal proceedings, particularly in designating the title of cases.

vulcanite (vul'kah-nīt) A hard material with a form of rubber as the base; formerly used for denture bases.

vulcanization (vul'kah-nĭ-zā-shun) The process of treating crude rubber to improve strength, hardness, etc. Usually consists of heating the rubber with sulfur in the presence of moisture, the sulfur uniting with the rubber to produce saturated double bonds.

vulcanize (vul'kah-nīz) To produce flexible or hard rubber, as desired, by subjecting caoutchouc, in the presence of sulfur, to heat and high-steam pressure in a vulcanizer.

VZ virus Varicella zoster virus, which causes chickenpox in humans.

wages The compensation agreed on by an employer to be paid to an employee hired to do work for him. waiting period The period of time between employment or enrollment in a dental program and the date when an insured person becomes eligible for benefits.

waiting period The period between employment or enrollment in a dental program and the date when a covered person becomes eligible for benefits.

waiver (wā′ver) **1:** Repudiation, abandonment, or surrender of a claim, right, or privilege. **2:** The intentional relinquishment of a known right.

wall The outside layer of material surrounding an object or space; a paries.

w., cavity One of the enclosing sides of a prepared cavity. It takes the name of the surface of the tooth adjoining the surface involved and toward which it is placed. Parts of a surrounding or peripheral wall are the cavosurface angle, the enamel wall, the dentinoenamel junction, and the dentin wall.

w., gingival cavity The peripheral wall that most closely approximates the apical end of the tooth.

w., peripheral cavity *See* wall, cavity, surrounding.

w., surrounding cavity (peripheral cavity wall) One of the external, bounding side walls of a cavity; one side forms a part of the cavosurface angle of the preparation.

w., enamel The portion of the wall of a prepared cavity that consists of enamel.

w., finish of enamel The planing of the enamel in finishing a cavity preparation; includes the treatment of the cavosurface angle.

w., incisal The wall of a prepared cavity in an anterior tooth that is closest to or in direct relation to the incisal edge of the tooth.

Walter Reed staging system An alternative classification system used to describe various stages of HIV infection. *See* Centers for Disease Control classification.

Wanscher's mask (vahn′sherz) *See* mask, Wanscher's.

ward A person, especially one under the age of majority, placed by authority of law under the care of a guardian.

warp Uncontrolled torsional change of shape or outline, such as that which may occur in swaging sheet metal,

in denture material, or in other materials exposed to varying temperatures.

wart *See* verruca vulgaris.

Warthin's tumor *See* cystadenoma, papillary, lymphomatosum.

wash, Karo syrup A mixture of Karo syrup in warm water (1 tbs.: ½ glass [4 ounces] warm water) used as a protective soothing rinse in the treatment of inflammatory lesions of the oral mucous membrane.

Wassermann test *See* test, Wassermann.

water A tasteless, odorless, colorless compound made of hydrogen and oxygen (H_2O), which freezes at 32° F (O° C) and bonds at 212° F (100° C). The autonomic nervous system regulates water balance in the body.

w. depletion Cellular dehydration through decreased water intake, dysphagia, excessive sweating, and diuresis.

w. need The amount of water needed to maintain metabolism, approximately 1000 ml/day.

w. syringe *See* syringe, water.

water:powder ratio *See* ratio, water:powder.

Waters extraoral radiographic examination *See* examination, Waters extraoral radiographic.

Waters view *See* examination, Waters extraoral radiograhic.

wave, electromagnetic Energy manifested by movements in an advancing series of alternate elevations and depressions.

wavelength The distance between the peaks of waves in any wave form, such as light, x rays, and other electromotive forms. In electromagnetic radiation, the wavelength is equal to the velocity of light divided by the frequency of the wave.

w., effective The wavelength that would produce the same penetration as an average of the various wavelengths in a heterogeneous bundle of x rays.

wax One of several esters of fatty acids with higher alcohols, usually monohydric alcohols. Dental waxes are combinations of various types of waxes compounded to provide the desired physical properties.

w., baseplate A hard pink wax used for making occlusion rims and baseplates for occlusion rims.

w., bone A plastic mixture that may contain antiseptic and hemostatic drugs, designed for temporary application to freshly cut bone to prevent hemorrhage and infection.

w., boxing A soft wax used for boxing impressions.

w. burnout *See* burnout, inlay; wax elimination.

w., carnauba (kar-now'bah) A hard, high-melting wax used for the control of the melting range of dental waxes.

w., casting A composition containing various waxes with controlled properties of thermal expansion and contraction; used in making patterns to determine the shape of metal castings.

w. elimination (wax burnout) The procedure of removing the wax from a wax pattern invested in a mold preparatory to the introduction of another material into the resulting cavity. May be done by dry heat alone or by irrigation with boiling water followed by use of dry heat.

w. expansion Expanding wax patterns to compensate for the shrinkage of gold during the casting process.

w., fluid A series of waxes, each having different physical properties, used for making a correctable impression of the foundation structures that are to support a denture base. The term indicates that the wax is applied in fluid form as required.

w. inlay *See* wax casting.

w. out *See* blockout.

w. pattern *See* pattern, wax.

w. template *See* template, wax.

waxing (waxing up) The contouring of a wax pattern or the wax base of a trial denture into the desired form.

WBC Abbreviation for white blood cell. *See also* leukocyte; white blood cell count.

wear A loss of substance or a diminishing through use, friction, etc.

w., interproximal A loss of tooth substance in contact areas through functional wear and friction, resulting in broadening and flattening of the contacts and a decrease of the mesiodistal dimension of the teeth and of the dentition as a whole.

w., occlusal Attritional loss of substance on opposing occlusal units or surfaces. *See also* abrasion.

w., abnormal occlusal Wear that exceeds the physiologic wear patterns associated with the attritional effects of food substances; the excessive wear of the teeth occurring as a result of continued afunctional gyrations of the mandible.

w. pattern *See* pattern, wear.

w., physiologic Attrition or abrasion of tooth substance occurring as a result of the abrasive consistency of the normal diet, the slight buccolingual movement of the teeth possible in the masticatory process, etc. It does not include the wear produced by habits, occlusal prematurities, etc.

Weber-Dimitri disease *See* disease, Sturge-Weber-Dimitri.

Weber's disease *See* telangiectasia, hereditary hemorrhagic.

Wedelstaedt chisel (věd'el-staht) *See* chisel, Wedelstaedt.

wedge A small, pointed, triangular, contoured piece of wood used to seal the gingival margin of a cavity preparation before placement of an amalgam restoration.

wedge, step *See* penetrometer.

wedging Packing or fixing tightly by driving in a wedge or wedges.

w. effect *See* effect, wedging.

weekly permissible dose *See* dose, weekly permissible.

weight The pull toward the center of the earth of a body at its surface; the force of gravity acting on a mass.

w., molecular (mō-lěk'ū-lar) The sum of atomic weights of all the atoms in a molecule.

w., rubber dam A piece of metal varying in shape and weight, attached to a clip that is hung on the bottom of a placed rubber dam to keep the field of operation clear.

Weil's disease (vīlz) *See* disease, Weil's.

welding A process used to join metals.

w., arc and gas *See* welding, fusion.

w., cold Property of welding at room temperature, when clean surfaces are pressed into contact. Exhibited to the highest degree by gold in the form of foil or crystals.

w., fusion (arc and gas welding) A process in which parts are melted and fused together.

w., pressure (resistance welding, spot welding) A welding process in which the parts are not melted, although heat is usually required. Recrystalization across the interface occurs. Gold foil is welded by pressure without temperature elevation.

w. property The characteristic of certain materials, especially metals, to unite together firmly when subjected to heat and/or pressure in a suitable environment.

w., resistance *See* welding, pressure.

w., spot *See* welding, pressure.

Werlhof's disease (verl'hofs) *See* purpura, thrombocytopenic.

Western blot A confimatory test for HIV exposure that identifies antibodies to HIV proteins and glycoproteins.

wet strength *See* strength, wet.

wetting agent *See* agent, wetting.

Wharton's duct *See* duct, Wharton's.

wheal (whēl) Edematous elevation of the skin or mucosa. *See also* urticaria.

wheel, Burlew *See* Burlew wheel.

wheel, lathe *See* stone, lathe.

wheel stone *See* stone, wheel.

wheeze A whistling sound made in breathing that is caused by a foreign body in the trachea or bronchus.

white blood cell count A diagnostic clinical laboratory test to determine the number and types of leukocytes present in a measured sample of blood. Overall the normal number of leukocytes ranges from 5,000 to 10,000/mm^3. A differential white blood cell count identifies, counts, and determines the ratios of the various types of leukocytes present in a sample of blood. *See also* leukopenia; leukocytosis.

white lesions A wide array of lesions found on the mucosa that have a white coating. They require differential diagnosis because they may indicate trauma, infection, or a cancerous process.

Widman procedure A surgical procedure in which a periodontal flap is made to gain better access to root surfaces for complete debridement and root planing.

wife A woman united to a man in lawful wedlock; a married woman whose husband is alive and from whom she is not divorced; a spouse.

will A legal document detailing one's wishes in the disposal of one's body and property and the care of one's minor children and/or dependents. **w., living** A document that details one's wishes regarding the degree and amount of health care desired if one becomes mentally incapacitated.

willfully Intentionally; purposefully.

Wilson, curve of A lateral curve of the occlusal table formed by the lingual inclination of the posterior teeth. Because the lingual cusps are lower than the buccal cusps, they form a curve with their antimeres. *See also* curve of Wilson theory.

winking, jaw *See* syndrome, jaw-winking.

wire Slender and pliable rod or thread of metal.
w., arch Wire used in orthodontics as a source of force to direct teeth to move in desired directions. According to the shape of its cross section, the wire may be described as ribbon, rectangular, round, etc.
w., diagnostic *See* wire, measuring.
w., Kirschner A surgical steel wire of heavy gauge with pointed ends; used in the reduction and fixation of bone fragments by being passed through the cancellous portion of the bone and spanning the fracture site.
w., ligature A soft, thin wire used to tie an arch wire to the band attachments.
w., measuring A wire or other similar metal placed in a root canal; made for the purpose of determining the length of the canal. A radiogram is used to make the determination.
w., orthodontic Stainless steel and wrought gold wire of various dimensions used in orthodontic treatment.
w., Risdon (rĭz'don) A wire arch bar tied in the midline.

w., separating Wires threaded interproximally between two adjacent teeth and tightened by twisting the ends together so as to wedge the teeth slightly apart. Used preparatory to adapting bands to teeth having tight contacts with adjacent teeth.
w., wrought 1: A wire formed by drawing a cast structure through a die. Used in dentistry for partial denture clasps and orthodontic appliances. **2:** A form of metal resulting from the swaging, rolling, and drawing of a metal ingot into a desired shape and size.

wiring An arrangement of a wire or wires.
w., circumferential To maintain mandibular and maxillofacial surgical appliances, the placement of a wire around a bone contiguous to the oral cavity, with the ends exiting in the oral cavity (e.g., circumferential mandibular wiring, circumzygomatic wiring).
w., continuous loop (multiple loop wire) A technique for wiring the teeth for the reduction and fixation of fractures.
w., craniofacial suspension A method of wiring using areas of bones not contiguous with the oral cavity for the support of fractured jaw segments (e.g., piriform aperture, zygomatic arch, zygomatic process of the frontal bone). **w., Ivy loop** A method using a wire around two adjacent teeth, providing a loop useful for fixation of a fracture.
w., multiple loop *See* wiring, continuous loop.
w., perialveolar (pĕr"ē-ăl-vē'ō-lar) A method of wiring a splint to the maxilla by passing a wire through the bone from the buccal plate to the palate.
w., piriform aperture (pir'ĭ-form) A method of wiring using that area of the nasal bones for the stabilizing of fractures of the jaws.

Witkop's disease A hereditary, benign intraepithelial dyskeratosis of the oral mucosa and conjunctiva characterized by white-cream asymptomatic plaques on the buccal mucosa, tongue, and floor of the mouth.

witness One who has knowledge of an event; a person whose declaration under oath is received as evidence for any purpose.
w., hostile Witness who manifests so much hostility or prejudice under examination (in chief, or direct) that the party who has called him or her, or his or her representative, is allowed to cross-examine the witness (i.e., to treat him or her as though he or she had been called by the opposite party).
w., marks The small hemispheric depressions that may be prepared in the bone surface in lieu of abutment grooves as a guide for seating the abutment posts of the implant.

Wolf's law *See* law, Wolf's.

Wolinella recta (wo"lĭ-nel'ah rek'tah) Also known as *Campylobacter rectus*; a microorganism associated with progressive periodontal destruction and refractory forms of periodontitis. A regimen using amoxicillin and clavulanic acid combined with metronidazole seems to suppress *W. recta* infections.

word processing (W/P) The handling, manipulating, or performing of some operation or sequence of operations by a dedicated machine (usually by a microprocessor) on free text.

work hardening *See* hardening, work.

work sheet The office form used for a complete planing program for the completion of dental services.

work simplification The application of the principles of the scientific method to increase the ability to produce without sacrificing quality.

working capital A firm's investment in short-term assets—cash, short-term securities, accounts receivable, and inventories. Gross working capital is defined as current assets minus current liabilities. If the term *working capital* is used without further qualification, it generally refers to gross working capital.

working contact *See* contact, working.

working occlusal surfaces *See* surface, working occlusal.

working occlusion *See* occlusion, working.

working side The lateral segment of a denture or dentition toward which the mandible is moved.

Workmen's Compensation Board of Industrial Commission An administrative body that receives claims for injuries and refers them to certain physicians or dentists for treatment, if indicated, with the express or implied assurance to the claimant that the expense will be defrayed by the employed under the Workmen's Compensation Law. The determination of the Industrial Commission is subject to an appeal to court. The federal agency for these matters is the Bureau of Employees Compensation.

wound An injury to the body of a person, especially one caused by violence.

    w., incised In medical jurisprudence, a cut or incision on a human body; a wound made by a cutting instrument.

writ of execution A mandatory precept in writing to implement that judgment or decree of a court.

writing Any written or printed paper or document (e.g., contract, deed).

wrong An injury; a tort; a violation of right or of law; an injustice; a violation of right resulting in damage to another.

wrought clasp (wraht) *See* clasp, wrought.

wrought metal *See* metal, wrought.

wrought wire *See* wire, wrought.

xanthines (xan'thin) A family of chemicals that include caffeine, theophylline, and theobromine that stimulate the central nervous system, act on the kidneys to produce diuresis, stimulate cardiac muscle, and relax smooth muscle.

xanthogranuloma (zăn"thŏn"ū-lō'mah) A benign lesion of infancy, usually solitary and composed of lipid-laden histiocytes with varying numbers of Touton giant cells. In the oral cavity the lesion occurs most often on the tongue and regresses spontaneously.

xanthoma (zăn-thō'mah) Small yellow nodules, composed of lipid-laden macrophages, which generally occur in subcutaneous tissue.

x. palpebrarum (păl-pĕ-brā'rŭm) **(xanthelasma palpebrarum)** Small yellowish plaques on the eyelids resulting from an accumulation of lipids in reticuloendothelial cells. They are a frequent occurrence in persons with diabetes.

xanthomatosis (zăn"thō-mah-tō'sĭs) A disease characterized by the accumulation of excess lipids. *See also* histiocytosis X.

X-bite *See* cross-bite.

xerodermosteosis (zē"rō-dĕrm-os"tē-o*See* syndrome, Sjögren's.

xerophthalmia (zē"rof-thăl'mē-ah) Dryness of the conjunctiva caused by functional or organic disorders of the lacrimal apparatus. It may be found in vitamin A deficiency or Sjögren's syndrome and may follow chronic conjunctivitis.

xerostomia (zē"rō-stō'mē-ah) Dryness of the month resulting from functional or organic disturbances of the salivary glands and lack of the normal secretion. Dryness and resultant overgrowth of oral microorganisms frequentiy lead to rampant caries. *See also* hyposalivation.

X-linkage *See* linkage, sex.

x-ray A type of electromagnetic radiation characterized by wavelengths between approximately 1000 Å and 10^{-4} Å, corresponding to photon energies of about 20 eV to 125 meV. They are invisible, penetrative, especially at higher photon energies, and travel with the same speed as visible light. They are usually produced by bombarding a target of high atomic number with fast electrons in a high vacuum; they are also emitted as a product of some radioactive disintegrations (specifically originating from the extranuclear part of the atom). X-rays were first discovered by Wilhelm C. Roentgen in 1895; hence the term *roentgen rays,* often applied to mechanically generated x-rays. Roentgen called them *x-rays* after the mathematic symbol "x" for an unknown.

x., monochromatic An x-ray that has a single wavelength or an extremely narrow band of wavelengths.

x-ray beam The spatial distribution of radiation emerging from an x-ray generator or source.

x. b., central The straight line passing through the center of the source and the center of the final beam-limiting diaphragm.

x. b., edges The lines joining the center of the anterior face of the source to the diaphragm edges farthest from the source.

x. b., field size The geometric projection, on a plane perpendicular to the central ray, of the distal end of the limiting diaphragm as seen from the center of the front surface of the source. The field is thus the same shape as the aperture of the collimator, and it can be defined at any distance from the source.

x. b., principal plane A plane that contains the central ray and, in the case of rectangular section beams, is parallel to one side of the rectangle.

x-ray film, full-mouth *See* survey, radiographic.

x-ray mount *See* mount, x-ray.

x-ray tube An electronic tube in which x-rays can be generated.

x. t., Coolidge A vacuum tube in which x-rays are generated when the target (integral with the anode) is bombarded by electrons that are emitted from a heated filament (on the cathode) and accelerated toward the anode across a high-potential difference. Modern x-ray tubes are of this type. *See also* tube, Coolidge.

x. t., Crookes' A vacuum discharge tube used by Sir William Crookes in early experimental work with cathode rays. Wilhelm C. Roentgen first discovered that in addition to the production of cathode rays, x-rays were emitted during the operation of these tubes.

x. t., gas An early type of x-ray tube in which electrons were derived from residual gases within the tube.

x-ray unit *See* unit, x-ray.

xylene (zī'lēn) **(xylol; $C_6H_4(CH_3)_2$ dimethylbenzene)** A colorless, flammable fluid used as a solvent and clarifying agent in the preparation of tissue sections for microscopic study.

Xylocaine *See* lidocaine.

xylol (zī'lol) *See* xylene.

Y axis *See* axis, Y.

yaws (yăwz) A disease caused by *Treponema pertenue*. It occurs in hot regions, and raspberry-like excrescences occur on the hands, face, feet, and external genitalia. Synonym: fambesia.

yield point *See* point, yield.

yield strength *See* strength, yield.

yoke 1: Something that connects or binds. **2:** Metal clamps with adjustable screws that secure the cylinders to the apparatus or reducing valves. They are equipped with nipples that fit snugly into the inlet socket or part of the cylinder valve.

Young's modulus *See* elasticity, modulus of.

Young's rule *See* rule, Young's.

Z A symbol for atomic number.

zidovudine (zi-do′-vu-dēn) A dideoxynucleoside, the first antiviral agent approved by the FDA for the treatment of HIV-positive patients. It acts to inhibit the replication of HIV. Brand name: Retrovir.

zinc (zĭngk) A bluish-white chemical element used in medicine in the form of various salts and as a component in some silver amalgams.

zinc oxide and eugenol (zĭngk ok′sīd ū′jē-nol) Two substances that react chemically to form a relatively hard mass. When modified by certain additives, the material is used for impression pastes, root canal fillings, surgical dressings, temporary filling materials, and cementing media.

zinc oxide–eugenol cement (zĭngk ok′sīd ū′jē-nol) *See* cement, dental, zinc oxide–eugenol.

zinc oxyphosphate (zĭngk ok″sē-fos-fāt) *See* cements.

zinc polycarbonate cement (zĭngk pol″ē-kar-bōn-āt) *See* cements.

zinc phosphate cement (zĭngk fos′fāt) *See* cement, zinc phosphate.

Zinsser-Engman-Cole syndrome *See* syndrome, Zinsser-Engman-Cole.

ZnOE Zinc oxide and eugenol.

zone (zōn) A region or area with specific characteristics or boundary.

   z. incubation An area that provides a favorable environment for growth of microorganisms and is thus conducive to initiation or perpetuation of a pathologic process (e.g., gingival flap over a partly erupted third molar).

   z., neutral The potential space between the lips and cheeks on one side and the tongue on the other. Natural or artificial teeth in this zone are subject to equal and opposite forces from the surrounding musculature.

   z. of reference The area of of perceived pain referred by the trigger point. *See also* trigger point.

Z-plasty A surgical procedure using the transposition of tissue flaps to ensure the release of contractures, as in ankyloglossia.

z-score (z) A standard score based on the normal distribution; the difference between the obtained score and the mean, divided by the standard deviation; standard scores computed for different variables are comparable; used to determine statistical significance in large samples.

zygomaxillare (zī″gō-măks′ĭl-ăr-ē) *See* ridge, key.

How Dental Terms Are Made and Read

Dental terminology is a hybrid speech. Most of the words are also common to medical terminology and as such are largely made up of Greek and Latin stems, prefixes, and suffixes. However, many words have been borrowed from other languages, as well. Dental terminology is also dynamic in the sense that many new words are coined as necessity demands. Generally, technical words can be analyzed for their meanings by dividing them into their component parts and determining the meaning of each part.

To build or analyze any vocabulary, it is necessary to understand the five elements that can be used to form words: the word root, combining vowel, combining form, prefix, and suffix.

WORD ROOT

The word root is the basic core of any word and gives it its major meaning. (Some compound words may be made up of more than one root.) For instance, in the words *stomatitis, adenitis,* and *pulpitis* the word roots are *stomat* (meaning "mouth"), *aden* (meaning "gland"), and *pulp* (meaning "the soft tissue within a tooth").

COMBINING VOWEL

Certain combinations of word roots are difficult to pronounce, especially when the first word root ends in a consonant and the second begins with a consonant. This awkwardness of pronunciation necessitates the insertion of a vowel called a *combining vowel.* Usually the combining vowel is an *o,* although *a, e, i, u,* and *y* may be encountered occasionally. Combining vowels are encountered in everyday words. Instead of joining the two word roots *speed* and *meter* directly, the combining vowel *o* is inserted to speed-o-meter. Another example is *megal* and *glossia,* which becomes megaloglossia.

COMBINING FORM

The combination of word root plus combining vowel is known as the *combining form.*

WORD ROOT	+	COMBINING VOWEL	=	COMBINING FORM
-gnath-		0		-gnatho-
-micr-		0		-micro-
-dent-		0		-dento-
-arthr-		0		-arthro-

SUFFIX

A suffix is a syllable or syllables added at the end of a word root or combining form to change the meaning of the root, give it grammatical function, or form a new word. *Play, read,* and *speak* are word roots; by adding the suffix-*er* (meaning "one who") the words are changed to "one who plays," "one who reads," and "one who speaks." If the suffix -*able* (meaning "capable of being") were added, the words mean "capable of being played," "capable of being read," and "capable of being spoken." In the words *microtome, dermatome,* and *arthrotome,-tome* is a suffix meaning "instrument for cutting." Notice that the suffix is added to the combining form rather than the word root:

WORD ROOT	+	COMBINING VOWEL	+	SUFFIX	=	MEANING
micr-		0		-tome		instrument to cut very fine sections
derm-		0		-tome		instrument to cut skin
arthr-		0		-tome		instrument to cut joints

PREFIX

A prefix is a syllable or syllables placed before a word or word root to alter its meaning or create a new word. If the prefixes *over-*, *re-*, and *out-* are added before the words *play*, *read*, and *speak*, three new words are created—*overplay, reread,* and *outspeak.* Any number of these five elements can be combined to form new words.

AUTO-BI-O-GRAPH-IC-AL		SUB-STRAT-O-SPHER-E		ELECTR-O-CARDI-O-GRAM	
auto-	prefix	sub-	prefix	electr-	word root
-bi-	word root	-strat-	word root	-o-	combining vowel
-o-	combining vowel	-o-	combining vowel	-cardi-	word root
-graph-	word root	-spher-	word root	-o-	combining vowel
-ic	suffix	-e	suffix	-gram	suffix
-al	suffix				

WORD AND ROOT ORDER

The order in which the various elements of compound words are placed is of great importance. Observe the consequences if the order of the elements in the following words were reversed:

leg iron	became	iron leg
motorboat	became	boat motor
snake poison	became	poison snake
pig iron	became	iron pig
zoo animal	became	animal zoo
eyeglass	became	glass eye
house dog	became	dog house

In all of the instances above, the order of the elements can be reversed and still arrive at a sensible word, although the subject in each example has changed. There are other compound words, such as the following, that would be nonsensical if the order of their elements were changed:

shoulder blade	cannot become	blade shoulder
nerve tonic	cannot become	tonic nerve
chickenpox	cannot become	pox chicken
headache	cannot become	achehead

The following is a list of combining forms for anatomic structures and body fluids, prefixes, suffixes, verbs, and adjectives. Although the combining form generally appears at the begnning of a term, it may appear within a term or at the end of it.*

---

*From Young CG, Austin MG: *Learning medical terminology step by step,* ed 4, St Louis, 1979, Mosby–Year Book.

adeno- gland
adreno- adrenal gland
angio- vessel
ano- anus
arterio- artery
arthro- joint
balano- glans penis
blepharo- eyelid
broncho- bronchus (windpipe)
cantho- canthus (angle at either end of slit between eyelids)
capit- head
cardi, cardio- heart
carpo- wrist
cephalo- head
cerebello- cerebellum (part of brain)
cerebro- cerebrum (part of brain)
cheilo- lip (mouth)
chole- bile (Note: *chole-* + *cyst* meaning "bladder," = gallbladder; *chole-* + *doch,* meaning "duct," = choledocho, or common bile duct.)
chondro- cartilage
chordo- cord or string (generally used in connection with the vocal cord or spermatic cord)
cilia- hair (Latin)
cleido- collarbone
coccygo- coccyx (end bone of the spinal column)
colpo- vagina
cordo- cord (usually vocal cord)
coxa- hip (Latin)
cranio- head
cysto- sac, cyst, or bladder (most often used in connection with the urinary bladder)
cyto- cell
dacryo- tear (used commonly in relation to tear duct or sac)
dento-, donto- tooth
derma- skin
duodeno- duodenum (part of small intestine)
emia- blood
encephalo- brain
entero- intestines
fascia- sheet or band of fibrous tissue (Latin)
fibro- fibers
gastro- stomach
genu- knee (Latin)
gingivo- gums
glomerulo- glomerulus (often a structure of the kidney)

glosso- tongue
gnatho- jaw
hem-, hema-, hemo-, hemato- blood
hepato- liver
hilus- pit or depression in an organ where vessels and nerves enter (Latin)
histio- tissue
hystero- uterus (NOTE: This term may also pertain to hysteria.)
ileo- ileum (part of small intestine)
ilio- flank or ilium (bone of pelvis)
jejuno- jejunum (part of small intestine)
kerato- cornea or horny layer of the skin
labio- lips (either of mouth or vulva)
lacrimo- tears (used also in connection with tear ducts or sacs)
laparo- loin or flank (also refers to abdomen)
laryngo- larynx
linguo- tongue
lympho- lymph
masto- breast
meningo- meninges (coverings of the brain and spinal cord)
metra-, metro- uterus
morpho- form
myelo- bone marrow and spinal cord (NOTE: Use of this term will determine which tissue is meant.)
myo- muscle (NOTE: The Latin word for muscle is *mus*.)
myringo- eardrum
naso- nose
nephro- kidney
neuro- nerve
oculo- eye
odonto- tooth
omphalo- navel or umbilicus
onycho- nails
oophoro- ovary
ophthalmo- eye
ora-, oro- mouth
orthio-, orchido- testis
os- bone or mouth
osteo- bone
oto- ear
ovario- ovary
palato- palate of mouth
palpebro- eyelid
pectus- breast, chest, or thorax (Latin)
pharyngo- pharynx
phlebo- vein
pilo- hair
pleuro- pleura of lung (relates also to side or rib)

pneumo-, pneumono- lungs (also used in referring to air or breath)
procto- rectum
pyelo- pelvis of kidney
pyloro- pylorus (part of stomach just before duodenum)
rhino- nose
sacro- sacrum
salpingo- fallopian tube or oviduct
sialo- saliva (used in connection with a salivary duct or gland)
splanchno- viscera
spleno- spleen
sterno- sternum
stoma- mouth
tarso- instep of foot; ankle (also edge of eyelid)

teno-, tenonto- tendon
thoraco- thorax or chest
thyro- thyroid
trachelo- neck, particularly the neck of the uterus or bladder
tracheo- trachea
unguis- nail
uretero- ureter
urethro- urethra
uro- urine, urinary
utero- uterus
vaso- vessel
veno- vein
ventriculo- ventricle of heart or brain
viscero- viscera

PREFIXES

Prefixes, the most frequently used elements in the formation of medical-dental words, are one or more syllables (prepositions or adverbs) placed before words or roots to show various kinds of relationships. They are never used independently, but when added before verbs, adjectives, or nouns, they modify the meaning. Most prefixes are a part of words in ordinary speech and do not refer specifically to medical-dental or scientific terminology, but there are many that occur frequently in medical terminology. Studying them is an important step in learning medical terms and building a medical-dental vocabulary.

PREFIX	TRANSLATION	EXAMPLES
a- (an before vowel)	Without, lack of	Apathy (lack of feeling), apnea (without breath), aphasia (without speech), anemia (lack of blood)
ab-	Away from	Abductor (leading away from), aboral (away from mouth)
ad-	To, toward, near to	Adductor (leading toward), adhesion (sticking to), adnexia (structures joined to), adrenal (near the kidney)
ambi-	Both	Ambidextrous (ability to use hands equally), ambilaterally (both sides)
amphi-	About, on both sides, both	Amphibious (living on both land and water)
ampho-	Both	Amphogenic (producing offspring of both sexes)
ana-	Up, back, again, excessive	Anatomy (a cutting up), anagenesis (reproduction of tissue), anasarca (excessive serum in cellular tissues of body)
ante-	Before, forward	Antecubital (before elbow), anteflexion (forward bending)
anti-	Against, opposed to, reversed	Antiperistalsis (reversed peristalsis), antisepsis (against infection)
apo-	From, away from	Aponeurosis (away from tendon), apochromatic (abnormal color)
bi-	Twice, double	Biarticulate (double joint), bifocal (two foci), bifurcation (two branches)

cata-	Down, according to, complete	Catabolism (breaking down), catalepsia (complete seizure), catarrh (flowing down)
circum-	Around, about	Circumflex (winding about), circumference (surrounding), circumarticular (around joint)
com-	With, together	Commissure (sending or coming together)
con-	With, together	Conductor (leading together), concrescence (growing together), concentric (having a common center)
contra-	Against, opposite	Contralateral (opposite side), contraception (prevention of conception), contraindicated (not indicated)
de-	Away from	Dehydrate (remove water from), decompensation (failure of compensation)
di-	Twice, double	Diplopia (double vision), dichromatic (two colors), digastric (double stomach)
dia-	Through, apart, across, completely	Diaphragm (wall across), diapedesis (ooze through), diagnosis (complete knowledge)
dis-	Reversal, apart from, separation	Disinfection (apart from infection), disparity (apart from equality), dissect (cut apart)
dys-	Bad, difficult, disordered	Dyspepsia (bad digestion), dyspnea (difficult breathing), dystopia (disordered position)
e-, ex-	Out, away from	Enucleate (remove from), eviscerate (take out viscera or bowels), exostosis (outgrowth of bone)
ec-	Out from	Ectopic (out of place), eccentric (away from center), ectasia (stretching out or dilation)
ecto-	On outside, situated on	Ectoderm (outer skin), ectoretina (outer layer of retina)
em-, en-	In	Empyema (pus in), encephalon (in the head)
endo-	Within	Endocardium (within heart), endometrium (within uterus), endodont (within tooth)
epi-	Upon, on	Epidural (upon dura), epidermis (on skin)
exo-	Outside, on outer side, outer layer	Exogenous (produced outside), exocolitis (inflammation of outer coat of colon)
extra-	Outside	Extracellular (outside cell), extrapleural (outside pleura)
hemi-	Half	Hemiplegia (partial paralysis), hemianesthesia (loss of feeling on one side of body)
hyper-	Over, above, excessive	Hyperemia (excessive blood), hypertrophy (overgrowth), hyperplasia (excessive formation)
hypo-	Under, below, deficient	Hypotension (low blood pressure), hypothyroidism (deficiency or underfunction of thyroid)
im-, in-	In, into	Immersion (act of dipping in), infiltration (act of filtering in), injection (act of forcing liquid into)
im-, in-	Not	Immature (not mature), involuntary (not voluntary), inability (not able)
infra-	Below	Infraorbital (below eye), infraclavicular (below clavicle or collarbone)

inter-	Between	Intercostal (between ribs), intervene (come between)
intra-	Within	Intracerebral (within cerebrum), intraocular (within eyes), intraventricular (within ventricles)
intro-	Into, within	Introversion (turning inward), introduce (lead into)
meta-	Beyond, after, change	Metamorphosis (change of form), metastasis (beyond original position), metacarpal (beyond wrist)
opistho-	Behind, backward	Opisthotic (behind ears), opisthognathous (behind jaws)
para-	Beside, by side	Paraplegia (paralysis of both sides), paracentesis (puncture along side of), parathyroid (beside thyroid)
per-	Through, excessive	Permeate (pass through), perforate (bore through), peracute (excessively acute)
peri-	Around	Periosteum (around bone), periatrial (around atrium), peribronchial (around bronchus)
post-	After, behind	Postoperative (after operation), postpartum (after childbirth), postocular (behind eye)
pre-	Before, in front of	Premaxillary (in front of maxilla), preoral (in front of mouth)
pro-	Before, in front of	Prognosis (foreknowledge), prophase (appear before)
re-	Back, again, contrary	Reflex (bend back), revert (turn again to), regurgitation (backward flowing, contrary to normal)
retro-	Backward, located behind	Retrocervical (located behind cervix), retrograde (going backward), retrolingual (behind tongue)
semi-	Half	Semicartilaginous (half cartilage), semilunar (half moon), semiconscious (half conscious)
sub-	Under	Subcutaneous (under skin), subarachnoid (under arachnoid), subungual (under nail)
super-	Above, upper, excessive	Supercilia (upper brows), supernumerary (excessive number), supermedial (above middle)
supra-	Above, upon	Suprarenal (above kidney), suprasternal (above sternum), suprascapular (on upper part of scapula)
sym-, syn-	Together, with	Symphysis (growing together), synapsis (joining together), synarthrosis (articulation of joints together)
trans-	Across, through	Transection (cut across), transduodenal (through duodenum), transmit (send beyond)
ultra-	Beyond, in	Ultraviolet (beyond violet end of spectrum), ultraligation (ligation of vessel beyond point of origin), ultrasonic (sound waves beyond the upper frequency of hearing by human ear)

SUFFIXES

Suffixes are the one or more syllables or elements added to the root, or stem, of a word (the part that indicates the essential meaning) to alter the meaning or indicate the intended part of speech.

To make it pronounceable the last letter or letters of the root to which the suffix is attached may be changed. the last vowel may be changed to an *o*, or *o* may be inserted if it is not already present before a suffix beginning with a consonant, as in *cardiology*. The final vowel in the root may be dropped before a suffix beginning with a vowel, as in *neuritis*.

Most suffixes are in common use in English, but some are peculiar to medical science. The suffixes most commonly used to indicte disease are -itis, meaning "inflammation," *-oma,* meaning "tumor," and *-osis,* meaning "a condition," usually morbid. The following suffixes occur often in medical-dental terminology, but they are also in use in ordinary language:

SUFFIX	USE	EXAMPLES
-ise, -ate	Added to nouns or adjectives to make verbs expressing to use and to act like; to subject to; make into	Visualize (able to see), impersonate (act like), hypnotize (put into state of hypnosis)
-ist, -or, -er	Added to verbs to make nouns expressing agent or person concerned or instrument	Anesthetist (one who practices the science of anesthesia), dissector (instrument that dissects or person who dissects), donor (giver)
-ent	Added to verbs to make adjectives or nouns of agency	Recipient (one who receives), concurrent (happening at the same time)
-sia, -y	Added to verbs to make nouns expressing action, process, or condition	Therapy (treatment), anesthesia (process or condition of feeling)
-ia, -ity	Added to adjectives or nouns to make nouns expressing quality or condition	Septicemia (poisoning of blood), disparity (inequality), acidity (condition of excess acid), neuralgia (pain in nerves)
-ma, -mata, -men, -mina, -ment, -ure	Added to verbs to make nouns expressing result of action or object of action	Trauma (injury), foramina (openings), ligament (tough fibrous band holding bone or viscera together), fissure (groove)
-ium, -olus, -olum, -culus, -culum, -cule, -cle	Added to nouns to make diminutive nouns	Bacterium, alveolus (air sac), follicle (little bag), cerebellum (little brain), molecule (little mass), ossicle (little bone)
-ible, -ile	Added to verbs to make adjectives expressing ability or capacity	Contractile (ability to contract), edible (capable of being eaten), flexible (capable of being bent)
-al, -c, -ious, -tic	Added to nouns to make adjectives expressing relationship, concern, or pertaining to	Neural (referring to nerve), neoplastic (referring to neoplasm), cardiac (referring to heart), delirious (suffering from delirium)
-id	Added to verbs or nouns to make adjectives expressing state or condition	Flaccid (state of being weak or lax), fluid (state of being fluid or liquid)

-tic	Added to verbs to make adjectives showing relationships	Caustic (referring to burn), acoustic (referring to sound or hearing)
-oid, -form	Added to nouns to make adjectives expressing resemblance	Polypoid (resembling polyp), plexiform (resembling a plexus), fusiform (resembling a fusion), epidermoid (resembling epidermis)
-ous	Added to nouns to make adjectives expressing material	Ferrous (composed of iron), serous (composed of serum), mucinous (composed of mucin)

The following verbs or combining forms of verbs are derived from Greek or Latin. They may be attached to other roots to form words, or suffixes and prefixes may be added to them to form words. In the following examples, the part or root of the word to which the verb is attached is underlined and the meaning, if not clear, is given in parentheses:

ROOT	TRANSLATION	EXAMPLES
-algia-	Pain	Cardialgia (heart), gastralgia (stomach), neuralgia (nerve)
-dynia-	Pain	Mastodynia (breast), pleurodynia (chest), esophagodynia (esophagus), coccygodynia (coccyx)
-audi-, -audio-	Hear, hearing	Audiometer (measure), audiophone (voice instrument for deaf)
-bio-	Live	Biology (study of living), biostatistics (vital statistics), biogenesis (origin)
cau-, -caus-	Burn	Caustic (suffic added to make adjective), cauterization; causalgia (burning pain), electrocautery
-centesis-	Puncture, perforate	Thoracentesis (chest), pneumocentesis (lung), arthrocentesis (joint), enterocentesis (intestine)
-clas-, -claz-	Smash, break	Osteoclasis (bone), odontoclasis (tooth)
-duct-	Lead	Ductal (suffix added to make adjective), oviduct (egg uterine tube or fallopian tube), periductal (peri means "around"), abduct (prefix meaning lead away from)
-ecta-, -ectas-	Dilate	Venectasia (dilation of vein), cardiectasis (heart), ectatic (suffix added for adjective)
-edem-	Swell	Myoedema (muscle), lymphedema (lymph) (a is a suffix added to make a noun)
-esthes-	Feel	Esthesia (suffix added to make noun), anesthesia (an is a prefix)
-flex-, -flec-	Bend	Flexion (suffix added to make noun), flexor (suffix added), anteflect (prefix added meaning "before" bending forward)
-fiss-	Split	Fissure, fission (suffixes added to make nouns)
-flu-, -flux-	Flow	Fluctuate, fluxion, affluent (abundant flowing)
-geno-, -genesis-	Produce, origin	Genotype, homogenesis (same origin), pathogenesis (disease, origin of disease) heterogenesis (prefix added meaning "other," alteration of generation)
-iatro-, -iatr-	Treat, cure	Geriatrics (old age), pediatrics (children)
-kine-, -kino-, -kineto-, -kinesio-	Move	Kinetogenic (producing movement), kinetic (suffix added to make adjective), kinesiology (study)

-liga-	Bind	Ligament (suffix added to make noun) ligate, ligature
-logy-	Study	Parasitology (parasites), bacteriology (bacteria), histology (tissues)
-lysis-	Breaking up, dissolving	Hemolysis (blood), glycolysis (sugar), autolysis (self-destruction of cells)
-morph-, -morpho-	Form	Morphology, amorphous (not definite form), pleomorphic (more, occurring in various forms), polymorphic (many)
-olfact-	Smell	Olfactophobia (fear), olfactory (suffix added to make adjective)
-op-, -opto-	See	Amblyopia (dull, dimness of vision), presbyopia (old, impairment of vision in old age), optic, myopia (myo, to wink, half close the eyes)
-palpit-	Flutter	Palpitation
-par-, -partus-	Labor	Postpartum (after birth), parturition (act of giving birth) (Note: para I, II, III, IV, etc., are symbols for number of births.)
-pep-	Digest	Dyspepsia (bad, difficult), peptic (suffix added to make adjective)
-phag-, -phago-	Eat	Phagocytosis (eating of cells), phagomania (madness, mad craving for food or to eat), dysphagia (difficult eating or swallowing)
-phan-	Appear, visible	Phanerosis (act of becoming visible), phantasia, phantasy
-pexy-	Fix	Mastopexy (fixation of breast), nephrosplenopexy (surgical fixation of kidney and spleen)
-phas-	Speak, utter	Aphasia (unable to speak), dysphasia (difficulty in speaking)
-phobia-	Fear	Hydrophobia (fear of water), photophobia (fear of light), claustrophobia (closeness, fear of close places)
-phil-	Like, love	Hemophilia (blood, a hereditary disease characterized by delayed clotting of blood), acidophilia (acid stain, liking or straining with acid stains), philanthropy (love of mankind)
-phrax-, -phrag-	Fence off, wall off	Diaphragm (across, partition separating thorax from abdomen), phragmoplast (formed)
-plas-	Form, grow	Neoplasm (new growth), rhinoplasty (nose operation for formation of nose), otoplasty (ear), choledochoplasty (common bile duct)
-plegia-	Paralyze	Paraplegia (paralysis of lower limbs), ophthalmoplegia (eye), hemiplegia (partial paralysis)
-pne-, -pneo-	Breathe	Dyspnea (difficult breathing), apnea (lack of breathing), hyperpnea (overbreathing)
-poie-	Make	Hematopoiesis (blood), erythropoiesis (red blood cells), leukopoiesis (making white cells)
-ptosis-	Fall	Proctoptosis (anus, prolapse of anuse), splanchnoptosis (viscera)
-rrhagia-	Burst forth, pour	Menorrhagia (abnormal bleeding during menstruation), menometrorrhagia (abnormal uterine bleeding), hemorrhage (blood)
-rrhaphy-	Suture	Herniorrhaphy (suturing or repair of hernia), hepatorrhaphy (liver), nephrorrhaphy (kidney)

-rrhea-	Flow, discharge	Leukorrhea (white discharge from vagina), galactorrhea (milk discharge), rhinorrhea (nasal discharge)
-rrhexis-	Rupture	Enterorrhexis (intestines), metrorrhexis (uterus)
-schiz-	Split, divide	Schizophrenia (mind, split personality), schizonychia (nails), schizotrichia (hair)
-scope-	Examine	Microscopic, cardioscope, endoscope (endo means "within," an instrument for examining the interior of a hollow internal organ)
-stasis-	Stop, stand still	Hematostatic (pertaining to stangation of blood), epistasis (checking or stopping of any discharge)
-stazien-	Drop	Epistaxis (nosebleed)
-teg-, -tect-	Cover	Tegmen, tectum (rooflike structure), integument (skin covering)
-therap-	Treat, cure	Therapy, neurotherapy (nerves), chemotherapy (chemicals), physiotherapy
-topo-	Place	Topography, toponarcosis (numbing, hence numbing of a part or localized anesthesia)
-tomy-	Cut, incise	Phlebotomy (incision of vein), arthrotomy (joint), appendectomy (ectomy, meaning "cutout," excision of appendix), oophorectomy (excision of ovary), ileocecostomy (ostomy, meaning "creation of an artifical opening," os, meaning "opening or mouth"; ileocecostomy is an anatomosis of ileum and cecum)
-tropho-	Nourish	Hypertrophy (enlargement or overnourishment), atrophy (undernourishment), dystrophy (difficult or bad)
-volv-	Turn	Involution, volvulus (twisting of an organ, as in intestinal obstruction with twisting of the bowel or twisting of the esophagus)

The following roots and combining forms are derived from Greek or Latin adjectives. Adjectives appear most often in compounds and are joined to nouns or verbs. Suffixes may be added to make them into nouns.

In the following examples, the part or root of the word that the adjective modifies is underlined, and the meaning, if not clear, is given in parentheses:

ROOT	TRANSLATION	EXAMPLES
-auto-	Self	Autoinfection, autolysis, autopathy (disease), autopsy (view, postmortem examination)
-brachy-	Short	Brachycephalia (head), brachydactylia (fingers), brachychelia (lip), brachygnathous (jaw)
-brady-	Slow	Bradypnea (breath), bradypragia (action), bradyuria (urine), bradypepsia (digestion)
-brevis-	Short	Brevity, breviflexor (short flexor muscle)
-cavus-	Hollow	Cavity, cavernous, vena cava (vein)
-coel-	Hollow	Coelarium (lining membrane of body cavity), coelom (body cavity of embryo)
-crypto-	Hidden, concealed	Cryptorchid (testis), cryptogenic (origin obscure or doubtful), cryptophthalmos (eye)
-cryo-	Cold	Cryotherapy, cryotolerant, cryometer

-dextro-	Right	Ambidextrous (using both hands with equal ease), dextrophobia (fear of objects on right side), dextrocardia (heart)
-dys-	Difficult, bad, disordered, painful	Dysarthria (speech), dyshidrosis* (sweat), dyskinesia* (motion), dystocia (birth), dysphasia (speech), dyspepsia (digestion)
-eu-	Well, good	Euphoria (well-being), euphagia, eupnea (breath), euthyroid (normal thyroid), eutocia (normal birth)
-eury-	Broad, wide	Eurycephalic (head), euryopia (vision), eurysomatic (body, squat thickset body)
-glyco-	Sugar, sweet	Glycohemia (sugar in blood), glycopenia (poverty of sugar, low blood sugar level)
-gravis-	Heavy	Gravida (pregnant woman), gravidism (pregnancy)
-haplo-	Single, simple	Haploid (having a single set of chromosomes), haplodont (teeth without simple crowns), haplopathy (simple uncomplicated disease)
-hetero-	Other, different	Heterogeneous (kind, dissimilar elements), heteroinoculation, heterology (abnormality of structure), heterointoxication
-homo-	Same	Homogeneous (same kind or quality throughout), homozygous (possessing identical pair of genes), homologous (corresponding in structure)
-hydro-	Wet, water	Hydronephrosis (kidney, collection of urine in kidney pelvis), hydropneumothorax (fluid in chest), hydrophobia (fear of water, water causes painful reaction in this disease)
-iso-	Equal	Isocellular (similar cells), isodontic (all teeth alike), isocytosis (equality of size of cells), isochromatic (having same color throughout)
-latus-	Broad	Latitude, latissimus dorsi (muscle adducting humerus)
-leio-	Smooth	Leiomyosarcoma (smooth muscle, fleshy malignant tumor), leiomyofibroma (tumor of muscle and fiber elements), leiomyoma (tumor of unstriped muscle)
-lepto-	Slender	Leptosomatic (body), leptodactylous (fingers)
-levo-	Left	Levocardia (heart), levorotation (turning to left)
-longus-	Long	Adductor longus (muscle of thigh), longitude
-macro-	Large, abnormal size	Macocephalic (head), macrocheiria (hands), macromastia (breast), macronychia (nails)
-magna-	Large, great	Magnitude, adductor magnus (thigh muscle)
-malaco-	Soft	Malacia (softening), osteomalacia (bones)
-malus-	Bad	Malady, malaise, malignant, malformation
-medius-	Middle	Median, medium, gluteus medius (femur muscle)
-mega-	Great	Megacolon (large colon), megacephaly (head)
-megalo-	Huge	Megalomania (delusion of grandeur), hepatomegaly (enlarged liver), splenomegaly (enlarged spleen)
-meso-	Middle, mid	Mesocarpal (wrist), mesoderm (skin), mesothelium (a lining membrane of cavities)
-micro-	Small	Microglossia (tongue), microblepharia (eyelids), microorganism, microphonia (voice)
-minimus-	Smallest	Gluteus minimus (smallest muscle of hip), adductor minimus (muscle of thigh)
-mio-	Less	Miolecithal (egg with little yolk), miopragia (perform), decreased activity)

-mono-	One, single, limited to one part	Monochromatic (color), monobrachia (arm)
-multi-	Many, much	Multipara (bear, woman who has borne many children), multilobar (numerous lobes), multicentric (many centers)
-necro-	Dead	Necrosed, necrosis, necropsy (postmortem examination), necrophobia (fear of death)
-neo-	New	Neoformation, neomorphism (form), neonatal (first 4 weeks of life), neopathy (disease)
-oligo-	Few, scanty, little	Oligophrenia (mind), oligopnea (breath), oliguria (urine), oligodipsia (thirst)
-ortho-	Straight, normal, correct	Orthodontic (teeth, normal), orthogenesis (progressive evolution in a given direction), orthograde (walk, carrying body upright), orthopnea (breath, unable to breathe unless in an upright position)
-oxy-	Sharp, quick	Oxyesthesia (feel), oxyopia (vision), oxyosmia (smell)
-pachy-	Thick	Pachyderm (skin), pachysulemia (blood), pachypleuritis (inflammation of pleura), pachycholia (bile), pachyotia (ears)
-paleo-	Old	Paleogenetic (origin in the past), paleopathology (study of diseases in mummies)
-platy-	Flat	Platybasia (skull base), platycoria (pupil), platycrania (skull)
-pleo-	More	Pleomorphism (forms), pleochromocytoma (tumor composed of different colored cells)
-poikilo-	Varied	Poikiloderma (skin mottling), poikilothermal (heat, variable body termperature)
-poly-	Many, much	Polyhedral (many bases or faces), polymastia (more than two breasts), polymelia (supernumerary limbs), polymyalgia (pain in many muscles)
-pseudo-	False, spurious	Pseudostratified (layered), pseudocirrhosis (apparent cirrhosis of liver), pseudohypertrophy
-pronus-	Face down	Prone, pronation
-sclero-	Hard	Sclerosis (hardening), arteriosclerosis (artery), scleronychia (nails), scleroderma (skin)
-scolio-	Twisted, crooked	Scoliodontic (teeth), scoliosis, scoliokyphosis (curvature of spine)
-sinistro-	Left	Sinistrocardia, sinistromanual (left handed), sinistraural (hearing better in left ear)
-supinus-	Face up	Supine, supination, supinator longus (muscle in arm)
-steno-	Narrow	Stenosis, stenostomia (mouth), mitral stenosis (mitral valve in heart)
-stereo-	Solid, three dimensions	Stereoscope, stereometer
-tachy-	Fast, swift	Tachycardia (heart), tachyphrasia (speech)
-tele-	End, far away	Telepathy, telecardiogram
-telo-	Complete	Telophase
-thermo-	Heat, warm	Thermal, thermometer, thermobiosis (ability to live in high temperature)
-trachy-	Rough	Trachyphonia (voice), trachychromatic (deeply staining)
-xero-	Dry	Xerophagia (eating of dry foods) xerostomia (mouth), xeroderma (skin)

PRONUNCIATION OF MEDICAL-DENTAL TERMS

Medical terms are hard to pronounce, especially if you have read them but never heard them spoken. Following are some helpful shortcuts:

ch is sometimes pronounced like *k*. Examples: chromatin, chronic.

ps is pronounced like *s*. Examples: psychiatry, psychology.

pn is pronounced with only the *n* sound. Example: pneumonia.

c and *g* are given the soft sound of *s* and *j*, respectively, before *e, i,* and *y* in words of both Greek and Latin origin. Examples: cycle, cytoplasm, giant, generic.

c and *g* have a harsh sound before other letters. Examples: gastric, gonad, cast, cardiac.

ae and *oe* are pronounced *ee*. Examples: coelom, fasciae.

i at the end of a word (to form a plural) is pronounced *eye*. Examples: alveoli, glomeruli, fasciculi.

e and *es,* when forming the final letters or letter of a word, are often pronounced as separate syllables. Examples: rete (reetee), nares (nayreez).

Plurals

In most English words the plurals are formed by merely adding an *s* or *es,* but in Greek and Latin the plural may be designated by changing the ending.

-ae, as in fasciae (singular form, fascia).*-ia,* as in crania (singular form, cranium).

-i, as in glomeruli (singular form, glomerulus). When the singular form ends in *us,* the plural form is made by adding *i* and dropping the *us.*

-ata, as in adenomata (singular form, adenoma).

Spelling

The aforementioned rules for pronunciation and the formation of plurals are essential for spelling, but it is important that you consult a medical dictionary if you are not sure. Phonetic spelling has no place in medicine, because a misspelled word may give the wrong meaning to a diagnosis. Furthermore, some terms are pronounced alike but spelled differently; for example, ileum is a part of the intestinal tract, but ilium is a pelvic bone.

Abbreviations

@ at

A amp

āā of each (F. ana)

a.c before meals (L., *ante cibum*)

ACTH adrenocorticotropic hormone

ad Latin preposition, -to, up to

a.d. alternating days (L., *alternis diebus*)

ad lib at pleasure, as needed or desired (L., *ad libitum*)

ADA American Dental Association

ADAMHA Alcohol, Drug Abuse, and Mental Health Administration

ADH antidiuretic hormone

adm admission

AFB acid-fast bacilli

AFDC Aid to Families with Dependent Children

A/G albumin-globulin (ratio)

Ag silver (L., *argentum)*

AIDS acquired immunodeficiency syndrome

alb albumin

alc alcoholism

alk alkaline

alt. dieb. every other day (L., *alternis diebus*)

alt. hor. every other hour (L., *alternis horis*)

alt. noct. every other night (L., *alternis noctibus*)

am, a, ag amalgam

AM, a.m. before noon (L., *ante meridiem*)

amp ampule

amt amount

anat anatomy, anatomic

anes anesthesia

ant anterior

AP anteroposterior

APF acidulated phosphate flouride

appl applicable, application, appliance

approx approximate

aq water (L., *aqua*)

ARC AIDS-related complex

av average

Av, avdp avoirdupois

AZT azidiothymidine

bact bacterium (-ia)

bar barometric

basos basophils

BCC basal cell carcinoma

BF bone fragment

BIA Bureau of Indian Affairs

bib drink (L., *bibe*)

b.i.d. twice a day (L., *bis in die*)

biol biologic, biology

BMR basal metabolic rate

BP blood pressure

BS blood sugar

BSA body surface area

BUN blood urea nitrogen

BW bite-wing radiograph

Bx biopsy

C centigrade, one hundred (L., *centum*)

c̄ with (L., *cum*)

C-1 to C-7 cervical vertebrae 1 to 7

CA cardiac arrest, chronologic age

Ca calcium, carcinoma

cal calorie

caps capsules

cav cavity

CBC complete blood count

CC chief complaint

cc cubic centimeter

CDC Centers for Disease Control

cent centigrade

CF complement fixation

cf compare, refer to (L., *confer*)

CFNP Community Food and Nutrition Programs

CFR Code of Federal Regulations

CFT complement fixation test

CHD childhood disease

CHF congestive heart failure

chr chronic

CM costal margin

cm centimeter

c.m. tomorrow morning (L., *cras mane*)

c/min cycles per minute

cm/s centimeters per second

CMV cytomegalovirus

CNS central nervous system

CO carbon monoxide, cardiac output

Co cobalt

CO₂ carbon dioxide

COD condition on discharge

comp compound

conc concentrated

cond condition

CP centric position

CPC Clinical Pathology Conference

cpd compound

c.p.s. cycles per second

Cs conscious, consciousness

CSF cerebrospinal fluid

Cu copper (L., *cuprum*)

cu cubic

cur curettage

CV cardiovascular

CVA cerebrovascular accident

Cx convex

CY calender year

cyl cylinder, cylindric

d dose (L., *dosis*)

D-1 to D-12 dorsal vertebrae 1 to 12

D, dist distal

D & C dilation and curettage

DA direct admission

DANA benzol-arginine napthylamide

db decibel

dbl double

dc direct current

DC & B dilation, curettage, and biopsy

DD differential diagnosis

d.d. let it be given to (L., *detur ad*)

DDC dideoxycytidine

DDI dideoxyinosine

DDT dichlorodiphenyltrichloroethane

DEA Drug Enforcement Administration

deg degree
dev develop, development
Dg, diag diagnosis
diam diameter
diff differential
dil dilute (L., *dilue*)
dim diminutive, diminish
dl deciliter
DO distocclusal
dis disease
disc discontinue
disch discharge
disp dispensary
dist distal
DMF decayed, missing, and filled (teeth)
DNA deoxyribonucleic acid
DOA dead on arrival
DOB date of birth
doz dozen
DPT diphtheria, pertussin, tetanus
Dr. doctor
DT delerium tremens
d.t.d. give of such a dose (L., *datur talis dosis*)
DTR deep tendon reflexes
D/W dextrose and water
dwt pennyweight
Dx diagnosis
EAC external auditory canal
EBL estimated blood loss
E. coli *Escherichia coli*
ECG electrocardiogram
ECT electric convulsive therapy
ed effective dose
EDTA ethylenediaminetetraacetic acid
EEG electroencephalogram
EENT ears, eyes, nose, and throat
EEO equal employment opportunity
EEOC Equal Employment Opportunity Commission
e.g. for example (L., *exempli gratia*)
EIA enzyme immunoassay
EKG elektrokardiogram (German)
ELISA enzyme-linked immunosorbent assay
emerg emergency
EMT emergency medical treatment
ENT ears, nose, and throat
EOM extraocular movements
eos eosinophil

EPA Environmental Protection Agency
epith epithelial
equiv equivalent
esp especially
est estimate, estimation
et Latin conjunction, and
et al. and others (L., *et alii*)
etc. and so on, and so forth, and others (L., *et cetera*)
EUA examination under anesthesia
evac evacuate, evacuation
eval evaluate, evaluation
ext extract, external
F Fahrenheit, female, field (of vision), formula
F & R force and rhythm (pulse)
FB fingerbreadth, foreign body
FBS fasting blood sugar
FD fatal dose
FDA Food and Drug Administration
ff following
FH family history
fl fluid
FLD full lower denture
fl. dr. fluid dram
fld field
fl. oz. fluid ounce
FMX full mouth x-ray examination
FNS Food and Nutrition Service
frac fracture
frag fragment
freq frequent, frequency
FSH follicle-stimulating hormone
FSQS Food Safety and Quality Service
ft foot, let it be made (L., *fiat/fiant*)
FTC Federal Trade Commission
FTSG full-thickness skin graft
FUD full upper denture
func function
FUO fever of undetermined origin
Fx fracture
g, gm gram
gal gallon
GB gallbladder
GC gonococcus, gonococcal
GH general hospital
GI gastrointestinal
GIF gastric intrinsic factor
ging gingiva, gingivectomy
glob globulin

GP general practitioner
gr grain
GSW gunshot wound
gt drop (L., *gutta*)
gtt drops (L., *guttae*)
GU genitourinary
G/W glucose and water
H, h, hr hour (L., *hora*)
H₂O water
Hb, hgb hemoglobin
HBD has been drinking
HBP high blood pressure
HC hospital course
HCA hydrocortisone acetate
HCFA Home Care Financing Administration
NCl hydrochloric acid
Hct hematocrit
h.d. at hour of lying down at bedtime (L., *hora decubitus*)
HDL high-density lipoprotein
Hdpc handpiece
HIAA Health Insurance Association of America
HIV-1 human immunodeficiency virus type 1
HIV-2 human immunodeficiency virus type 2
HIV-G human immunodeficiency virus gingivitis
HIV-P human immunodeficiency virus periodontitis
hosp hospital
hpf high-power field
HPI history of present illness
h.s. hour of sleep (L., *hora somni*)
HSA Health Services Administration
ht height
HVD hypertensive vascular disease
Hx history
I & D incision and drainage
IA incurred accidentally
ibid. in the same place (L., *ibidem*)
ICS intercostal space
ICSH interstitial cell–stimulating hormone
ICT inflammation of connective tissue
ICU intensive care unit
id the same (L., *idem*)
i.e. that is (L., *id est*)
IH infectious hepatitis

IM intramuscular
imp impression
in inch
inc incisal, incisive, incise
in d. daily (L., *in dies*)
inf infected, inferior, infusion
INH isonicotinic hydrazide
inj injection, injury
inoc inoculate
inop inoperable, inoperative
int internal
IP intercuspal position, initial pressure (spinal fluid)
IPPB intermittent positive pressure breathing
IQ intelligence quotient
i.q. the same as (L., *idem quod*)
IS interspace, inventory of systems
it joint
ITP idiopathic thrombocytopenic purpura
IU international unit
IV intravenous
JCAHO Joint Commission on the Accreditation of Health Care Organizations
K Elvin (scale), potassium (L., *kalium*)
kc kilocycle
kg, kgm, kilo kilogram
KS Kaposi's sarcoma
kV kilovolt
L Latin
L, l liter
L & W living and well
L-1 to L-5 lumbar vertebrae 1 to 5
lab laboratory
lac laceration
lap laparotomy
LASER (laser) light amplification by stimulated emission of radiation
lat lateral
lb pound
LBP low back pain
LD lethal dose
LDH lactic dehydrogenase
LE lupus erythematosus
lig ligament
ling lingual
liq liquid, liquor
LJP localized juvenile periodontitis
LMD local medical doctor

LN lymph node
lpf low-power field
LSH lutein-stimulating hormone
lt left
lymphs lymphocytes
m murmur, meter
M male, mix (L., *misce*)
M, mes mesial
MA mental age, moderately advanced
ma milliampere
MAL midaxillary line
mand mandibular
MASER (maser) microwave amplification by stimulated emission of radiation
max maximum, maxillary
Mc megacurie, megacycle
mc millicurie
mcg microgram
MCH mean corpuscular hemoglobin
MCHC mean corpuscular hemoglobin concentration
MCV mean corpuscular volume
m. dict. as directed (L., *modo dictu*)
MDR minimum daily requirement
MDS temporomandibular joint pain-dysfunction syndrome
med medical, medicine
MED minimal effective dose
MEDLARS medical literature analysis and retrieval system
mEq milliequivalent
mg, mgm milligram
MHB maximum hospital benefit
micro microscopic
min minute, minimum
MIST Medical Information Service via Telephone
ML midline
ml milliliter
MLD minimal lethal dosage
mm millimeter
MM mucous membrane
MO mesiocclusal
mo month
MOD mesiocclusodistal
monos monocytes
MS multiple sclerosis
msec millisecond
MSH melanocyte-stimulating hormone

mV millivolt
N$_2$O nitrous oxide
NAD no appreciable disease
NaPent thiopental sodium (Pentothal)
narc narcotic, narcotism
NAS National Academy of Science
nc no change
NDF no disease found
neg negative
NIH National Institutes of Health
NLM National Library of Medicine
NMR nuclear magnetic resonance
non. rep. do not repeat
norm normal
NP neuropsychiatry
NPC no previous complaint
NPH no previous history
NPN nonprotein nitrogen
n.p.o. nothing by mouth (L., *nil per os*)
NR normal record
n.r. not to be repeated (L., *non repetatur*)
NRC Nuclear Regulatory Commission, National Research Council
N/S normal saline
NS not significant
NSA no significant abnormality
NTP normal temperature and pressure
N/V nausea and/or vomiting
O oxygen
O$_2$ oxygen gas
OB obstetrics
OB-GYN obstetrics and gynecology
obl oblique
occ occlusal
OCD Office of Child Development
OCSE Office of Child Support Enforcement
o.d. every day (L., *omni die*), right eye
ODC oral disease control
OH oral hygiene
OHD Office of Human Development
o.h. every hour (L., *omni hora*)
OHI Office for Handicapped Individuals
OHMO Office of hazardous Materials Operations

o.m. every morning (L., *omni mane*)

o.n. every night (L., *omni nocte*)

op operation

OPC outpatient clinic

OPD outpatient department

Ophth ophthalmology

opp opposite, opposed

OPS outpatient section or service

OR operating room

org organism, organic

o.s. left eye

OSHA Occupational Safety and Health Administration

OT occupational therapy

OYD Office of Youth Development

oz ounce

P pulse

P̄ after (L., *post*)

p- para-

p 1, p 2, etc. para 1, para 2, etc.

P & A percussion and auscultation

PA posteroanterior

PAB, PABA paraaminobenzoic acid

PAHO Pan American Health Organization

Pan panoral x-ray examination

PAS, PASA paraaminosalicylic acid

path pathology

PATH pituitary adrenotropic hormone

PBCM particulate bone and cancellous marrow grafts

PBI protein-bound iodine

p.c. after meal (L., *post cibum*)

PCN penicillin

PCP *Pneumocystis carinii* pneumonia

pcpt perception

PDR *Physician's Desk Reference*

PE physical examination

Ped pediatrics

pen penetrating

perf perforating

PH past history

pH negative logarithm of hydrogen ion concentration

PI present illness

PID pelvic inflammatory disease

PLD partial lower denture

PM, p.m. after noon (L., *post meridiem*)

PM after death (L., *post mortem*)

PMB polymorphonuclear basophil leukocytes

PME polymorphonuclear eosinophil leukocytes

PMH past medical history

PMN polymorphonuclear neutrophil leukocytes

PMP previous menstrual period

PN percussion note

p.o. by mouth (L., *per os*)

PO postoperative

POD 1, 2, etc. postoperative day, first, second, etc.

POH personal oral hygiene

polys polymorphonuclear leukocytes

pos positive

postop postoperative

pp postpartum

PPBS postprandial blood sugar

PPLO pleuropneumonia-like organism

PPO Preferred Provider Organization

ppt precipitate

prep preparation, prepare (for surgery)

p.r.n. as required, as the occasion arises (L., *pro re nata*)

PRO Peer Review Organization

prog prognosis

pt patient

PT physical therapy, physiotherapy

PTT partial thromboplastin time

PUD partial upper denture

pulm pulmonary, pulmonic

Px prophylaxis

q every (L., *quaque*)

q.d. every day (L., *quaque die*)

q.h. every hour (L., *quaque hora*)

q1.2h every second hour (L., *quaque secunda hora*)

q.i.d. four times a day (L., *quater in die*)

q.l. as much as pleased (L., *quantum libet*)

q.n. every night (L., *quaque nocte*)

q.p. at will (L., *quantum placeat*)

q.q.h. every 4 hours (L., *quaque quarta hora*)

q.s. a sufficient quantity

qt quart

q.v. as much as liked (L., *quantum vis*)

R respiration

r roentgen

R & R rate and rhythm

RA rheumatoid arthritis

rad radiograph

RAI radioactive iodine

RBC red blood cells

RC retruded contact position, root canal

reg regular

rem(s) roentgen-equivalent-man

rep(s) roentgen-equivalent-physical

req requires, required

resp respiration

Rh Rh factor in blood (L., *Rhesus*)

RHD rheumatic heart disease

RN registered nurse

RNA ribonucleic acid

R/O rule out

ROH alcohol

ROM range of motion

ROS review of systems

RQ respiratory quotient

RR & E round, regular, and equal (pupils)

RSA Rehabilitation Services Administration

rt right

R$_x$ take (thou) a recipe

Rx treatment (L., *recipe*)

s̄ without (L., *sine*)

S-1 to S-5 sacral vertebrae 1 to 5

SBE subacute bacterial endocarditis

SD sterile dressing

sec second, secondary

sed rate sedimentation rate

segs segmented cells

SG skin graft, specific gravity

SGOT serum glutamic-oxaloacetic transaminase

SGPT serum glutamic pyruvic transaminase

SI seriously ill

Sig. write on label

SIL seriously ill list

sol solution

spec specimen

sp. fl. spinal fluid

sp. gr. specific gravity

SR systems review

s̄s̄ one half signs and symptoms (L., *semis*)

S/S signs and symptoms
SSA Social Security Administration
st let it stand (L., *stet*)
ST sedimentation rate
stat immediately (L., *statim*)
std standard
stim stimulator, stimulate
Strep *Streptococcus*
STS serologic test for syphilis
STSG split-thickness skin graft
SUD skin unit dose
sup superior
surg surgeon, surgery
Sx symptom
sym symmetric
symp symptom
sys system
T temperature
T & A tonsils and adenoids; tonsillectomy and adenoidectomy
T-1 to T-12 thoracic vertebrae 1 to 12
tab tablet
TAT tetanus antitoxin
TB, TBC tuberculosis
tbsp tablespoon
TC treatment completed
TE tracheoesophageal
TEFRA Tax Equity and Fiscal Responsibility Act of 1982

temp temperature
TIBC total iron-binding capacity
t.i.d. three times a day (L., *ter in die*)
tinc tincture
TLC tender loving care
TM temporomandibular
TMJ temporomandibular joint
TNF tumor necrosis factor
TPR temperature, pulse, respiration
TSH thyroid-stimulating hormone
tsp teaspoon
TSP total serum protein
TUR transurethral resection
U, u unit
UCHD usual childhood diseases
UGA under general anesthesia
UIBC unsaturated iron-binding capacity
UIS Unemployment Insurance Service
ung ointment (L., *unguentum*)
unk unknown
URI upper respiratory tract infection
USP *United States Pharmacopoeia*
ut. dict. as directed
V, v volt

VA Veterans Administration
vag vaginal
VC vital capacity
VD venereal disease
VDH valvular disease of the heart
VDRL Venereal Disease Research Laboratory
vert vertebra, vertical
visc viscous
VIT vitamin
viz that is, namely (L., *videlicet*)
VLDL very low-density lipids
VO verbal order
vol volume
v.s. see above (L., *vide supra*)
vs versus
VZ varicella zoster virus
WBC white blood cells
WD ward
w-d well-developed
WF white female
wh white
WHO World Health Organization
WM white male
w-n well-nourished
wnd wound
WNL within normal limits
wt weight

Symbols

& and
* birth
† death
↓ decrease
° degree
= equal
′ feet, minutes
♀ female
> greater than, or indicating increase
″ inches; seconds

↑ increase
< less than, or indicating decrease
♂ male
− minus, negative
number, pound
i, ii, iii one, two, or three (as in number of grams, etc.)
℥ ${\overline{iss}}$ one and one-half drams
℥ ${\overline{i}}$ one ounce
℥ ss one-half ounce

/ per
% percent
+ plus, positive
x times: 4 ×, four times; × 4, times four yard
xt extract, extracted
xyl, xylo Xylocaine
yd yard
YOB year of birth
yr year
z unknown quantity

Code on Dental Procedures and Nomenclature

COUNCIL ON DENTAL CARE PROGRAMS

The Council on Dental Care Programs* has approved the seventh revision of the *Code on Dental Procedures and Nomenclature*. The Code was developed in 1969 and was published in the *Journal of the American Dental Association (J Am Dent Assoc* 79:814, 1969). The seventh edition of the *Code* is a result of the work of the Council on Dental Care Programs in consultation with an Advisory Committee of the Code comprised of Council members and representation from the Blue Cross and Blue Shield Association, the Delta Dental Plans Association, the Health Insurance Association of America, the Health Care Financing Administration, and the dental specialty organizations.

Procedures covered

Although the Code includes primarily the dental services most frequently provided in a dentist's office, it also lists dental services performed in a hospital. Diagnostic services common to most categories of treatment are grouped under a separate diagnostic listing. These include oral examinations, radiographs, tests, and laboratory examinations. Dental services frequently performed by dental specialists are grouped and listed according to treatment sequence. To avoid duplication, other procedures that are performed by general practitioners and specialists alike have been grouped under the specialty category with which the procedures are most frequently identified. The groupings according to specialty categories are solely for convenience in using the *Code* and should not be interpreted as excluding general practitioners from performing such procedures.

Coding system

The *Code* is a five-digit system to identify dental procedures and services. The first digit is a zero throughout the code, and it identifies all procedures as being dental as contrasted to medical, hospital, or surgical services. The second digit designates the category of dental service. The third digit indicates the class of service within the dental category, and the fourth digit designates the subclass of specific procedure. The fifth digit allows for further expansion of the code when necessary.

New procedure *Code* numbers added to the seventh edition are identified with the symbol ● placed before the Code number. In instances where a code has been revised, the symbol ▲ is placed before the code number.

Guideline for use of the code

1. The existence of a code does not mean that the procedure is a covered or reimbursable benefit in a dental benefits plan. It is not easy for an office to become familiar with the

---

*From Council on Dental Care Programs: *CDT-1,* ed 1, Chicago, 1990-1995, American Dental Association.

details of every dental plan it deals with. It is, of course, the responsibility of the patient, not the dental office, to know what is covered and what is excluded in the dental plan. Certain dental benefits plans require predetermination when covered charges are expected to exceed a certain amount.

2. The dental procedure codes are divided into 12 categories of service. Procedures that are performed by general practitioners and specialist have been grouped under the category with which the procedures are most frequently identified. The categories are solely for convenience in using the *Code* and should not be interpreted as excluding general practitioners from performing or reporting such procedures.

3. Any procedure not accurately described in this *Code* should be reported using the appropriate unspecified (999) code with a narrative description. Unspecified codes are included for each category, with the exception of the preventive section. Every office will find occasions when a narrative report should be used. When reporting a procedure that is unusual, of which is accompanied by unusual circumstances, a narrative description (by report), with reference to the proper ''999'' number, may be the most appropriate way of explaining treatment to the third-party payer.

Coding system

The *Code* is set up in a five-digit system that identifies procedures and services. The categories are:

CATEGORY OF SERVICE		CODE SERIES
I.	Diagnostic	00100- 00999
II.	Preventive	01000- 01999
III.	Restorative	02000- 02999
IV.	Endodontics	03000- 03999
V.	Periodontics	04000- 04999
VI.	Prosthodontics, removable	05000- 05899
VII.	Maxillofacial prosthetics	05900- 05999
VIII.	Implant services	06000- 06199
IX.	Prosthodontics, fixed	06200- 06999
X.	Oral surgery	07000- 07999
XI.	Orthodontics	08000-08999
XII.	Adjunctive general services	09000-09999

Additional coding systems that may be used in a dental office are ICD-9, and HCFA's *Common Procedure Coding System (HCPCS)*. For more specific information, please contact:

1. ICD-9- CM
   Commission on Professional Hospital Activities
   Coding Assistance
   P.O. Box 1809
   Ann Arbor, MI 48106
   (313) 769- 6511
2. CPT
   American Medical Association
   Coding Assistance
   P.O. Box 10946
   Chicago, IL 06010
   (312) 464- 5000
3. HCPCS
   HCFA
   Superintendent of Documents
   U.S. Government Printing Office
   (202) 783-3238

Clinical Oral Examinations

00110   initial oral examination

No distinction made between initial exam performed by general practitioner or specialist; each subsequent practitioner (general practitioner or specialist) may report an initial exam, per episode, the first time a patient visits the office, or after a prolonged absence.

00120   periodic oral examination

Refers to exams performed subsequent to the initial examination(s) on a patient of record. Often performed with recall prophylaxis.

00130   emergency oral examination

Reported when it is necessary to relieve pain and suffering on an episodic basis. Not used in conjunction with a regular appointment; can be patient of record or a new patient; often reported together with 09110. Specific treatment should be reported separately with appropriate codes.

Radiographs

00210   intraoral—complete series (including bitewings)
00220   intraoral—periapical—first film
00230   intraoral—periapical—each additional film
00240   intraoral—occlusal film
00250   extraoral—first film
00260   extraoral—each additional film
00270   bitewing—single film
00272   bitewings—two films
00274   bitewings—four films
00290   posterior-anterior or lateral skull and facial bone survey film
▲ **00310   sialography**
00320   temporomandibular joint arthogram, including injection
00321   other temporomandibular joint films, by report
● **00322   tomographic survey**
00330   panoramic film
00340   cephalometric film

Tests and Laboratory Examinations

▲ **00415   bacteriologic studies for determination of pathologic agents**

May include, but is not limited to, tests for susceptibility to periodontal disease.

00425   caries susceptibility tests
00460   pulp vitality tests

Report by quadrant; includes contralateral comparison(s), as indicated.

00470   diagnostic casts

Also known as *diagnostic models* or *study models*.

00471   diagnostic photographs
00501   histopathologic examinations

Refers to gross and microscopic examination of presumptively abnormal tissue(s).

00502   other oral pathology procedures, by report

See 00501.

00999   unspecified diagnostic procedure, by report

Used for procedure which is not adequately described by a code. Describe procedure fully—what was done, and why.

Dental Prophylaxis

01110 **prophylaxis-adult**

Refers to a routine dental prophylaxis performed on transitional dentition or permanent dentition. Includes scaling and polishing procedure performed on dental patients in normal or good periodontal health to remove coronal plaque, calculus and stains. Since pockets are absent in a completely normal periodontium, scaling and polishing are performed on the anatomic or clinical crowns and into very shallow, healthy sulci. Some patients may require more than one appointment or one extended appointment to complete a prophylaxis; you may report for each appointment, but document need for additional time fully. "04345-Scaling performed in the presence of gingival inflammation" should not be reported with an adult prophylaxis at the same visit.

01120 **prophylaxis-child**

Refers to a routine dental prophylaxis performed on primary or transitional dentition only.

Topical Fluoride Treatment (Office Procedure)

Fluoride must be applied separately from prophylaxis paste.

01201 **topical application of fluoride (including prophylaxis)—child**

Used to report combined procedures of prophylaxis and fluoride treatment.

01203 **topical application of fluoride (excluding prophylaxis)—child**

This code is used when reporting prophylaxis and fluoride procedures separately.

01204 **topical application of fluoride (excluding prophylaxis)—adult**

This code is used when reporting prophylaxis and fluoride procedures separately.

01205 **topical application of fluoride (including prophylaxis)—adult**

This code is used to report combined procedures of prophylaxis and fluoride treatment.

Other Preventive Services

▲ **01310** **nutritional counseling for control of dental disease**

Counseling on food selection and dietary habits can be a significant part of treatment and control of periodontal disease and caries.

01330 **oral hygiene instructions**

Requires documentation of the type of instructions, number of appointments and content of instructions.

01351 **sealant—per tooth**

Application of pit and fissure sealant has been recognized by the ADA as an effective means of caries prevention since May, 1983.

Space Maintenance (Passive Appliances)

"Passive" means there is no tooth movement.

01510 **space maintainer—fixed—unilateral**
01515 **space maintainer—fixed—bilateral**
01520 **space maintainer—removable—unilateral**
01525 **space maintainer—removable—bilateral**
01550 **recementation of space maintainer**

02000-02999
III. RESTORATIVE*

A one- surface posterior restoration is one in which the restoration involves only one of the five surface classifications (mesial, distal, occlusal, lingual, or buccal).

A two-surface posterior restoration is one in which the restoration extends to two of the five surface classifications.

A three-surface posterior restoration is one in which the restoration extends to three of the five surface classifications.

A four-or-more surface posterior restoration is one in which the restoration extends to four or more of the five classifications.

A one-surface anterior proximal restoration is one in which neither the lingual nor labial margins of the restoration extends beyond the line angle.

A two-surface anterior proximal restoration is one in which either the lingual or labial margin of the restoration extends beyond the line angle.

A three-surface anterior proximal restoration is one in which both the lingual and labial margins of the restorations extend beyond the line angle.

A four-or-more surface anterior restoration is one in which both the lingual and labial margins extend beyond the line angle and the incisal angle is involved.

Amalgam Restorations (Including Polishing)
02110 amalgam—one surface, primary*
02120 amalgam—two surfaces, primary*
02130 amalgam—three surfaces, primary*
▲ 02131 amalgam—four or more surfaces, primary*
02140 amalgam—one surface, permanent*
02150 amalgam—two surfaces, permanent*
02160 amalgam—three surfaces, permanent*
02161 amalgam—four or more surfaces, permanent*

Silicate Restorations
02210 silicate cement—per restoration

Resin Restorations
Resin refers to a broad category of materials including but not limited to composites. May also be called *bonded composite, light-cured composite* or *acid etched composite.* There is no separate code for light curing or acid etching—include as part of restoration. Presently also includes glass ionomer restoration with narrative description. Pins should be reported separately (see 02951).
02330 resin—one surface, anterior*
02331 resin—two surfaces, anterior*
02332 resin—three surfaces, anterior*
▲ 02335 resin—four or more surfaces or involving incisal angle (anterior)*
● 02336 composite resin crown, anterior- primary
    Full composite resin coverage of tooth.
02380 resin—one surface, posterior- primary*
    Includes preventive resin restoration with narrative description.
02381 resin—two surfaces, posterior-primary*
▲ 02382 resin—three or more surfaces, posterior-primary*
02385 resin—one surface, posterior-permanent*
    Includes preventive resin restoration with narrative description.
02386 resin—two surfaces, posterior- permanent*
▲ 02387 resin—three or more surfaces, posterior- permanent*

Gold Foil Restorations
02410 gold foil—one surface
02420 gold foil—two surfaces
02430 gold foil—three surfaces

Inlay Restorations

Metallic inlays—no distinction made for type of metal. Describe metal used when reporting.

02510 **inlay—metallic—one surface**
> For onlay, see 02540.

02520 **inlay—metallic—two surfaces**
02530 **inlay—metallic—three surfaces**
02540 **onlay—metallic—per tooth (in addition to inlay)**
> Report with appropriate inlay code.

Porcelain/ceramic inlays presently include either *all* ceramic or porcelain inlays.

02610 **inlay—porcelain/ceramic—one surface**
02620 **inlay—porcelain/ceramic—two surfaces**
02630 **inlay—porcelain/ceramic—three surfaces**
● 02640 **onlay—porcelain/ceramic—per tooth (in addition to inlay)**
> Report with appropriate inlay code.

Composite/resin inlays must be laboratory processed.

● 02650 **inlay—composite/resin—one surface (laboratory processed)**
● 02651 **inlay—composite/resin—two surfaces (laboratory processed)**
● 02652 **inlay—composite/resin—three surfaces (laboratory processed)**
● 02660 **onlay—composite/resin—per tooth (in addition to inlay—laboratory processed)**
> Report with appropriate inlay code.

Crowns—Single Restorations Only

**Classification of metals—the noble metal classification system has been adopted as a more precise method of reporting various alloys used in dentistry. The alloys are defined on the basis of the percentage of noble metal content: high noble—Gold (Au), Palladium (Pd), and or Platinum (Pt) ≥ 60% (with at least 40% Au); noble—Gold (Au), Palladium (Pd), and or Platinum (Pt) ≥ 25%; predominantly base—Gold (Au), Palladium (Pd), and/or Platinum (Pt) < 25%.

02710 **crown—resin (laboratory)**
02720 **crown—resin with high noble metal****
02721 **crown—resin with predominantly base metal****
02722 **crown—resin with noble metal****
02740 **crown—porcelain/ceramic substrate****
> Includes porcelain jacket crowns, as well as ceramic substrate crowns. If latter reported, include narrative.

02750 **crown—porcelain fused to high noble metal****
02751 **crown—porcelain fused to predominantly base metal****
02752 **crown—porcelain fused to noble metal****
02790 **crown—full cast high noble metal****
02791 **crown—full cast predominantly base metal****
02792 **crown—full cast noble metal****
02810 **crown—¾ cast metallic**
> No distinction made for type of metal. Describe metal used when reporting.

Other Restorative Services

02910 **recement inlay**
02920 **recement crown**
02930 **prefabricated stainless steel crown—primary tooth**
02931 **prefabricated stainless steel crown—permanent tooth**
02932 **prefabricated resin crown**
● 02933 **prefabricated stainless steel crown with resin window**
> Open-face stainless steel crown with esthetic resin facing.

02940 **sedative filling**
> Temporary restoration intended to sedate pulp.

▲ 02950   **core buildup, including any pins**
Refers to building up of anatomical crown when restorative crown will be placed, whether or not pins are used.

02951   **pin retention—per tooth, in addition to restoration**
Specify number of pins.

02952   **cast post and core in addition to crown**
Cast post and core is separate from crown.

02954   **prefabricated post and core in addition to crown**
Core is not prefabricated but is built up around a prefabricated post.

02960   **labial veneer (laminate)—chairside**
Includes bonded veneer with narrative.

02961   **labial veneer (porcelain laminate)—laboratory**
Note if done as repair (rather than esthetic) procedure.

02970   **temporary crown (fractured tooth)**
A preformed artificial crown, usually made of stainless steel or resin, which is fitted over a damaged tooth as an immediate protective device in tooth injury.

02980   **crown repair, by report**
Includes removal of crown, if necessary. Describe procedure fully—what was done and why (i.e. materials, time, difficulty).

02999   **unspecified restorative procedure, by report**
Use for procedure which is not adequately described by a code. Describe procedure fully—what was done, and why.

Pulp Capping

03110   **pulp cap—direct (excluding final restoration)**
Procedure in which the exposed pulp is covered with a dressing or cement that protects the pulp and promotes healing and repair. American Dental Association sets no standard for appropriate time to place direct and indirect pulp caps (i.e., same day as restoration or different day.)

03120   **pulp cap—indirect (excluding final restoration)**
Procedure in which the nearly exposed pulp is covered with a protective dressing to protect the pulp from additional injury and to promote healing and repair via formation of secondary dentin. Should not be reported unless all caries are eventually removed.

Pulpotomy

03220   **therapeutic pulpotomy (excluding final restoration)**
Performed on primary or permanent teeth.

Root Canal Therapy (Including Treatment Plan, Clinical Procedures, and Follow-Up Care)
Note: includes primary and permanent teeth.

▲ 03310   **anterior (excluding final restoration)**
Complete root canal therapy in an anterior tooth. Pulpectomy is part of root canal therapy. Includes all appointments necessary to complete treatment; also includes intraoperative radiographs. Does not include diagnostic examination—see 00110-00120.

▲ 03320   **bicuspid (excluding final restoration)**
See 03310. Complete root canal therapy in a bicuspid tooth.

▲ 03330   **molar (excluding final restoration)**
See 03310. Complete root canal therapy in a molar tooth.

● 03346   **retreatment—anterior, by report**
This procedure may include the removal of a post, pin(s), old root canal filling material, and the procedures necessary to prepare and place the new material. This includes complete root canal therapy. See also 03310.

● 03347   **retreatment—bicuspid, by report**
                    See 03310 and 03346.

● 03348   **retreatment—molar, by report**
                    See 03346.

▲ 03351   **apexification/recalcification—initial visit (apical closure/calcific repair of perforations, root resorption, etc.)**
                    Includes opening tooth, pulpectomy, preparation of canal spaces, first place-ment of medication and necessary radiographs. (This procedure includes first phase of complete root canal therapy.)

▲ 03352   **apexification/recalcification—interim medication replacement (apical clo-sure/calcific repair of perforations, root resorption, etc.)**
                    For visits in which the intracanal medication is replaced with new medication and necessary radiographs. There may be several of these visits.

▲ 03353   **apexification/recalcification—final visit (includes completed root canal ther-apy—apical closure/calcific repair of perforations, root resorption, etc.)**
                    Includes removal of intracanal medication and procedures necessary to place final root canal filling material including necessary radiographs. (This proce-dure includes last phase of complete root canal therapy.)

Apicoectomy/Periradicular Services

Periradicular surgery is a term used to describe surgery to the root surface (i.e. apicoectomy, repair of a root perforation or resorptive defect, exploratory curettage to look for root fractures, removal of extruded filling materials or instruments, removal of broken root fragments, sealing of accessory canals). This does not include retrograde fill-ing material placement.

▲ 03410   **apicoectomy/periradicular surgery*—anterior**
                    For surgery on root of anterior tooth. Does not include placement of retrograde filling material.

● 03421   **apicoectomy/periradicular surgery*—bicuspid (first root)**
                    For surgery on one root of a bicuspid. If more than one root is treated, see 03426.

● 03425   **apicoectomy/periradicular surgery—molar (first root)**
                    For surgery on one root of a molar tooth. See 03426 if more than one root is treated.

▲ 03426   **apicoectomy/periradicular surgery (each additional root)**
                    Typically used for bicuspids and molar surgeries when more than one root is treated during the same procedure. This does not include retrograde filling ma-terial placement.

03430   **retrograde filling—per root**
                    For placement of retrograde filling material during periradicular surgery proce-dures. If more than one filling placed in one root, report as 03999 and de-scribe.

03450   **root amputation—per root**
                    Removal of a root of a multirooted tooth. Often it is necessary to remove (am-putate) a root from a multirooted tooth to retain the remaining portion of the tooth without extensive damage to the remaining structure. See 03920.

03460   **endodontic endosseous implant**
                    Placement of implant material that extends from a pulpal space into the bone beyond the end of the root.

● 03470   **intentional replantation (including necessary splinting)**
                    For the intentional removal, inspection, and treatment of the root and replace-ment of a tooth into its own socket. This does not include necessary retrograde filling material placement.

Other Endodontic Procedures
03910   **surgical procedure for isolation of tooth with rubber dam**

03920 **hemisection (including any root removal), not including root canal therapy**
Includes separation of a multirooted tooth into separate sections containing the root and the overlying portion of the crown. It may also include the removal of one or more of those sections.

03950 **canal preparation and fitting of preformed dowel or post**
Same practitioner should not report 03950 in conjunction with 02952 or 02954.

03960 **bleaching of discolored tooth**
Specify whether tooth is vital or nonvital; report per treatment visit; includes microabrasion.

03999 **unspecified endodontic procedure, by report**
Used for procedure which is not adequately described by a code. Describe procedure fully—what was done and why.

Periodontal Case Types

The following are the American Academy of Periodontology's definitions of periodontal case types used for diagnostic identification. Please note that there are no ADA numeric codes associated with these case types, as the ADA's *Code on Dental Procedures and Nomenclature* is intended to classify treatment, not diagnoses.

Case type I *Gingivitis.* Inflammation of the gingiva characterized clinically by changes in color, gingival form, position, surface appearance, and presence of bleeding, and/or exudate.

Case type II *Slight periodonitis.* Progression of the gingival inflammation into the deeper periodontal structures and alveolar bone crest, with slight bone loss. The usual periodontal probing depth is 3 to 4 mm with slight loss of connective tissue attachment and slight loss of alveolar bone.

Case type III **Moderate periodontitis.** A more advanced stage of the above condition with increased destruction of the periodontal structures and noticeable loss of bone support, possibly accompanied by an increase in tooth mobility. There may be furcation involvement in multirooted teeth.

Case type IV **Advanced periodontitis.** Further progression of periodontitis with major loss of alveolar bone support usually accompanied by increased tooth mobility. Furcation involvement in multirooted teeth is likely.

Case type V **Refractory progressive periodontitis.** This category includes patients with multiple disease sites that continue to demonstrate attachment loss after apparently appropriate therapy. These sites presumably continue to be infected by periodontal pathogens no matter how thorough or frequent the therapy is provided. It also includes patients with recurrent disease at a few or many sites.

04000-04999
V. PERIODONTICS

Surgical services (including usual postoperative care)

04210 **gingivectomy or gingivoplasty—per quadrant**
Involves the excision of the soft tissue wall of the periodontal pocket which may be accomplished by an external or an internal bevel. They are performed in shallow to moderate suprabony pockets after adequate initial preparation, for suprabony pockets that need access for restorative dentistry, when moderate gingival enlargements or aberration are present, and when there is asymmetrical or unesthetic gingival topography.

04211 **gingivectomy or gingivoplasty, per tooth**
See 04210.

▲ 04220 **gingival curettage, surgical, per quadrant, by report**

The surgical procedure of debriding the soft tissue wall of the periodontal pocket by means of curette. Root instrumentation is routinely accomplished with the procedure, which usually is performed under local anesthesia. Gingival curettage often is appropriate in the treatment of compromised patients, debridement of localized sites of recalcitrant periodontitis, treatment of juvenile periodontitis, treatment of other types of periodontitis, and when esthetics is of concern. Report should include diagnosis, treatment needs, and teeth to be treated.

04240 **gingival flap procedure, including root planing—per quadrant**

Surgical debridement of the root surface and the removal of granulation tissue after the resection of soft tissue flap. Osseous recontouring is not accomplished with this procedure. Aesthetic modifications of this approach have been reported under the title of open flap curettage, reverse bevel flap surgery, modified Kirkland flap procedure, Widman surgery, and modified Widman surgery. This procedure is performed in the presence of moderate to deep probing depths, loss of probing attachment, need to maintain esthetics, and need for increased access to the root surface and alveolar bone. It heals with a long junctional epithelium (repair).

● 04249 **crown lengthening—hard and soft tissue, by report**

Often, the crown of a tooth is lost through trauma or decay, leaving little or no sound tooth structure exposed to the oral cavity. It is impossible to carry out restorative dental procedures in these cases without impinging on the biologic width of the gingiva or the alveolar bone itself. Sound tooth structure must be exposed by removal and contouring of healthy supporting alveolar bone and/or gingival tissue so that other dental procedures can be carried out. It is performed in a healthy periodontal environment as opposed to osseous surgery, which is performed in the presence of periodontal disease.

● 04250 **mucogingival surgery—per quadrant**

Plastic surgical procedure designed to correct defects in the morphology, position, and/or amount of gingiva surrounding the teeth. This procedure is designed to maintain and/or enhance the dental gingival junction because defects in the morphology of the gingival and alveolar mucosa can cause periodontal disease, accelerate its course, or interfere with the successful outcome of periodontal treatment.

04260 **osseous surgery (including flap entry and closure)—per quadrant**

This procedure modifies the bony support of the teeth by reshaping of the alveolar process to achieve a more physiologic form without the removal of the alveolar (supporting bone) (osteoplasty) or by the removal of some alveolar bone, thus changing the position of crestal bone on the tooth root (ostectomy). It is a common requirement in effective treatment of the more involved periodontal lesions. In some instances, the bony support of the tooth assumes an unusual configuration as a result of the even progression of the disease. When this occurs, modification of the altered bone support may be indicated.

▲ 04261 **bone replacement graft—single site (including flap entry and closure)**

May involve the use of osseous autografts, osseous allografts, and nonosseous grafts to stimulate bone formation or periodontal regeneration when the disease process has led to deformity of the bone. Healing may occur by repair, regeneration, reattachment, or new attachment. Identify specific site and type of material used for graft.

▲ 04262 **bone replacement graft—multiple sites (including flap entry and closure)**

See 04261.

● 04268 **guided tissue regeneration (includes the surgery and re-entry)**

This procedure is used to regenerate lost or injured periodontal tissue through differential tissue responses. A membrane is placed over the root surface of surgically exposed and debrided areas. The mucoperiosteal flaps are then adapted over the membrane and sutured. The membrane excludes epithelium and gingival connective tissue from the healing wound, thus allowing the area to be repopulated with cells originating from the periodontal ligament. A new periodontal ligament-cementum complex is formed, varying in extent from complete coverage to formation of only a limited amount of new cementum. New alveolar bone also may be formed. Use of this procedure may be complicated by the need for a second surgical procedure to remove the membrane and/or to correct the gingival contours. A similar procedure is used when placing an endosseous implant into an immediate extraction site or an area with inadequate buccal-lingual bone width.

04270   pedicle soft tissue graft procedure

A pedicle flap of gingiva can be raised from an edentulous ridge, from the adjacent teeth, or from the existing gingiva on the tooth and moved laterally or coronally to become marginal tissue when the tooth has alveolar mucosa as marginal tissue. Such a pedicle flap also can be used to cover an exposed root or to eliminate a gingival defect if the root is not too prominent in the arch. Identify tooth/teeth involved and donor site.

04271   free soft tissue graft procedure (including donor site)

This graft is used to create or augment the gingiva and may be accomplished with or without root coverage. It also eliminates the pull of frena and muscle attachments to extend the vestibular fornix and to correct localized gingival recession. Gingiva or masticatory mucosa are suitable for grafting, and the hard palate is usually the source of donor material. Identify specific tooth (teeth) for graft and donor site.

Adjunctive Periodontal Service

04320   provisional splinting—intracoronal

This is a temporary (interim) stabilization of mobile teeth. A variety of methods and appliances may be used for this purpose. Identify the teeth involved and the nature of the splint, by report.

04321   provisional splinting—extracoronal

This is a temporary (interim) stabilization of mobile teeth. A variety of methods and appliances may be used for this purpose. Identify the teeth involved and the nature of the splint, by report.

04341   periodontal scaling and root planing, per quadrant

Periodontal scaling is a treatment procedure involving instrumentation of the crown and root surfaces of the teeth to remove plaque, calculus, and stains from these surfaces. It is performed on patients with periodontal disease and is therapeutic, not prophylactic in nature. Periodontal scaling precedes root planing, which is a definitive, meticulous treatment procedure designed to remove cementum and/or dentin that is rough, and may be permeated by calculus, or contaminated with toxins or microorganisms. When done in a thorough fashion, some unavoidable soft tissue removal occurs. This procedure is used as a definitive treatment in some stages of periodontal disease and is part of presurgical procedures in others. Debriding the root surface is a critical element in establishing periodontal health. Periodontal scaling and root planing are arduous and time consuming. They may need to be repeated and may require local anesthetic.

04345   periodontal scaling performed in presence of gingival inflammation

Gingivitis can be characterized clinically by marked changes in color, gingival form, position, surface appearance, presence of bleeding, and/or exudate. With no loss of attachment or bone loss in gingivitis, this scaling treatment procedure is more precise in describing therapy for generalized gingivitis and is not meant to be performed on a routine basis. On completion of treatment the gingival tissues should be normal and can be maintained by adult prophylaxis on a regular basis. This is a scaling-only procedure; it may require single or multiple visits. Should not be reported in conjunction with an adult prophylaxis; for reporting periodontal scaling performed with root planing, see 04341.

Other Periodontal Services

04910   periodontal maintenance procedures (following active therapy)

Successful periodontal therapy with regular periodic maintenance care can sustain periodontal health and reduce tooth loss. After active periodontal treatment, an interval is established for periodic ongoing care. This is under the supervision of the dentist and includes an update of the medical and dental histories, radiographic review, extraoral and intraoral soft tissue examination, dental examination, periodontal evaluation, removal of the bacterial flora from crevicular and pocket areas, scaling and root planing where indicated, polishing of the teeth, and a review of the patient's plaque control efficiency. An interval of 3 months between appointments appears to be an effective treatment schedule, but this can vary depending on the clinical judgment of the dentist. When new or recurring periodontal disease appears, additional diagnostic and treatment procedures must be considered. The successful long-term control of periodontal disease depends on active maintenance care through supportive periodontal treatment. Active periodontal therapy may consist of surgical, nonsurgical services, or both. Periodic maintenance treatment after active therapy is not synonymous with a prophylaxis.

04920   unscheduled dressing change (by someone other than treating dentist)

Must be dentist other than dentist of record or can be appropriately licensed dental auxiliary.

04999   unspecified periodontal procedure, by report

Use for procedure not adequately described by a code. Describe procedure fully—what was done and why.

05000- 05899
VI. PROSTHODONTICS
(REMOVABLE)

Complete Dentures (Including Routine Postdelivery Care)

If denture is metal- based, use this code for the denture itself and include a narrative description (by report) to describe the type of metal used.

05110   complete upper

05120   complete lower

05130   immediate upper

Includes limited follow-up care only; does not include required future rebasing/relining procedure(s) or a complete new denture.

05140   immediate lower

See 05130.

Partial Dentures (Including Routine Postdelivery Care)

▲ **05211   upper partial—resin base (including any conventional clasps, rests and teeth)**

All partials include major connectors and framework. Note specific number of clasps and rests. No code number for immediate partial dentures. For precision partial dentures, report precision attachments with code 05862 by report. Partial dentures for pediatric use are also included in this category.

▲ **05212   lower partial—resin base (including any conventional clasps, rests and teeth)**

Includes acrylic resin base denture with acrylic resin clasps. See 05211.

▲ 05213   upper partial—cast metal base with resin saddles (including any conventional clasps, rests and teeth)
    Cast metal base alloys have less than 60% Au, Pd, or Pt content. See 05211.

▲ 05214   lower partial—cast metal base with resin saddles (including any conventional clasps, rests and teeth)
    See 05213.

▲ 05281   removable unilateral partial denture—one-piece cast metal (including clasps and pontics)

Adjustments to Dentures

05410   adjust complete denture—upper
05411   adjust complete denture—lower
05421   adjust partial denture—upper
05422   adjust partial denture—lower

Repairs to Complete Dentures

Note: Include a description of what was done.

05510   repair broken complete denture base
05520   replace missing or broken teeth (complete denture)—each tooth

Repairs to Partial Dentures

▲ 05610   repair resin saddle or base
05620   repair cast framework
05630   repair or replace broken clasp
05640   replace broken teeth—per tooth
05650   add tooth to existing partial denture
05660   add clasp to existing partial denture

Denture Rebase Procedures

Rebase—process of refitting a denture by replacing the base material.

05710   rebase complete upper denture
05711   rebase complete lower denture
05720   rebase upper partial denture
05721   rebase lower partial denture

Denture Reline Procedures

Reline—process of resurfacing the tissue side of a denture with new base material

05730   reline complete upper denture (chairside)
05731   reline complete lower denture (chairside)
05740   reline upper partial denture (chairside)
05741   reline lower partial denture (chairside)
05750   reline complete upper denture (laboratory)
05751   reline complete lower denture (laboratory)
05760   reline upper partial denture (laboratory)
05761   reline lower partial denture (laboratory)

Other Removable Prosthetic Services

A provisional prosthesis designed for use over a limited time, after which it is to be replaced by a more definitive restoration.

▲ 05810   interim complete denture (upper)
▲ 05811   interim complete denture (lower)
▲ 05820   interim partial denture (upper)
    Includes any necessary clasps and rests.
▲ 05821   interim partial denture (lower)
▲ 05850   tissue conditioning, upper—per denture unit
● 05851   tissue conditioning, lower—per denture unit

05860   **overdenture—complete, by report**

Includes overdenture and associated components. Describe procedures performed by reporting the materials used (i.e., precision attachments, copings).

05861   **overdenture—partial, by report**

Includes overdenture and associated components. Describe procedures performed by reporting the materials used (i.e., precision attachments, copings).

05862   **precision attachment, by report**

Each set of male and female components should be reported as one precision attachment. Describe the type of attachment used.

05899   **unspecified removable prosthodontic procedure, by report**

Use for a procedure not adequately described by a code. Describe procedure fully—what was done and why (i.e., materials, complications, etc).

**05900-05999
VII. MAXILLOFACIAL
PROSTHETICS**

05911   **facial moulage (sectional)**

A sectional facial moulage impression is a procedure used to record the soft tissue contours of a portion of the face.

Occasionally several separate sectional impressions are made and then reassembled to provide a full facial contour cast.

05912   **facial moulage (complete)**

Synonymous terminology: facial impression, face mask impression. A complete facial moulage impression is a procedure used to record the soft tissue contours of the whole face.

The impression is used to create a facial moulage and generally is not reusable.

05913   **nasal prosthesis**

Synonymous terminology: artificial nose.

A removable prosthesis attached to the skin that artificially restores part or all of the nose.

Fabrication of a nasal prosthesis requires creation of an original mold. Additional prostheses usually can be made from the same mold, and assuming no further tissue changes occur, the same mold can be used for extended periods. When a new prosthesis is made from the existing mold, this procedure is termed a *nasal prosthesis replacement*.

05914   **auricular prosthesis**

Synonymous terminology: artificial ear, ear prosthesis.

A removable prosthesis that artificially restores part or all of the natural ear.

Usually, replacement prostheses can be made from the original mold if tissue bed changes have not occurred. Creation of an auricular prosthesis requires fabrication of a mold, from which additional prostheses usually can be made, as needed later (auricular prosthesis, replacement).

05915   **orbital prosthesis**

A prosthesis that artificially restores the eye, eyelids, and adjacent hard and soft tissue lost as a result of trauma or surgery.

Fabrication of an orbital prosthesis requires creation of an original mold. Additional prostheses usually can be made from the same mold, and assuming no further tissue changes occur, the same mold can be used for extended periods. When a new prosthesis is made from the existing mold, this procedure is termed an *orbital prosthesis replacement*.

05916   **ocular prosthesis**

Synonymous terminology: artificial eye, glass eye.

A prosthesis that artificially replaces an eye missing as a result of trauma, surgery, or congenital absence. The prosthesis does not replace missing eyelids or adjacent skin, mucosa, or muscle.

Ocular prostheses require semiannual or annual cleaning and polishing. Also, occasional revisions to re-adapt the prosthesis to the tissue bed may be necessary. Glass eyes are rarely made and cannot be re-adapted.

▲ 05919 **facial prosthesis**
Synonymous terminology: prosthetic dressing.
    A removable prosthesis that artificially replaces a portion of the face lost because of surgery, trauma, or congenital absence.
    Flexion of natural tissues may preclude adaptation and movement of the prosthesis to match the adjacent skin. Salivary leakage, when communicating with the oral cavity, adversely affects retention.

● 05922 **nasal septal prosthesis**
Synonymous terminology: Septal plug, septal button.
    Removable prosthesis to occlude (obturate) a hole within the nasal septal wall. Adverse chemical degradation in this moist environment may require frequent replacement. Silicone prostheses are occasionally subject to fungal invasion.

● 05923 **ocular prosthesis, interim**
Synonymous terminology: Eye shell, shell, ocular conformer, conformer.
    A temporary replacement generally made of clear acrylic resin for an eye lost resulting from surgery or trauma. No attempt is made to reestablish esthetics. Fabrication of an interim ocular prosthesis generally implies subsequent fabrication of an esthetic ocular prosthesis.

● 05924 **cranial prosthesis**
Synonymous terminology: Skull plate, cranioplasty prosthesis, cranial implant.
    A biocompatible, permanently implanted replacement of a portion of the skull bones; an artificial replacement for a portion of the skull bone.

● 05925 **facial augmentation implant prosthesis**
Synonymous terminology: facial implant.
    An implantable biocompatible material generally onlayed on an existing bony area beneath the skin tissues to fill in or selectively raise portions of the overlaying facial skin tissues to create acceptable contours.
    Although some forms of premade surgical implants are commercially available, the facial augmentation is usually custom made for surgical implantation for each individual because of the irregular or extensive nature of the facial deficit.

● 05926 **nasal prosthesis, replacement**
Synonymous terminology: replacement nose.
    An artificial nose produced from a previously made mold.
    A replacement prosthesis does not require fabrication of a new mold. Generally, several prostheses can be made from the same mold assuming that no changes occur in the tissue bed resulting from surgery or age-related topographical variations.

● 05927 **auricular prosthesis, replacement**
Synonymous terminology: replacement ear.
    An artificial ear produced from a previously made mold.
    A replacement prosthesis does not require fabrication of a new mold. Generally, several prostheses can be made from the same mold assuming that no changes occur in the tissue bed resulting from surgery or age-related topographical variations.

● 05928 **orbital prosthesis, replacement**
    A replacement for a previously made orbital prosthesis.
    A replacement prosthesis does not require fabrication of a new mold. Generally, several prostheses can be made from the same mold assuming that no changes occur in the tissue bed resulting from surgery or age-related topographical variations

● 05929 **facial prosthesis, replacement**
    A replacement facial prosthesis made from the original mold.
    A replacement prosthesis does not require fabrication of a new mold. Generally, several prostheses can be made from the same mold assuming that no changes occur in the tissue bed resulting from further surgery or age-related topographical variations.

▲ 05931   **obturator prosthesis, surgical**
Synonymous terminology: Obturator, surgical stayplate, immediate temporary obturator.

A temporary prosthesis inserted during or immediately after surgical or traumatic loss of a portion or all of one or both maxillary bones and contiguous alveolar structures (i.e., gingival tissue, teeth).

Frequent revisions of surgical obturators are necessary during the ensuing healing phase (approximately 6 months). Some dentists prefer to replace many or all teeth removed by the surgical procedure in the surgical obturator, whereas others do not replace any teeth. Further surgical revisions may require fabrication of another surgical obturator (i.e., an initially planned small defect may be revised and greatly enlarged after the final pathologic report indicates that margins are not free of tumor).

▲ 05932   **obturator prosthesis, definitive**
Synonymous terminology: obturator.

A prosthesis that artificially replaces part or all of the maxilla and associated teeth lost resulting from surgery or trauma.

A definitive obturator is made when it is deemed that further tissue changes or recurrence of tumor are unlikely and a more permanent prosthetic rehabilitation can be achieved; it is intended for long-term use.

▲ 05933   **obturator prosthesis, modification**
Synonymous terminology: adjustment, denture adjustment, temporary or office reline.

Revision or alteration of an existing obturator (surgical o., interim o., or definitive o.); possible modifications include relief of the denture base resulting from tissue compression, augmentation of the seal, or peripheral areas to affect adequate sealing or separation between the nasal and oral cavities.

▲ 05934   **mandibular resection prosthesis with guide flange**
Synonymous terminology: resection device, resection appliance.

A prosthesis that guides the remaining portion of the mandible, left after a partial resection, into a more normal relationship with the maxilla. This allows for some tooth-to-tooth or an improved tooth contact. It may also artificially replace missing teeth and thereby increase masticatory efficiency.

▲ 05935   **mandibular resection prosthesis without guide flange**
A prosthesis that helps guide the partially resected mandible to a more normal relation with the maxilla allowing tooth or increased tooth contact. It does not have a flange or ramp, however, to assist in directional closure. It may replace missing teeth and thereby increase masticatory efficiency.

Dentists who treat mandibulectomy patients may prefer to replace some, all, or none of the teeth in the defect area. Frequently, the defect's margins preclude even partial replacement. Use of a guide (a mandibular resection prosthesis with a guide flange) may not be possible because of anatomical limitations or poor patient tolerance. Ramps, extended occlusal arrangements, and irregular occlusal positioning relative to the denture foundation frequently preclude stability of the prostheses, and thus some prostheses are poorly tolerated under such adverse circumstances.

● 05936   **obturator prosthesis, interim**
Synonymous terminology: immediate postoperative obturator.

A prosthesis made after completion of the initial healing after a surgical resection of a portion or all of one or both the maxillae; frequently many or all teeth in the defect area are replaced by this prosthesis. This prosthesis replaces the surgical obturator, which is usually inserted at or immediately after the resection.

Generally, an interim obturator is made to facilitate closure of the resultant defect after initial healing has been completed. Unlike the surgical obturator, which usually is made before surgery and frequently revised in the operating room during surgery, the interim obturator is made when the defect margins are clearly defined and further surgical revisions are not planned. It is a provisional prosthesis that may replace some or all lost teeth and other lost bone and soft tissue structures. Also, it frequently must be revised (termed an *obturator prosthesis modification*) during subsequent dental procedures (i.e., restorations, gingival surgery, etc.), as well as to compensate for further tissue shrinkage before a definitive obturator prosthesis is made.

● 05937 **trismus appliance (not for TMD treatment)**
Synonymous terminology: occlusal device for mandibular trismus dynamic bite opener.

A prosthesis that assists the patient in increasing the oral aperture width to eat and maintain oral hygiene.

Several versions and designs are possible, all intending to ease the severe lack of oral opening experienced by many patients immediately after extensive intraoral surgical procedures. Occasionally helpful in patients suffering from lye burns.

05951 **feeding aid**
Synonymous terminology: feeding prosthesis.

A prosthesis that maintains the right and left maxillary segments of an infant cleft palate patient in their proper orientation until surgery is performed to repair the cleft. It closes the oral-nasal cavity defect, thus enhancing sucking and swallowing.

Used on an interim basis, this prosthesis achieves separation of the oral and nasal cavities in infants born with wide clefts necessitating delayed closure. It is eliminated if surgical closure can be affected or, alternatively, with eruption of the deciduous dentition, a pediatric speech aid may be made to facilitate closure of the defect.

▲ 05952 **speech aid prosthesis, pediatric**
Synonymous terminology: nasopharyngeal obturator, speech appliance, obturator, cleft palate appliance, prosthetic speech aid, speech bulb.

A temporary or interim prosthesis used to close a defect in the hard and/or soft palate. It may replace tissue lost because of developmental or surgical alterations. It is necessary for the production of intelligible speech.

Normal lateral growth of the palatal bones necessitates occasional replacement of this prosthesis. Intermittent revisions of the obturator section can assist in the maintenance of palatalpharyngeal closure (termed a *speech aid prosthesis modification*). Frequently, such prostheses are not fabricated before the deciduous dentition is fully erupted because clasp retention is often essential.

▲ 05953 **speech aid prosthesis, adult**
Synonymous terminology: prosthetic speech appliance, speech aid, speech bulb.

A definitive prosthesis that can improve speech in adult cleft palate patients by obturating (sealing off) a palatal cleft or fistula or occasionally by assisting an incompetent soft palate. Both mechanisms are necessary to achieve velopharyngeal competency. Generally, this prosthesis is fabricated when no further growth is anticipated and the objective is to achieve long-term use; hence, more precise materials and techniques are used. Occasionally, such procedures are accomplished with precision attachments in crown work undertaken on some or all maxillary teeth to achieve improved esthetics.

▲ 05954 **palatal augmentation prosthesis**
Synonymous terminology: Superimposed prosthesis, maxillary glossectomy prosthesis, maxillary speech prosthesis, palatal drop prosthesis.

A removable prosthesis that alters the hard and/or soft palate's topographical form adjacent to the tongue.

▲ 05955 **palatal lift prosthesis, definitive**
A prosthesis that elevates the soft palate superiorly and aids in restoration of soft palate functions, which may be lost resulting from an acquired, congenital, or developmental defect.

A definitive palatal lift is usually made for patients whose experience with diagnostic palatal lifts has been successful, especially if surgical alterations are deemed unwarranted.

● 05958   **palatal lift prosthesis, interim**

Synonymous terminology: diagnostic palatal lift.

A prosthesis that elevates and assists in restoring soft palate function, which may be lost resulting from clefting, surgery, trauma, or unknown paralysis. It is intended for interim use to determine its usefulness in achieving palatalpharyngeal competency or enhancing swallowing reflexes.

This prosthesis is intended for interim use as a diagnostic aid to assess the level of possible improvement in speech intelligibility. Some clinicians believe use of a palatal lift on an interim basis may stimulate an otherwise flaccid soft palate to increase functional activity, subsequently lessening its need.

● 05959   **palatal lift prosthesis, modification**

Synonymous terminology: revision of lift, adjustment.

Alterations in the adaptation, contour, form or function of an existing palatal lift necessitated because of tissue impingement, lack of function, poor clasp adaptation, or the like.

● 05960   **speech aid prosthesis, modification**

Synonymous terminology: adjustment, repair, revision.

Revision of a pediatric or adult speech aid not necessitating its replacement.

Frequently, revisions of the obturating section of any speech aid is required to facilitate enhanced speech intelligibility. Such revisions or repairs do not require complete remaking of the prosthesis, thus extending its longevity.

05982   **surgical stent**

Synonymous terminology: periodontal stent, skin graft stent, columellar stent.

Named for the dentist who first described their use, stents are used to apply pressure to soft tissues to facilitate healing and prevent cicatrization or collapse.

A surgical stent may be required in surgical and postsurgical revisions to achieve close approximation of tissues. Usually, such materials as temporary or interim soft denture lines, gutta percha, or dental modeling impression compound may be used.

05983   **radiation carrier**

Synonymous terminology: radiotherapy prosthesis, carrier prosthesis, radiation applicator, radium carrier, intracavity carrier, intracavity applicator.

A device used to administer radiation to confined areas by means of capsules, beads, or needles of radiation-emitting materials such as radium or cesium. Its function is to hold the radiation source securely in the same location during the entire period of treatment.

Radiation oncologists occasionally request these devices to achieve close approximation and controlled application of radiation to a tumor deemed amiable to eradication.

05984   **radiation shield**

Synonymous terminology: radiation stent, tongue protector, lead shield.

An intraoral prosthesis designed to shield adjacent tissues from radiation during orthovoltage treatment of malignant lesions of the head and neck region.

▲ 05985   **radiation cone locator**

Synonymous terminology: docking device, cone locator.

A prosthesis used to direct and reduplicate the path of radiation to an oral tumor during a split course of irradiation.

▲ 05986   **fluoride gel carrier**

Synonymous terminology: fluoride applicator.

A prosthesis that covers the teeth in either dental arch and is used to apply topical fluoride in close proximity to tooth enamel and dentin for several minutes daily.

Generally considered essential for all patients with any natural dentition who undergo oral radiation therapy to assist in prevention of extensive secondary dental decay.

● **05987   commissure splint**

Synonymous terminology: lip splint.

A device placed between the lips which assists in achieving increased opening between the lips.

Use of such devices enhances opening where surgical, chemical or electrical alterations of the lips has resulted in severe restriction or contractures.

● **05988   surgical splint**

Synonymous terminology: Gunning splint, modified Gunning splint, labiolingual splint, fenestrated splint, Kingsley splint, cast metal splint.

Splints are designed to use existing teeth and/or alveolar processes as points of anchorage to assist in stabilization and immobilization of broken bones during healing. They are used to re-establish, as much as possible, normal occlusal relationships, during immobilization. Frequently, existing prostheses (i.e., complete dentures) can be modified to serve as surgical splints. Frequently, surgical splints have arch bars added to facilitate intermaxillary fixation. Rubber elastics may be used to assist in this process. Circummandibular eyelet hooks can be used for enhanced stabilization with wiring to adjacent bone.

05999   unspecified maxillofacial prosthesis, by report

Used for procedure not adequately described by a code. Describe procedure fully—what was done and why.

**06000-06199
VIII. IMPLANT
SERVICES**

Report surgical implant procedure using appropriate codes; these presently include fixture exposure and abutment connection. Prosthetic devices should be reported using existing overdenture or fixed prosthodontic codes. If fixed bridgework is performed, the crown over the implant is considered the abutment.

● **06030   endosseous implant (in the bone)**

A biocompatible alloplastic device surgically inserted into alveolar and/or basal bone to furnish support or retention for a dental prosthesis. Previously code 05974.

● **06040   subperiosteal implant**

A framework of a biocompatible material made to fit on the surface of the bone of the mandible or maxilla with permucosal extensions that provide support and attachment of a prosthesis. This may be a complete arch or unilateral appliance. Subperiosteal implants rest on the bone and under the periosteum. Previously code 05973.

● **06050   transosseous implant**

A biocompatible device with threaded posts penetrating the superior and inferior cortical bone plates of the mandibular symphysis and exiting through the permucosa, providing support and attachment for a dental prosthesis. Transosteal implants are placed completely through the bone and into the oral cavity from extraoral or intraoral. Previously code 05976.

● **06055   implant connecting bar**

A device attached to transmucosal abutments to stabilize and anchor a removable overdenture prosthesis.

● **06080   implant maintenance procedures, including removal of prosthesis, cleansing of prosthesis and abutments, reinsertion of prosthesis**

Those procedures necessary to provide periodic maintenance for implants and their prosthodontic components. This procedure includes prophylaxis to provide active debriding of the implant and examination of all aspects of the implant system, including the occlusion and stability of the superstructure. The patient is also instructed in thorough daily cleansing of the implant. Guidance is provided in the selection of the proper oral hygiene aids and their implementation in removal of bacterial masses (plaque) and their toxins, food debris, and foreign matter from the implant.

● **06090   repair implant, by report**

This procedure involves the repair or replacement of any part of the implant system. It may also include periodontal surgical procedures to remove granulation tissue and gain reattachment to the implant device.

● **06100   implant removal, by report**

Failing implants may require surgical removal. It may also necessitate soft or hard tissue grafting. Hard tissue grafting with autogenous or alloplastic materials will correct osseous defects associated with implant failure. Soft tissue grafting is used to repair soft tissue disturbances caused by a failed dental implant.

● **06199   unspecified implant procedure, by report**

Use for procedure not adequately described by a code. Describe procedure fully—what was done and why.

06200-06999 IX. PROSTHODONTICS, FIXED (EACH ABUTMENT AND EACH PONTIC CONSTITUTES A UNIT IN A BRIDGE)

**Classification of Metals—The noble metal classification system has been adopted as a more precise method of reporting various alloys used in dentistry. The alloys are defined on the basis of the percentage of noble metal content: high noble—Gold (Au), Au, Pd, and/or $Pt \geq 60\%$ (with at least 40% Au); noble—Au, Pd, and/or $Pt \geq 25\%$; and predominantly base—Au, Pd, and/or $Pt < 25\%$.

Bridge Pontics

06210   pontic—cast high noble metal**
06211   pontic—cast predominantly base metal**
06212   pontic—cast noble metal**
06240   pontic—porcelain fused to high noble metal**
06241   pontic—porcelain fused to predominantly base metal**
06242   pontic—porcelain fused to noble metal**
06250   pontic—resin with high noble metal**
06251   pontic—resin with predominantly base metal**
06252   pontic—resin with noble metal**

Retainers

06520   inlay—metallic—two surfaces

No distinction made between types of alloy. Describe type of metal used.

06530   inlay—metallic—three or more surfaces

See 06520.

▲ 06540   onlay—metallic—per tooth (in addition to inlay)

See 06520.

▲ 06545   retainer—cast metal for acid etched fixed prosthesis

Report pontics separately with appropriate code from the 06200 series.

Bridge Retainers—Crowns

06720   crown—resin with high noble metal**
06721   crown—resin with predominantly base metal**
06722   crown—resin with noble metal**
06750   crown—porcelain fused to high noble metal**
06751   crown—porcelain fused to predominantly base metal**
06752   crown—porcelain fused to noble metal**
06780   crown—¾ cast high noble metal**
06790   crown—full cast high noble metal**

06791   crown—full cast predominantly base metal**
06792   crown—full cast noble metal**

Other Fixed Prosthetic Services
06930   recement bridge
06940   stress breaker
         A non-rigid connector.
06950   precision attachment
         Report attachment separately from crown; each male and female component
         constitutes one precision attachment. Describe type of attachment used.
06970   cast post and core in addition to bridge retainer
06971   cast post as part of bridge retainer
06972   prefabricated post and core in addition to bridge retainer
● 06973   core build up for retainer, including any pins
● 06975   coping—metal
         A thin covering of the coronal portion of the tooth usually without anatomic
         conformity. It can be used as a definitive restoration or as part of a transfer
         procedure.
06980   bridge repair, by report
06999   unspecified fixed prosthodontic procedure, by report
         Used for procedure not adequately described by a code. Describe procedure
         fully—what was done and why (i.e., materials, complications, etc.).

07000-07999 X. ORAL SURGERY

Extractions (Includes Local Anesthesia and Routine Postoperative Care)
07110   single tooth
07120   each additional tooth
07130   root removal—exposed roots

Surgical Extractions (Including Local Anesthesia and Routine Postoperative Care)
     It is the American Association of Oral and Maxillofacial Surgeons' (AAOMS) position that classification of an impacted tooth may be based on the anatomical relationship of the impacted tooth to bony and soft tissue structures, to another tooth, or to the surgical procedures required for removal.
07210   surgical removal of erupted tooth requiring elevation of mucoperiosteal flap and removal of bone and/or section of tooth
         Includes cutting of gingiva and bone, removal of bone and/or tooth, and closure.
07220   removal of impacted tooth—soft tissue
         Tooth is embedded in soft tissue.
07230   removal of impacted tooth—partially bony
         Crown of tooth is partially covered by bone.
07240   removal of impacted tooth—completely bony
         Crown of tooth is completely covered by bone.
07241   removal of impacted tooth—completely bony, with unusual surgical complications
         Crown of tooth is completely covered by bone. Unusual complications may include but are not limited to nerve involvement and/or tooth location (e.g., maxillary sinus).
07250   surgical removal of residual tooth roots (cutting procedure)

Other Surgical Procedures

07260   oral antral fistula closure
Closing of space between sinus and mouth. Note unusual circumstances with a narrative report.

07270   tooth reimplantation and/or stabilization of accidentally evulsed or displaced tooth and/or alveolus
Includes splinting and/or stabilization.

07271   tooth implantation
Includes splinting and/or stabilization.

07272   tooth transplantation
Includes splinting and/or stabilization.

07280   surgical exposure of impacted or unerupted tooth for orthodontic reasons (including orthodontic attachments)
Occasionally, a tooth fails to erupt because of overlying dense fibrous connective tissue. An incision is made and this tissue is reflected to expose the crown of the tooth. An orthodontic attachment is placed on the crown, allowing activation of an eruptive force.

07281   surgical exposure of impacted or unerupted tooth to aid eruption
The dense fibrous connective tissue overlying an impacted or unerupted tooth is reflected to allow the tooth to erupt unaided into the mouth. Orthodontic appliances may be needed at that time to guide the tooth into its proper position.

07285   biopsy of oral tissue—hard
For surgical removal of specimen only. For surgical oral pathology procedures, See 00502.

07286   biopsy of oral tissue—soft
For surgical oral pathology procedures, See 00501 or 00502.

07290   surgical repositioning of teeth

07291   transseptal fiberotomy
This procedure is used to reduce relapse after orthodontic tooth movement. Because the incisions are within the gingival tissue and the root surface is not touched, this procedure heals by the reunion of connective tissue with the root surface on which viable periodontal tissue is present (reattachment).

Alveoloplasty—Surgical Preparation of Ridge for Dentures

07310   alveoloplasty in conjunction with extractions—per quadrant
Usually in preparation for prostheses; often reported on a quadrant basis.

07320   alveoloplasty not in conjunction with extractions—per quadrant
No extractions—patient is edentulous. See 07310.

Vestibuloplasty

07340   vestibuloplasty-ridge extension (secondary epithelialization)

07350   vestibuloplasty—ridge extension (including soft tissue grafts, muscle re-attachment, revision of soft tissue attachment and management of hypertrophied and hyperplastic tissue)
More complex than 07340.

Surgical Excision of Reactive Inflammatory Lesions (Scar Tissue or Localized Congenital Lesions)

07410   radical excision—lesion diameter up to 1.25 cm
Lesion is about ½′ or smaller.

07420   radical excision—lesion diameter greater than 1.25 cm
Lesion is larger than ½′.

Removal of Tumors, Cysts, and Neoplasms

07430   excision of benign tumor—lesion diameter up to 1.25 cm
Lesion is about ½′ or smaller.

07431 **excision of benign tumor—lesion diameter greater than 1.25 cm**
Lesion is larger than ½'.

07440 **excision of malignant tumor—lesion diameter up to 1.25 cm**
Lesion is about ½' or smaller.

07441 **excision of malignant tumor—lesion diameter greater than 1.25 cm**
Lesion is larger than ½'.

07450 **removal of odontogenic cyst or tumor—lesion diameter up to 1.25 cm**
Lesion is about ½' or smaller.

07451 **removal of odontogenic tumor or cyst—lesion diameter greater than 1.25 cm**
Lesion is larger than ½'.

07460 **removal of nonodontogenic cyst or tumor—lesion diameter up to 1.25 cm**
Lesion is about ½' or smaller.

07461 **removal of nonodontogenic cyst or tumor—lesion diameter greater than 1.25 cm**
Lesion is larger than ½'.

▲ 07465 **destruction of lesion(s) by physical or chemical methods, by report**
Includes destruction of lesion by using chemicals, intense cold, intense light, or electricity.

Excision of Bone Tissue

07470 **removal of exostosis—maxilla or mandible**
Includes removal of tori, tuberosity and other protuberances. The overlying soft tissue is reflected and sufficient bone removed to provide an acceptable tissue contour.

07480 **partial ostectomy (guttering or saucerization)**
May also be known as *osteotomy*.

07490 **radical resection of mandible with bone graft**

Surgical Incision

07510 **incision and drainage of abscess—intraoral soft tissue**
Soft tissue abscess found in the mouth.

07520 **incision and drainage of abscess—extraoral soft tissue**
Soft tissue abscess found outside the mouth.

07530 **removal of foreign body, skin, or subcutaneous areolar tissue**

07540 **removal of reaction- producing foreign bodies—musculoskeletal system**
May include but is not limited to removal of splinters, pieces of wire, etc., from muscle and/or bone.

07550 **sequestrectomy for osteomyelitis**
Removal from healthy bone of loose or sloughed-off dead bone caused by infection or reduced blood supply.

07560 **maxillary sinusotomy for removal of tooth fragment or foreign body**

Treatment of Fractures—Simple

07610 **maxilla—open reduction (teeth immobilized, if present)**
Teeth may be wired, banded, or splinted together to prevent movement.

07620 **maxilla—closed reduction (teeth immobilized, if present)**
See 07610.

07630 **mandible—open reduction (teeth immobilized, if present)**
Teeth may be wired, banded, or splinted together to prevent movement.

07640 **mandible—closed reduction (teeth immobilized, if present)**
See 07630.

07650 **malar and/or zygomatic arch—open reduction**

07660 **malar and/or zygomatic arch—closed reduction**

07670 **alveolus—stabilization of teeth, open reduction splinting**
Teeth may be wired, banded or splinted together to prevent movement.

07680 **facial bones—complicated reduction with fixation and multiple surgical approaches**
> Facial bones include upper and lower jaw, cheek, and bones around eyes, nose, and ears.

Treatment of Fractures—Compound
07710 **maxilla—open reduction**
07720 **maxilla—closed reduction**
07730 **mandible—open reduction**
07740 **mandible—closed reduction**
07750 **malar and/or zygomatic arch—open reduction**
07760 **malar and/or zygomatic arch—closed reduction**
07770 **alveolus—stabilization of teeth, open reduction splinting**
> Fractured bone(s) are exposed to mouth or outside the face; see 07670.

07780 **facial bones—complicated reduction with fixation and multiple surgical approaches**

Reduction of Dislocation and Management of Other Temporomandibular Joint Dysfunctions
07810 **open reduction of dislocation**
> Access to TMJ via surgical opening.

07820 **closed reduction of dislocation**
> Joint manipulated into place; no surgical exposure.

07830 **manipulation under anesthesia**
> Usually done via general anesthesia.

07840 **condylectomy**
> Surgical removal of a condyle (the most superior portion of the ramus or the mandible which articulates with the skull) or a portion thereof. If bilateral, report twice.

▲ 07850 **surgical discectomy; with/without implant**
> Excision of the intraarticular disk of a joint.

● 07852 **disc repair**
> Repositioning and/or sculpting of disk; repair of perforated posterior attachment.

● 07854 **synovectomy**
> Excision of a portion or all of the synovial membrane of a joint.

● 07856 **myotomy**
> Cutting of a muscle.

● 07858 **joint reconstruction**
> Reconstruction of osseous components, including or excluding soft tissues of the joint with autogenous homologous or alloplastic materials.

07860 **arthrotomy**
> Cutting into a joint.

● 07865 **arthoplasty**
> Reduction of osseous components of the joint to create a pseudoarthrosis or eliminate an irregular remodeling pattern (osteophytes).

07870 **arthrocentesis**
> Withdrawal of fluid from a joint space by aspiration.

● 07872 **arthroscopy—diagnosis, with or without biopsy**
● 07873 **arthroscopy—surgical: lavage and lysis of adhesions**
> Removal of adhesions using the arthroscope and lavage of the joint cavities.

● 07874 **arthroscopy—surgical: disk repositioning and stabilization**
> Repositioning and stabilization of disk using arthroscopic techniques.

● 07875 **arthroscopy—surgical: synovectomy**
> Removal of inflamed and hyperplastic synovium (partial/complete) via an arthroscopic technique.

● 07876 **arthroscopy—surgical: discectomy**
Removal of disc and remodeled posterior attachment via the arthroscope.

● 07877 **arthroscopy—surgical: debridement**
Removal of pathologic hard and/or soft tissue using the arthroscope.

07880 **occlusal orthotic device, by report**
Presently includes splints provided for treatment of temporomandibular joint dysfunction.

● 07899 **unspecified TMD therapy, by report**
Used for procedure that is not adequately described by a code. Describe procedure fully—what was done and why.

Repair of Traumatic Wounds

07910 **suture of recent small wounds up to 5 cm**
Wound is about 2′ or smaller.

Complicated Suturing (Reconstruction Requiring Delicate Handling of Tissues and Wide Undermining for Meticulous Closure)

▲ 07911 **complicated suture up to 5 cm**
Wound is about 2′ or smaller.

▲ 07912 **complicated suture greater than 5 cm**
Wound is larger than 2′.

Other Repair Procedures

07920 **skin grafts (identify defect covered, location, and type of graft)**

07940 **osteoplasty—for orthognathic deformities**
A surgical procedure that modifies or changes the configuration of a bone.

07941 **osteotomy—ramus, closed**
Intraoral.

07942 **osteotomy—ramus, open**
Extraoral

07943 **osteotomy—ramus, open with bone graft**
See 07942.

07944 **osteotomy—segmented or subapical-per sextant or quadrant**

07945 **osteotomy—body of mandible**

07946 **LeFort I (maxilla—total)**

07947 **LeFort I (maxilla—segmented)**

07948 **LeFort II or LeFort III (osteoplasty of facial bones for midface hypoplasia or retrusion)—without bone graft**

07949 **LeFort II or LeFort III—with bone graft**
Same as 07948, with bone graft.

07950 **osseous, osteoperiosteal, periosteal, or cartilage graft of the mandible-autogenous or nonautogenous**

07955 **repair of maxillofacial soft and hard tissue defects**
Various soft tissue grafting procedures may be used alone or with alloplastic hard tissue materials.

07960 **frenulectomy (frenectomy or frenotomy)—separate procedure**
The frenum may be excised when the tongue has limited mobility; for large diastemas between teeth; or when the frenum interferes with a prosthetic appliance.

07970 **excision of hyperplastic tissue—per arch**

07971 **excision of pericoronal gingiva**
Also see 04211.

07980 **sialolithotomy**
Surgical procedure by which a stone within a salivary gland or its duct is removed intraorally or extraorally.

07981 **excision of salivary gland**

07982 **sialodochoplasty**
Surgical procedure for the repair of a defect and/or restoration of a portion of a salivary gland duct.

07983 **closures of salivary fistula**
Surgical closure of an opening between a salivary duct and/or gland and the cutaneous surface, or an opening into the oral cavity through other than the normal anatomic pathway.

07990 **emergency tracheotomy**
Surgical formation of a tracheal opening usually below the cricoid cartilage to allow for respiratory exchange.

07991 **coronoidectomy**
Surgical removal of the coronoid process of the mandible.

07993 **implant—facial bones (homologous, heterologous, or alloplastic)**
Presently includes ridge augmentation with synthetic or nonsynthetic materials.

07994 **implant—other than facial bones**
See 07993.

07999 **unspecified oral surgery procedure, by report**
Used for procedure not adequately describe by a code. Describe procedure fully—what was done and why.

08000-08999 XI. ORTHODONTICS

Minor Treatment for Tooth Guidance

08110 **removable appliance therapy**
Removable indicates that patient can remove appliance. Does not include comprehensive treatment.

08120 **fixed appliance therapy**
Fixed indicates that patient cannot remove appliance.

Minor Treatment to Control Harmful Habits

08210 **removable appliance therapy**
Removable indicates that patient can remove appliance; includes appliances for thumb sucking and tongue thrusting.

08220 **fixed appliance therapy**
Fixed indicates that patient cannot remove appliance; includes appliances for thumb sucking and tongue thrusting.

Interceptive Orthodontic Treatment

NOTE: Orthodontic treatment, usually involving the primary or transitional dentition and frequently occurring as a first phase of treatment preceding comprehensive treatment.

08360 **removable appliance therapy**
Removable indicates that patient can remove appliance; includes functional appliance (e.g., Frankel appliance).

08370 **fixed appliance therapy**
Fixed indicates that patient cannot remove appliance; see 08360.

Comprehensive Orthodontic Treatment—Transitional Dentition

NOTE: *Transitional* refers to a combination of primary and permanent teeth in the mouth. Comprehensive treatment may include:

A. Banded and/or bonded orthodontic appliances in one or both dental arches.

B. Functional jaw orthopaedic therapy using removable or banded and/or bonded orthodontic appliances.

C. Treatment using a combination of A and B.

Comprehensive treatment is aimed at resolving malocclusion that involves the entire dentition. Comprehensive treatment may begin in any stage of dental development and is followed by retention until appropriate stability has been achieved.

08460   Class I malocclusion
08470   Class II malocclusion
08480   Class III malocclusion

Comprehensive Orthodontic Treatment—Permanent Dentition

NOTE: *Permanent dentition* refers to a dentition in which the primary teeth have exfoliated and their permanent successors may have erupted.

Comprehensive treatment is aimed at resolving malocclusion that involves the entire dentition. Comprehensive treatment may begin in any stage of dental development and is followed by retention until appropriate stability has been achieved.

08560   Class I malocclusion
08570   Class II malocclusion
08580   Class III malocclusion

Other Orthodontic Services

08650   treatment of the atypical or extended skeletal case
08750   posttreatment stabilization
        Refers to *retainer*.
08999   unspecified orthodontic procedure, by report
        Used for procedure not adequately described by a code. Describe procedure fully—what was done and why.

**09000-09999 XII.
ADJUNCTIVE GENERAL
SERVICES**

Unclassified Treatment

09110   palliative (emergency) treatment of dental pain—minor procedures
        May be reported in conjunction with 00130.

Anesthesia

09210   local anesthesia not in conjunction with operative or surgical procedures
09211   regional block anesthesia
09212   trigeminal division block anesthesia
09215   local anesthesia
09220   general anesthesia—first 30 minutes
09221   general anesthesia—each additional 15 minutes
09230   analgesia
        Includes nitrous oxide.
09240   intravenous sedation
        Includes pharmacological management (sedation).

Professional Consultation

▲ 09310   consultation—(diagnostic service provided by dentist or physician other than practitioner providing treatment)
        Includes specialist consultation; should not be reported to describe discussion of treatment plan.

Professional Visits

09410   house call
        Includes nursing home visits, in addition to reporting appropriate code numbers for actual services performed.
09420   hospital call
        May be reported when providing treatment in hospital, in addition to reporting appropriate code numbers for actual services performed.
09430   office visit for observation (during regularly scheduled hours)—no other services performed
09440   office visit—after regularly scheduled hours

Drugs
09610 therapeutic drug injection, by report
Includes antibiotic or injection of sedative.

09630 other drugs and/or medicaments, by report
Includes but is not limited to oral antibiotics, oral analgesics, oral sedatives, and topical fluoride dispensed in the office for home use; does not include writing prescriptions.

Miscellaneous Services
09910 application of desensitizing medicaments
Includes (in-office) topical fluoride treatment for root sensitivity.

09920 behavior management, by report
May be reported in addition to treatment provided. Should be reported in 15-minute increments.

09930 treatment of complications (postsurgical)—unusual circumstances, by report

09940 occlusal guards, by report
Removable dental appliances designed to minimize the effects of bruxism (clenching and grinding) and other occlusal factors.

09941 fabrication of athletic mouthguards

09950 occlusion analysis—mounted case
Includes, but is not limited to, facebow, interocclusal records tracings, and diagnostic wax-up; for diagnostic casts, see 00470.

09951 occlusal adjustment—limited
May also be known as *equilibration;* reshaping the occlusal surfaces of teeth by grinding to create harmonious contact relationships between the upper and lower teeth. Presently includes disking/odontoplasty/enamelplasty.

09952 occlusal adjustment—complete
Occlusal adjustment may require several appointments of varying length, and sedation may be necessary to attain adequate relaxation of the musculature. Study casts mounted on an articulating instrument may be used for analysis of occlusal disharmony. It is designed to achieve functional relationships and masticatory efficiency with restorative treatment, orthodontics, orthognathic surgery, or jaw trauma when indicated. Occlusal adjustment enhances the healing potential of tissues affected by the lesions of occlusal trauma.

09999 unspecified adjunctive procedure, by report
Used for procedure not adequately described by a code. Describe procedure fully—what is done and why.

Explanation of the American Dental Association Tooth Numbering Systems and Explanation for Mounting Radiographs

TOOTH NUMBERING

According to a resolution passed by the 1968 American Dental Association House of Delegates, teeth should be numbered as follows:

Permanent dentition

1-32, starting with the patient's upper right third molar (1), following around the upper arch to the patient's upper left third molar (16), descending to the patient's lower left third molar (17), and following around the lower arch to the patient's lower right third molar (32).

Primary dentition

In the same manner as described for permanent dentition, primary teeth should be lettered, with upper case letters, A-T, with A being the patient's upper right second primary molar and T being the patient's lower right second primary molar.

MOUNTING RADIOGRAPHS

According to the same resolution from the 1968 ADA House of Delegates, radiographs should be mounted as follows:

Looking at the teeth from outside the mouth, radiographs should be viewed in the same manner, and so mounted.

NOTE: The raised dot in the film should be toward you when mounting radiographs.

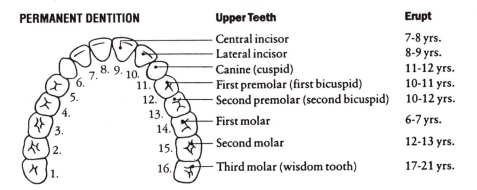

PERMANENT DENTITION

Upper Teeth	Erupt
Central incisor	7-8 yrs.
Lateral incisor	8-9 yrs.
Canine (cuspid)	11-12 yrs.
First premolar (first bicuspid)	10-11 yrs.
Second premolar (second bicuspid)	10-12 yrs.
First molar	6-7 yrs.
Second molar	12-13 yrs.
Third molar (wisdom tooth)	17-21 yrs.

Lower Teeth	Erupt
Third molar (wisdom tooth)	17-21 yrs.
Second molar	11-13 yrs.
First molar	6-7 yrs.
Second premolar (second bicuspid)	11-12 yrs.
First premolar (first bicuspid)	10-12 yrs.
Canine (cuspid)	9-10 yrs.
Lateral incisor	7-8 yrs.
Central incisor	6-7 yrs.

PRIMARY DENTITION

Upper Teeth	Erupt	Shed
Central incisor	8-12 mos.	6-7 yrs.
Lateral incisor	9-13 mos.	7-8 yrs.
Canine (cuspid)	16-22 mos.	10-12 yrs.
First molar	13-19 mos.	9-11 yrs.
Second molar	25-33 mos.	10-12 yrs.

Lower Teeth	Erupt	Shed
Second molar	23-31 mos.	10-12 yrs.
First molar	14-18 mos.	9-11 yrs.
Canine (cuspid)	17-23 mos.	9-12 yrs.
Lateral incisor	10-16 mos.	7-8 yrs.
Central incisor	6-10 mos.	6-7 yrs.

Dental Claim Form

ITEM-BY-ITEM DESCRIPTION OF THE DENTAL CLAIM FORM

The following is an item-by-item description of the questions appearing on the new form. All questions in the Billing Dentist Section should be answered as completely as possible to facilitate prompt and accurate reimbursement and to reduce follow-up inquiries. Special completion and mailing instructions, which may vary from company to company, will be printed on the form and will not be addressed here.

Dentist's pretreatment estimate or statement of actual services By checking the appropriate box, the form may be processed more quickly and with less chance of error.

Carrier name and address The name and address of the carrier where the claim is to be sent. On carrier-supplied claim forms, this information ordinarily will be preprinted at the top of the form.

1. *Patient name:* This should be completed in full for proper identification purposes.
2. *Relationship to employee:* Employee here refers to the insured person and his or her relationship to the patient. This relationship sometimes affects the patient's eligibility, as well as level of benefits available.
3. *Sex:* This is requested for identification purposes and for statistical analysis.
4. *Patient birthdate:* Very important for determination of eligibility.
5. *If full-time student:* Eligibility of the dependent patient may be affected if he or she is over a certain age and is still a full-time student.
6. *Employee/subscriber name and address:* Refers to the insured person and is not necessarily the patient.
7. *Employee/subscriber social security or ID number:* The social security number (SSN) is commonly used for computer and manual processing of claims. Some carriers use an identification number different than the SSN. This number may not necessarily be the patient's SS or ID number.
8. *Employee/subscriber birthday:* Very important for determination of coordination of benefits.
9. *Employer (company) name and address:* Refers to employer of person in *#8.*
10. *Group number:* Refers to master contract policy number assigned to the employer group.
11. *Is patient covered by another dental plan? Is patient covered by a medical plan?* This is to determine multiple coverage. The information contained in *#11-15* is very important to determine which other carriers, if any, have primary liability for treatment rendered.
12. *Name and address of carrier(s):* Refers to carrier(s) in *#11.*
12b. *Group number:* Refers to *#11.*
13. *Name and address of other employer(s):* Refers to employer offering plan in *#11.*
14a. *Employee/subscriber name (if different than patient's):* Refers to employee from *#13.*
14b. *Employee/subscriber social security or ID number:* Refers to Employee in *#14a.*

Dental Claim Form

Check one:	Carrier name and address
☐ Dentist's pre-treatment estimate	
☐ Dentist's statement of actual services	

P A T I E N T　C O V E R A G E　I N F O R M A T I O N

1. Patient name first　　　　m.i.　　　　last	2. Relationship to employee ☐ self　☐ child ☐ spouse　☐ other_____	3. Sex m　f	4. Patient birthdate MM　DD　YYYY	5. If full time student school city

6. Employee/subscriber name and mailing address	7. Employee/subscriber soc. sec. or I.D. number	8. Employee/subscriber birthdate MM　DD　YYYY	9. Employer (company) name and address	10. Group number

11. Is patient covered by another dental plan? ☐ yes　☐ no If yes, complete 12-a. Is patient covered by a medical plan?　☐ yes　　☐ no	12-a. Name and address of carrier(s)	12-b. Group no.(s)	13. Name and address of other employer(s)

14-a. Employee/subscriber name (if different than patient's)	14-b. Employee/subscriber soc. sec. or I.D. number	14-c. Employee/subscriber birth date MM　　DD　　YYYY	15. Relationship to patient ☐ self　　☐ parent ☐ spouse　☐ other _____

I have reviewed the following treatment plan. I authorize release of any information relating to this claim. I understand that I am responsible for all costs of dental treatment.

► _____
Signed (Patient, or parent if minor)　　　　　Date

I hereby authorize payment of the dental benefits otherwise payable to me directly to the below named dental entity.

► _____
Signed (Insured person)　　　　　　　　　Date

B I L L I N G　D E N T I S T

16. Name of Billing Dentist or Dental Entity	24. Is treatment result of occupational illness or injury?	No	Yes	If yes, enter brief description and dates.
17. Address where payment should be remitted	25. Is treatment result of auto accident?			
City, State, Zip	26. Other accident?			

18. Dentist Soc. Sec. or T.I.N.	19. Dentist license no.	20. Dentist phone no.	27. If prosthesis, is this initial placement?	(If no, reason for replacement).	28. Date of prior placement
21. First visit date current series	22. Place of treatment Office　Hosp.　ECF　Other	23. Radiographs or models enclosed?　No　Yes　How many?	29. Is treatment for orthodontics?	If services already commenced enter:	Date appliances placed	Mos. treatment remaining

Identify missing teeth wiht "x"

Tooth # or letter	Surface	30. Examination and treatment plan—List in order from no.1 through tooth no 32—Use charting system shown. Description of service (including x-rays, prophylaxis, materials used, etc.)	Date service performed Mo. Day Year	Procedure number	Fee	For administrative use only

31. Remarks for unusual services

I hereby certify that the procedures as indicated by date have been completed and that the fees submitted are the actual fees I have charged and intend to collect for those procedures.

	Total Fee Charged	

► _____
Signed (Treating Dentist)　　　License　　　　Date

Max. Allowable	
Deductible	
Carrier %	
Carrier pays	
Patient pays	

©American Dental Association, 1990

14c. *Employee/subscriber birthdate:* Refers to employee in *#14a.* Necessary for co-ordination of benefits.

15. *Relationship to patient:* Refers to employee in *#14a.*

Patient signature block: Self explanatory.

Insured person's signature block: This block must be completed if the patient and/or the dentist wish to have benefits paid directly to the provider.

16. *Name of billing dentist, or dental entity:* The individual dentist's name or the name of the group practice/corporation responsible for billing. This may differ from the actual treating dentist's name. This is the name that should appear on any payments or correspondence that will be remitted to the billing dentist.

17. *Address where payment should be remitted:* Self explanatory.

18. *Dentist's social security number or tax identification number (TIN):* These numbers are frequently used as individual provider identification numbers. The Internal Revenue Service requires that the SSN or TIN of the billing dentist or dental entity be supplied only if the provider accepts assignment.

19. *Dentist's license number:* Frequently used as a means of provider identification. This should be the license number of the billing dentist. This may differ from that of the treating dentist, which appears in the dentist's signature block at the bottom of the form.

20. *Dentist's phone number:* Self explanatory. Include area code also.

21. *First visit date current series:* Important to determine what services are covered when a patient becomes eligible in the middle of an active treatment plan.

22. *Place of treatment:* Depending on where treatment is rendered, medical and or hospital coverage including dental benefits may be activated. *ECF* stands for "extended care facility."

23. *Radiographs or models enclosed:* Indicates whether diagnostic materials were submitted. Aids in return of proper number of materials to dentist.

24. *Is treatment result of occupational illness or injury?* Refers to possible application of workmen's compensation, which would alter coverage available and carrier involved. Important for coordination of benefits and accurate claims processing.

25. *Is treatment result of auto accident?* Will affect reimbursement in no-fault auto cases. Indicates whether another party's insurance may be responsible. Also important for coordination of benefits.

26. *Other accident?* Similar to *#24* and *#25.*

27. *If prosthesis, is this initial placement?* Most dental contracts have specific limitations on replacement of dentures, partials, crowns, and bridges. This is used to determine eligibility and liability.

28. *Date of prior placement:* Contracts specify time limitations concerning the replacement of prosthetic devices.

29. *Is treatment for orthodontics?* When orthodontics are covered, dates and months of treatment remaining will affect the prorated monthly reimbursement made to the dentist.

30. *Examination and treatment plan:* Self-explanatory. Use the American Dental Association's *Current Dental Terminology (CDT-I)* for appropriate procedure codes.

31. *Remarks for unusual services:* Use to indicate any information that you feel may help in determining the most appropriate benefit for the treatment. If space is inadequate, use unused portion of *#30* or attach a separate sheet.

For administrative use only: Area where carrier calculates benefits.

Dentist's signature block: The treating dentist's signature and license number.

Payment itemization: The spaces under "total fee charged" will be completed by the carrier and may vary from carrier to carrier.

Selected Craniofacial Anatomy Illustrations

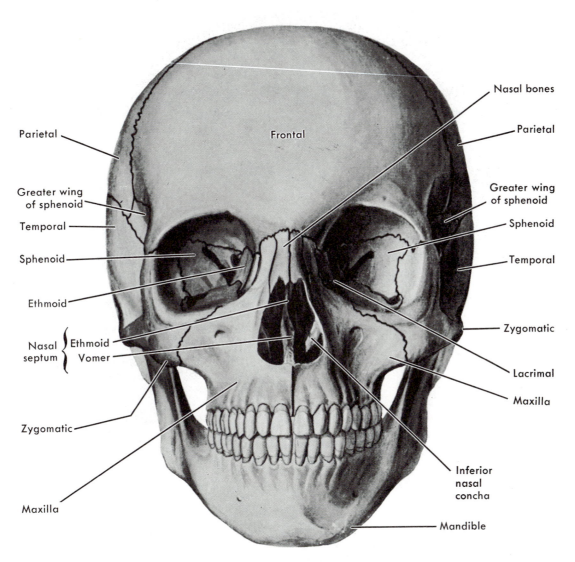

Anterior view of skull.

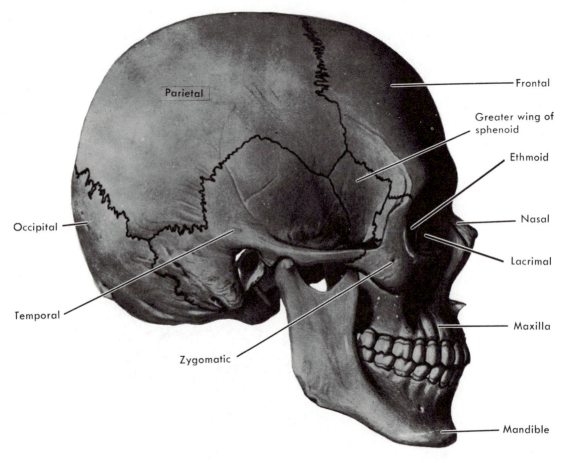

Lateral view of skull.

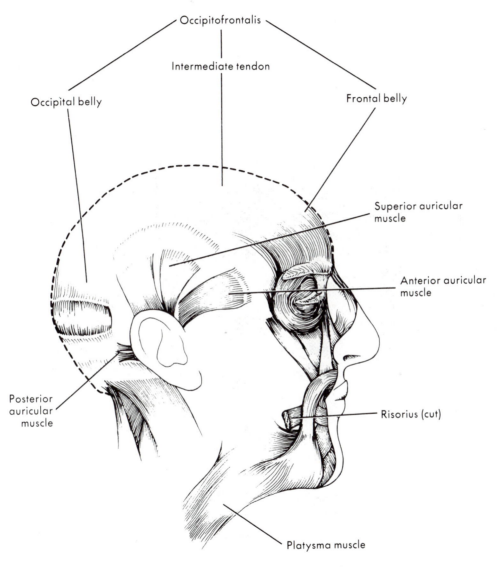

Occipitofrontalis

Intermediate tendon

Occipital belly

Frontal belly

Superior auricular
muscle

Anterior auricular
muscle

Posterior
auricular
muscle

Risorius (cut)

Platysma muscle

Three groups of auricular muscles around the ear.

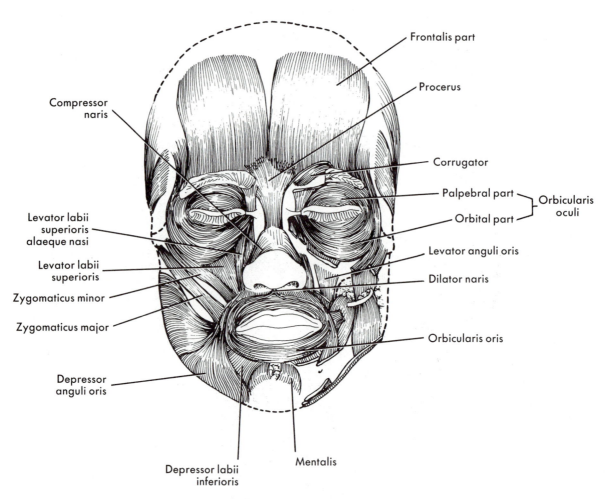

Muscles of eye, nose, and mouth.

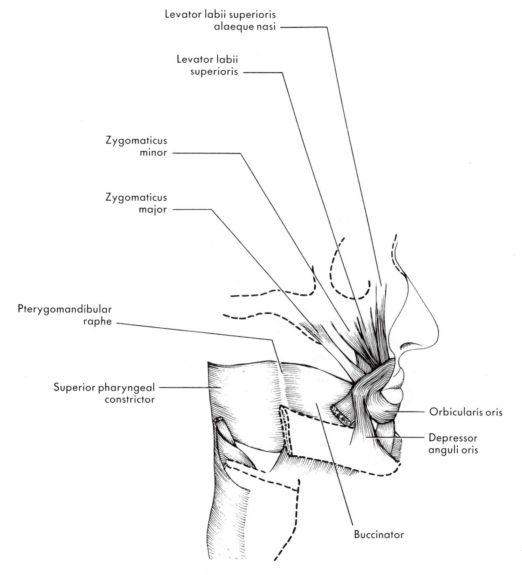

Levator labii superioris
alaeque nasi

Levator labii
superioris

Zygomaticus
minor

Zygomaticus
major

Pterygomandibular
raphe

Superior pharyngeal
constrictor

Orbicularis oris

Depressor
anguli oris

Buccinator

Muscles of the mouth.

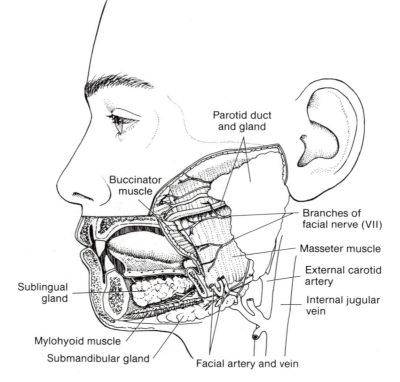

Location of salivary glands.

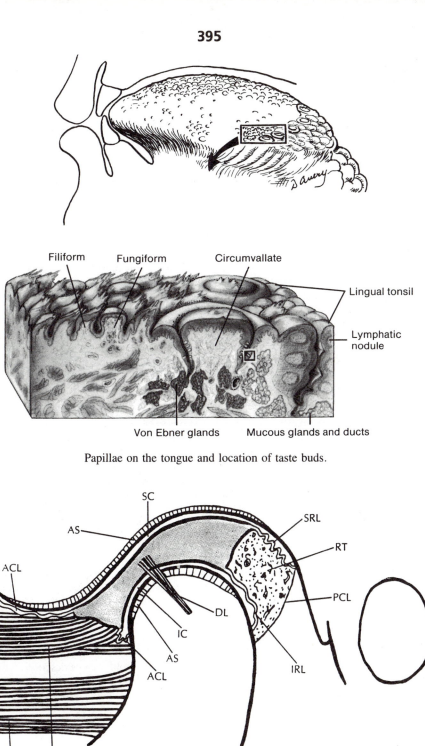

Papillae on the tongue and location of taste buds.

Temporomandibular joint.

Biochemical Profiling in Diagnostic Medicine*

INTRODUCTION

During the past 4 years many physicians have become familiar with the concept of Biochemical Profiles, owing in large part to the widespread use of the SMA 12/60 analyzer. The diagnosic advantages of the 12-test biochemical panels are well known. Routine screening of hospital admissions yields evidence of biochemical abnormalities leading to significant unexpected diagnoses in about 4% of admissions. In addition, biochemical panels often lead the physician to early diagnoses of disorders with either vague or absent symptoms, i.e., hyperparathyroidism, pernicious anemia, anicteric hepatitis, occult neoplasms and their metastases, silent myocardial infarctions, etc. Furthermore, these profiles provide the physician with a record of the patient's own normal chemical values against which subsequent changes may be compared.

PATTERN RECOGNITION

Use of the chemistry panel requires a different approach in the clinician's interpretation of laboratory data. As physicians have been trained to take a careful medical history, perform a thorough physical examination, and then order those tests from the laboratory that will either confirm or exclude our provisional diagnosis. However, with the SMA 12/60 biochemical profile, we are confronted with 12 different biochemical test results from which we must deduce a diagnosis or differential diagnosis. From the analysis of large numbers of chemistry profiles, certain patterns of abnormalities have emerged that are sufficiently characteristic to suggest a specific diagnosis or groups of differential diagnoses. It is the purpose of this monograph to stress the recognition of these diagnostic patterns as a means of increasing the diagnostic value of the SMA 12/60 chemistry profile. The graphic display of the biochemical data, unique to the SMA 12/60, permits *pattern recognition*. This is analogous to the pathologist's recognition of tissue patterns as he examines biopsy material, and in fact, the SMA 12/60 profile may be thought of as a "biochemical biopsy."

METHODOLOGY AND DETERMINATIONS

Before studying the actual biochemical profile, let us describe briefly how the results are obtained on an SMA 12/60 analyzer. Each serum sample (approximately 2 ml), is aspirated into the system, split into 12 portions, and subjected to specific chemical reactions. Results of each such reaction are recorded on a strip-chart recorder. Approximately 8 minutes are required to process a single sample. Complete 12-test profiles are recorded at the rate of one a minute.

---

*From Preston JA, Troxel DB: *Biochemical profiling in diagnostic medicine,* Tarrytown, NY, 1971, Technicon Instruments.

Nineteen different tests are available for the SMA 12/60, of which the following 12 represent determinations done in our lab on a standard SMA 12/60 survey instrument.

1. SGOT
2. LDH
3. Uric acid
4. Inorganic phosphorus
5. Urea nitrogen
6. Glucose
7. Albumin
8. Alkaline phosphatase
9. Total protein
10. Bilirubin
11. Cholesterol
12. Calcium

THE SERUM CHEMISTRY GRAPH

Results from determinations performed by the SMA 12/60 analyzer are recorded on a Serum Chemistry Graph (Fig. 1). They appear in the same sequence that tests are performed on the instrument. Each test shows a concentration range *(A)* and includes a shaded area *(B)* representing the values normal for that particular determination within any population. The pen tracing *(C)* represents the actual concentration of material detected by the instrument for each test, drawn across the concentration scale for that test. This type of presentation enables the physician to scan all 12 chemistries rapidly and to see immediately which results fall outside the normal range.

In this monograph we want to explore the interrelationship among various abnormal chemistry results. Before we can do this, we must define *normal* as applied to the data derived.

THE NORMAL RANGE

The shaded areas on the SMA 12/60 Serum Chemistry Graph represent the normal range for each of the particular test values. The normal range, as we define it, is based on a simple statistical concept—the normal distribution or the Gaussian curve (Fig. 2). Any population will characteristically show this curve for a particular measurement. There will be scatter around a mean or average value. The characteristic bell-shaped curve defines mathematically the spread of a population around the mean or average value. It has been shown that 66% of a population will fall within one standard deviation of the mean and 95% within two standard deviations.

Normal in the statistical sense we employ here does not necessarily mean healthy. The word merely describes the typical range of values we might anticipate in any given population. One out of 20 results will always be outside the two standard deviation range. The farther from the average value a particular physiological value falls, the more certain one becomes of its clinical significance. The probability becomes greater and greater that a value outside the 95% limits reflects a definite clinical problem.

In Fig. 3 we have superimposed the typical Gaussian curve on the normal range. As one can see, the farther the result lies from the center of this normal range, the more significant it can become diagnostically.

Since these ranges are generated from the total population, regardless of age, sex, or race, the "normal range" is a very broad indicator. It must be understood in terms of the individual patient.

This fact brings us to one of the most intriguing possibilities afforded clinicians by routine profiling: the determination of an individual's personal normal range or baseline. As data are accumulated for a patient over several years, a deviation in a given determination may indicate a radical change in the individual, although the result never deviates from the "normal" population range.

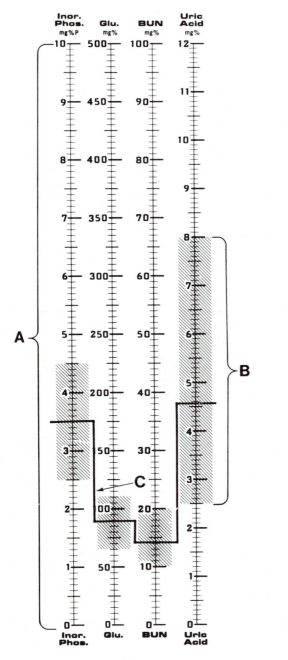

Fig. 1

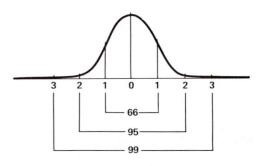

Fig. 2

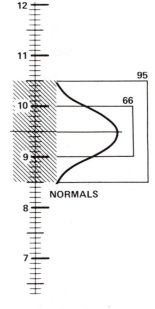

Fig. 3

**CLINICAL
SIGNIFICANCE OF
DETERMINATIONS**

To understand fully the relevance of the biochemical profiles that follow, we should examine briefly the clinical significance of elevated or diminished values for the various determinations included in the 12-test panel.*

SGOT

SGOT elevation may be indicative of several disease states, most commonly heart or liver disease. Elevations of this enzyme are typical in the conditions listed below; slight elevations occur during normal pregnancy:
1. Acute hepatitis
2. Acute myocardial infarction
3. Active cirrhosis
4. Infectious mononucleosis with hepatitis
5. Hepatic necrosis chemically and drug induced
6. Hepatic metastases
7. Acute pancreatitis
8. Trauma to skeletal muscle; irradiation of skeletal muscle
9. Pseudohypertrophe muscular dystrophy
10. Dermatomyositis
11. Acute hemolytic anemia
12. Acute renal disease
13. Severe burns
14. Cardiac catheterization and angiography
15. Recent brain trauma with brain necrosis
Reduced levels of SGOT may be seen in certain conditions.
1. Beriberi
2. Uncontrolled diabetes mellitus with acidosis
3. Liver disease (occasionally)

LDH

LDH is an intracellular enzyme, and increases in the reported value usually indicate cellular death and leakage of enzyme from the cell. Elevation occurs when neoplastic cells proliferate. Increased levels of this enzyme are also found after strenuous exercise, including the muscular exertion involved in childbirth. Causes for elevated *LDH* include the following:
1. Acute myocardial infarction
2. Acute leukemia
3. Hemolytic anemia of any type
4. Acute pulmonary infarction
5. Malignant neoplasms
6. Acute renal infarction
7. Hepatic disease
8. Skeletal muscle necrosis
9. Sprue
10. Shock with necrosis of minor organs

Uric acid

Uric acid levels may increase as a result either of overproduction or the patient's inability to excrete the substance produced. The following are possible causes:
1. Renal failure (most common cause in hospital patients)
2. Gout
3. Eclampsia of pregnancy with hepatic necrosis

---

*For a detailed discussion of clinical significance of various tests, see Wolf PL et al: Utilization of SMA 12/60 and SMA 6/60 Charts as a Teaching Aid in Laboratory Medicine, *Advances in Automated Analysis: Proceeding of the Technicon International Congress,* vol 1, Mount Kinso, NY, 1970, Futura.

4. Leukemias or lymphomas
5. Metabolic acidosis
6. Starvation
7. Thiazide diuretics, salicylates, ethanol, and other drugs
8. Lead poisoning
9. Infectious mononucleosis
10. Chemotherapy for cancer

Reduced levels of *uric acid* are encountered in patients being treated with a uricosuric drug.

Inorganic phosphorus

Inorganic phosphorus is inversely related to calcium, and therefore many of the causes of elevated calcium are also causes of hypophosphatemia. Phosphorus levels are normally elevated in youth and adolescence. Abnormal elevations may result from several causes, including the following:

1. Renal failure (most common cause in a hospital population)
2. Healing bone fractures
3. Diabetic ketosis
4. Hypoparathyroidism
5. Hypervitaminosis D
6. Acromegaly (early sign)

Reduced *inorganic phosphorus* levels derive from a variety of causes:

1. Continuous use of intravenous (IV) glucose in a nondiabetic
2. Negative nitrogen balance
3. Rickets
4. Some hepatic disorders
5. Osteomalacia
6. Fanconi syndrome
7. Ingestion of antacids

Urea nitrogen

Urea nitrogen elevations are associated with renal failure, with or without obstructive uropathy from any cause:

1. Dehydration (mild to moderate elevation)
2. Gastrointestinal hemorrhage

Reduced levels of *BUN* are also symptomatic

1. Liver failure (e.g., from acute atrophy or toxicity)
2. Negative nitrogen balance
3. Excessive use of IV fluids
4. Physiologic hydremia in pregnancy

Glucose

Hyperglycemia is related to several disease states:

1. Diabetes mellitus (most common cause; unlikely diagnosis in cases in which phosphorus values are depressed)
2. Cushing's disease (and other conditions related to excess production of adrenal corticoids)
3. Pheochromocytoma
4. Brain trauma

Hypoglycemia also has several possible causes:

1. Excess insulin administered to a diabetic
2. Addison's disease
3. Bacterial sepsis
4. Islet cell adenoma of the pancreas
5. Mesenchymal neoplasm that consumes glucose

6. Massive hepatic necrosis
7. Psychogenic

Albumin

Hyperalbuminemia is generally not observed. *Low albumin* readings are usually caused by multiple and diverse conditions:
1. Inadequate protein intake
2. Severe liver disease
3. Malabsorption
4. Diarrhea
5. Nephrosis
6. Exfoliative dermatitis
7. Burns
8. Dilution by excessive intravenous infusion of glucose in water

Alkaline phosphatase

Alkaline phosphatase levels are higher in children and adolescents and also in pregnant women. Levels are somewhat higher in the male than in the female. Levels may also be elevated if serum is retained for several hours at 20° C before it is processed on the SMA 12/60. Abnormal elevations have several causes:
1. Metastatic carcinoma involving the bones
2. Primary malignant neoplasms
3. Infusion of 5% human albumin
4. Healing fractures
5. Obstructive liver disease
6. Hyperparathyroidism, primary or secondary
7. Paget's disease of the bone
8. Pulmonary infarct
9. Acute or chronic liver disease
Reduced levels of the enzyme may indicate malnutrition.

Total protein

The causes of *hyperproteinemia* are actually the causes for hyperglobulinemia:
1. Lupus erythematosus
2. Rheumatoid arthritis
3. Other collagen diseases
4. Chronic infections
5. Multiple myeloma (and other malignant tumors)
6. Acute liver disease
Low *total protein* values derive from the same causes as are listed above for hypoalbuminemia.

Bilirubin

Bilirubin elevations and jaundice have many causes, generally falling into three major categories: hepatic, obstructive, and hemolytic.
Elevation of nonconjugated bilirubin
1. Hemolytic anemia
2. Trauma with the presence of a large hematoma
3. Hemorrhagic pulmonary infarct
4. Crigler-Najjar syndrome (rare)
5. Gilbert's disease (rare)
Conjugated and nonconjugated bilirubin elevated, conjugated more elevated
1. Hepatic metastases
2. Hepatitis
3. Lymphoma
4. Cholestasis secondary to drugs
5. Decompensated cirrhosis

Elevated conjugated bilirubin
1. Carcinoma of the head of the pancreas
2. Choledocholithiasis
3. Dubin-Johnson syndrome

Cholesterol

Cholesterol elevations are attributable to several causes:
1. Cardiovascular disease
2. Obstructive jaundice
3. Hypothyroidism
4. Nephrosis
5. Uncontrolled diabetes
6. Pregnancy

Low *cholesterol* values occur when cholesterol is not absorbed from the gastrointestinal tract:
1. Malabsorption
2. Severe liver disease
3. Hyperthyroidism
4. Anemia
5. Sepsis
6. Stress and drug therapy

Calcium

Causes for *calcium* elevations are well understood:
1. Primary hyperparathyroidism
2. Secondary hyperparathyroidism associated with chronic renal failure
3. Bony metastases from carcinomas
4. Sarcoidosis with bone involvement
5. Bone involvement from lymphoma or multiple myeloma
6. Carcinoma of the lung and kidney parathormone production
7. Hypervitaminosis D
8. Long-term use of diuretics
9. Milk-alkali syndrome
10. Acidosis

Low *calcium* values are also of interest. Causes include the following:
1. Low albumin
2. Hypoparathyroidism (usually surgically induced)
3. Chronic renal failure
4. Steatorrhea or malabsorption syndrome
5. Pancreatitis
6. EDTA anticoagulation therapy
7. Alkalosis

Clinical examples

We shall now look at a few biochemical profiles from our own clinical studies, arranged in six categories reflecting particular states, ranging from normal variations to specific pathologies (Figs. 4 to 6).

Please note that differential diagnosis is enhanced by simple ancillary determinations such as protein and LDH isoenzyme electrophoresis and heat stability studies of alkaline phosphatase.

Another factor that must always be considered in reviewing patient test data is the possible effect of therapeutic agents. The medication a patient receives can influence either the quantity of the compound measured owing to a physiological response or can cause an interference in the analytical measurement itself. For further information on this subject, we recommend reading Elking MP, Kabat HF: *Am J Hosp Pharm* 25:485, 1968; and Christian DG: *Am J Clin Path* 54:118, 1970.

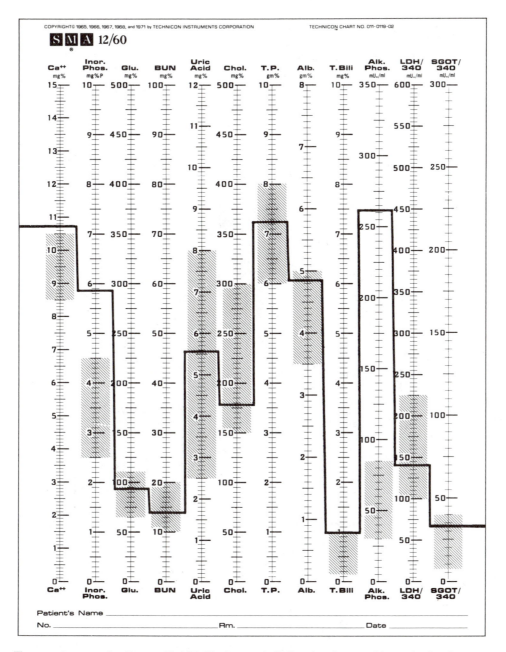

The normal pattern of a 12-year-old child. The increased alkaline phosphatase and inorganic phosphorus are due to bone growth. The alkaline phosphatase is heat labile and therefore bone in origin.

S M A 12/60

Pattern of normal pregnancy, last trimester. There is a slight but distinct elevation in glucose, cholesterol, bilirubin, and alkaline phosphatase. Fifty percent of the alkaline phosphatase is heat stable. It is therefore both placental and bone in origin.

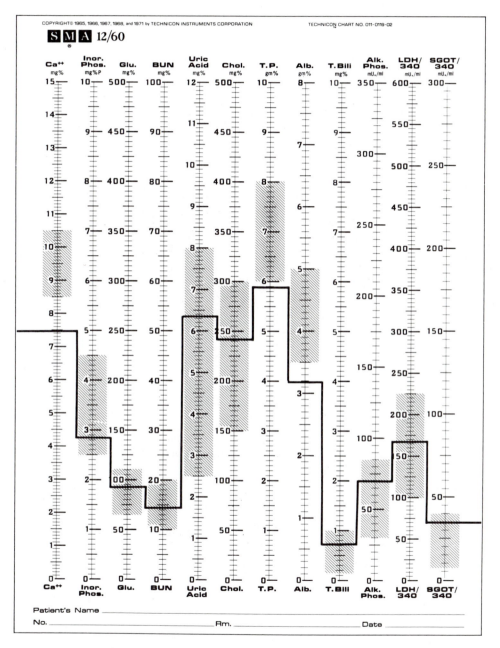

Normal pattern of old age with hypoproteinemia and calcemia.

Daily dietary guide—the basic four food groups

Food group	Main nutrients	Daily amounts*
Milk		
Milk, cheese, ice cream, or other products made with whole or skimmed milk	Calcium Protein Riboflavin	Children under 9: 2-3 cups Children 9-12: 3 or more cups Teenagers: 4 or more cups Adults: 2 or more cups Pregnant women: 3 or more cups Nursing mothers: 4 or more cups (1 cup = 8 oz fluid milk or designated milk equivalent†)
Meats		
Beef, veal, lamb, pork, poultry, fish, eggs	Protein Iron Thiamin	2 or more servings Count as 1 serving 2-3 oz of lean, boneless, cooked meat, poultry, or fish 2 eggs
Alternates: dry beans, dry peas, nuts, peanut butter	Niacin Riboflavin	1 cup cooked dry beans or peas 4 tbsp peanut butter
Vegetables and fruits		4 or more servings Count as 1 serving ½ cup of vegetable or fruit or a portion such as 1 medium apple, banana, orange, potato, or ½ a medium grapefruit or melon Include
	Vitamin A	Dark-green or deep-yellow vegetable or fruit rich in vitamin A at least every other day
	Vitamin C (ascorbic acid)	Citrus fruit or other fruit or vegetable rich in vitamin C daily
	Smaller amounts of other vitamins and minerals	Other vegetables and fruits including potatoes
Bread and cereals	Thiamin Niacin Riboflavin Iron Protein	4 or more servings of whole grain, enriched or restored Count as 1 serving 1 slice of bread 1 oz (1 cup) ready to eat cereal, flake or puff varieties ½-¾ cup cooked cereal ½-¾ cup cooked pastes (macaroni, spaghetti, noodles) Crackers: 5 saltines, 2 squares graham crackers

*Use additional amounts of these foods or added butter, margarine, oils, sugars, etc., as desired or needed.
†Milk equivalents: 1 oz cheddar cheese, 3 servings cottage cheese, 1 cup fluid skimmed milk, 1 cup buttermilk, ½ cup dry skimmed milk powder, 1 cup ice milk, 1⅔ cups ice cream, ½ cup evaporated milk.

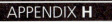

Medical Tables

Conversion formulas

Temperature	To convert Fahrenheit to centigrade, subtract 32 from °F, multiply by⅝.		
	To convert centigrade to Fahrenheit, multiply °C by ⅞ and add 32.		
Weight	1 kg = 2.2 pounds	1 pound = 0.45 kg.	
	1 g = 15.43 grains	1 grain = 0.065 g	
Length	1 inch = 2.54 cm	1 cm = 0.3937 inch	
Approximate household measures	1 Teaspoonful		5 ml
	1 Dessertspoonful		8 ml
	1 Tablespoonful	½ fl oz	15 ml
	1 Jigger	1½ fl oz	45 ml
	1 Wineglassful	2 fl oz	60 ml
	1 Teacupful	4 fl oz	120 ml
	1 Glassful	8 fl oz	240 ml

From *Pocket book of medical tables,* ed 25, Philadelphia, 1980, Smith Kline.

Nomenclature and synonyms for coagulation factors

Roman numeral	Preferred descriptive name	Synonyms
I	Fibrinogen	
II	Prothrombin	
III	Tissue factor	Thromboplastin
IV	Calcium ions	
V	Proaccelerin	Labile factor, accelerator globulin (AcG), thrombogen
VII	Proconvertin	Stable factor, serum prothrombin conversion accelerator (SPCA), autoprothrombin I, cothromboplastin
VIII	Antihemophilic factor (AHF)	Antihemophilic globulin (AHG), antihemophilic factor A, platelet cofactor 1, thromboplastinogen
IX	Plasma thromboplastin component (PTC)	Christmas factor, antihemophilic factor B, autoprothrombin II, platelet cofactor 2
X	Stuart-Prower factor	Stuart factor, autoprothrombin III, thrombokinase
XI	Plasma thromboplastin antecedent (PTA)	Antihemophilic factor C
XII	Hageman factor	Glass factor, contact factor
XIII	Fibrin stabilizing factor (FSF)	Laki-Lorand factor (LLF), fibrinase, plasma transglutaminase

From Wintrobe MM: *Clinical hematology,* ed. 7, Philadelphia, 1974, Lea & Febiger.

Desirable weights for men and women according to height and frame (age 25 and over)

Men

Weight in pounds (in indoor clothing; for nude weight deduct 5 to 7 pounds)

Height (with shoes)

Feet	Inches	Small frame	Medium frame	Large frame
5	2	112-120	118-129	126-141
5	3	115-123	121-133	129-144
5	4	118-126	124-136	132-148
5	5	121-129	127-139	135-152
5	6	124-133	130-143	138-156
5	7	128-137	134-147	142-161
5	8	132-141	138-152	147-166
5	9	136-145	142-156	151-170
5	10	140-150	146-160	155-174
5	11	144-154	150-165	159-179
6	0	148-158	154-170	164-184
6	1	152-162	158-175	168-189
6	2	156-167	162-180	173-194
6	3	160-171	167-185	178-199
6	4	164-175	172-190	182-204

Women

Weight in pounds (in indoor clothing; for nude weight deduct 2 to 4 pounds)

Height (with shoes)

Feet	Inches	Small frame	Medium frame	Large frame
4	10	92-98	96-107	104-119
4	11	94-101	98-110	106-122
5	0	96-104	101-113	109-125
5	1	99-107	104-116	112-128
5	2	102-110	107-119	115-131
5	3	105-113	110-122	118-134
5	4	108-116	113-126	121-138
5	5	111-119	116-130	125-142
5	6	114-123	120-135	129-146
5	7	118-127	124-139	133-150
5	8	122-131	128-143	137-154
5	9	126-135	132-147	141-158
5	10	130-140	136-151	145-163
5	11	134-144	140-155	149-168
6	0	138-148	144-159	153-173

From Society of Actuaries: *The build and blood pressure study,* New York, 1959, Metropolitan Life Insurance Co.

Hematology

RBC measurements	Diameter	5.5-8.8 μ (newborn: 8.6)
	Mean corpuscular volume	82-92 cuμ (newborn: 106)
	Mean corpuscular Hb	27-31 μm (newborn: 38)
	Mean corpuscular Hb Conc.	32%-36%
	Color, saturation, and volume indices	1
Miscellaneous	Bleeding time	1-4 min (Duke)
		1-9 min (Ivy)
	Circulation time, arm to lung (ether)	4-8 sec
	Circulation time, arm to tongue (sodium dehydrocholate)	9-16 sec
	Clot retraction time	2-4 hr
	Coagulation time (venous)	6-10 min (Lee & White)
		10-30 min (Howell)
	Fragility, erythrocyte (hemolysis)	0.44%-0.35% NaCl
	Partial thromboplastin time	68-82 sec (standard)
		32-46 sec (activated)
	Sedimentation rate:	
	Men	0-9 mm/hr (Wintrobe)
	Women	0-20 mm/hr (Wintrobe)

From *Pocket book of medical tables,* ed 25, Philadelphia, 1980, Smith Kline.

Blood chemistry

Constituent	Material*	mg/dl (mg %)—or as noted†
Aldolase	S	0.8-3 ImU/ml
Ammonia	P	20-150 μg/dl
Amylase	S	60-160 units (Somogyi)
		0.06-0.34 ImU/ml
α-1-Antitrypsin	S	210-500
Ascorbic acid	B	0.4-1.5
Bilirubin		
Direct	S	Up to 0.4
Indirect	S	0.4-0.8
Total	S	Up to 1.2
Bromide	S	Toxic level about 15 mEq/L
Bromsulphalein (5 mg/kg)	S	5% dye or less at 45 minutes
Calcium (ionized)	S	4.5-5.5 mEq/L
		2.4-2.9 mEq/L (at pH 7.4)
Carbon dioxide content	S	24-30 mM/L
Carotene	S	50-300 μg/dl
Ceruloplasmin	S	23-50
Chloride	S	98-109 mEq/L
Cholesterol, total	S	150-250
Cholesterol esters	S	60%-75% of total
Cholinesterase	S	0.5 pH unit/hour or more
		2-5.3 IU/ml
Creatine		
Males	S	0.2-0.6
Females	S	0.6-1.0

*B, whole blood; P, plasma; S, serum. † IU, International units; ImU, International milliunits.
From *Pocket book of medical tables,* ed 25, Philadelphia, 1980, Smith Kline.   *Continued.*

Blood chemistry—cont'd

Constituent	Material*	mg/dl (mg %)—or as noted†
Creatine phosphokinase (CPK)		
Males	S	5-50 ImU/ml
Females	S	5-30 ImU/ml
Creatinine	S	0.8-1.2
Ferritin		
Males	S	27-329 ng/ml
Females	S	9-125 ng/ml
Fibrinogen	P	160-415
Folate	S	5-21 ng/ml
Gastrin	S	0-20 pg/ml
Glucose	S	60-100 (Nelson-Somogyi)
Glucose-6-phosphate dehydrogenase (G6PD)	Red cells	5-10 IU/g Hb/30° C
γ-Glutamyl transpeptidase		
Males	S	<28 ImU/ml
Females	S	<18 ImU/ml
α-Hydroxybutyric dehydrogenase	S	0-180 ImU/ml
17-Hydroxycorticosteroids		7-19 μg/dl
Males	P	9-21 μg/dl
Females	P	
After 25 units ACTH, IM		35-55 μg/dl
Immunoglobulins		
IgG	S	800-1500
IgA	S	50-200
IgM	S	40-120
Iodine, protein-bound	S	4-8 μg/dl
Iron	S	50-150 μg/dl
Iron-binding capacity	S	250-410 μg/dl
Isocitric dehydrogenase	S	50-260 units
17-Ketosteroids		
Males	P	40-150 μg/dl
Females	P	38-130 μg/dl
Lactic acid	B	6-20
Lactic dehydrogenase (LDH)	S	0-300 ImU/ml
Isozymes		

American	European	Myocardium	Liver	Muscle	RBC
5	1	4+	±	±	3+
4	2	4+	±	±	3+
3	3	+	+	+	+
2	4	±	2+	2+	±
1	5	±	4+	4+	±

Constituent	Material*	mg/dl (mg %)—or as noted†
Lipase	S	0.2-1.5 units/ml (N/20 NaOH)
Lipids, total	S	400-800
Cholesterol		
Total	S	115-340
Esterified	S	70%
Free fatty acids	S	0.3-0.8 mEq/L
Phospholipids	S	130-380
Triglycerides (neutral fat)	S	10-190
Lithium (therapeutic level)	S	0.5-1.0 mEq/L

Blood chemistry—cont'd

Constituent	Material*	mg/dl (mg %)—or as noted†
Magnesium	S	1.5-2.4 mEq/L
Nonprotein nitrogen	S	25-40
Osmolality	S	280-290 mOsm/kg plasma water
pH	P	7.35-7.45 glass electrode method
Phenylalanine	S	0-2
Phosphatase, acid	S	0.1-1.0 units (Bodansky)
		0-11 ImU/ml
Phosphatase, alkaline		
Children	S	5-14 units (Bodansky)
		15-20 units (King-Armstrong)
Adults	S	1.4-4.1 units (Bodansky)
		4-13 units (King-Armstrong)
		20-48 ImU/ml
Phosphorus		
Children	S	2.3-3.8 mEq/L
Adults	S	1.45-2.76 mEq/L
Potassium	S	3.6-5.5 mEq/L
Proteins (electrophoresis)		
Albumin	S	3.2-5.6 g/dl
α_1 Globulin	S	0.1-0.4 g/dl
α_2 Globulin	S	0.4-1.2 g/dl
β Globulin	S	0.5-1.1 g/dl
γ Globulin	S	0.5-1.6 g/dl
Renin activity by RIA	P	(EDTA) 0.4-4.5 ng/ml/hr
Salicylates (therapeutic level)	S	20-25 (toxic >30)
Sodium	S	135-145 mEq/L
Transaminase		
Glutamic oxaloacetic (SGOT)	S	6-40 units (Karmen)
		0-15 ImU/ml
Glutamic pyruvic (SGPT)	S	6-36 units (Karmen)
		0-15 ImU/ml
Urea	S	17-42
Urea nitrogen	S	8-20
Uric acid		
Males	S	2.1-7.8
Females	S	2.0-6.4
Vitamin A	S	65-275 IU/dl
Vitamin B_{12}	S	330-1025 pg/ml

Stool

Fat	
Total	10%-25% of dry matter and <5 g/24 hr
Neutral	1%-5% of dry matter
Free fatty acids	5%-13% of dry matter
Combined fatty acids	5%-15% of dry matter
Urobilinogen	40%-200 mg/24 hr

From *Pocket book of medical tables,* ed 25, Philadelphia, 1980, Smith Kline.

Urine

Specific gravity: 1.015-1.025
pH: 4.8-8.5
Volume: 600-2500 ml/24 hr

Constituent	24-hour excretion or as noted		
Aldosterone	2-10 µg		
Ammonia nitrogen	20-70 mEq		
Amylase	35-260 Somogyi units/L		
Calcium			
200 mg diet	<7.5 mEq		
Catecholamines			
Free, epinephrine and norepinephrine	<100 µg		
Metanephrine	<1.3 mg		
VMA	<8 mg		
Chloride	110-250 mEq		
Coproporphyrin	100-300 µg		
Cortisol	2-10 mg		
Free cortisol	7-25 mg, male		
	4-15 mg, female		
Creatine			
Adult male	<50 mg		
Adult female	<100 mg		
Higher in children and pregnancy			
Creatinine	1-1.6 g (15-25 mg/kg)		
	Estrone	**Estradiol (µg)**	**Estriol**
Estrogens			
Female postpubertal	5-20	2-10	5-30
Female postmenopausal	0.3-2.4	0-14	2.2-7.5
Male			
Female prepubertal	0-15	0-5	0-10
5-HIAA	2-9 mg		
Lead	<120 µg		
Phosphorus	0.9-1.3 g		
Porphobilinogen	<2 mg		
Potassium	25-100 mEq		
Protein	<50 mg		
Sodium	100-260 mEq		
Urea nitrogen	6-15 g		
Uric acid	0.2-0.6 g		
Urobilinogen	1-3.5 mg		

From Beeson P, McDermott W: *Textbook of medicine,* ed. 14, Philadelphia, 1979, Saunders; modified from Thorn GW et al: *Harrison's principles of internal medicine,* ed 8, New York, 1977, McGraw-Hill.

POISONING

The following notes are intended to provide the physician with a brief guide to the general management of acute poisoning, and specific antidotal measures for a wide range of potentially toxic substances.

General management

Emetics When someone has swallowed poison, giving an emetic is usually the quickest and most handy way of cleaning out the stomach. However, there are many patients who should *not* be given an emetic—unconscious patients and those who have been poisoned by strong acid or alkali. Also, emetics may be ineffective in patients poisoned by *anti*emetics (for example, phenothiazine derivatives).

An easy emetic to improvise is a saline solution consisting of 3 heaping teaspoonfuls of salt in a glass of hot water (at 37° to 40° C). In treating a child, though, syrup of ipecac (15 to 20 ml followed by at least 200 ml of fluid) is preferable because hypertonic saline may cause severe hypernatremia if the child does not vomit. However, ipecac should not be used if the child is in shock. Furthermore, if the child is given ipecac and does not vomit, gastric lavage or the instillation of activated charcoal is imperative.

Apomorphine, a good emetic for adults and children, may be administered *intramuscularly* at a dose of 1 mg/10 Kg for adults and 1 or 2 mg for children. Nalorphine or levallorphan should be given later to counteract the emetic effect.

Gastric lavage Gastric lavage is useful if it is done within 3 or 4 hours after the poison has been taken. It should not be done, however, on patients poisoned by a strong acid, alkali, or strychnine. Nor should it be done on patients poisoned by iron—taken perhaps in the form of iron tablets—if the iron has been taken more than 1 hour previously. (The danger here is that, because iron poisoning causes gastric necrosis, the lavage tube might perforate the stomach.) Gastric lavage is also usually not performed on patients who have swallowed gasoline or other petroleum distillates because of the risk of chemical pneumonitis. (One cooperative study, however, has shown no such increased risk.)

These procedures should be followed in gastric lavage:
1. Aspirate as much of the stomach contents as possible before starting the lavage.
2. Lavage the unconscious patient while he or she is lying on the side, the head lower than his body, instilling 200-300 ml fluid over 1 to 2 minutes.
3. Use gastric tubes of ample caliber (34 French).
4. Use normal saline solution instead of tap water to lavage children—no more than 50 ml per lavage.
5. Repeat procedure until the return fluid is clear—usually about 10 times.

Certain antidotes can be administered through the gastric tube. Egg white and milk, for example, will help capture iron; sodium bicarbonate (1% solution) will convert iron to a less soluble form so that it will not be absorbed by the body. Activated charcoal is an antidote that is indicated for some poisons; however, when the poison is unknown, activated charcoal should be administered—about 15 to 30 g mixed with water to form a thin paste.

If the poison is fat soluble, do not administer milk or castor oil because they will cause the poison to be more easily absorbed. Liquid paraffin or mineral oil, which are not absorbable, will help prevent further absorption of fat-soluble substances. After lavage, replace lost fluids, lost blood or plasma, and correct any electrolyte imbalance.

Other types of poisons A number of poisons are easily absorbed through the skin (for example, cholinesterase-inhibiting insecticides and halogenated hydrocarbons). To treat this type of poisoning, remove contaminated clothing and thoroughly wash the affected areas with soap and water. Do not use phenothiazine derivatives to treat emesis in these patients because phenothiazines may delay the recovery of enzyme activity.

If the patient has *injected* the poison into an arm or leg, tie off the extremity and apply ice locally. Some inhalants may cause pulmonary edema. This condition calls for the administration of oxygen and a rapid-acting corticosteroid.

SPECIFIC ANTIDOTES*   **BAL**—For the treatment of heavy metal poisoning *except* that resulting from lead, iron or cadmium. 2.5 to 3.0 mg/Kg *intramuscularly* q4h for 2 days; q6h for the third day; bid for next 10 days.

---

*From *Pocket book of medical tables*, ed. 25, Philadelphia, 1980, Smith Kline Corp.

Atropine sulfate—For the treatment of cholinesterase-inhibiting insecticide poisoning, 2 to 3 mg per injection repeated every few minutes as necessary. As much as 50 to 70 mg may be required.

Protopam chloride—For the treatment of organic phosphorus insecticide poisoning. 500 mg *intravenously* as a 0.1% solution is the initial dose.

Lorfan, Narcan, or Nalline—For the treatment of poisoning resulting from morphine, codeine, heroin, other semisynthetic and synthetic narcotic analgesics as well as propoxyphene.

Lorfan—1 mg *intravenously* followed by 1 or 2 doses of 0.5 mg at 3-minute intervals.

Nalline—5 to 10 mg *intravenously* repeated every few minutes as necessary.

Narcan—0.01 mg/kg *intravenously, intramuscularly* or *subcutaneously* repeated as necessary.

Calcium disodium versenate—For the treatment of lead poisoning. It forms a soluble lead chelate, which is excreted by the kidneys. *For adults:* 1 g in 250 ml or 500 ml of 5% glucose in water or saline administered by *intravenous* drip over a 1-hour period. Two courses daily for 3 to 5 days, followed by a 2 to 14-day rest period. *For children:* 50 to 75 mg/kg daily. Repeat as necessary.

Desferal—For the treatment of iron poisoning. When a patient is in cardiovascular collapse, 1 g *intravenously* at a rate not to exceed 15 mg/Kg/hr. This may be followed with 0.5 g q4h for two doses. Depending on the response, subsequent doses of 0.5 g may be given every 4 to 12 hours. Do not exceed 6 g in 24 hours. As soon as the patient's condition improves, administer the drug *intramuscularly*. For less severely affected patients, administer the drug *intramuscularly* at the beginning, following the same schedule.

Sodium nitrite and sodium thiosulfate—For the treatment of cyanide poisoning, 0.3 to 0.5 g of sodium nitrite, dissolved in 10 to 15 ml of water, is given *intravenously* over 3 to 4 minutes. After this, 12.5 g of sodium thiosulfate dissolved in 50 ml of water is given over a 10 minutes. If the drugs must be administered a second time, *halve* the dose.

ROUTINE IMMUNIZATION FOR INFANTS AND YOUNG CHILDREN (UNDER 6 YEARS OF AGE)*

	AGE
First dose IM	2 mos
Second dose IM	4 mos
Third dose IM	6 mos
Fourth dose IM	12 to 18 mos or preschool

Pertussis need not be given children 7 years of age or older.

Adult type of combined tetanus-diphtheria toxoids with adjuvant is recommended for children over 6 years of age.

Poliomyelitis vaccine The recommended preparation contains types I, II, and III of live attenuated poliovirus. Infants may be given three oral doses along with the DPT injections starting at 2 months of age. A fourth dose should be given at 15 to 18 months of age and another booster dose at ages 4 to 6.

Mumps vaccine The mumps vaccine is seldom indicated in younger children except as combined with other vaccines.

Measles (rubeola) vaccine (live attenuated virus) A single subcutaneous or intramuscular injection of 0.5 ml is given to children who are at least 15 months of age.

German measles (rubella) vaccine (live attenuated virus) A single 0.5 ml subcutaneous dose is injected into children 1 year of age or older.

Other vaccines Vaccines are available for cholera, plague, Rocky Mountain spotted fever, smallpox, typhoid fever, paratyphoid, typhus fever, and tuberculosis.

American Academy of Pediatrics: *Report of the Committee on Infectious Diseases,* ed 18, Elk Grove Village, Ill, 1977, The Academy.

Sample Prescription Form

(Heading)
Dentist's Name and Degree
Street Address
City, State, Zip Code
Telephone

Date: _____

Patient Name: _____.   Age: (optional for adults) _____.
Address: _____.   Telephone: _____.
(Body) Rx
      Name of drug, dosage, and form
      Amount to be dispensed
      Signature: instructions to patient
(Closing) Label as to contents
      Refill ___ times.
      Brand ___.Generic:___.
DEA Number _____   _____ D.D.S./D.M.D.
                            (Doctor's Signature)

Latin Terminology Used in Prescriptions

Term or Phrase	Contraction	Meaning
ana	aa.	of each
ante	a.	before
ante cibum	a.c.	before meals
aqua	aq.	water
bis	b.	twice
bis in die	b.i.d.	twice a day
capsula	caps.	a capsule
collutorium	collut.	a mouthwash
cum	c̄.	with
dies	d.	a day
dispensa	disp.	dispense
gargarisma	garg.	a gargle
gutta	gtt.	a drop
hora somni	h.s.	at bedtime
non repetatur	non. rep.	do not repeat
peractus	p.o.	by mouth
post cibum	p.c.	after meals
pro re nata	p.r.n.	as occasion arises, if needed
quantum satis	q.s.	a sufficient quantity
quaque	q.	each, every
quaque die	q.d.	every day
quaque hora	q.h.	every hour
quartros in die	q.i.d.	four times a day
quaque quarta hora	q.4h.	every 4 hours
recipe	Rx.	take
semi, semis	s.s.	a half
signa, signetur	sig.	label
statim	stat.	immediately, at once
tabella	tab.	a tablet
ter in die	t.i.d.	three times a day
ut dictum	ut.dict.	as directed

Directory of American Dental Association, Constituent Societies, Boards of Dental Examiners, and Accredited Dental Schools

American Dental Association
211 E Chicago Ave
Chicago, IL 60611-2678
312/440-2500
Career guidance   Ex. 2788
Code of ethics   Ex. 2889
Delta dental plans   Ex. 2760
Dental practice acts   Ex. 2877
Dental student research   Ex. 2556
National board examinations   Ex. 7465
Product testing   Ex. 2508
Young dentists   Ex. 2937

Alabama Dental Association
Executive Director
Mr. Wayne McMahan
836 Washington St
Montgomery, AL 36104-3893
205/265-1684
Fax: 205/262-6218

Alaska Dental Society
Executive Director
Ms. Martha Reinbold
3400 Spenard Rd #10
Anchorage, AK 99503-3783
907/277-4675
Fax: 907/274-2960

Arizona State Dental Association
Executive Director
Mr. Greg McFarland
4131 N 36th St
Phoenix, AZ 85018-4761
602/957-4777
Fax: 602/957-1342

Arkansas State Dental Association
Executive Director
Mr. Kelley Erstine
920 W 2nd St #103
Little Rock, AR 72201-2125
501/372-3368
Fax: 501/372-7981

California Dental Association
Executive Director
Dr. Dale F Redig
PO Box 13749
Sacramento, CA 95853-4749
916/443-0505
Fax: 916/443-2943

Colorado Dental Association
Executive Director
Mr. Jeffrey Thompson
7535 E Hampden Ave, Ste 505
Denver, CO 80231-4844
303/671-6600
Fax: 303/671-0499

Connecticut State Dental Association
Executive Director
Mr. Noel Bishop
62 Russ St
Hartford, CT 06106-1589
203/278-5550
Fax: 203/522-6587

Delaware State Dental Society
Executive Director
Ms. Margaret Novak
1925 Lovering Ave
Wilmington, DE 19806-2147
302/654-4335
Fax: 302/427-9412

District of Columbia Dental Society
Executive Director
Mr. C. Jay Brown
502 C St NE
Washington, DC 20002-5810
202/547-7613
Fax: 202/546-1482

Florida Dental Association
Executive Director
Mr. Dan Buker
3021 W Swann Ave
Tampa, FL 33609-4098
813/877-7597
Fax: 813/876-3225

Georgia Dental Association
Executive Director
Mrs. Martha S Phillips
2951 Flowers Rd S #112
Atlanta, GA 30341-5533
404/458-6166
Fax: 404/454-8543

Hawaii Dental Association
Executive Director
Mr. Daniel Park
1000 Bishop St, Ste 805
Honolulu, HI 96813-4281
808/536-2135
Fax: 808/536-2137

Idaho State Dental Association
Executive Director
Mr. A Jerry Davis
1220 W Hays St
Boise, ID 83702-5315
208/343-7543
Fax: 208/383-9631

Illinois State Dental Society
Executive Director
Mr. Robert Rechner
PO Box 376
Springfield, IL 62705-0376
217/525-1406
Fax: 217/525-8872

Indiana Dental Association
Executive Director
Mr. Gale Coons
1 Virginia Ave, Ste 402
Indianapolis, IN 46204-3697
317/634-2610
Fax: 317/634-2612

Iowa Dental Association
Executive Director
Mr. Robert W Harpster
333 Insurance Exchange
Des Moines, IA 50309-2322
515/282-7250
Fax: 515/282-7256

Kansas Dental Association
Executive Director
Mr. Carl Schmitthenner, Jr.
5200 SW Huntoon St
Topeka, KS 66604-2398
913/272-7360
Fax: 913/272-2301

Kentucky Dental Association
Executive Director
Mr. Detlef B. Moore
1940 Princeton Dr
Louisville, KY 40205-1873
502/459-5373
Fax: 502/458-5915

Louisiana Dental Association
Executive Director
Mr. Gerard J Haddican
3031 22nd St
Metairie, LA 70002-4918
504/835-1612
Fax: 504/835-1614

Maine Dental Association
Executive Director
Ms. Frances Miliano
PO Box 215
Manchester, ME 04351-0215
207/622-7900
Fax: 207/622-6210

Maryland State Dental Association
Executive Director
Ms. Elza Harrison
6470 Dobbin Rd
Columbia, MD 21045-4767
410/964-2880
Fax: 410/964-0583

Massachusetts Dental Society
Executive Director
Mr. Matthew E Boylan, Jr.
83 Speen St
Natick, MA 01760-4125
508/651-7511
Fax: 508/653-7115

Michigan Dental Association
Executive Director
Ms. Gerri Cherney
230 Washington Sq N, Ste 208
Lansing, MI 48933-1392
517/372-9070
Fax: 517/372-0008

Minnesota Dental Association
Executive Director
Mr. Robert A. Harder
2236 Marshall Ave
Saint Paul, MN 55104-5792
612/646-7454
Fax: 612/646-8246

Mississippi Dental Association
Executive Director
Ms. Carolyn Simmons
2630 Ridgewood Rd
Jackson, MS 39216-4920
601/982-0442
Fax: 601/366-3050

Missouri Dental Association
Executive Director
Mr. Roger A. Weis
PO Box 1707
Jefferson City, MO 65102-1707
314/634-3436
Fax: 314/635-0764

Montana Dental Association
Executive Director
Mr. William Zepp
PO Box 1154
Helena, MT 59624-1154
406/443-2061
Fax: 406/443-1546

Nebraska Dental Association
Executive Director
Mr. Tom Bassett
3120 O St
Lincoln, NE 68510-1533
402/476-1704
Fax: 402/476-2641

Nevada Dental Association
Executive Director
Dr. William L. Thomason
PO Box 80360
Las Vegas, NV 89180-0360
702/258-4230
Fax: 702/258-4232

New Hampshire Dental Society
Executive Director
Mr. Henry Dougherty
PO Box 2229
Concord, NH 03302-2229
603/225-5961
Fax: 603/226-2548

New Jersey Dental Association
Executive Director
Mr. Philip Cocuzza
NJDA One Dental Plaza
North Brunswick, NJ 08902-4311
908/821-9400
Fax: 908/821-1082

New Mexico Dental Association
Executive Director
Ms. Marjorie Nelson
3037 San Patricio Pl NW
Albuquerque, NM 87107-2932
505/345-9135
Fax: 505/344-7930

Dental Society of the State of New York
Executive Director
Mr. Roy Lasky
7 Elk St
Albany, NY 12207-1023
518/465-0044
Fax: 518/427-0461

North Carolina Dental Society
Executive Director
Mr. Thomas V. Bennett
PO Box 12047
Raleigh, NC 27605-2047
919/832-1222
Fax: 919/833-7666

North Dakota Dental Association
Executive Director
Dr. Jack H. Pfister
419 Dakota Ave
Wahpeton, ND 58075-4413
701/642-1881
Fax: 701/642-1881

Ohio Dental Association
Executive Director
Ms. Nancy Quinn
1370 Dublin Rd
Columbus, OH 43215-1098
614/486-2700
Fax: 614/486-0381

Oklahoma Dental Association
Executive Director
Mr. Bob Berry
629 W Interstate 44 Service Rd
Oklahoma City, OK 73118-6032
405/848-8873
Fax: 405/840-7741

Oregon Dental Association
Executive Director
Mr. Barry Rice
17898 SW McEwan Ave
Portland, OR 97224-7798
503/620-3230
Fax: 503/620-4169

Panama Canal Dental Society
Executive Director
Dr. Steve Olson
PSC #02, Box 2016
APO AA 34002
011/507/843009

Pennsylvania Dental Association
Executive Director
Mrs. Esther F. Richwine
PO Box 3341
Harrisburg, PA 17105-3341
717/234-5941
Fax: 717/232-7169

Colegio de Cirujanos Dentistas de Puerto Rico
Executive Director
Mr. Carlos A. Joglar
Ave Domenech 200
Hato Rey PR 00918-0000
809/764-1969
Fax: 809/763-6335

Rhode Island Dental Association
Executive Director
Ms. Valerie Donnelly
200 Centerville Rd
Warwick, RI 02886-4369
401/732-6833
Fax: 401/732-9351

South Carolina Dental Association
Executive Director
Mr. James H. Zorn
120 Stonemark Lane
Columbia, SC 29210-3841
803/750-2277
Fax: 803/750-1644

South Dakota Dental Association
Executive Director
Ms. Trudy Feigum
PO Box 1194
Pierre, SD 57501-1194
605/224-9133
Fax: 605/224-9168

Tennessee Dental Association
Executive Director
Mr. David S. Horvat
PO Box 120188
Nashville, TN 37212-0188
615/383-8962
Fax: 615/383-0214

Texas Dental Association
Executive Director
Mr. Ben White
PO Box 3358
Austin, TX 78764-3358
512/443-3675
Fax: 512/443-3031

Utah Dental Association
Executive Director
Mr. Monte Thompson
1151 E 3900 S # 160B
Salt Lake City, UT 84124-1216
801/261-5315
Fax: 801/265-8560

Vermont State Dental Society
Executive Director
Mr. Peter Taylor
132 Church St
Burlington, VT 05401-8495
802/864-0115

Virgin Islands Dental Association
Executive Director
Dr. Henry E. Karlin
PO Box 10422
Charlotte Amalie, VI 00801-3422
809/775-9110

Virginia Dental Association
Executive Director
Ms. Patricia K. Watkins
PO Box 6906
Richmond, VA 23230-0906
804/358-4927
Fax: 804/353-7342

Washington State Dental Association
Executive Director
Ms. Anne Hecker
2033 6th Ave, Ste 333
Seattle, WA 98121-9982
206/448-1914
Fax: 206/443-9266

West Virginia Dental Association
Executive Director
Mr. Richard D. Stevens
1002 Kanawha Valley Building
300 Capitol St
Charleston, WV 25301-1794
304/344-5246
Fax: 304/344-5316

Wisconsin Dental Association
Executive Director
Mr. Dennis McGuire
633 W Wisconsin Ave
Milwaukee, WI 53203-1918
414/276-4520
Fax: 414/276-8431

Wyoming Dental Association
Executive Director
Ms. Linda Skorcz
PO Box 4630
Casper, WY 82604-0630
307/234-0777
Fax: 307/234-7133

Air Force Dental Corps
Executive Director
Dr. Donald J. Butz
Hq Usaf/Sgd Bolling Afb
Washington, DC 20332-0000
202/767-5070

Navy Dental Corps
Executive Director
Dr. Milton C. Clegg
Bur Of Medicine & Sur
Department Of The Navy
Washington, DC 20372-0001
202/653-0093

Army Dental Corps
Executive Director
Dr. Thomas R. Tempel
U.S. Army Dental Corps
5109 Leesburg Pike
Falls Church, VA 22041-3201
703/756-0029

Public Health Service
Executive Director
Dr. Robert Collins
Parklawn Building
5600 Fishers Ln #3
Rockville, MD 20857-0001
301/443-1993

Department of Defense
Executive Director
Dr. Edward T. Herbold
Off Asst Sec Of Defense
Pentagon Health Affairs
Washington, DC 20310-0000
202/695-7116

American Association of Dental Examiners
Suite 844
211 E Chicago Ave, Chicago, IL 60611
312/440-7464

JURISDICTION	EXECUTIVE SECRETARY/ADMINISTRATOR
Alabama	
State Board of Dental Examiners of Alabama	Ms. Dianne E. Pool 2308-B Starmount Circle Huntsville, AL 35801 205/533-4638 Fax: 205/533-4638 (Call before sending fax)
Alaska	
State of Alaska Board of Dental Examiners	Ms. Carol Whelan Licensing Examiner Dept. of Commerce & Econ. Dev. PO Box 110806 Juneau, AK 99811-0806 907/465-2542 Fax: 907/465-2974
Arizona	
Arizona State Board of Dental Examiners	Ms. Cynthia J. Witting Interim Executive Director 5060 N 19th Ave, #406 Phoenix, AZ 85308 602/255-3696 Fax: 602/255-4289
Arkansas	
Arkansas State Board of Dental Examiners	Ms. Judith Safly Executive Director The Tower Bldg., Ste 1200 323 Center St Little Rock, AR 72201 501/682-2085 Fax: 501/682-3543
California	
State of California Board of Dental Examiners	Ms. Georgetta Coleman Executive Officer 1432 Howe Ave, #85B Sacramento, CA 95825 916/920-7197 Fax: 916/920-6865
Central Regional Dental Testing Service, Inc. (CRDTS)	Ms. Cynthia G. Barrett Administrative Secretary 1725 Gage Blvd. Topeka, KS 66604 913/273-0380
Colorado	
Colorado State Board of Dental Examiners	Ms. Brenda L. Handy Program Administrator 1560 Broadway, Ste 1310 Denver, CO 80202 303/894-7758 Fax: 303/894-7764

JURISDICTION	EXECUTIVE SECRETARY/ADMINISTRATOR

Connecticut

Connecticut Dental
Commission

Ms. Debra Turcotte
Board Liaison
Dept. of Health Services
Div. of Med. Qual. Assur.
150 Washington St
Hartford, CT 06106
203/566-4068

Delaware

Delaware State Board
of Dental Examiners

Ms. Sheila H. Wolfe
Administrative Assistant
PO Box 1401
O'Neill Bldg.
Dover, DE 19903
302/739-4522
Fax: 302/739-6148

District of Columbia

District of Columbia
Board of Dentistry

Mr. Andres Izaguirre
Contact Representative
Dept. of Consumer & Reg. Affairs
614 H St NW, Rm 904
Washington, DC 20001
202/727-7463
Fax: 202/727-8030

Florida

Florida Board of
Dentistry

Mr. Bill Buckhalt
Executive Director
North Center
1940 N Monroe St
Tallahassee, FL 32399-0765
904/488-6015
Fax: 904/922-3040

Georgia

Georgia Board of
Dentistry

Dr. Frederick J. Meadows
Executive Director
166 Pryor St SW
Atlanta, GA 30303
404/656-3925
Fax: 404/651-9532

Hawaii

Hawaii State Board
of Dental Examiners

Mr. Michael D. Machado
Dept. of Commerce & Consumer Affairs
PO Box 3469
Honolulu, HI 96801
808/586-2701
Fax: 808/586-2689

JURISDICTION	EXECUTIVE SECRETARY/ADMINISTRATOR

Idaho

Idaho State Board of
Dentistry

Ms. Sylvia C. Boyle
Administrator
Statehouse Mail
Boise, ID 83720-6000
208/334-2369

Illinois

Illinois State Board of
Dentistry

Ms. Mary Wright
Board Liaison
Dept. of Prof. Reg.
320 W Washington, 3 Fl
Springfield, IL 62786
217/785-0872
Fax: 217/782-7645

Indiana

Indiana State Board
of Dental Examiners

Ms. Barbara Marvel McNutt
Board Director
Health Professions Bureau
402 W Washington, Rm 041
Indianapolis, IN 46204
317/233-4406
Fax: 317/233-4236

Iowa

Iowa Board
of Dental Examiners

Mrs. Constance L. Price
Executive Director
Executive Hills West
1209 E Ct
Des Moines, IA 50319
515/281-5157

Kansas

Kansas Dental Board

Ms. Carol L. MacDonald
4301 Huntoon, Ste 4LL
Topeka, KS 66604
913/273-0780

Kentucky

Kentucky Board of
Dentistry

Dr. R. Bruce Thompson
Executive Director
2106 Bardstown Rd
Louisville, KY 40205
502/451-6832

Louisiana

Louisiana State Board
of Dentistry

Mr. C. Barry Ogden, Esq.
Executive Director
1515 Poydras St, #1850
New Orleans, LA 70112
504/568-8574
Fax: 504/568-8598

JURISDICTION	EXECUTIVE SECRETARY/ADMINISTRATOR
Maine	
Maine Board of Dental Examiners	Ms. Irene Boucher Executive Secretary 2 Bangor St State House Station 143 Augusta, ME 04333 207/289-3333
Maryland	
Maryland State Board of Dental Examiners	Mr. Larrie Bennett Administrator Metro-Executive Center 4201 Patterson Ave. Baltimore, MD 21215-2299 410/764-4730 Fax: 410/764-5987
Massachusetts	
Massachusetts Board of Registration in Dentistry	Ms. Janet Selwitz Assistant Secretary 100 Cambridge St, Rm 1514 Boston, MA 02202 617/727-9928 Fax: 617/727-7378
Michigan	
Michigan Board of Dentistry	Ms. Doris Foley Licensing Administrator Dept. of Commerce-BOPR PO Box 30018 Lansing, MI 48909 517/335-0918 Fax: 517/373-2179
Minnesota	
Minnesota Board of Dentistry	Ms. Karen Ramsey Acting Executive Director 2700 University Ave W, Ste 70 St. Paul, MN 55114-1055 612/642-0579 Fax: 612/643-3021
Mississippi	
Mississippi State Board of Dental Examiners	Ms. June C. Harris Executive Secretary 580 Springridge Rd, Se C PO Box 1960 Clinton, MS 39060 601/924-9622

JURISDICTION	EXECUTIVE SECRETARY/ADMINISTRATOR
Missouri	
Missouri Dental Board	Mr. Alden Henrickson Executive Director PO Box 1367 Jefferson City, MO 65102 314/751-0040 Fax: 314/751-8216
Montana	
Montana Board of Dentistry	Ms. Lisa F. Casman Administrative Assistant Arcade Building, Lower Level 111 N Jackson Helena, MT 59620-0407 406/444-3745 Fax: 406/444-1667
Nebraska	
Nebraska Board of Examiners in Dentistry	Ms. Becky Wisell Board Coordinator 301 Centennial Mall S PO Box 95007 Lincoln, NE 68509-5007 402/471-2115 Fax: 402/471-0383
Nevada	
Nevada State Board of Dental Examiners	Dr. William L. Thomason 6769 W Charleston Blvd, Ste D Las Vegas, NV 89102 702/258-4230 Fax: 702/258-4232
New Hampshire	
New Hampshire Board of Dental Examiners	Dr. Raymond J. Jarvis Health & Welfare Bldg. 6 Hazen Dr Concord, NH 03301 603/271-4561
New Jersey	
New Jersey State Board of Dentistry	Ms. Agnes Clarke Executive Director 124 Halsey St PO Box 45005 Newark, NJ 07101 201/648-7087 Fax: 201/648-3481
New Mexico	
New Mexico Board of Dentistry	Ms. Karen Valdez Administrator PO Drawer 8397 Santa Fe, NM 87504 505/827-7165 Fax: 505/827-7095

JURISDICTION	EXECUTIVE SECRETARY/ADMINISTRATOR

New York

New York State
Board of Dentistry

Dr. Martin A. Rubin
Rm 3023
Cultural Education Center
Albany, NY 12230
518/474-3838
Fax: 518/473-0578

North Carolina

North Carolina State
Board of Dental Examiners

Mrs. Christine H. Lockwood
Executive Secretary
3716 National Dr, Ste 221
PO Box 32270
Raleigh, NC 27622-2270
919/781-4901
Fax: 919/571-8457

North Dakota

North Dakota
Board of Dentistry

Dr. Robert McKibben
Box 179
Valley City, ND 58072
701/845-3708

**Northeast Regional
Board of Dental
Examiners, Inc (NERB)**

Dr. William K. Collins
4645 Burroughs Ave NE
3rd Fl
Washington, DC 20019
202/398-6196
Fax: 202/398-4709

Ohio

Ohio State Dental Board

Mr. Omar P. Whisman
Executive Director
77 S High St, 18th Fl
Columbus, OH 43266-0306
614/466-2580
Fax: 614/752-8995

Oklahoma

Board of Governors of
Registered Dentists

Ms. Linda C. Campbell
Executive Director
2726 N Oklahoma Ave
Oklahoma City, OK 73105
405/521-2350
Fax: 405/521-6389

Oregon

Oregon Board of Dentistry

Ms. Betty Reynolds
Executive Director
1515 SW Fifth Ave
Ste 400
Portland, OR 97201
503/229-5520
Fax: 503/229-5120

JURISDICTION	EXECUTIVE SECRETARY/ADMINISTRATOR
Pennsylvania	
Pennsylvania State Board of Dentistry	Ms. June L. Barner Administrative Assistant PO Box 2649 Harrisburg, PA 17105 717/783-7162 Fax: 717/787-7769
Puerto Rico	
Puerto Rico Board of Dental Examiners	Mr. Carlos Santana Rabell Director, Examining Boards Dept of Health Call Box 10200 San Juan, PR 00908 809/725-8161 Fax: 809/725-3090
Rhode Island	
Rhode Island State Board of Examiners in Dentistry	Mr. Robert W. McClanaghan Administrator 3 Capitol Hill, Rm 404 Providence, RI 02908-5097 401/277-2151 Fax: 401/277-1250
South Carolina	
South Carolina State Board of Dentistry	Mr. H. Rion Alvey Executive Director 1315 Blanding St Columbia, SC 29201 803/734-8904 Fax: 803/734-8958
South Dakota	
South Dakota State Board of Dentistry	Ms. Anita Aker 1708 Space Ct Rapid City, SD 57701 605/342-3026
Southern Regional Testing Agency, Inc. (SRTA)	Mr. Robert W. Minnich 1072 Laskin Rd, Ste 203 Virginia Beach, VA 23451 804/428-1003
Tennessee	
Tennessee Board of Dentistry	Ms. Anita VanTries Regulatory Brds. Admin. 283 Plus Park Blvd Nashville, TN 37247-1010 615/367-6228

JURISDICTION	EXECUTIVE SECRETARY/ADMINISTRATOR
Texas	
Texas State Board of Dental Examiners	Mr. C. Thomas Camp Executive Director 327 Congress Ave, Ste 500 Austin, TX 78701 512/477-2985 Fax: 512/477-0879
Utah	
Utah Board of Dentists and Dental Hygienists	Ms. Diane Blake, RN, MPA Assoc. Bureau Manager Div. of Occup. & Prof. Lic. PO Box 45805 Salt Lake City, UT 84145-0805 801/530-6767 Fax: 801/530-6511
Vermont	
Vermont Board of Dental Examiners	Ms. Diane W. Lafaille Secretary of State's Office 109 State St Montpelier, VT 05609-1106 802/828-2390 Fax: 802/828-2496
Virginia	
Virginia Board of Dentistry	Mrs. Nancy T. Feldman Executive Director 1601 Rolling Hills Dr Richmond, VA 23229-5005 804/662-9906 Fax: 804/662-9943
Virgin Islands	
Virgin Islands Board of Dental Examiners	Mrs. Jane Aubain Dept of Health 48 Sugar Estate St. Thomas, VI 00802 809/774-0117 Fax: 809/776-0610
Washington	
Washington Dental Health Care Boards	Ms. Judy E. Mayo Executive Director 1300 SE Quince St Mail Stop EY-26 Olympia, WA 98504 206/753-2461 Fax: 206/586-7774

JURISDICTION	EXECUTIVE SECRETARY/ADMINISTRATOR

West Virginia

West Virginia Board
of Dental Examiners

Mr. James G. Anderson, III
PO Drawer 1459
65 Stamm Circle
Beckley, WV 25802-1459
304/252-8266
Fax: 304/256-1617

**Western Regional
Examining Board
(WREB)**

Ms. Linda Paul
Executive Administrator
10040 N 25th Ave, #116
Phoenix, AZ 85021
602/944-3315

Wisconsin

Wisconsin Dentistry
Examining Board

Mr. Patrick D. Braatz
Bureau Director
PO Box 8935
1400 E. Washington Ave
Madison, WI 53708
608/266-2811 or 608/266-0483

Wyoming

Wyoming Board of
Dental Examiners

Ms. Shirley Thomas
PO Box 1270
Powell, WY 82435
307/754-3476

**ACCREDITED DENTAL
SCHOOLS:
COMMISSION
ON DENTAL
ACCREDITATION**

Dental schools that have approval, conditional approval or provisional approval status are listed here. All programs have approval status except those designated with a dagger (†) or an asterisk (*). A dagger (†) indicates that the program has conditional approval status. An asterisk (*) indicates that the program has provisional approval status. The year appearing adjacent to the address of the institution identifies the year in which the next regularly scheduled on-site evaluation of the program(s) will be conducted. This identification does not preclude the commission from authorizing a site evaluation before the designated year. Definitions of accreditation classifications appear in the addendum.

Alabama
School of Dentistry
University of Alabama (1993)
UAB Station
Birmingham, AL 35294

California
School of Dentistry
Loma Linda University (1995)
Loma Linda, CA 92350

School of Dentistry
University of California at Los Angeles
  (1997)
Center for the Health Sciences
Los Angeles, CA 90024

California—cont'd
School of Dentistry
University of Southern California (1994)
University Park, MC 0641
Los Angeles, CA 90089-0641

School of Dentistry
University of California, San Francisco
 (1998)
513 Parnassus Ave, S-630
San Francisco, CA 94145

School of Dentistry
University of the Pacific (1993)
2155 Webster St
San Francisco, CA 94115

Colorado
School of Dentistry
University of Colorado Medical Center
 (1994)
4200 E Ninth Ave, Box C-284
Denver, CO 80262

Connecticut
School of Dental Medicine
The University of Connecticut (1994)
263 Farmington Ave
Farmington, CT 06032

District of Columbia
College of Dentistry
Howard University (1995)
600 W Street NW
Washington, DC 20059

Florida
College of Dentistry
University of Florida (1994)
Box J-405, JHMHC
Gainesville, FL 32610

Georgia
School of Dentistry
Medical College of Georgia (1997)
1459 Laney Walker Blvd
Augusta, GA 30912-0200

Illinois
College of Dentistry
University of Illinois at Chicago (1999)
801 S Paulina St
Chicago, IL 60612

School of Dental Medicine
Southern Illinois University (1998)
2800 College Ave
Alton, IL 62002

Illinois—cont'd
Northwestern University Dental School
 (1998)
240 E Huron St
Chicago, IL 60611
School of Dentistry

Indiana
School of Dentistry
Indiana University (1992)
1121 W Michigan St
Indianapolis, IN 46202

Iowa
College of Dentistry
The University of Iowa (1997)
Iowa City, IA 52242

Kentucky
College of Dentistry
University of Kentucky (1997)
800 Rose St
Lexington, KY 40536-0084

School of Dentistry
University of Louisville (1994)
Health Sciences Center
Louisville, KY 40292

Louisiana
School of Dentistry
Louisiana State University (1994)
1100 Florida Ave, Bldg 101
New Orleans, LA 70119

Maryland
Baltimore College of Dental Surgery
Dental School
University of Maryland at Baltimore
 (1997)
666 W Baltimore St
Baltimore, MD 21201

Massachusetts
Harvard School of Dental Medicine
 (1998)
188 Longwood Ave
Boston, MA 02115

School of Dental Medicine
Tufts University (1994)
1 Kneeland St
Boston, MA 02111

Massachusetts—cont'd
Goldman School of Graduate Dentistry
Boston University
Medical Center (1998)
100 E Newton St
Boston, MA 02118

Michigan
School of Dentistry
The University of Michigan (1995)
1234 Dental Building
Ann Arbor, MI 48109-1078

School of Dentistry
University of Detroit (1993)
2985 E Jefferson Ave
Detroit, MI 48207

Minnesota
School of Dentistry
University of Minnesota (1992)
515 Delaware St, SE
Minneapolis, MN 55455

Mississippi
School of Dentistry
The University of Mississippi (1996)
Medical Center
2500 N State St
Jackson, MS 39216-4505

Missouri
School of Dentistry
University of Missouri-Kansas City
  (1996)
650 E 25th St
Kansas City, MO 64108

Nebraska
College of Dentistry
University of Nebraska Medical Center
  (1993)
40th and Holdrege Streets
Lincoln, NE 68583-0740

School of Dentistry
Creighton University (1998)
2500 California St
Omaha, NE 68178

New Jersey
University of Medicine and
Dentistry of New Jersey, New Jersey
  Dental School (1999)
110 Bergen St
Newark, NJ 07103-2425

New York
School of Dental Medicine,
State University of New York at Buffalo
  (1996)
325 Squire Hall
Buffalo, NY 14214

School of Dental Medicine
State University of New York at Stony
  Brook (1992)
Health Science Center
Stony Brook, NY 11794-8700

School of Dental and Oral Surgery
Columbia University (1995)
630 W 168th St
New York, NY 10032

College of Dentistry
New York University (1997)
345 East 24th St
New York, NY 10010-4099

North Carolina
School of Dentistry
University of North Carolina (1996)
CB#7450, 104 Brauer Hall
Chapel Hill, NC 27599-7450

Ohio
School of Dentistry
Case Western Reserve University (1995)
2123 Abington Rd.
Cleveland, OH 44106

College of Dentistry
The Ohio State University (1999)
305 W 12th Ave
Columbus, OH 43210

Oklahoma
College of Dentistry
University of Oklahoma (1994)
Health Sciences Center
PO Box 26901
1001 NE Stanton L. Young
Oklahoma City, OK 73190

Oregon
School of Dentistry
The Oregon Health Sciences University
  (1995)
611 SW Campus Dr
Sam Jackson Park
Portland, OR 97201

Pennsylvania

School of Dental Medicine
University of Pennsylvania (1993)
4001 Spruce St
Philadelphia, PA 19104

School of Dentistry
Temple University (1997)
3223 N Broad St
Philadelphia, PA 19140

School of Dental Medicine
University of Pittsburgh (1996)
C-333 Salk Hall
3501 Terrace St
Pittsburgh, PA 15261

Puerto Rico

School of Dentistry
University of Puerto Rico (1999)
GPO Box 5067
San Juan, PR 00936

South Carolina

College of Dental Medicine
Medical University of South Carolina
  (1996)
171 Ashley Ave
Charleston, SC 29425

Tennessee

College of Dentistry
University of Tennessee (1996)
875 Union Ave
Memphis, TN 38163

†School of Dentistry
Meharry Medical College (1993)
1005 DB Todd Blvd.
Nashville, TN 37208

Texas

Baylor College of Dentistry (1997)
3302 Gaston Ave
Dallas, TX 75246

The University of Texas
Health Science Center at Houston
Dental Branch (1998)
PO Box 20068
Houston, TX 77225

The University of Texas
Health Science Center at San Antonio
  Dental School (1998)
7703 Floyd Curl Dr
San Antonio, TX 78284-7906

Virginia

School of Dentistry
Medical College of Virginia (1996)
Virginia Commonwealth University
PO Box 566
Richmond, VA 23298

Washington

School of Dentistry
University of Washington (1995)
Health Sciences Bldg, SC62
Seattle, WA 98195

West Virginia

School of Dentistry
West Virginia University (1995)
Health Sciences Center North
Morgantown, WV 26506

Wisconsin

School of Dentistry
Marquette University (1993)
604 N 16th St
Milwaukee, WI 53233

Canada

Reciprocal agreement between the Council on Education of the Canadian Dental Association and the Commission on Dental Accreditation of the American Dental Association was made to recognize as accredited:

Faculty of Dentistry
University of Alberta
Dentistry Pharmacy Building
Edmonton, Alberta T6G-2N8

Faculty of Dentistry
Dalhousie University
5981 University Ave
Halifax, Nova Scotia B3H-3J5

Faculty of Dentistry
University of Manitoba
780 Bannatyne Ave
Winnipeg, Manitoba R3E-0W3

Faculte de Medecine Dentaire
Universite de Montreal
2900 Boulevard Edouard Montpeit
Montreal, Quebec H3C-3J7

Faculty of Dentistry
University of Toronto
124 Edward St.
Toronto, Ontario M5G-1G6

Faculty of Dentistry
University of British Columbia
350-2194 Health Sciences Mall
Vancouver, British Columbia
V67-1W5

Ecole De Medicine Dentaire
Universite Laval
Ste-Foy, Quebec G1K-7P4

Faculty of Dentistry
McGill University
740 Docteur Penfield
Montreal, Quebec H3A-1A4

College of Dentistry
University of Saskatchewan
Saskatoon, Saskatchewan S7N-0W0

Faculty of Dentistry
The University of Western Ontario
London, Ontario N6A-5C1